Orthopedics Quick Review

Seventh Edition

Conferred As '**Magic Book of Orthopedics**' by Students

Apurv Mehra
MBBS MAMC MS ORTHO (UCMS)
DNB ORTHO DIP. SICOT (BELGIUM)
FELLOWSHIP COMPUTER NAVIGATION JOINT REPLACEMENT
FROM GERMANY, AUSTRALIA AND MALAYSIA

Consultant Orthopedic Surgeon
Computer Navigation Joint Replacement
and Arthroscopy Surgeon

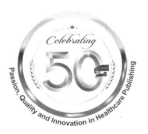

JAYPEE BROTHERS MEDICAL PUBLISHERS
The Health Sciences Publisher
New Delhi | London | Panama

Jaypee Brothers Medical Publishers (P) Ltd

Headquarters
Jaypee Brothers Medical Publishers (P) Ltd.
4838/24, Ansari Road, Daryaganj
New Delhi 110 002, India
Phone: +91-11-43574357
Fax: +91-11-43574314
E-mail: jaypee@jaypeebrothers.com

Overseas Offices
JP Medical Ltd.
83, Victoria Street, London
SW1H 0HW (UK)
Phone: +44-20 3170 8910
Fax: +44(0)20 3008 6180
E-mail: info@jpmedpub.com

Jaypee-Highlights Medical Publishers Inc.
City of Knowledge, Bld. 235, 2nd Floor, Clayton
Panama City, Panama
Phone: +1 507-301-0496
Fax: +1 507-301-0499
E-mail: cservice@jphmedical.com

Jaypee Brothers Medical Publishers (P) Ltd.
Bhotahity, Kathmandu, Nepal
Phone: +977-9741283608
E-mail: kathmandu@jaypeebrothers.com

Website: www.jaypeebrothers.com
Website: www.jaypeedigital.com

© 2019, Jaypee Brothers Medical Publishers

The views and opinions expressed in this book are solely those of the original contributor(s)/author(s) and do not necessarily represent those of editor(s) of the book.

All rights reserved. No part of this publication may be reproduced, stored or transmitted in any form or by any means, electronic, mechanical, photocopying, recording or otherwise, without the prior permission in writing of the publishers.

All brand names and product names used in this book are trade names, service marks, trademarks or registered trademarks of their respective owners. The publisher is not associated with any product or vendor mentioned in this book.

Medical knowledge and practice change constantly. This book is designed to provide accurate, authoritative information about the subject matter in question. However, readers are advised to check the most current information available on procedures included and check information from the manufacturer of each product to be administered, to verify the recommended dose, formula, method and duration of administration, adverse effects and contraindications. It is the responsibility of the practitioner to take all appropriate safety precautions. Neither the publisher nor the author(s)/editor(s) assume any liability for any injury and/or damage to persons or property arising from or related to use of material in this book.

This book is sold on the understanding that the publisher is not engaged in providing professional medical services. If such advice or services are required, the services of a competent medical professional should be sought.

Every effort has been made where necessary to contact holders of copyright to obtain permission to reproduce copyright material. If any have been inadvertently overlooked, the publisher will be pleased to make the necessary arrangements at the first opportunity. The **CD/DVD-ROM** (if any) provided in the sealed envelope with this book is complimentary and free of cost. **Not meant for sale**.

Inquiries for bulk sales may be solicited at: jaypee@jaypeebrothers.com

Orthopedics Quick Review

First Edition: 2012
Second Edition: 2013
Revised Reprint: 2014
Third Edition: 2015
Fourth Edition: 2016
Fifth Edition: 2017
Sixth Edition: 2018
Seventh Edition: 2019

ISBN 978-93-5270-931-1

Printed at Rajkamal Electric Press, Kundli (Haryana)

Believe to Achieve

Dedicated to

My Daughter, Vrinda Mehra

My Patients and My Students who have helped me evolve as an Orthopedic Surgeon and a Teacher.

— *Dr. Apurv Mehra*

"People are often unreasonable and self-centered. Forgive them anyway. If you are kind, people may accuse you of ulterior motives. Be kind anyway. If you are honest, people may cheat you. Be honest anyway. If you find happiness, people may be jealous. Be happy anyway. The good you do today may be forgotten tomorrow. Do good anyway. Give the world the best you have and it may never be enough. Give your best anyway. For you see, in the end, it is between you and God.

— Mother Teresa

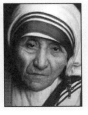

FOREWORD

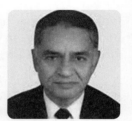

Despite the availability of more lucrative opportunities to the current generation in business and technology, the brightest of the young generation of any country opts for medicine as a career. Orthopedics happens to be one of the most sought after clinical discipline, fully aware of the long years of arduous training involved for success in the profession. It is just natural that the best amongst the admission seekers would be able to enroll themselves for the limited seat available in Orthopedics in the teaching and training institute. To maintain objectivity and transparency, admissions based upon objective MCQ type of questions is the best of all assessment systems, granting that no assessment system is really "perfect". This book is intended to help the student to quickly review the subject for MCQ examinations. The table of contents of the book covers the wide landscape of orthopedic discipline.

Dr Apurv Mehra over the last 14 years has been trying to analyse the system of MCQ type examinations, collate and organise the material for understanding at the graduate level. This book would help the prospective candidates to channelise their thinking process for the admission tests. The question-answer style of various sections would also help the prospective faculty (who compose the MCQs) to standardise the frame word for constructing the question with least ambiguity and for appropriate level of MBBS graduates. It is a laudable effort by Dr Apurv Mehra, and it is a must-read for the admission seekers.

SM Tuli
MBBS MS PhD FAMS
Formerly: Director
Institute of Medical Sciences
Banaras Hindu University Varanasi, Uttar Pradesh, India
Senior Consultant Spinal Disorder and Orthopedic
VIMHANS Hospital, Nehru Nagar, New Delhi

FOREWORD

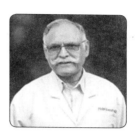

Orthopedics today has become one of the most sought after branches in medicine and similar is the representation of number of questions in PG entrance examinations. Clear concepts and crisp knowledge is often required to solve MCQs irrespective of the type and format of questions.

Orthopedics Quick Review comes with a complete package for PG aspirants to have a concept based knowledge, important points to remember and recollect at the time of examination. Illustrative diagrams, images, flowcharts and summary have been made keeping in mind the need of students today. **This book is not one for the shelf but is for the last minutes specially chapters like Complete Summary of Orthopedics.**

Dr Apurv Mehra has carefully included questions and topics keeping in mind that the whole spectrum of Orthopedics is covered and retained by students.

Orthopedics Quick Review is a must-read for Orthopedics MCQs.

Sudhir Kumar
Head of Department
Department of Orthopedics
Sharda Hospital
School of Medical Sciences and Research
Greater Noida, Uttar Pradesh, India

FOREWORD

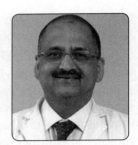

Dr Apurv Mehra has put forth a new volume for the aspiring postgraduates in orthopedic surgery. While there is an ocean of knowledge and texts available this volume comes from the heart of a young orthopedic surgeon who has himself faced the pleasures and difficulties of acquiring knowledge.

Many a texts are available to the examinees and seekers of information and each has a flavour of its own. In this case Apurv has a refreshing approach towards imparting information.

The text comes with useful pictorial diagrams and X-rays to illustrate concepts. Whilst putting forward a multiple choice questions the author has given an elaborate reasoning for the best choice answer. He has classified the chapters with good deal of thought.

It makes a simple read for those revising for examinations and subtly adds information to the candidates knowledge bank. In fact the volume will be an asset in the collection of all those learning and teaching the art of Orthopedic surgery.

SKS Marya
Chairman
Bone and Joint Institute
Medanta the Medicity
Gurgaon, Haryana, India

ABOUT THE EDITORS

Anil Arora

Dr (Prof) Anil Arora holds an experience of more than 20 years in Orthopedics. He has been **Senior Orthopedic Surgeon** and Professor of Orthopedics at University College of Medical Sciences, New Delhi. He is an Internationally known figure in Orthopedics. He is a Joint Replacement Surgeon, currently he is Head of the Department of Orthopedics at Max Superspeciality Hospital and Institute of Joint Replacement, Patparganj, New Delhi. He is known for his brilliant clinical skills and knowledge.

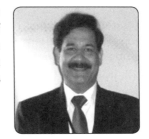

He has many **International and National Achievements and Awards** to his credit like:
- SIROT Award in USA (First Indian to win this award from a body of 85 countries),
- Weller Gold Medal
- AA Mehta Gold Medal of Indian Orthopaedic Association
- "Silver Jubilee Oration" Award of Indian Orthopaedic Association
- He has also delivered White Paper of Indian Orthopaedic Association
- He has published about 50 research papers in various International, National and Regional Journals
- He has about 20 Chapters in International and National Orthopedic Textbooks

Prof Anil Arora has carefully edited the contents of this book and has given valuable feedbacks in the making of this book.

Thameem Saif

Dr Thameem Saif, MD (Medicine), is a renowned teacher held in very high regard by medicos both in India and the US. He is an intellect of high order with brilliant teaching skills. His inputs have been found to be very valuable by his students across the country and he has helped lots of students achieve their dreams of clearing the tough Indian Medical PG Entrance Exams and The USMLE. Most of the toppers in the country today thank him in their heart for playing an important role in their success. He is well known for solving MCQs in an organized approach to reach towards the answer. His Orientation about how to approach MCQs with latest patterns proposed for National Eligibility Entrance Test is an important aspect of his sessions.

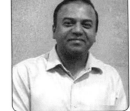

He has carefully gone through the book and his suggestion has given birth to a chapter on **'Complete Summary of Orthopedics'** for students to revise in last minutes.

PREFACE

Ortho Pedics Quick Review (OPQR) is a concise MCQ book having to the point information to be read in the shortest possible time with high degree of retention and maximum output.

OPQR was first released in 2012. The tremendous response the book received in its first year itself came as a surprise. Since then OPQR has become the popular choice and is the Best Selling Book for Orthopedics across the globe for those preparing for Entrance Exams.

In last few years OPQR has evolved and gained recognition, matching the current trend in examinations.

OPQR has now been adopted by all PG Institutes as No.1 MCQ book for Orthopedics.

Students who have achieved good ranks strongly recommend reading OPQR and have named it as "Magic Book of Orthopedics".

— Apurv Mehra

Mail Your Queries @ drapurv@medmiracle.in
Lets Connect @ Facebook: Apurv Mehra
Get Inspired : www.drapurv.com

GOOD THINGS TAKE TIME ...

Here Are Answers To Few Questions I Am Often Asked By My Students...

Q. 1. Why didn't I achieve a rank when I worked so hard...?

My Answer: I would like to share with you, when most of my friends qualified in the first attempt and I didn't, it was a heartbreak and quite unbelievable. That is when I realized that our so called failure in entrance exams is not a failure but is the inability to plan a strategy and identify our areas of lacunae.

I analyzed my lacunas and came to this conclusion:
- Group all 19 subjects into 4 parts
    - Part 1: First year subjects
    - Part 2: Second Year Subjects
    - Part 3: Final year subjects including PSM
    - Part 4: Short subjects that include skin, Psychiatry, Radio, Anesthesia, ENT, Ophtha, Ortho and Forensic Medicine
- After assessing last 5 year papers, on the basis of my MCQ knowledge I noted
    - My weak subjects, Strong Subjects and Relatively Strong Subjects
    - In my weak subjects, I made a list of topics to be covered and
    - In my relatively better subjects, I made a list of topics I was weak in.

This is a point that we need to understand and accept that even in our strong subjects there will be areas we are weak in.

A good player of cricket is the one who needs to be a good runner but if his running is weak then he'll be run out, so he needs to work on his running. As well at the same time he needs to keep practicing his batting skills too.

Through this I wish to convey that you should keep revising your strengths otherwise soon they become your short comings.

Q. 2. Why do we keep forgetting what we learn...?

My Answer: In your first reading itself, make it a habit to highlight important points to be read in your second reading. This helps you a lots. In the second reading as it gives you a feel that you have already read this earlier and also saves your time.

I also advice to make 2 schedules:
1. Main schedule for preparation for the whole day.
2. Revision Schedule in which you have 90 minutes each day to revise volatile subjects, for example for me - Pharma was one such subject.

Q. 3. Why do we lag behind in our schedule ...?

My Answer: **You can never complete 100% of any subject. Selective Study is the best way to prepare for Medical Entrance Exams.** Read each subject in the order of importance of the topics so that in case you exceed your time allotted to each subject, you move on to the next subject but don't miss on vital things. Here our aim is to complete all 19 subjects. But if you till the end don't follow this advice of sticking with your schedule, you will end up with a catastrophe of leaving a subject which no one can never compensate.

Also keep practicing MCQs every day, preferably in the morning hours, at the same time when the exams are conducted, so that your internal clock is tuned.

Q. 4. Negative Thoughts- What if I study properly and still don't make it this time then what ...???

My Answer: There is a self belief which tells you to take chances. I agree there will be doubts but you must at the same time realize that even Rank 1 of any exam, will have doubts but even then the power to conquer the fears is more. So the basic thing you can do to counter this is - to develop a habit of surrounding yourself with positivity and positive human beings and to my brain, they are your parents- talk to them, they will always show you the positive aspect.

Q. 5. Sir, when will my time come...?

My Answer: This is a big question and I can just tell you one simple thing. 'Time never comes, you need to create it.' God will write your destiny according to your efforts, and only hard work can beat any talent and I know it surely will.

My batchmates in MAMC were very talented and intelligent but I always had this habit called as hard work, which I gradually realized is the biggest asset, which if nurtured and fed well, can take you everywhere. Those who work hard can do good not only with themselves but also to lots of people around. Just as I have learnt from my Grandmother, 'To live like a king, we need to work like a slave.'

So to summarise:

- Right approach to examination is the most important step, so start as early as you can.
- Select the right books with updated pretexts in latest editions.
- Your preparation decides your fate, analyze and evaluate your current preparation.
- Accordingly start with a combo of strong and weak subjects. Prepare list of important topics, shortlist topics in weak subjects and weak topics in strong subjects.
- Be consistent and keep revising your strong topics too at the same time managing your time well.
- Practice MCQs daily, preferably from the topics you have read.
- Plan your day in advance to bring in effectiveness.
- Prepare a schedule where you also give 90 minutes to revision each day.
- Stick to your time table and don't neglect any subject–completing all subjects is more important than trying to complete 100 percent of a subject.
- Keep talking to your parents, they are the sea of positivity and will always stand by you.
- Hard work can beat talent, it surely will, so work hard like a slave and then live like a king.

FOR MY PATRIOTS

A MESSAGE FROM MY HEART...

First of all, pat your back and be proud to be a 'Doctor' the most noble profession on earth. You are an achiever and are now preparing for a bigger challenge...Indian PG Medical Entrance Exam which is bound to become more difficult with each passing year with the rise in the number of individuals appearing for these entrance exams every year. I, Dr Apurv Mehra, Your Teacher, take it as my responsibility to guide and help you achieve what you desire.

First and Foremost

To turn your dreams into reality, there is NO SHORT CUT, instead all you need to do is:
- Draw a plan for the next day before you sleep so that by the time you get up, you already have a target to achieve.
- Study **SIX hours** per day without your mobile phone, for a period of six months.
- Always remember, selections in Entrance Exams are not based on intelligence or knowledge, but on more number of revisions of important topics and following a proper strategy
- Prepare notes, crisp and easy for you to understand, only if you are going to use them for revision. Otherwise it is just a waste of time.!!
- Go for selective reading of important topics (follow General Rule), practice MCQs, do refer to standard textbooks for concepts/doubts/controversies.
- Prepare your own small diary of mnemonics, powerful enough for you to remember.

A combined approach is a must to prepare for all Entrance Exams (NEET DNB /AIIMS/ PGI / JIPMER)
- It is advisable to go through last 7 years AIIMS papers, 6–8 PGI papers and 3–4 DNB papers.
- Memorize the Important topics of last 5 years All India questions. Don't forget to check recent updates.
- Revise your notes you have made and also course notes if you had joined any coaching institute.
- No need to waste time on finding answers to controversial questions just decide an answer you will mark if asked in exam.
- Your knowledge and presence of mind are equally important on the day of the exam.
- Make use of every single day. (Read, Practice, Revise)
- Keep a positive attitude throughout.

Do not count the days make the days count!

---

10 lessons I learnt in my journey of starting from nowhere...just nowhere...

1. **Attitude...**
   Life may not have given you enough reasons but smile and also laugh and do both every often. After this just pause and think the difference between smile and laugh...

2. **Struggle...**
   The fight for the victory is more precious than the victory and most important is the attitude in handling the fight and the victory...

3. **Supporters...**
   The supporters are like noose around your neck that can only constrict you or stop you just untie and release them as soon as possible....and then jump and fly...

4. **Success...**
   First success is just the declaration of your arrival and then progress on your journey...

5. Failure...
Everyone knows how to handle success, precious is to handle failure with the same grace and then just announce you failed …but have the courage to turn it into success…have the courage to standup for yourself…

6. Planning...
Plan and also most importantly execute the plan…

7. Innovative...
Be innovative and be conceptual….and have the courage to follow your conceptual innovation…

8. Thoughts about business...
Refusal in any business is to reject a possible growth plan and acceptance in business is about the expenditure whereas success is about the precarious balance between the refusal and acceptance…

9. My career...
Most felt I was not good enough to do MS Orthopedics, Most felt I could not teach as they claimed that I was not gifted with that talent…. but they did not measure my hard work and determination and with those I could defeat the talent. Most importantly they did not realize it was my dream and I wanted to live that dream badly and there was good God above …rest was history…

10. Always remember these two most important things—Thrust and Hunger are for your soul, so take care that it is fed well…

FEW VALUABLE PEARLS THAT SHALL HELP YOU ALWAYS

A Day Before The Examination

Every time we would go to write an exam our seniors (at MAMC) would guide us...
1. Sleep on time and sleep well a night before.
2. Before sleeping preferably speak to your closest family member or your wise friend and do promise that you will give your best and keep a positive attitude.
3. Reading few jokes from a joke book has been found as a stress reliever by some.
4. On the morning of the exam, never go empty stomach, never eat too much, take a balanced fruit, a sandwich and a cup of coffee/tea is preferred by most.
5. Always get ready on time and wear your most comfortable clothes and shoes. Trying out a new footwear is not advisable.
6. Most prefer some music in morning hours to de-stress themselves.
7. Leave early from house for the center and avoid driving at any cost.
8. Make sure to carry your Photo Identity proof, Admit card and Stationery.
9. At the center preferably involve yourself in some meditation or stay with your family or friend accompanying you. Avoid mingling with groups.
10. Please do all the formalities before the exam on time to avoid any last minute panic.
11. Follow instructions of the examiners or invigilators at the center dare not involve in any of them.

On The Day Of The Exam

TELL YOURSELF ... IF I CAN'T NO ONE CAN...

Remember to take up challenges...

Each day the heart has fear, each day the mind has doubts, for most of us it is a big issue... but for few it is a challenge...
- Outside the examination hall there are three different kinds of student personalities..
  - Category 1: Geared and charged up, discussing things in over excited manner. You will find them discussing all the important things and their BMR too is toned up –that's the **Hyper Group**.
  - Category 2: **The Quiet Group** revising and reading in a corner. On their faces you will find serenity and shine, they are not talking or mingling with anyone, they are just with their notes.
  - Category 3: **The Analyst Group** is calm and quiet. They have no book in their hand and are just sitting in a corner planning their exam strategy, reminding themselves that they have actually worked hard for this exam and now they need to carefully select out the questions.
- Category of questions asked in every entrance exam:
  - The first category of questions are the ones you already know about (Repeat Questions) and you should try to get all of them correct–Please read carefully and go slow on them.
  - The second category of questions will be the ones which will require you to make educated guesses, questions which you already will have some idea about. Such questions require time –PAY ATTENTION and CAREFULLY ANSWER THEM.
  - The third category of questions will be the new ones which most of the students will find tough to answer but if you try to find out the answer by carefully ruling out the options it might help.

The Analyst is the group that understands their preparation can never be completed 100 percent so studying outside the examination hall will not make much of a difference (Just Like category 1 or category 2 students).

- Outside the hall is the place to fill yourself with positivity and encouragement along with a well-planned strategy.(Category 3)
- Remember strategy is always more powerful than knowledge and talent.
- Stay calm, even those who Top don't know everything, but they apply all the knowledge that they know, they plan their strategies and they plan well.

Finally your results will depend on the strategies you followed...

So enter the examination hall with positivity, well planned strategy and self belief...

If I can't no one else can... Believe in yourself...it really works...

During The Exam...
- Start the paper and read each question very carefully.
- One liners should be read at least 3 times and message should be very clear what the examiner is asking and then read all 4 choices.
- One by one try to rule out options so that you have more probability of getting the answers correct for e.g: If you select one answer out of 4 then your success probability is 25% but if you rule out one option then your success probability is 33% and if you are able to rule out 2 options then you have to mark from the remaining 2 choices thus your success probability is 50%.
- Do not make a mistake of marking the first answer without reading all 4 choices. Most of the examiners set 3 to 4% questions on the principle that student marks the first answer on reflex.
- This makes a total of about 10 to 12 questions in your exam thus can make a huge difference.
- Please do not try to find mistakes in questions. For all practical reasons try to answer questions accepting them as correctly framed .
- Multiple lines or clinical questions should be answered on remembering the following points:
    - Age of the patient may help you decide the answer.
    - Unilateral or bilateral may help you rule out few choices.
    - Normal features mentioned helps rule out few choices.
    - Please make a note of important radiological findings .
    - Give very high importance to histopathological or biopsy features to arrive at diagnosis and always give tissue diagnosis more importance than radiological findings because radiological finding can be non-specific.
    - Always make a note whether most common finding is asked or most characteristic finding is asked.
    - Similarly observe that whether investigation of choice is asked or gold standard investigation is asked.
    - If you look at questions, investigation of choice refers to next investigation and gold standard refers to best investigation usually.
- Each question is highly valuable and do not take any question lightly no matter how much confident you are.
- It is very strange that students try to save time on the questions that they have knowledge about and give more time to questions they are not aware of. Actually you must focus strongly on topics you know and answer their questions carefully rather than giving more time to topics you are unaware of. Most Toppers get the repeat topics correct as compared to scoring high on new topics.

My Grandmother used to recite these Lines from Guru Granth Sahib......which I often read out to all My students..

"Teri kismat da likha
Tere toh koi kho nahin sakda
Tu shram (Karam) kara chal bande...
Je usdi meher hove ta tenu o v mil jauga jo tera ho nahin sakda"

Go Chase Your Dreams, I Pray To Almighty To Grant It...!!!

— Dr Apurv Mehra

your queries – orthodhoomdhadaka@gmail.com

Let's Connect @ Apurv Mehra (Profile 1, 2 or 3) OR Apurv Mehra

Get Inspired @ www.drapurv.com

Dr. Apurv Mehra

For Any Doubt Academic / Nonacademic write to drapurv@medmiracle.in

Dr. Apurv Mehra – The Orthopedic Surgeon

Dr. Apurv Mehra is an Internationally Trained & Experienced Computer Navigation Joint Replacement & Arthroscopy Surgeon
He is an Orthopedic Consultant at Max Institute of Bone & Joint Care at Patparganj, New Delhi
Dr. Apurv Mehra is the Founder & Director of Vidya Jeevan Ortho Pedics Centre, New Delhi – India's most Trusted Orthopedic Centre as per Leading Clinicians.
He has exceptional academic skills, his clear logical thoughts & approach to complex surgical issues makes him a standout in Knee Arthoplasty & Ligament Reconstructions. His surgical skills & compassionate behavior helps his patients to return back to routine activities & lead a normal life. His clinical skills are exemplary, he achieves good outcomes, and his patients love him.

Dr. Apurv Mehra—Renowned Author, Leading Faculty, Inspirational & Motivational Speaker

Dr. Apurv Mehra is The Leading Faculty of Orthopedics & is recognized Nationally & Internationally as an outstanding teacher, world class scholar & dedicated mentor. Dr. Apurv Mehra is also Co-Founder of MedMiracle—Online Platform To Guide Students Preparing for Medical Entrance Exams. He is best known for his stupendous efforts in teaching, motivating & inspiring budding doctors.
The quality that sets him apart is his unique style of teaching with fun & passion. He is the Author of many International Bestsellers across South East Asia. His books are being appreciated across the globe.
Dr. Apurv Mehra is a youth icon, guide, mentor & role model for aspiring doctors. He is known for his highly inspirational & motivational Speeches.
He has a vision & aims to provide high content resources needed to take students to the next level of education.
Thousands of students have been benefitted by his His Leading Orthopedic Lectures named Ortho Dhoom Dhadaka. His lectures are highly recommended by PG Toppers since Dr. Apurv inspires students to work hard, he builds trust in them & helps them to achieve their goals.
 Inspired from his lectures, students not only learn but also follow his advice & guidance in their day to day lives.

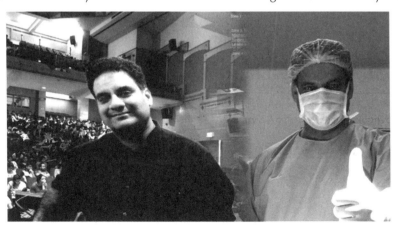

Dr Apurv Mehra's
Vidya Jeevan Orthopedics Super Speciality Centre,
Indias Most Trusted Centre For Ethical Practice As Per Clinicians
28, Vigyan Vihar, Near Yamuna Sports Complex, (Gate No. 2), Delhi-110092.
Timing: Monday to Saturday: 9 am to 9 pm
For Clinical / Surgical Appointments: **8800222008, 011-41512008**

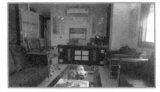

MedMiracle – The Learning App To Help Excel In Exams

Under The Guidance of Dr.Thameem Saif & Dr. Apurv Mehra

MedMiracle is an initiative FOR THE DOCTORS BY THE DOCTORS - NEET & AIIMS PG Toppers from Top Institutes like AIIMS Delhi, MAMC Delhi, KEM Mumbai, MMC Chennai & GMC Trivandrum with a Team of 19 Subject Specialists (Gold Medalists in PG) for the benefit of their Juniors.

Precise Content @ Lowest Price

- Q. Bank
- Unlimited Tests
- Notes
- Video Lectures
- Audio Lessons
- Pearl of the day
- Talk to MedMiracle Mentors- for personlized counselling

MedMiracle Subscriptions

- 6 Months @ Rs.7000/- (Actual Cost Rs.9000)
- 12 Months @ Rs.12000/- (Actual Cost Rs.18000)
- 18 Months @ Rs.18000 (Actual Cost Rs.27000)
- 24 Months @ Rs.20000 (Actual Cost Rs.36000)

Special Discount For ODD Students / Toppers / Gold Medalists in MBBS

Special Offer (for OPQR 7th Ed. Buyer)
Get Rs 2000 discount on MedMiracle Subscriptions

To Avail Discount Coupon
Call / Whatsapp: 9999664864 / 8800222009

Download MedMiracle:
Mail Your Queries to drapurv@medmiracle.in / help@medmiracle.in

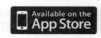

UNIQUE SELLING PREPOSITION OF OPQR

- Exam Oriented authentic and concise content
- Emphasis on concept building and focused learning
- Self explanatory flowcharts
- Diagrams and images to supplement the text to enable students to understand basic concepts in a better way
- Easy to grasp and retain mnemonics
- Each chapter is followed by potential questions for Retro Analysis
- 'Summary of Ortho' – For Review at a glance
- Ortho is a Rank Deciding Subject and OPQR is a must-read book for every student aspiring for Top Ranks in PGMEE
- Important points highlighted in each topic
- High Yield Authentic Questions marked for Quick Revision

CONTENTS

1. Imaging for Orthopedics — 1
2. Infection of Bone and Joints***** — 10
3. Tuberculosis of Bone and Joints — 22
4. Orthopedics Oncology — 30
5. Fracture and Fracture Healing — 58
6. Advanced Trauma Life Support — 68
7. Upper Limb Traumatology***** — 70
8. Spinal Injury — 104
9. Pelvis and Hip Injury — 112
10. Lower Limb Traumatology — 127
11. Fracture Management — 139
12. Amputations — 150
13. Sports Injury — 154
14. Neuromuscular Disease — 168
15. Peripheral Nerve Injury***** — 183
16. Joint Disorders***** — 203
17. Metabolic Disorders of Bone — 232
18. Pediatric Orthopedics — 256
19. Osteochondritis and Avascular Necrosis — 284
20. DNB CET Questions — 292
21. Complete Summary of Orthopedics***** — 317

All the chapters are important because they are under MCI curriculum. But the starred marked chapters hold maximum importance as per recent exam trend.

CHAPTER 1: Imaging for Orthopedics (Including Normal X-rays)

Orthopedics: The term was coined by Nicolas Andry. Ortho means straight and pedics means child so **orthopedics means Straight child.**

Definition of orthopedics: The branch of surgery that deals with the prevention or correction of injuries or disorders of the skeletal system and associated muscles, joints and ligaments.

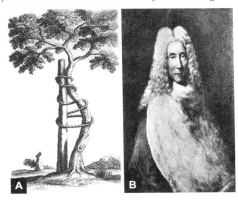

Figs. 1.1A and B: (A) Orthopedics emblem crooked tree (B) Nicolas Andry

- **Father of Orthopedics—Nicolas Andry.**
- **Father of Modern Orthopedics—Robert Jones.**
- Father of Arthroplasty—John Charnley.
- Father of Arthroscopy—Kenji Takagi and Masaki Watanabe
- Father of Orthopedic Oncology—Enneking
- Plaster of Paris ($CaSO_4 \cdot 1/2\ H_2O$): Mathysen.

ROLE OF IMAGING IN ORTHOPEDICS

X-rays are usually the first radiological investigation done in orthopedics and its uses involve screening of Cortex and Marrow. **X-rays are the first investigations in traumatic disorders.**

Soft tissue planes (muscle and fat planes) are visualized on X-rays and often students forget this!

(Loss of soft tissue planes is earliest X-ray changes in infection/swelling in limb and it is seen after 24–48 hours of onset of disease they are more useful for infections than tumors).

- Glass pieces are visualized on X-rays due to presence of lead in them.
- **Cartilage is not seen on X-ray.**

Note: Joint space is a misnomer. Actually there is no space in areas of joints, it is the cartilage occupied area which is not visualized on X-ray. Thus whenever joint is destroyed, cartilage is destroyed. Hence joint space is reduced on X-rays.

Reduction of Joint space means arthritis.

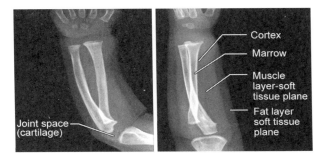

Fig. 1.2: X-ray of forearm with wrist and elbow

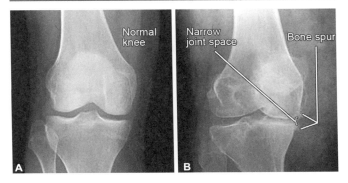

Figs. 1.3A and B: X-ray knee (A) Normal (B) Knee arthritis (Reduced Medial Joint Space)

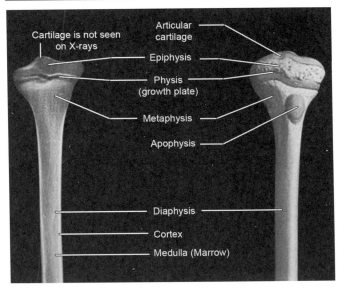

Fig. 1.4: Relationship of bone parts on X-ray

Ossified tissue (Live bone) is like a brick wall! (Fig. 1.5A)	Calcified tissue/dead bone is like a chalk! (Fig. 1.5A)
Properly laid down Architecture of haversian and volkmann's Canal with calcified hydroxyapatite crystals.	Deposition of calcium salts without bony architecture/trabeculae.
Live bone looks less white on X-rays and is strong in strength.	Dead bone looks more white on X-rays as compared to surrounding normal bone.

Live bone (e.g. Brick wall) is stronger, heavier but less white on X-rays (osteopenia or rarefaction) and dead bone (e.g. chalk) is light and white (Sclerosed on X-ray) (Figs. 1.5A to C).

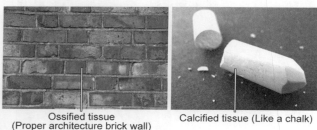

Fig. 1.5A: Comparison between live and dead bone

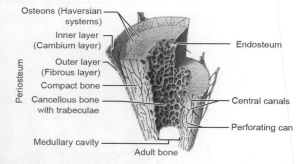

Fig. 1.5B: Architecture of bone

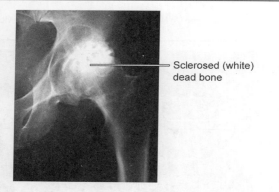

Fig. 1.5C: X-ray showing necrotic (dead) bone

Periosteum has two layers outer Fibrous layer (non-functional layer) and inner Cambium layer (Cellular layer/active layer). It does not contain dense regular connective tissue as seen in tendon, ligament and aponeurosis. Roles of cambium layer are:

1. **Bone union:** Cambium layer has important role in bone union at fracture site by providing the osteoprogenitor cells. If cambium layer is deficient bone union is difficult, e.g. neck of femur cambium layer is universally absent hence this is one of the causes of higher rates of non-union in femoral neck fractures.

2. **Origin of bone tumors:** Since cambium layer is cellular layer it is more prone to give origin to bone tumors, e.g. **osteochondroma**. Treatment principle of any bone tumor is to remove the tumor along with cells of origin so in such tumors surgical management consists of tumor excision along with periosteum and failure to remove the periosteum would cause recurrence of the tumor.

3. **Periosteal reaction:** Whenever a disease pathology destroys the bone cambium layer is irritated and responds by periosteal reaction, that is bone formation under the periosteum. Thus periosteal reaction is an indicator that disease is destroying the bone.

Types of Periosteal Reaction

- *No reaction:* **Tuberculosis of bones do not usually have a periosteal reaction.**
- Narrow zone of activity, e.g. Solid periosteal reaction (single layer of periosteal elevation) is seen in benign lesion like, **Benign tumors or Pyogenic Osteomyelitis.**
- In case of osteomyelitis the periosteal reaction is seen on day 7 to 10th (or 2nd week or day 10th).

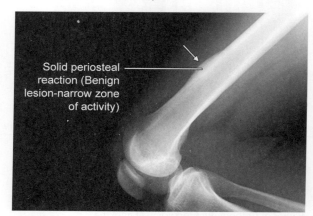

Fig. 1.6: Solid periosteal reaction

In **malignant lesions** there is wide area of activity, e.g. Onion peel/Codman's triangle and sunray appearance (all are indicative of wide area of activity).

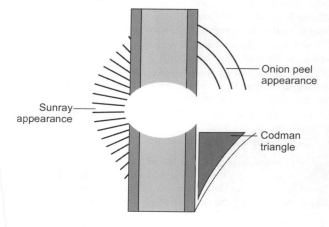

Fig. 1.7: Wide area of activity

Onion peel or lamellated appearance—Seen in any malignant or chronic lesions (e.g. chronic osteomyelitis) but usually **Ewing's sarcoma**.

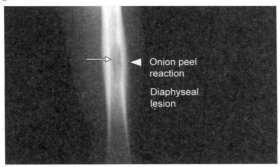

Fig. 1.8: Onion peel reaction

Codman Triangle—Triangular bony growth seen at angle of lifting of periosteum, it can be seen in any **malignant lesion** but usually **osteosarcoma**.

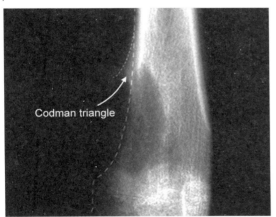

Fig. 1.9: Codman triangle

Sunray appearance/sunburst/spiculated appearance – Calcification along the Sharpey's fibers, can be seen in **any malignant lesion** but usually **osteosarcoma**.

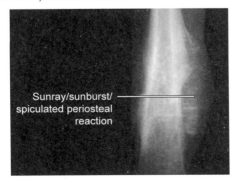

Fig. 1.10: Sunray appearance

Osteophytes—(Osteo means bone and phytes means growth) They are seen in case of joint damage.

Note: Reduced Joint Space also indicates joint damage as joint space is cartilage.

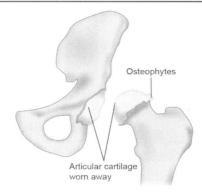

Fig. 1.11: Osteophytes

Syndesmophytes indicates Spine destruction (Osteophyte of spine) but they bridge across the joint as compared to osteophytes which are non-bridging.

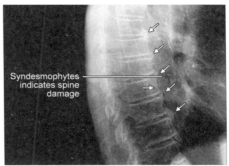

Fig. 1.12: X-ray spine

Ultrasound (USG): Now-a-days there is increasing role of USG in assessment of various joint and soft tissue pathologies.
1. High frequency transducers are used (5–12 MHz).
2. It provides the benefit of real-time imaging and evaluation of soft tissue near a metallic orthopedic hardware without the artifact that limits MR imaging.
3. USG is specially useful in evaluation of muscles and tendons.
4. Due to subjective variations in ultrasound results, MRI has replaced its use for many indications.

CT Scan: CT scan is the investigation for cortex and calcification.

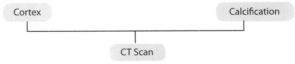

Any **new bone formation or 3D image**—CT Scan is preferred investigation.

MRI is investigation of choice for Marrow, Soft tissues (Brain/Spinal cord/Ligaments/Tendons/nerves/vessels) and Cartilage.

Basic Images in MRI are T_1 and T_2

- T_1 – 1st professional subject anatomy—so in T_1 image anatomy is seen.
- T_2 – 2nd professional subject pathology—so in T_2 image Pathology is seen.

'Water is white on T_2'

Water is any body fluid example, synovial fluid/CSF/inflammatory or traumatic edema.

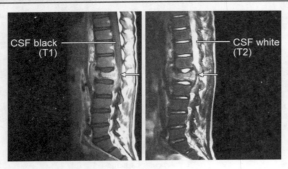

Fig. 1.13: MRI of spine (T_1 and T_2 images)

Please Note:

Any <u>occult fracture</u> (not visualized on X-ray) e.g. <u>Fracture neck femur</u> ~ MRI is investigation of choice.

Any fracture in which there is marrow edema example <u>stress fracture – MRI</u> is investigation of choice.

Osteomyelitis starts in marrow of metaphysis—**MRI** is best radiological investigation.

Tumors with marrow involvement, any micrometastasis or soft tissue component—**MRI** can aid in diagnosis.

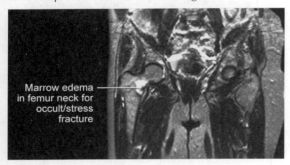

Fig. 1.14: MRI pelvis

Avascular Necrosis/Perthes disease (avascular necrosis of femoral epiphysis)-MRI is investigation of choice.

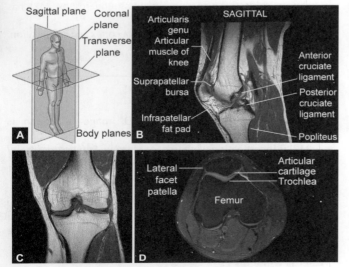

Figs. 1.15A to D: (A) Body planes MRI (B) Sagittal (C) Coronal and (D) Axial sections of the knee

Note: CT scan can principally show only the bony structures whereas MRI can show the soft tissues very well.

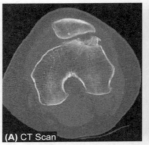 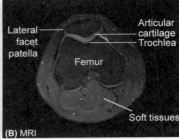

Figs. 1.16A and B: (A) CT Scan mainly shows the bony structure whereas (B) MRI Shows Bone, Soft tissues and cartilage

T_C **labeled bone scan:** Can pick-up—Blastic (Osteoblastic) activity—methylene diphosphonate is taken up by osteoblasts on scanning the whole skeleton.

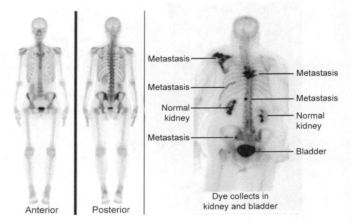

Fig. 1.17: Bone scan

Bone scan show activity in areas with increased osteoblastic activity example tumors, infection or fracture. Thus in cases with bilateral stress fractures bone scan is preferred investigation.

Note: Investigation of choice for unilateral stress fracture is MRI and bilateral is Bone Scan.

It can pick-up tumors that go from one bone to other, i.e. bone to bone metastasis.

BONE: **B**one to bone/**O**steosarcoma/**N**euroblastoma/**E**wing sarcoma (maximum incidence)

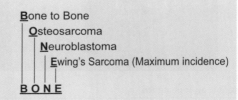

Limitation: Bone Scan cannot identify the source of unknown primary.

Note: Lesions with lytic activity do not show activity on bone scan, e.g. multiple myeloma.

PET CT: Position emission tomography + CT Scan for whole body. It is a combination of 2 modalities.

18 F Deoxy glucose uptake by tumor cells (as they have anaerobic metabolism) and CT scan for all viscera so it can identify unknown primary. (Bone Scan the uptake is by osteoblast and PET Scan by tumor cells)

Thus **PET–CT is more useful than Bone Scan** as it can identify primary and is more specific for tumor cells.

Limitation: Osteoblastic lesions have limited uptake on PET so bone scan may be more valuable.

Metastasis
• Single lesion: MRI
• Multiple Osteoblastic metastasis: Bone Scan
• Multiple Metastasis: PET Scan

Remember that radiological diagnosis in cases of infection and tumors is suggestive never diagnostic.

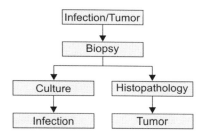

Diagnostic is always Tissue Diagnosis

Tumors and infection can mimic each other (clinically and radiologically), e.g. Osteosarcoma and Ewings sarcoma are two tumors that mimic osteomyelitis. (Both have accompanying fever and increased local temperature).

Tumors and bone infections are usually metaphyseal and both need tissue diagnosis for differentiation.

- **Thus, Culture is gold standard for infection**
- **Histopathology is gold standard for tumors**
- So rule is <u>Culture all biopsies, biopsy all cultures</u>. That is whenever you obtain any sample from a suspected case of tumor or infection divide it into two parts send one for culture and other for histopathology.

Osteomyelitis

- **Pyogenic Osteomyelitis on X-rays will show loss of soft tissue planes after 24–48 hours (1st change).**
- **Day 7 to 10-solid periosteal reaction is identified.** (1st Bony change)
- **In tuberculosis there is no periosteal reaction.**
- Chronic osteomyelitis—sclerosed dead bone (sequestrum) is important for diagnosis and onion peel appearance is the usual periosteal reaction.
- **MRI can pick-up marrow changes in metaphysis. (Best radiological investigation for Osteomyelitis and Tuberculosis).**
- **Bone scan is next in preference to MRI** to pick up infections by picking osteoblastic activity at the site of infection.
- **Culture and growth of organism is most definitive diagnostic modality for Osteomyelitis.**

Bone Tumors

- X-ray is to localize the tumor.
- CT scan is for extent and cortical lesion.
- MRI is for Marrow extent, micrometastasis and soft tissue involvement (Most preferred investigation for most tumors).
- PET-CT and Bone scan for multiple lesions (PET-CT is better than Bone Scan).
- **Biopsy is definitive diagnostic modality for any tumor.**

MRI in Developmental Dysplasia of Hip (DDH)

- T1W images display exact position of the cartilage which is useful when position of the same is uncertain on X-rays or serial follow-up is required, thereby reducing radiation exposure.
- Useful in patients with or without plaster casts.
- When ossific nucleus is not visible on plain X-ray or CT.
- **T2W images are useful for complications like ischemic necrosis and effusions which are not demonstrated with USG or X-ray.**
- 3D MR rendering for complex femoral head and acetabular special relationships and dysplasias.

USG in DDH

- Evaluation of cartilaginous femoral head prior to appearance of ossific nucleus, subluxation, dislocation, pulvinar or inverted labrum, hypoplastic ossific nucleus, acetabular dysplasia and ossification. The findings in USG are subjective and are not as specific as MRI.

Thus if the question is asked for screening of neonatal hip or hip instability then USG is investigation of choice.

If the question is asked about Investigation of choice for <u>DDH</u> than <u>MRI >USG</u> will be the order as MRI will be more useful for assessment of complete disease spectrum, management and complications of DDH.

Reference: MRI in Orthopedics and Sports Medicine. David W Stoller. 3rd edition Vol 1.

MULTIPLE CHOICE QUESTIONS

1. Which investigation is not useful for Osteomyelitis evaluation: *(PGI Nov 2018)*
   - A. X-ray
   - B. MRI
   - C. CT Scan
   - D. Bone Scan
   - E. Culture

Ans. is 'C' CT Scan

CT Scan is the least preferred investigation out of given options. Although it is done in selective cases of chronic Osteomyelitis.

2. Intraosseous skeletal tumor is best detected by: *(JIPMER MAY 2017)*
   - A. Bone scan with CT
   - B. X-ray
   - C. Bone scan
   - D. MRI

Ans. is 'D' MRI

3. X-ray appearance of sequestrum is: *(NEET DEC 2016)*
   - A. Unnatural radiodense fragments
   - B. Osteopenic fragment
   - C. Fragment with honeycomb loculated appearance
   - D. Radiolucent area with speckled calcification

Ans. is 'A' Unnatural radiodense fragments

Orthopedics Quick Review

4. Most sensitive investigation for early bone infections is: *(NEET DEC 2016)*
   A. X-ray B. CT scan
   C. Bone scan D. USG
   Ans. is 'C' Bone scan
   MRI > Bone scan is the preferred answer for investigation in osteomyelitis

5. Onion skin periosteal reaction is seen in: *(DNB JUNE 2017)*
   A. Ewings sarcoma B. Osteosarcoma
   C. Wilms tumor D. Osteoblastoma
   Ans. is 'A' Ewings sarcoma

6. Which of the following is not an aggressive periosteal reaction? *(NEET DEC 2016)*
   A. Spiculated B. Laminated
   C. Thick and irregular D. Interrupted
   Ans. is 'C' Thick and irregular
   Non-aggressive reactions are thin, Solid, thick and irregular.
   Aggressive reactions are Spiculated, Laminated, Hair on End, Sun burst, disorganised, Interrupted and Codman's triangle.

7. Stress fractures are diagnosed by:
   (JIPMER May 2016, AIIMS May 2015, AI 2004)
   A. X-ray B. CT
   C. MRI D. Bone scan
   Ans. is 'C' MRI (Investigation of choice for unilateral stress fracture is MRI and for bilateral is Bone Scan), when it is not mentioned unilateral or bilateral, MRI is preferred answer.

8. Image of knee joint, which investigation is being done? *(AI 2016)*

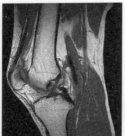

   A. MRI Coronal section B. MRI Sagittal section
   C. CT Coronal section D. CT Sagittal section
   Ans. is 'B' MRI Sagittal section

9. Acute Osteomyelitis, earliest bone change can be best seen by? *(AI 2016)*
   A. PET CT B. MRI
   C. Bone Scan D. X-ray
   Ans. is 'B' MRI > 'C' Bone Scan

10. Identify the marked structure: *(AI 2016)*

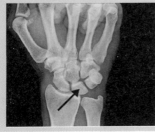

   A. Trapezium B. Lunate
   C. Trapezoid D. Capitate
   Ans. is 'B' Lunate

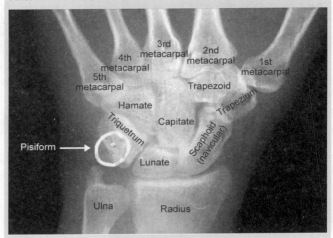

11. Which of the following is the investigation of choice for Perthes disease of the bone? *(JIPMER 2015)*
    A. MRI B. CT
    C. X-ray D. USG
    Ans. is 'A' MRI

12. Occult fracture of neck femur is best diagnosed by
    A. CT Scan B. Bone scan *(PGM-CET 2015)*
    C. MRI D. None of the above
    Ans. is 'C' MRI

13. Sunray appearance in osteosarcoma is due to:
    (AIIMS Nov 2014)
    A. Periosteal reaction B. Muscle fiber calcification
    C. Blood vessel calcification D. Bone resorption
    Ans. is 'A' Periosteal reaction

14. A child with injury in hand with glass pieces next investigation would be: *(AIIMS Nov 2014)*
    A. X-ray B. USG
    C. MRI D. CT Scan
    Ans. is 'A' X-ray

15. Dense regular connective tissue fibers are seen in all except:
    A. Periosteum B. Tendon *(AIIMS Nov 2014)*
    C. Ligament D. Aponeurosis
    Ans. is 'A' Periosteum

16. Developmental Dysplasia of Hip (DDH) best diagnostic modality is: *(Neet Pattern 2014, May AIIMS 2012)*
    A. Clinical B. X-ray
    C. MRI D. CT
    Ans. is 'C' MRI

17. A 4-year-old girl with fever and mass in thigh, on her X-ray there is periosteal reaction and destruction of bone. Next investigation to be done in this girl is: *(AIIMS Nov 2013)*
    A. Bone biopsy B. Bone scan
    C. Blood culture D. CT Scan
    Ans. is 'A' Bone biopsy
    (Order is X-ray → MRI → Bone biopsy)

18. A 10-year-old obese child from endocrinology department was referred to emergency for a painful limp with hip pain which of the following investigation is not required: *(AIIMS Nov 2013)*
    A. X-ray of the hip
    B. MRI of the hip
    C. CT scan of hip
    D. USG of hip

Ans. is 'C' CT scan of hip

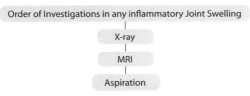

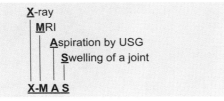

This is an Obese Limping child with hip pain the possible differential diagnosis will be
Osteomyelitis (X-MAS)
Septic arthritis (X-MAS)
Slipped capital femoral epiphysis (X-MRI)
Transient synovitis (X-MAS)
Hence CT will be least preferred. Previously CT Scan was carried out for SCFE but now MRI has replaced its indication.

19. 4-year-old child complains of pain and swelling of right tibia on evaluation patient has high ESR, leucocytosis and on X-ray tibial lesion best investigation is: *(AIIMS Nov 2012)*
    A. Blood C/S   B. Pus C/S
    C. MRI   D. Biopsy

Ans. is 'D' Biopsy

20. Screening of neonatal hip instability most commonly used modality is: *(NEET Pattern 2012)*
    A. USG   B. X-ray
    C. MRI   D. CT

Ans. is 'A' USG

21. Bilateral stress fractures are diagnosed by: *(NEET Pattern 2012)*
    A. X-ray   B. CT
    C. MRI   D. Bone scan

Ans. is 'D' Bone Scan

22. 45-year-old female has history of slip in bathroom complaints of pain right hip, tenderness in scarpas triangle and normal X-ray. Next investigation is: *(May AIIMS 2012)*
    A. USG guided aspiration   B. CT
    C. MRI   D. Bone scan

Ans. is 'C' MRI

This case refers to post-traumatic pain in proximal femur, scarpas triangle refers to area of femoral neck and for stress or occult fracture of neck femur where traumatic marrow edema is seen – MRI is investigation of choice.

23. Tuberculosis of spine best diagnostic modality is: *(May AIIMS 2012)*
    A. Clinical
    B. X-ray
    C. MRI
    D. CT guided biopsy

Ans. is 'D' CT guided biopsy

Tissue diagnosis is always preferred over any radiological diagnosis hence CT guided biopsy to obtain tissue and then further investigations to grow the organisms is the preferred approach. Many make a mistake of marking MRI as the answer please remember that MRI is best radiological investigation but best investigation overall for infections or tumors is always biopsy.

24. Multiple Bone metastasis are diagnosed by: *(AI 2011/AIIMS Nov 2010)*
    A. X-ray
    B. CT
    C. MRI
    D. Bone scan

Ans. is 'D' Bone Scan

25. Best investigations for multiple bone metastasis: *(NEET Pattern 2012)*
    A. PET CT
    B. CT
    C. MRI
    D. Bone scan

Ans. is 'A' PET CT

For bone metastasis PET CT is better than bone scan.

26. What is the earliest change of osteomyelitis on X-rays: *(AIIMS May 2010)*
    A. Loss of soft tissue planes
    B. Periosteal reaction
    C. Sequestrum
    D. Lytic defects

Ans. is 'A' Loss of soft tissue planes

27. What is the earliest bony change of osteomyelitis on X-rays? *(AIIMS Nov 2009)*
    A. Loss of soft tissue planes
    B. Periosteal reaction
    C. Sequestrum
    D. Lytic defects

Ans. is 'B' Periosteal reaction

Pyogenic osteomyelitis on X-ray in 24–48 hours will show loss of soft tissue planes **(earliest change on X-ray)**.
Day 7 to 10-solid periosteal reaction **(earliest bony change on X-ray)**.

28. The father of joint replacement surgery is: *(NEET Pattern 2013)*
    A. Manning
    B. Girdlestone
    C. Charnley
    D. Ponseti

Ans. is 'C' Charnley

NORMAL X-RAYS

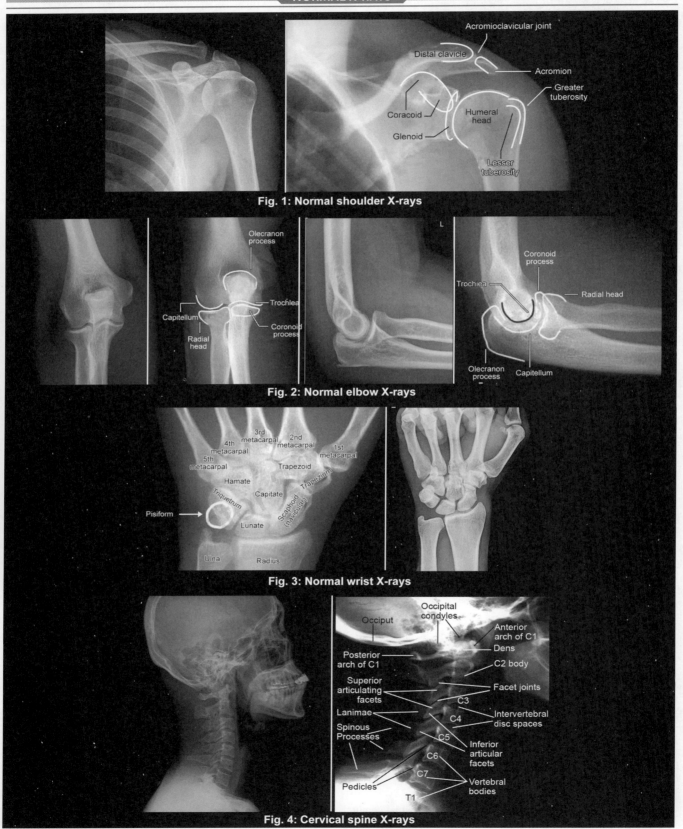

Fig. 1: Normal shoulder X-rays

Fig. 2: Normal elbow X-rays

Fig. 3: Normal wrist X-rays

Fig. 4: Cervical spine X-rays

NORMAL X-RAYS

Imaging for Orthopedics (Including Normal X-rays)

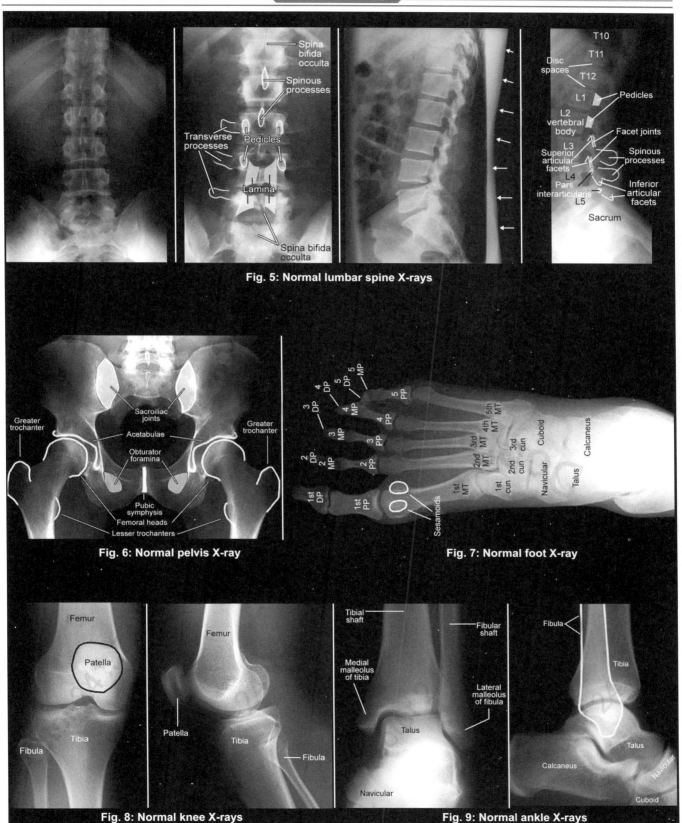

Fig. 5: Normal lumbar spine X-rays

Fig. 6: Normal pelvis X-ray

Fig. 7: Normal foot X-ray

Fig. 8: Normal knee X-rays

Fig. 9: Normal ankle X-rays

CHAPTER 2: Infection of Bone and Joints

OSTEOMYELITIS

Acute Osteomyelitis

- Acute osteomyelitis is infection of bone.

Etiology

- **Staphylococcus aureus is the most common organism in all age groups**
- **Salmonella is the commonest organism in sickle cell anemia patients (diaphyseal)**
- **Pseudomonas aeruginosa is the commonest organism in drug abusers**
- Animal bite – Pasteurella multocida
- Human bite – Eikenella corrodens
- Diabetic ulcer and fight bites – Anaerobes
- Immunocompromised (HIV) – **Staphylococcus aureus**
- Post-traumatic osteomyelitis/Post-surgical osteomyelitis – S. aureus
- Open injuries – Staphylococcus
- Foot injuries – Pseudomonas.

Pathology

- Most common mode of infection is **hematogenous**
- In children metaphysis of long bone (usually **lower end femur > upper end tibia**) is earliest and most commonly involved site
- **In adults the commonest site of infection is thoracolumbar spine.**

Starts in Metaphysis because of:

- **Defective phagocytosis** in metaphysis (Inherently depleted Reticuloendothelial System)
- Rich blood supply
- **Hair pin bend** of metaphyseal vessels (leads to vascular stasis)
- Metaphyseal hemorrhage due to repeated trauma (acts as culture media).

Pathophysiology

i. *Metaphyseal Abscess is formed initially and* it spreads Subperiosteally in children because periosteum is loosely attached to bone in children and in adults pus spreads to Medullary cavity involving the diaphysis.
ii. Infection rarely crosses growth plate because it has no blood vessels and periosteum is firmly attached to the plate at this level.
iii. Joint involvement can take place if—metaphysis is intracapsular (e.g. hip, shoulder, elbow).
iv. The pathological sequence is inflammation, suppuration, necrosis, reactive new bone formation and ultimately resolution and healing. **(Same sequence is seen in HIV positive patient also).**

Clinical Feature and Investigation

- Presenting complaints are Fever (>38.3°C), swelling of the limb, pain, systemic symptoms and increased levels of Total leucocyte counts, ESR and CRP. **(Toxic child)**

Note: Systemic signs are absent in immunocompromised and neonates.

- **Absent movements of a limb after ruling out trauma in pediatric population is osteomyelitis till proved otherwise.**
- X-rays in <24 hours is normal.
- 1st change on X-rays is loss of soft tissue planes.
- **1st bony change is periosteal reaction seen on day 7–10 (2nd week or day 10) Solid Periosteal Reaction.**
- Later, features of bone destruction appear.
- MRI is considered the best radiological investigation for bone infections because it can identify marrow edema (seen within 6 hours) and soft tissue extension in bone infections.
- Tc99-MDP, Ga-67—citrate or Indium 111 labeled leucocytes (Best out of 3) are the 2nd best radiological investigation.
- *Gold standard is always tissue diagnosis (from the lesion) hence growth of organism on culture media is the best investigation for infections.*
- Blood Culture is positive in 60% cases.
- Note: Order of investigation done in case of osteomyelitis is X-ray→MRI→Bone scan.
- In osteomyelitis order of investigation that show positive changes are in the following order MRI→Bone scan→X-ray.

Criteria for Diagnosis of Osteomyelitis

A. **Morrey and Peterson's criterion:**
   - *Definite:* Pathogen isolated from bone or adjacent soft tissue or there is histologic evidence of osteomyelitis.
   - *Probable:* Blood culture positive + Clinical (absent movements of the limb) + Radiological diagnosis.
   - *Likely:* Typical clinical findings and definite radiographic evidence of OM + Response to antibiotics.

B. **Peltola and Valvanen's criteria:**
   Diagnosis when 2/4 are present
   1. Pus from bone
   2. Bone/blood culture
   3. Clinical diagnosis
   4. Radiological diagnosis

Remember: Clinical suspicion of bone and joint infections is most important indication for treatment.

Treatment

- If osteomyelitis is suspected on clinical grounds, blood and fluid sample should be taken and **treatment started immediately without waiting for final confirmation of diagnosis.**

Osteomyelitis < 24 Hours

- X-ray – No Loss of Soft tissue planes.
- MRI – Marrow changes in metaphysis.
- Bone scan – Increased activity.
- Treatment is started with, IV antibiotics until condition begins to improve or CRP values return to normal, usually for 2 weeks. Thereafter antibiotics are given orally for another 4 weeks.
- Peak elevation of the ESR occurs at 3–5 days after infection and returns to normal approximately 3 weeks after treatment is begun. The CRP increases within 6 hours of infection, reaches a peak elevation 2 days after infection, and returns to normal within 1 week after adequate treatment has begun. So CRP is better indicator of infection as compared to ESR.
- If antibiotics are given early (<24 hours), drainage is often unnecessary.
- Change of antibiotics or surgery is considered, if no improvement occurs with in 48 hours of antibiotics.

Osteomyelitis > 24 Hours

- X-ray – Loss of soft tissue planes.
- MRI – Marrow changes in metaphysis.
- Bone scan – Increased activity.
- Treatment evacuation and exploration of pus.

Drainage is followed by antibiotics course of antibiotics is same as Osteomyelitis < 24 Hours, i.e. for 2 weeks IV and 4 weeks oral. The antibiotics that cover Staphylococcus aureus are preferred and ones that have both oral and injectable preparation are preferred, e.g. Amoxyclavulanic or Linezolid (reserved drug).

```
Reduced Movements of Limb, Toxic Child
and Metaphysis Tender (Clinical Diagnosis)
        |
   -----+-----
   |         |
Osteomyelitis < 24 hours     Osteomyelitis > 24 hours
   |                           |
X-ray – No loss of soft      X-ray – Loss of soft
tissue planes                tissue planes
   |                           |
MRI – Marrow changes in      MRI – Marrow changes in
metaphysis                   metaphysis
   |                           |
Bone scan – Increased        Bone scan – Increased
activity                     activity
   |                           |
Treatment is started with    Treatment is evacuation and
IV antibiotics               exploration of pus and antibiotics
   |                         for 6 weeks
Once condition begins to
improve or CRP values return to
normal, (usually for 2 weeks) then
antibiotics are given orally for
another 4 weeks.
```

The Important Complications of Acute Osteomyelitis are:

i. **Chronic osteomyelitis (most common complication)**
ii. Septicemia and pyemia
iii. Septic arthritis
iv. Metastatic infection to other body parts
v. Pathological fracture
vi. Altered growth from damage to epiphyseal growth plate
vii. Recurrence.

Osteomyelitis in Newborn

1. More susceptible than older children.
2. Early diagnosis difficult due to paucity of clinical signs.
3. More common in males and preterm.
4. **Hematogenous** spread, **metaphysis** of long bones.
5. **S. Aureus** most common organism > Group B Streptococci > Gram negative.
6. 2 presentations
   i. Benign form with little or no evidence of infection
   ii. Sepsis like syndrome (multifocal >50% cases involve ≥ 2 bones).
7. Prognosis is poor.

SUBACUTE OSTEOMYELITIS

Brodie's Abscess: Seen in Immunocompetent Host!

- It is long standing localized pyogenic abscess in the bone (long standing because of **strong defence mechanism** of body).
- It usually involves long bones (metaphysis or diaphysis), e.g. **Upper end tibia.**

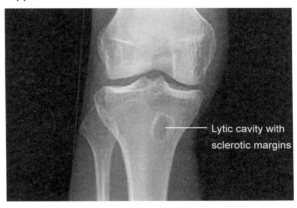

Fig. 2.1: Brodie's abscess

- Classical Brodie's abscess looks like a small walled off (Sclerotic margins) cavity in bone with little or no periosteal reaction.
- Usual isolated organism is **Staphylococcus aureus** (although most cultures are negative).

Treatment

Trial of injectable antibiotics is given if it fails curettage of the cavity is carried out.

CHRONIC OSTEOMYELITIS: USUALLY A SEQUELAE OF INADEQUATELY TREATED ACUTE OSTEOMYELITIS

Causative Organism; Staphylococcus Aureus

1. **Sequestrum: Avascular piece of bone** surrounded by granulation tissue, it is pathognomic of chronic osteomyelitis.
   - It acts as nidus of infection and is most common cause of non-healing sinus in chronic osteomyelitis.
   - Chronic persistent neutrophilic discharge can be seen.
2. Involucrum is dense sclerotic new bone surrounding the sequestrum formed from deep layers of stripped periosteum (usually obvious by the end of 2nd week). At least 2/3rd surface

of sequestrum should be surrounded by involucrum before carrying out sequestrectomy (Removal of Sequestrum).
3. If infection persists, pus and tiny sequestrated spicules of bone may continue to discharge through **perforations in involucrum (cloacae)**.
4. **Cierny and Mader classification** is used for chronic osteomyelitis.

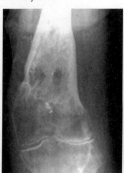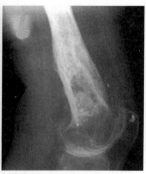

Fig. 2.2: Chronic osteomyelitis (Lower end femur)

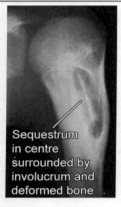

Fig. 2.3: Chronic osteomyelitis (Upper end humerus)

Rim Sign is seen on MRI

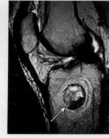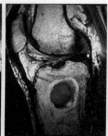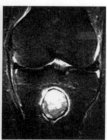

Fig. 2.4: Rim sign in chronic osteomyelitis seen on MRI

TREATMENT

1. Remove the sequestrum from cavity or saucerization of cavity (Leaving the cavity open).

Note: Paprika sign is appearance of live bone after removal of sequestrum.

2. **Identify the organism and control the infection (most important step).**

3. Fill the gap in cavity with Bone graft/Bone cement (Polymethyl Methacrylate) e.g.
   i. *PMMA beads + occlusive dressing*: Bead pouch technique
   ii. *Bone transport*: (Ilizarov method)—If large gaps are present
   iii. Papineau **technique of bone grafting**.
4. Provide a good soft tissue coverage—**Local closure or by Myoplasty or composite graft of bone, Muscle and skin.**
   Instillation-suction technique for the treatment of chronic bone infection is described in which infected bone is first exposed and all sequestra removed. Two drainage tubes are inserted. One tube is connected to a drip containing antibiotic solution and the second to a continuous suction pump. Closed continuous steady flow instillation-suction is established to do lavage of cavity.
5. Negative pressure wound therapy/vacuum-assisted closure
   Negative pressure wound therapy is used to heal chronic or non-healing wounds. Air tight environment is created and vacuum applied to it. This technique is used continuously or intermittently and develops a good granulation tissue. The pressures are between –75 to –125 mm Hg.

Complications of Chronic Osteomyelitis
i. Acute exacerbation
ii. Growth abnormalities due to damage to adjacent growth plate
iii. Pathological fracture
iv. Joint stiffness
v. *Sinus tract malignancy (very rare): Squamous cell carcinoma*
vi. *Amyloidosis*

Garre's Osteomyelitis

It is non-suppurative sclerosing, chronic osteomyelitis characterized by marked sclerosis and cortical thickening.
There is no abscess, only a diffuse enlargement of the bone at affected Site usually **mandible** or diaphysis of tubular bone.
Treatment is excision of fragment.
Infection of the bone (classification based on time period of osteomyelitis) – Was used earlier
- Acute (< 2 weeks)
- Chronic (> 3 weeks)
- Subacute (2–3 weeks)

Multifocal Osteomyelitis They are Two Varieties in Which this topic can be asked:

1. Chronic Recurrent Multifocal Osteomyelitis (CRMO) is an autoimmune/auto inflammatory disease involving multiple bone with lesions, inflammation and pain. There is no infection. It is a diagnosis of exclusion. Some relate it to SAPHO syndrome.
   - SAPHO Syndrome (Synovitis, Acne, Pustulosis palmo-plantar, Hyperostosis and Osteitis).
   - Treatment is NSAIDs/Steroids/Disease Modifying Anti-Rheumatoid Drugs (DMARD).

2. Sickle cell anemia can involve multiple bones hence it can cause multifocal osteomyelitis and causative organism is Salmonella.

MULTIPLE CHOICE QUESTIONS

1. Multifocal osteomyelitis is associated with?
   (NBE Pattern 2018)
   A. SAPHO syndrome   B. Sickle cell anemia
   C. Thalassemia   D. Salmonella infection
   Ans. is 'B' Sickle cell anemia

2. A boy presented with multiple nonsuppurative osteomyelitis with sickle cell anemia, what will be the causative organism? *(NBE Pattern 2018)*
   A. Salmonella
   B. S. aureus
   C. H. influenzae
   D. Enterobacter species

Ans. is 'A' Salmonella

3. True about acute osteomyelitis? *(PGI MAY 2018)*
   A. Cannot be detected on X-ray before 2 weeks
   B. Bone scan detect after 2 weeks
   C. Severe pain
   D. Secondary osteomyelitis associated with compound fracture is more common than primary variety
   E. Limitation of movements

Ans. is 'C' Severe pain; 'E' Limitation of movements

4. A child presents with fever and discharging pus from right thigh × 3 months. Following is the X-ray. Identify the labeled structured: *(AIIMS Nov 2018)*

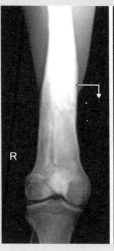
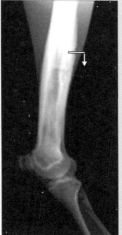

   A. Sequestrum
   B. Cloacae
   C. Involucrum
   D. Worsen Bone

Ans. is 'C' Involucrum

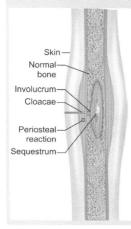
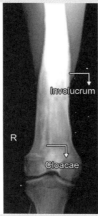
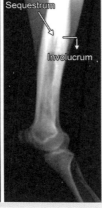

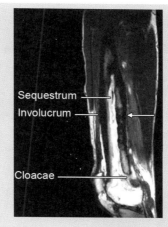

5. 12 years male came with swelling of lower end tibia which is surrounded by rim of reactive bone. What is most likely diagnosis? *(AIIMS Nov 2018)*
   A. Giant cell tumor (GCT)   B. Brodie's Abscess
   C. Hyperparathyroidism   D. Osteomyelitis

Ans. is 'B' Brodie's Abscess

Brodie's Abscess: Seen in Immunocompetent Host!

- It is long-standing localized pyogenic abscess in the bone (long-standing because of **strong defence mechanism** of body).
- It usually involves long bones (metaphysis or diaphysis), e.g. **Upper end tibia.**

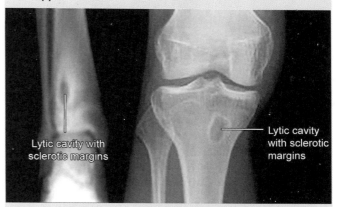

Fig. 2.1: Brodie's abscess

- Classical Brodie's abscess looks like a small walled off (Sclerotic margins) cavity in bone with little or no periosteal reaction.
- Usual isolated organism is **Staphylococcus aureus** (although most cultures are negative).

6. Multifocal nonsuppurative Osteomyelitis is seen in:
   A. Infantile cortical hyperostosis   *(NEET 2018)*
   B. Thalassemia   C. Salmonella
   D. SAPHO syndrome

Ans. is 'D' SAPHO syndrome

7. A 22 yr male presents with pain and deformity in right lower limb. He sustained trauma in the same limb 2 years back. The X-ray of the patient is suggestive of: *(NEET 2018)*

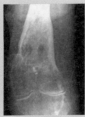 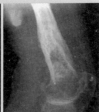

A. Osteogenic sarcoma B. Ewings sarcoma
C. Chronic osteomyelitis D. Stress fracture

Ans. is 'C' Chronic osteomyelitis
Another variety of same question.

8. A 25 years old male having pain and deformity of the tibia as shown in X-ray. He had history of trauma 2 years back. What is the most probable diagnosis?
 (NBE Pattern 2018)

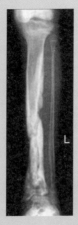

A. Ewing's Sarcoma B. Chronic osteomyelitis
C. Osteosarcoma D. Stess fracture tibia

Ans. is 'B' Chronic osteomyelitis

9. Paprika sign during debridement is crucial in management of which of the following condition? *(DNB JUNE 2017)*
A. Chronic osteomyelitis B. Osteosarcoma
c. Osteoid osteoma d. Brodies abscess

Ans. is 'A' Chronic osteomyelitis

10. Negative pressure wound therapy false is:
 (DNB JUNE 2017)
A. Necrotic tissue with eschar in wound is a contraindication to its use
B. Pressure is 30 mm Hg
C. Gives good granulation tissue
D. Used intermittently or continuously

Ans. is 'B' Pressure is 30 mm Hg

11. Osteomyelitis in sickle cell anemia is due to.
 (NEET DEC 2016)
A. Salmonella B. Streptococcus
C. Haemophilus D. Neisseria

Ans. is 'A' Salmonella
 – Musculoskeletal abnormalities in Sickle cell disease.
 1. Dactylitis or hand-foot syndrome is swelling, tenderness and warmth of hands and feet (< 5 years age group).
 2. Sterile joint effusion and periarticular pain in sickle cell crisis (knee and elbow are usually involved).
 3. Diaphyseal osteomyelitis of long tubular bone esp. Salmonella infections, also it can involve multiple bones.
 4. Infarction of bone marrow and avascular necrosis.

12. Which of the following is not true regarding acute pyogenic osteomyelitis: *(PGI Nov 2017)*
A. MC site in bone is diaphysis of bone
B. Sequestrum is the new bone formation surrounding involucrum
C. Is most commonly caused by Staphylococcus aureus
D. MC mode of Infection is direct inoculation due to trauma
D. Cloacae are discharging sinus

Ans. is 'A' MC site in bone is diaphysis of bone; 'B' Sequestrum is the new bone formation surrounding involucrum; 'D' MC mode of Infection is direct inoculation due to trauma

13. Osteomyelitis most commonly starts at:
 (NEET Pattern 2016, 2012)
A. Epiphysis B. Metaphysis
C. Diaphysis D. None

Ans. is 'B' Metaphysis

14. X-ray shoulder of the patient with following image shows:
 (AIIMS Nov 16)

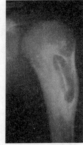

A. Ewing's sarcoma B. Osteosarcoma
C. Callus D. Chronic osteomyelitis

Ans. is 'D' Chronic osteomyelitis

15. An 18-year-old male presents with a draining sinus on his left leg with pus discharge and discharge of bony pieces since 3 months. The diagnosis is: *(CET July 16)*
A. Chronic osteomyelitis B. Ewing's sarcoma
C. Osteoid osteoma D. Cellulitis

Ans. is 'A' Chronic osteomyelitis

16. Total duration of antibiotics in acute osteomyelitis is:
A. 4 weeks B. 2 weeks *(CET Nov 15)*
C. 6 weeks D. 8 weeks

Ans. is 'C' 6 weeks

17. True regarding osteomyelitis in newborn: *(JIPMER 2015)*
A. Most common in diaphysis
B. The infection is unifocal
C. Organisms are derived from maternal genital tract
D. Most common organism is E. coli

Ans. is 'C' Organisms are derived from maternal genital tract.

18. All are true about septic arthritis except: *(PGI May 2015)*
A. Staph. aureus is most common causative organisms
B. Common in children
C. Affect growth plate
D. E. coli is the commonest causative organism
E. Aspiration of joint fluid is used for diagnosis

Ans. is 'D' E. coli is the commonest causative organism

19. Brodie's abscess is a terminology for: *(PGM-CET 2015)*
    A. Subungual infection B. Chronic osteomyelitis
    C. Web space infection D. Infected hematoma
Ans. is 'B' Chronic osteomyelitis
    (Better answer would have been subacute osteomyelitis but since it is not mentioned second best answer is chronic osteomyelitis)

20. Commonest cause of acute osteomyelitis: *(PGI Nov 2014)*
    A. Trauma   B. Surgery
    C. Fungal infection D. Hematogenous route
    E. Tubercular infection
Ans. is 'D' Hematogenous route

21. Post-traumatic osteomyelitis causing organism is: *(AIIMS May 2014)*
    A. Staphylococcus aureus B. Staphylococcus pyogenes
    C. E. coli   D. Pseudomonas
Ans. is 'A' Staphylococcus aureus

22. Osteomyelitis of spine most common organism is: *(AIIMS May 2014)*
    A. Staphylococcus aureus B. Pseudomonas
    C. Tuberculosis   D. Streptococcus
Ans. is 'A' Staphylococcus aureus, Overall, Worldwide Staphylococcus aureus is commonest organism. In India Tuberculosis is commonest.

23. All are true about chronic osteomyelitis except: *(NEET Pattern 2013)*
    A. Reactive new bone formation
    B. Cloaca is an opening in involucrum
    C. Involucrum is dead bone
    D. Sequestrum is hard and porous
Ans. is 'C' Involucrum is dead bone

24. Brodie's abscess is: *(NEET Pattern 2013)*
    A. Acute osteomyelitis   B. Subacute osteomyelitis
    C. Chronic osteomyelitis D. Septic arthritis
Ans. is 'B' Subacute osteomyelitis

25. Most common organism causing infection after open fracture: *(NEET Pattern 2012)*
    A. Pseudomonas   B. Staphylococcus aureus
    C. Klebsiella   D. Gonococcus
Ans. is 'B' Staphylococcus aureus

26. Postsurgical osteomyelitis most common organism is: *(NEET Pattern 2012)*
    A. Staphylococcus B. Pseudomonas
    C. Streptococcus   D. E. coli
Ans. is 'A' Staphylococcus

27. Brodie's abscess at upper end tibia is: *(NEET Pattern 2012)*
    A. Acute osteomyelitis   B. Subacute osteomyelitis
    C. Chronic osteomyelitis D. Septic arthritis
Ans. is 'B' Subacute osteomyelitis

28. Acute osteomyelitis of long bones commonly affects the: *(AIIMS 2009 May 09, PGI 1998, AP 97, JIPMER 95)*
    A. Epiphysis   B. Diaphysis
    C. Metaphysis D. Articular surface
Ans. is 'C' Metaphysis
    – Metaphysis of long bone is the earliest and most common site involved in osteomyelitis.

29. Chronic osteomyelitis is diagnosed mainly by: *(PGI Nov 2009, Manipal 1997, Bihar 91, AMU 89)* *(PGI 1998) (Manipal 1998)*
    A. Sequestrum B. Bone fracture
    C. Deformity   D. Brodie's abscess
Ans. is 'A' Sequestrum
    – **Sequestrum:** Avascular piece of bone surrounded by granulation tissue-pathognomic of chronic osteomyelitis.

30. Which of the following is NOT TRUE regarding tubercular osteomyelitis? *(AI 08)*
    A. It is a secondary TB
    B. Periosteal reaction is seen
    C. Sequestration is uncommon
    D. Inflammation is minimum
Ans. is 'B' Periosteal reaction is seen. Periosteal reaction is usually not seen in tubercular osteomyelitis

31. Complications of acute osteomyelitis: *(PGI June 05)*
    A. Malignancy
    B. Fracture of the affected bone
    C. Sepsis
    D. Chronicity
Ans. is 'B' Fracture of the affected bone; 'C' Sepsis; 'D' Chronicity.
    – Malignancy can be seen in chronic osteomyelitis.

32. An 8-year-old boy presents with a gradually progressing swelling and pain since 6 months over the upper tibia. On X-ray, there is a lytic lesion with sclerotic margins in the upper tibial metaphysis. The diagnosis is: *(AIIMS May 2001)*
    A. Osteogenic sarcoma B. Osteoclastoma
    C. Brodie's abscess   D. Ewing's sarcoma
Ans. is 'C', Brodie's abscess
    – Lytic lesion with sclerotic margin in upper end of tibia in an 8-year-old suggests the diagnosis of Brodie's abscess. Lytic lesions with sclerotic margins is seen in:
       i. Simple bone cyst
       ii. Brodie's abscess
       iii. Osteoblastoma
       iv. Chondroblastoma

33. All are associated with chronic osteomyelitis except: *(All India 1999)*
    A. Amyloidosis   B. Sequestrum
    C. Metastatic abscess D. Myositis ossificans
Ans. is 'D' Myositis ossificans

34. True about HIV, osteomyelitis is all except: *(AIIMS June 1997)*
    A. Necrosis absent
    B. Often bilateral
    C. Periosteal new bone formation
    D. Most common cause is Staphylococcus aureus
Ans. is 'A' Necrosis absent

Osteomyelitis in AIDS
– Osteomyelitis, which rarely develops in patients with AIDS, is monomicrobial in 50 percent of patients and polymicrobial in 35 percent with the remaining showing no organism.
– Staphylococcus is the most common organism and often it is bilateral.
– As pathophysiology of osteomyelitis is not altered, all the pathological changes seen in other osteomyelitis are seen in AIDS also.
    i. Dead necrotic bone (necrosis is present)
    ii. Periosteal reaction (periosteal new bone formation).

35. The most common organism causing osteomyelitis in drug abusers is: (PGI 1997)
    A. E. coli
    B. Pseudomonas
    C. Klebsiella
    D. Staphylococcus aureus

Ans. is 'B' Pseudomonas
- Pseudomonas aeruginosa is most common organism in intravenous drug users and Salmonella in sickle cell anemia patients.

36. Instillation treatment in osteomyelitis is: (JIPMER 94)
    A. Continuous suction + continuous drainage
    B. Intermittent suction + continuous drainage
    C. Continuous suction + intermittent drainage
    D. Intermittent suction + intermittent drainage

Ans. is 'A' Continuous suction + continuous drainage
- Continuous instillation of antibiotics followed by continuous drainage to cure chronic osteomyelitis is instillation treatment.

37. The ideal treatment for acute osteomyelitis of long bones is: (UP 93, Kerala 89, PGI 88)
    A. Antibiotics only
    B. Drilling of bone
    C. Decompression
    D. Antibiotics and if indicated decompression

Ans. is 'D' Antibiotics and if indicated decompression

38. When does the bony lesion of osteomyelitis appear on X-ray?
    A. 2 hours
    B. 24 hours (Delhi 1990)
    C. 1 week
    D. 2 weeks

Ans. is 'D' 2 weeks

39. Non-healing sinus is a common clinical feature is chronic osteomyelitis. The most common frequent cause for this presentation is: (Karnataka 1988)
    A. Resistant organisms
    B. Retained foreign body
    C. Presence of sequestrum
    D. Intraosseous cavities

Ans. is 'C' Presence of sequestrum
- Due to necrosis pieces of dead bone separate as sequestra varying in size from spicule to large segment. It is lighter than live bone and normal pattern of bone is lost. It acts as nidus and is most common cause of non healing sinus in chronic osteomyelitis.

SEPTIC ARTHRITIS

Septic (Pyogenic) Arthritis

Refers to Infection of Joint. Septic arthritis word is a **misnomer** as initially there is only infection of joint and if not treated early than Arthritis (joint destruction) develops. Thus all sepsis of joints do not cause arthritis only inadequately treated ones do.

Etiology and Pathology

- The hematogenous route of infection is the most common route in all age groups.

Epidemiology

- S. aureus – is the most common organism.

(Absent movements of a joint after ruling out trauma in pediatric population is septic arthritis till proved otherwise).

Diagnosis: X-rays are usually normal or may indicate soft tissue swellings, MRI may show effusion, synovitis or cartilage destruction and aspiration of joint will help to confirm the diagnosis by culture and sensitivity and can also help to differentiate from transient synovitis. Aspiration also decreases intra-articular pressure and reduces chances of Avascular necrosis (AVN) of femoral head.

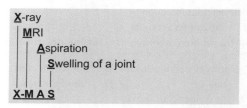

X-ray
MRI
Aspiration
Swelling of a joint
X-M A S

- Aspiration shows > 50,000 cells/mL and > 75% polymorphoneutrophils in septic arthritis.
- Culture of the aspirate is the gold standard for diagnosis.

Septic arthritis with negative cultures – Diagnostic Criterion (Morrey and associates criterion)

5 out of 6 must be present
1. > 38.3°C temperature
2. Swelling of suspected joint
3. Pain in joint that increases with movement
4. Systemic symptoms
5. No other pathologic process
6. Satisfactory response to antibiotics therapy.

Clinically

1. Knee (most commonly affected joint) – Position is flexion
2. Hip—Position is flexion, Abduction and external rotation as this is the position of maximum capacity of joint to accommodate pus.

Treatment

Arthrotomy (opening the joint capsule), surgical drainage (decompression) synovectomy and antibiotics. (2 weeks IV and 4 weeks oral). Duration of antibiotics is same as osteomyelitis as usually focus is from the bone.

Non-operative treatment is not considered in joint infections as cartilage destruction occurs very rapidly and can cause permanent joint destruction.

Septic arthritis results in bony ankylosis and it is the most common cause of bony ankylosis.

Ankylosis is the pathological fusion of bones in a joint leading to stiffness of the joint.

Ankylosis may be:
1. **Fibrous ankylosis:** Two articular surfaces are fused by fibrous tissue. The features are:
   - Some movement of joint is possible (though just a jog of movement)
   - Movements are painful
   - *Most common cause is tubercular arthritis of hip and knee*
2. **Bony ankylosis:** There is bony union between two articular surfaces. The features are:
   - No movements possible
   - Joint is painless

– Most common cause is acute suppurative arthritis (septic arthritis) > Pott's spine (TB of spine).

TOM SMITH ARTHRITIS

Tom Smith Arthritis is septic arthritis of hip in infants which may **destroy the cartilaginous femoral head rapidly and completely (chondrolysis).** So child presents with limp, unstable gait, shortening of limb, telescopy and increased hip movements in all direction. Treatment includes procedures to stabilize the hip.

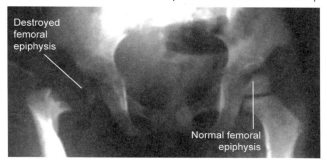

Fig. 2.5: Tom Smith Arthritis

TRANSIENT (TOXIC) SYNOVITIS OF HIP

- It is self-limiting, inflammatory condition of synovium. It is common cause of hip pain and limping in children 6 to 12 years of age. It is also known as irritable hip, observation hip, coxitis serosa and coxalgia fugax.
- Boys are affected 2–3 times as often as girls. 95% cases are unilateral, right and left hips are affected equally.
- A recent history of an upper respiratory tract infection, of viral origin is usually present.
- In any type of synovitis, the joint is held in Flexion, abduction and external rotation because in this position the joint capacity is maximum (so stretching due to effusion is minimal), thus causing least pain.
- Physical examination is characterized by guarded rotation of hip joint. Pain can be elicited at the extreme of motion.
- The patient is nontoxic rarely have temperature above 38°C or indications of systemic illness. The white blood cells (WBC) count, C-reactive protein level, and erythrocyte sedimentation rate (ESR) usually are within normal limits.
- Radiographs are normal or have slightly widened joint space medially.
- Ultrasound reveals mild effusion and widening of joint space.
- Joint aspiration usually reveal a WBC count between 5,000 and 15,000 cells/mL, with more than 25% polymorphonuclear leukocytes.
- The primary aim of treatment is to expedite spontaneous resolution with brief period of bed rest and non-weight bearing, light traction and use of oral NSAIDs. When the pain subsides, the patient should be mobilized. The long-term outcome is generally favorable.

Difference between Septic Arthritis and Transient Synovitis (Both have flexion abduction and external rotation at hip)

	Transient Synovitis	Septic Arthritis
1. Symptoms	Mild	Severe (Toxic child)
2. Movements	Mild reduction	Absent
3. Age	6–12 years	0–5 years
4. ESR	(n) to mild increase	Markedly increased
5. WBC	(n) to mild increase	Markedly increased

Ultrasonographic guided aspiration of hip joint (for cytological, histological evaluation and culture sensitivity of aspirate) is the best way of making definitive diagnosis and differentiating septic arthritis and transient synovitis.

MULTIPLE CHOICE QUESTIONS

1. Tom Smith septic arthritis affects: *(DNB Pattern 2018)*
   A. Neck of infants
   B. Hip joint of infants
   C. Elbow joint of children
   D. Shoulder joint in children

   Ans. is 'B' Hip joint of infants

2. All are true about septic arthritis except: *(PGI MAY 2018)*
   A. Staph. aureus is the most common cause
   B. Most common cause is E. coli
   C. Common in children
   D. Affects growth plate
   E. Aspiration of joint fluid used for diagnosis

   Ans. is 'B' Most common cause is E. coli

3. Tom Smith arthritis is infectious arthritis destroying: *(NEET 2018)*
   A. Femur neck
   B. Acetabular roof
   C. Greater trochanter
   D. Capital epiphyses femur

   Ans. 'D' Capital epiphyses femur

4. Tom Smith arthritis is: *(CET July 2016, JIPMER 2014, PGI 1999)*
   A. Tuberculous involvement of hip joint
   B. Tuberculous involvement of knee joint
   C. Syphilitic involvement of hip joint
   D. Septic arthritis of hip joint in infants

   Ans. 'D' Septic arthritis of hip joint in infants

5. In case of suspected septic arthritis, best way to confirm the diagnosis is by: *(Maharashtra PG 2016)*
   A. Aspiration of joint
   B. CT scan (computerized tomography)
   C. MRI scan (magnetic resonance imaging)
   D. Blood investigations

   Ans. is 'A' Aspiration of joint

6. Which of the following is an orthopedic emergency?
   A. Intra-articular fracture *(NEET Pattern 2013)*
   B. Septic arthritis
   C. Fracture lateral condyle humerus
   D. Fracture neck femur

   Ans. is 'B' Septic arthritis

7. Most common joint involved in septic arthritis:
   A. Knee
   B. Flip *(NEET Pattern 2013)*
   C. Shoulder
   D. Elbow

   Ans. is 'A' Knee

8. Aspirated synovial fluid in septic arthritis will have:
   A. Clear color *(NEET Pattern 2013)*
   B. High viscosity
   C. Markedly increased polymorphonuclear leukocytes
   D. None of the above

   Ans. is 'C' Markedly increased polymorphonuclear leukocytes

9. Deformity in transient synovitis of hip: *(NEET Pattern 2013)*
   A. Abduction
   B. Flexion
   C. External rotation
   D. All of the above

   Ans. is 'D' All of the above

10. Septic arthritis is diagnosed by: (NEET Pattern 2012)
    A. X-ray B. Joint aspiration
    C. USG D. MRI
Ans. is 'B' Joint aspiration

11. A 4-year-old male complaints of high grade fever, decreased appetite and pain right hip. On examination he has dehydration/tenderness in Scarpa's triangle/ swelling in right hip region, flexion, abduction and external rotation at hip/absent movements in right hip region. on X-ray there is mild increase in medial joint space. Diagnosis is: (AIIMS May 2009)
    A. Septic arthritis B. Transient synovitis
    C. Tubercular arthritis D. Dislocation hip
Ans. is 'A' Septic arthritis

12. A 7-year-old male complains of fever and pain right hip. On examination he has swelling in right hip region, flexion, abduction and external rotation at hip and there is mild reduction in movements in right hip region. On X-ray there is mild increase in medial joint space. Diagnosis is: (AIIMS May 2009)
    A. Septic arthritis B. Transient synovitis
    C. Tubercular arthritis D. Dislocation hip
Ans. is 'B' Transient synovitis

13. A 7-year-old boy with abrupt onset of pain in hip with hip held in abduction. Hemogram is normal. ESR is raised. What is the next line of management? (AIIMS May 09)
    A. Hospitalize and observe B. Ambulatory observation
    C. Intravenous antibiotics D. USG guided aspiration of hip
Ans. is 'D' USG guided aspiration of hip

14. Transient synovitis (toxic synovitis) of the hip is characterized by all of the following, except: (AIIMS May 2006)
    A. May follow upper respiratory infection
    B. ESR and white blood cell counts are usually normal
    C. Ultrasound of the joint reveals widening of the joint space
    D. The hip is typically held in adduction and internal rotation
Ans. is 'D' The hip is typically held in adduction and internal rotation
    - In any type of synovitis, the joint is held in Flexion, abduction and external rotation because in this position the joint capacity is maximum (so stretching due to effusion is minimal), thus causing least pain.

15. Tom Smith arthritis manifests as: (AI 96)
    A. Increase hip mobility and instability
    B. Hip stiffness
    C. Ankylosis
    D. Lengthening of limb
Ans. is 'A' Increase hip mobility and instability

16. Septic arthritis in a 2-year-old child is often caused by: (AIIMS May 1994)
    A. Haemophilous influenzae B. Staphylococcus aureus
    C. Gonococci D. Pneumococci
Ans. is 'B' Staphylococcus aureus
    - Staphylococcus aureus is the most common cause of septic arthritis in all ages.

17. Most common cause of bony ankylosis is: (AIIMS May 1993) (PGI 94) (PGI 87, 85)
    A. Rheumatoid arthritis B. Pyogenic arthritis
    C. Tubercular arthritis D. Osteoarthritis
Ans. is 'B' Pyogenic arthritis

18. Chondrolysis occurs commonly in: (PGI 92)
    A. TB arthritis
    B. Syphilitic arthritis
    C. Chondrosarcoma only
    D. Septic arthritis of infancy
Ans. is 'D' Septic arthritis of infancy

ACTINOMYCOSIS OVER CERVICOFACIAL REGION USUALLY!

- Mycetoma is chronic granulomatous infection of subcutaneous tissue
1. Multiple discharging sinuses
2. Discharge of granules   } Triad
3. Swelling (painless)
- X-ray: Sunray appearance: or Codman's Δ
- MRI: Dot in circle sign

Treatment
- **Actinomycetoma: Usually medically managed**
- **Eumycetoma: Usually surgically managed**

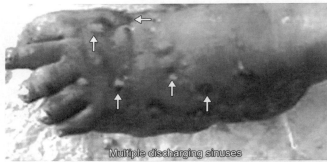
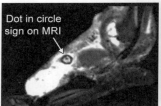
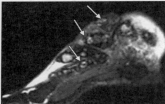

Fig. 2.6: Mycetoma

Actinomycosis

- It is caused by anaerobic or microaerophilic gram positive bacilli primarily Actinomyces israelii. The sinus tract may spontaneously resolve and recur.
- It frequently occurs at an oral, cervical or facial site, usually as a soft tissue swelling, abscess or mass that is often mistaken for neoplasm. Angle of jaw is most commonly involved.
- Involvement of bone is usually due to adjacent soft tissues. Mandible is most commonly involved. Vertebrae (spreading from lung or gut) or pelvis (spreading from cecum or colon) may also be involved. Infection of an extremity is uncommon. Cutaneous sinus tract frequently develops.
- X-ray show cystic areas of bone destruction with concomitant bone formation and bone destruction.
- Treatment is penicillin G, tetracycline or erythromycin for several months.

Swelling with Multiple Discharging Sinus

Over mandible (or head - neck region) — **Actinomycosis**
On Foot-Madura foot/Madura mycosis.

MULTIPLE CHOICE QUESTIONS

1. A patient with swelling foot, pus discharge, multiple sinuses. KOH smear shows filamentous structures. Diagnosis is: *(AIIMS May 2012, Sept 199, Dec 95, AI 95, UPSC 1990) (Karnataka 1997)*
   A. Osteomyelitis
   B. Madura mycosis
   C. Anthrax
   D. Actinomycosis

Ans. is 'B' Madura mycosis

2. In actinomycosis of the spine, the abscess usually erodes: *(AI 2003)*
   A. Intervertebral disc
   B. Into the pleural cavity
   C. Into the retroperitoneal space
   D. Towards the skin

Ans. is 'D' Towards the skin
   – Actinomycosis of spine is characterized by granulomatous lesions or osteomyelitis. Cutaneous sinus tracts frequently develop.

3. Most common site of actinomycosis amongst the following is: *(AI 1999)*
   A. Tibia   B. Rib
   C. Mandible   D. Femur

Ans. is 'C' Mandible
   – Most common type of actinomycosis is oro-cervico-facial.
   – Angle of the jaw is the most common site.

FASCIAL SPACES OF THE PALM

- These are potential spaces filled with loose connective tissue and their boundaries limit the spread of infection in the palm.
- The triangular palmar aponeurosis fans out from the lower border of the flexor retinaculum. From its medial and lateral borders a fibrous septum passes backward and is attached to the anterior border of 5th and 3rd metacarpal bones respectively.
- These septum divides palm into three compartments.

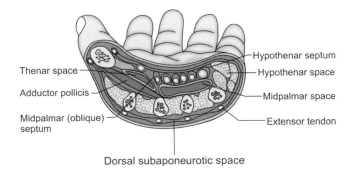

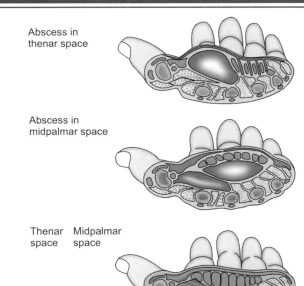

Fig. 2.7: Fascial space of hand and abscess in hand spaces

Thenar Space: It is lateral to lateral septum and must not be confused with the fascial compartment containing the thenar muscles. It lies posterior to the long flexor tendons to the index finger and in front of the adductor pollicis muscle and contains the first lumbricals muscles.

Midpalmar Space

- It lies between medial and lateral septum.

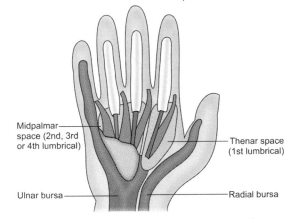

Fig. 2.8: Bursae and spaces of hand

- It contains 2nd, 3rd and 4th lumbrical muscles and lies posterior to the long flexor tendons to the middle, ring, and little fingers. It lies in front of the interossei and 3rd, 4th, and 5th metacarpal bones.
- Space medial to medial septum contain hypothenar muscles. This space is clinically unimportant.
- Proximally thenar and mid-palmar spaces are closed off from the forearm by the walls of the carpal tunnel. Distally, the two spaces are continuous with appropriate lumbrical canals. (Lumbrical canal is a potential space surrounding tendon of each lumbrical muscle).

Web Space Infection (Collar Button Abscess)

Web space infection usually localizes in one of the three fat-filled interdigital spaces just proximal to the superficial transverse ligament at the level of the metacarpophalangeal joints. Typically, the infection begins beneath palmar calluses in laborers. It may begin near the palmar surface, but because the skin and fascia here are less yielding, it may localize to drain dorsally.

Infections of Radial and Ulnar Bursae

The radial and ulnar bursae are the tenosynovial sheaths of the flexor tendons at the wrist. The proximal prolongation of the thumb flexor sheath is the radial bursa. The flexor sheaths communicate from the proximal palmar crease to the level of the pronator quadratus and extend distally as the tendon sheath of the little finger to form the ulnar bursa. Often the two bursae communicate with each other and allow infection to spread from one to the other in a "horseshoe abscess."

TENOSYNOVITIS

An infection within the flexor tendon sheath may be the result of the spread of adjacent pulp infections or puncture wounds in the flexor creases. Although the flexor sheath is usually involved, the radial and ulnar bursae may be involved as well.

Kanavel's Sign

Kanavel considered **tenderness** over the involved sheath, (most significant) rigid positioning of the **finger in flexion, pain on attempts** to **hyperextend** the fingers, and **swelling of the involved part** to be the four cardinal signs of suppurative tenosynovitis. Most common organism is *S. aureus*.

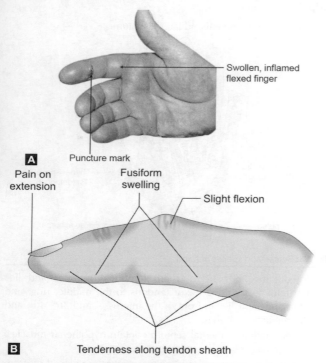

Figs. 2.9A and B: Infectious tenosynovitis (A) and (B) Kanavel's Sign

When early tenosynovitis is suspected, immediate treatment with antibiotics and splinting may abort spread of the infection, if the patient's symptoms have been present for less than 48 hours.

If drainage is required, an open or closed irrigation technique can be used. If an open technique is used, healing and rehabilitation are prolonged, and full motion may not be regained.

Felon

A felon is an abscess in the subcutaneous tissues of distal pulp of Most Commonly **Thumb** > index finger. The distal digital pulp is divided into tiny compartments by strong fibrous septa that traverse it from skin to bone. A transverse fibrous curtain also is present at the distal flexor finger crease. *S. aureus* is the organism most commonly isolated from fingertip infections. Swelling, redness, and pain, typical of cellulitis, initially are present. Abscess formation may follow rapidly.

Treatment consists of antibiotics and longitudinal incision for drainage.

Complications are Osteomyelitis >Tenosynovitis.

Paronychia

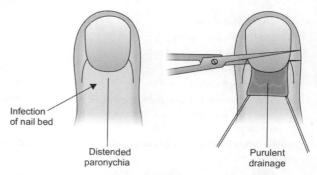

Fig. 2.10: Incision and drainage of paronychia

A paronychia ("runaround") infection usually caused by the *S. aureus* into the soft-tissue fold around the fingernail (eponychium) associated with poor nail hygiene. It usually begins at one corner of the horny nail and travels under either the eponychium or the nail toward the opposite side. Treatment is incision and drainage and antibiotics.

MULTIPLE CHOICE QUESTIONS

FASCIAL SPACE

1. Correct statement about hand infection: *(PGI Nov 2016)*
   A. Opening of Felon by fish month incision is preferred incision technique
   B. Felon is middle volar pulp infection
   C. Apical subungual infection- V-shaped piece is removed from the center of the free edge of the nail along with a little wedge of the full thickness of the skin overlying the abscess
   D. When the pus extends beneath the nail, it is necessary to remove some part of nail for adequate drainage of pus
   E. Felon is most common infection of hand

   Ans. is 'C' Apical subungual infection- V-shaped piece is removed from the center of the free edge of the nail along with a little wedge of the full thickness of the skin overlying the abscess, 'D' When the pus extends beneath the nail, it is necessary to remove some part of nail for adequate drainage of pus.

2. Index finger infection spreads to: (NEET 2015)
   A. Thenar space
   B. Mid palmar space
   C. Hypothenar space
   D. Flexion space

Ans. is 'A' Thenar space

3. Felon most common complication: (NEET Pattern 2012)
   A. Osteomyelitis
   B. Subungual hematoma
   C. Infective arthritis
   D. None

Ans. is 'A' Osteomyelitis

4. Felon is: (NEET Pattern 2012)
   A. Infection of nail fold
   B. Infection of ulnar bursa
   C. Infection of pulp space
   D. Infection of DIP joint

Ans. is 'C' Infection of pulp space

5. True about felon all except: (NEET Pattern 2012)
   A. Affects pulp space of finger
   B. Staphylococcus is the causative organism
   C. Transverse incision is usually used
   D. All septae should be broken

Ans. is 'C' Transverse incision is usually used

6. Most common finger infected with felon is: (NEET Pattern 2012)
   A. Thumb
   B. Index finger
   C. Middle finger
   D. Ring finger

Ans. is 'A > B' Thumb > Index finger

TENOSYNOVITIS

1. Synovial Tenosynovitis of flexor tendon. What is the correct option? (NEET Pattern 2019)
   A. The affected finger is extended at all joints
   B. It has to be conservatively managed
   C. Little finger infection can spread to thumb but not to index finger
   D. Patient present with minimal pain

Ans. is 'C' Little finger infection can spread to thumb but not to index finger

An infection within the flexor tendon sheath may be the result of the spread of adjacent pulp infections or puncture wounds in the flexor creases. Although the flexor sheath usually is involved, the radial and ulnar bursae may be involved as well.

Kanavel's Sign

Kanavel considered **tenderness** over the involved sheath, (most significant) rigid positioning of the **finger in flexion, pain on attempts** to **hyperextend** the fingers, and **swelling of the involved part** to be the four cardinal signs of suppurative tenosynovitis. Most common organism is *S. aureus*.

Infections of Radial and Ulnar Bursae

The radial and ulnar bursae are the tenosynovial sheaths of the flexor tendons at the wrist. The proximal prolongation of the thumb flexor sheath is the radial bursa. The flexor sheaths communicate from the proximal palmar crease to the level of the pronator quadratus and extend distally as the tendon sheath of the little finger to form the ulnar bursa. Often the two bursae communicate with each other and allow infection to spread from one to the other in a "horseshoe abscess."

2. Infection of ulnar bursa is diagnosed by: (NEET 2015)
   A. Kanavel's sign
   B. Chvostek's sign
   C. Gower's sign
   D. Ludloff's sign

Ans. is 'A' Kanavel's sign

3. Kanavel's sign is positive in: (AIIMS 2012 Nov 07)
   A. Tenosynovitis
   B. Carpal tunnel syndrome
   C. Trigger finger
   D. Dupuytren's contracture

Ans. is 'A' Tenosynovitis

CHAPTER 3

Tuberculosis of Bone and Joints

TUBERCULOSIS OF SPINE—POTT'S SPINE

The **spine is the most common site of skeletal tuberculosis**, accounting for 50% of cases followed by hip (15%) and knee (10%). **Spina ventosa** is tuberculosis of short bones of hand. Tuberculosis of shoulder is dry (no effusion)—**caries sicca (dry)**.

Tuberculosis with polyarthritis is called as **Poncet's disease**.

The tubercular spread to spine usually takes place from Lungs > lymph nodes that is usually secondary.

The route of spread is mostly **hematogenous** (through artery and Bateson's plexus). The initial focus of infection usually begins in the cancellous bone of vertebral body near the disc **(paradiscal type)**. According to blood supply of somites—as lower part of upper vertebra and upper part of lower vertebra develop from same mesodermal somites and thus have same blood supply thus spread is paradiscal.

"The Lesions are Paucibacillary"

Most common infective pathology of **spine in India is tuberculosis**. Acute pyogenic infections of spine are uncommon and mostly caused by *Staphylococcus aureus*.

Any level of the spine may be involved, the lower thoracic region being the most common; next in decreasing order of frequency are the lumbar, upper dorsal, cervical and sacral region. So dorsolumbar region is the most commonly involved segment. (Remember it is **dorsolumbar region** and **not dorsolumbar junction**)

- **Regional distribution:**
  - Cervical   12%
  - Cervicodorsal junction   0.5%
  - Dorsal   42%
  - Dorsolumbar junction   12%
  - Lumbar   26%
  - Lumbosacral   3%
- 7% patients can have more than one region of spine involved.
- The most common type is infection in paradiscal region and least common is in the posterior area. **The paradiscal type is most common** > central type (central part of vertebral body) > anterior type (anterior surface of vertebral body) > appendiceal type (involving pedicle, lamina, and less commonly transverse process, **2nd least common is spinous process and rarest variety is synovitis of facet joints**).
- The prominence of single spinous process is called as knuckle and this is usually not seen in tubercular spine, prominence of 2–3 spinous process is angular kyphosis which is commonest in tuberculosis because of 2 contiguous vertebra involved with paradiscal destruction and prominence of more than 3 spinous process is called as rounded kyphosis which is usually seen in osteoporotic spine and can be seen in tuberculosis.

- In the thoracic region kyphosis is most marked because of normal kyphotic curvature. **Tuberculosis is the most common cause of kyphosis in males**. The deformity being maximum in dorsal spine > lumbar spine > cervical spine.

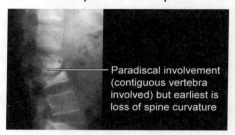

Fig. 3.1: Paradiscal involvement (contiguous vertebra involved) but earliest is loss of spine curvature!

- Tuberculosis is the most common cause of cold abscess.
- **Psoas abscess can give rise to pseudo-hip flexion deformity.** The flexion deformity of hip joint due to spasm of iliopsoas muscle does not show any limitation of rotation of hip joint when tested in the position of flexion deformity. Ipsilateral flexion of hip joint (more than the deformity) relieves pain and extension increases pain (by stretching muscle).

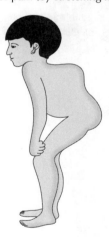

Fig. 3.2: Kyphosis most commonly involves thoracic region

- **Paraplegia occurs most often in upper thoracic region,** where kyphosis is most acute, the spinal canal is narrow and spinal cord is relatively large.
- Early onset paresis is due to inflammatory edema, granulation tissue an abscess, caseous material. It has good prognosis. Late onset: paresis is due to increasing deformity or reactivation of disease, bony sequestrum, stenosis of the vertebral canal, fibrosis or vascular insufficiency and has poor prognosis.
- Sequelae of TB spine is usually bony ankylosis.

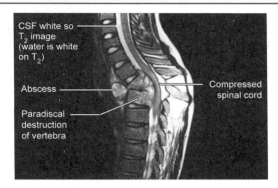

Fig. 3.3: MRI spine (Possibly tuberculosis)

Clinical Features

- **Back pain,** Usually minimal, is the **commonest symptom.** (1st symptom).
- **Tenderness** is the **earliest sign.** Twist tenderness for Anterior elements is more significant as disease is anteriorly involving the vertebral body (paradiscal).
- Paravertebral muscle spasm resulting in stiffness in the affected region is a constant early finding. The spine is held rigid. When picking an object up from floor, there is flexion at hips and knees and the spine is in extension, (Coin test).
- Earliest sign in patient with neurological deficit—**Increased deep tendon reflexes** or clonus or extensor plantar response (twitching of muscles can be seen even earlier).

Radiological Image Features

- **The Earliest X-ray feature is loss of Curvature due to paravertebral spasm.**
- The next radiological feature of spinal tuberculosis is reduction of intervertebral disk space and osteoporosis of two adjacent vertebrae sometimes with fuzziness of the endplates.
- Paraspinal abscess appears as fusiform shadows along vertebral column.
- X-rays can show scalloping effect or aneurysmal appearance or saw tooth appearance due to erosions by abscess or aortic pulsations.
- **Prof Rajsekaran** has described radiographic signs of spine at risk.
- MRI is one of the best radiological investigation for Pott's Spine (showing soft tissues, cartilage and marrow changes). Remember that radiological picture always lags behind the biological process which is already more progressive.

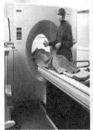 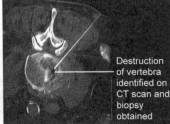

Fig. 3.4: CT guided biopsy

Note: TB usually involves vertebral body and malignancy usually involves posterior elements.

- Disk space collapse is typical of infection; disk preservation is typical of metastatic disease. Metastasis causes vertebral body collapse, but in contrast to TB, the disk space is usually preserved.
- **CT Guided biopsy** through the transpedicular route is a good procedure to obtain tissue from the lesion as Gold standard is always growth of organism on culture medium by biopsy thus it will be more reliable than radiological investigations.
- Culture of tuberculosis is by automated radiometric technique – **BACTEC method (Middle Brook media)** gives result in 3 weeks.

Stages of TB Spine with Neural Deficit

- **Stage 1:** Patient has no neural complaint clinician elicits increased reflexes.
- **Stage 2:** Patient has weakness but can walk with support.
- **Stage 3:** Patient is non-ambulatory or has sensory loss <50%.
- **Stage 4:** Patient has bowel/bladder involvement or sensory loss >50%.

Treatment of Pott's Spine

- **Middle path regimen is used in India**
- Patient is treated by antitubercular therapy (ATT), spinal brace and rest. Patient is followed on with complete neural examination and if progress is good then continued on non-operative management but if indications of surgery exist then he needs to be operated.

  Stage-wise treatment of Pott's spine
- **Stage 1:** ATT + rest + monthly Neural Examination
- **Stage 2:** ATT + rest + weekly Neural Examination
- **Stage 3:** ATT + rest + daily Neural Examination
- **Stage 4: ATT + Decompression and bone grafting**

  ATT: Rifampicin is always a part of all regimens. Minimum duration is 9–12 months in spinal TB and may be given up to 18–24 months depending upon clinical, radiological (MRI) and hematological (ESR) healing (in non-spinal TB the duration of ATT is 6 months–1 year).

  Indications of surgery in any disease of spine (These are for all pathologies of spine—trauma, tumor, TB, disc prolapse)
- Bowel bladder involvement.
- Deterioration in neural or clinical status on treatment
- No improvement in neural or clinical status after conservative trial of 3–4 weeks or

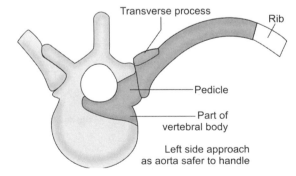

Fig. 3.5: Structures removed in anterolateral decompression

Surgical options for most of the cases are—anterior decompression + bone grafting or anterolateral decompression + bone grafting and both have similar success rates.
- Hong Kong operation is also carried out for Pott's spine.

Structures removed in anterolateral decompression are part of rib, one side transverse process, one pedicle and small part of vertebral body (intercostal nerves are exposed).

Posterior structures like lamina are never removed in tuberculosis because disease destroys anteriorly and if surgeon destroys posteriorly then there will be instability.

These surgeries are carried out in right lateral position (right side down and left side up) approaching the spine from left side as the vessel handled is aorta on left side which is thick muscular vessel with more resilience to handling pressure as compared to vena cava on right side which is friable to handle.

Prognostic Factor

Feature	Better prognosis	Poor prognosis
Degree of cord involvement	Partial	Complete (grade IV)
Duration of cord involvement	Shorter	Longer (>12 months)
Speed onset	Slow	Rapid
Type	Early onset	Late onset
Age	Younger	Older
General condition	Good	Poor
Vertebral disease	Active	Healed
Kyphotic deformity	<60 degree	>60 degree
Cord on MRI	Normal	Myelomalacia/syrinx (cord damaged)
Preoperative	Wet lesion	Dry lesion

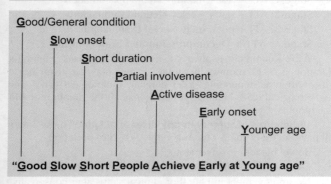

"**G**ood **S**low **S**hort **P**eople **A**chieve **E**arly at **Y**oung age"

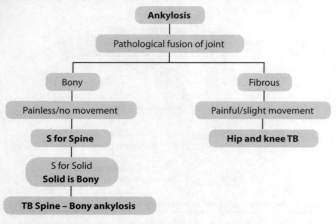

Immunomodulation (Prof SM Tuli)

In case response to ATT is not on the expected ground and it is suspected that patient's immune system is not controlling the disease then immunomodulation is done to enhance the immune response. In immunomodulation the following sets of bacilli are attacked—dormant/resistant/persistent/slow grower/atypical m TB.

Drugs given are:

1. Levamisole
2. BCG
3. DPT

MULTIPLE CHOICE QUESTIONS

1. Good Prognostic Factors for TB spine are: *(PGI Nov 2018)*
   A. Young
   B. Active
   C. Early Onset Weakness
   D. Spinal Cord Changes
   E. Rapid Onset

   Ans. is 'A' Young; 'B' Active 'C' Early Onset Weakness

2. Which of the following is not true about the management of Pott's paraplegia? *(NEET Dec 2016)*
   A. Chemotherapy is the mainstay of conservative management
   B. Paraplegia not improving with conservative treatment even after 3–6 weeks is an indication for operative intervention
   C. Decompression via anterolateral approach is most preferred
   D. Posterior decompression and instrumentation can be used to correct the deformity

   Ans. is 'D' Posterior decompression and instrumentation can be used to correct the deformity

3. True about spinal tuberculosis is/are: *(PGI May 2017)*
   A. Middle path regimen is used in management
   B. Cervical spine is most commonly affected
   C. Commonly spread by hematogenous route from lung
   D. Acute onset early paraplegia has good prognosis
   E. Lower thoracic vertebra is most commonly involved

   Ans. is 'A' Middle path regimen is used in management; 'C' Commonly spread by hematogenous route from lung; 'D' Acute onset early paraplegia has good prognosis; and 'E' Lower thoracic vertebra is most commonly involved

4. About TB spine choose the correct statement: *(PGI Nov 2016)*
   A. Most common in thoracic spine
   B. Long standing paraplegia carries poor prognosis
   C. Has hematogenous spread
   D. Middle path regime is used for treatment in our country
   E. Involves posterior complex commonly

   Ans. is 'A' Most common in thoracic spine; 'B' Long standing paraplegia carries poor prognosis; 'C' Has hematogenous spread; 'D' Middle path regime is used for treatment in our country

5. The earliest radiological sign in Pott's disease is:
   A. Erosion of vertebral bodies *(APPG 2015)*
   B. Collapse and destruction of vertebra
   C. Narrowing of intervertebral disc space
   D. Paraspinal soft tissue shadow

   Ans. is 'C' Narrowing of intervertebral disc space

6. Most common site of TB: *(NEET 2015, 2012)*
   A. Spine
   B. Knee
   C. Hip
   D. Shoulder

   Ans. is 'A' Spine

Tuberculosis of Bone and Joints

7. All are true about Pott's spine except: *(PGI Nov 2014)*
   A. Thoracic vertebrae T_6-T_8 is most commonly affected site
   B. Paradiscal is commonest variety
   C. Muscular rigidity and stiffness is common
   D. Posterior part of vertebrae is more affected than anterior part
   E. Back pain is the commonest presenting symptom

Ans. is 'A' Thoracic vertebrae T_6-T_8 is most commonly affected site (lower thoracic is most common T_9-T_{12}), and 'D' Posterior part of vertebrae is more affected than anterior part

8. A patient with tuberculosis of spine first neurological sign is: *(AIIMS May 2014)*
   A. Motor loss   B. Sensory loss
   C. Increased deep tendon reflexes
   D. Bladder involvement

Ans. is 'C' Increased deep tendon reflexes

9. Patient with D_7 D_8 Koch spine with paraplegia, treatment of choice: *(NEET Pattern 2013)*
   A. ATT
   B. Anterior decompression + ATT
   C. Laminectomy
   D. Posterior decompression

Ans. is 'B' Anterior decompression + ATT
   – Since patient has paraplegia with Dorsal Kochs, Decompression will be performed.

10. Investigation of choice for spinal tuberculosis usually is: *(NEET Pattern 2013)*
    A. X-ray   B. CT-Scan
    C. Open biopsy   D. MRI

Ans. is 'D' MRI

11. What causes both destruction of bone and reduction of joint space? *(NEET Dec 2016, AIIMS Nov 2013)*
    A. Tuberculosis   B. Metastasis
    C. Multiple myeloma D. Lymphoma

Ans. is 'A' Tuberculosis

TB in spine involves
   – 2 Vertebra (Bone) + Disk (Cartilage)
   – Paradiscal
   – Anterior (to spinal cord)

Note: Involvement of posterior elements and single vertebra is relatively rare in TB.

12. Caries sicca is seen in: *(DNB, June 2017, NEET Pattern 2013; 2012) (Rohtak 96)*
    A. Hip   B. Shoulder
    C. Knee   D. None of the above

Ans. is 'B' Shoulder

13. Poor prognostic indicator of Pott's paraplegia: *(NEET Pattern 2013)*
    A. Early onset   B. Active disease
    C. Healed disease D. Wet lesion

Ans. is 'C' Healed disease

14. All are true about spinal tuberculosis except: *(NEET Pattern 2013)*
    A. Back pain earliest symptom
    B. Dorsolumbar spine commonest site
    C. Exaggerated lumbar lordosis
    D. Secondary to lung infection

Ans. is 'C' Exaggerated lumbar lordosis

15. False about Pott's spine: *(NEET Pattern 2015, 2012)*
    A. Commonest at dorsolumbar junction
    B. Always heals by chemotherapy
    C. Back pain is an early symptom
    D. There is disk space narrowing on X-ray

Ans. is 'B' Always heals by chemotherapy

16. TB hand: *(NEET Pattern 2012)*
    A. Spina ventosa   B. Caries sicca
    C. Pott's disease D. None

Ans. is 'A' Spina ventosa

17. Most common site of TB: *(NEET Pattern 2012)*
    A. Spine   B. Knee
    C. Hip   D. Shoulder

Ans. is 'A' Spine

18. Tuberculosis spine; most common site is: *(NEET Pattern 2012)*
    A. Sacral   B. Cervical
    C. Dorsolumbar   D. Lumbosacral

Ans. is 'C' Dorsolumbar

19. Anterolateral decompression is done for: *(NEET Pattern 2012)*
    A. Spinal tuberculosis B. Chest TB
    C. Hand TB   D. Foot TB

Ans. is 'A' Spinal tuberculosis

20. Tuberculosis with polyarthritis is called as: *(NEET Pattern 2012)*
    A. Poncet's disease B. Barton's disease
    C. Von Gierke disease D. Gordon's disease

Ans. is 'A' Poncet's disease

21. Indication of steroids in Pott's spine: *(NEET Pattern 2012)*
    A. Pain   B. Deformity
    C. Meningitis   D. Fever

Ans. is 'C' Meningitis

22. Hong Kong's operation is done for? *(NEET Pattern 2012)*
    A. Tuberculosis   B. Leprosy
    C. Septic arthritis D. Osteomyelitis

Ans. is 'A' Tuberculosis

23. Tuberculosis of spine best diagnostic modality is:
    A. Clinical   B. X-ray *(MAY AIIMS 2012)*
    C. MRI   D. CT guided biopsy

Ans. is 'D' CT guided biopsy

24. Tuberculosis in Bone is due to: *(AIPG 2012)*
    A. Paucibacillary and hematogenous
    B. Multibacillary and hematogenous
    C. Paucibacillary and lymphatic
    D. Multibacillary and lymphatic

Ans. is 'A' Paucibacillary and hematogenous

25. A 35-year-old lady with chronic backache. On X-ray she had a D12 collapse. But intervertebral disk space is maintained. All are possible except: *(AIIMS Nov 2010)*
    A. Multiple myeloma B. Osteoporosis
    C. Metastasis   D. Tuberculosis

Ans. is 'D' Tuberculosis
   – Characteristic radiological feature of Pott's spine is obliteration of disk space with destruction of two adjacent vertebrae.
   – This feature differentiate TB spine from other diseases causing vertebral destruction (like metastasis) in which disk space is preserved.

26. Poor prognostic factors in Pott's paraplegia:
    A. Acute onset of paraplegia *(PGI Dec 08, Dec 03, June 2K)*
    B. Sudden progression of paraplegia
    C. Motor paralysis alone
    D. Longstanding paraplegia
    E. Paraplegia in children
Ans. is 'A Acute onset of paraplegia; 'B' Sudden progression of paraplegia; 'D' Longstanding paraplegia

27. Earliest feature of spinal tuberculosis is:
    (PGI June 2006-04-03, AIIMS May 1995, Orissa 1992, CUPGEE 99)
    A. Gibbus   B. Muscle spasm
    C. Pain   D. Psoas abscess
Ans. is 'C' Pain

28. The most common sequelae of tuberculous spondylitis in an adolescent is: *(AI 2005)*
    A. Fibrous ankylosis   B. Bony-ankylosis
    C. Pathological dislocation   D. Chronic osteomyelitis
Ans. is 'B' Bony-ankylosis
    - *The usual outcome of healed tuberculosis in spine is the bony ankylosis and in peripheral joints like Hip and Knee Fibrous ankylosis is seen.*

29. Tuberculosis of the spine commonly affects all of the following parts of the vertebra except: *(AI 2004)*
    A. Body   B. Lamina
    C. Spinous process D. Pedicle
Ans. is 'C' Spinous process
    Least common is facet joints and 2nd least common is spinous process.

30. A 46-year-old, known alcoholic, presented with pain in the dorsal spine. On examination there is tenderness at the dorsolumbar junction. Radiograph shows destruction of the 12th dorsal vertebra and L1 vertebra with loss of disk space between D12 - L1 vertebra. The most probable diagnosis is: *(AIIMS Nov 2004)*
    A. Metastatic spine disease   B. Pott's spine
    C. Missed trauma   D. Multiple myeloma
Ans. is 'B' Pott's spine

31. In tuberculosis of spine, which one of the following is not a cause for Paraplegia? *(NIMS 2000)*
    A. Stretching of spinal cord in gibbus deformity
    B. Spinal artery compression
    C. Compression by granulation tissue
    D. Edema of spinal cord
Ans. is 'B' Spinal artery compression
    - Early onset paresis is due to inflammatory edema, granulation tissue, an abscess, caseous material. It has good prognosis. Late onset paresis is due to increasing deformity or reactivation of disease, or bony sequestrum, stenosis of the vertebral canal, fibrosis or vascular insufficiency and has poor prognosis.

32. The 1st sign of TB is: *(NIMS 2K, CUPGEE 95 Bihar 88)*
    A. Narrowing of intervertebral space
    B. Rarefaction of vertebral bodies
    C. Destruction of laminae
    D. Fusion of spinous processes
Ans. is 'A' Narrowing of intervertebral space
    - The earliest feature is loss of curvature due to paravertebral spasm.
    - The next radiological feature of spinal tuberculosis is reduction of intervertebral disk space and osteoporosis of two adjacent vertebrae sometimes with fuzziness of the endplates.

33. Cold abscess in chest wall is most common due to:
    A. TB spine   B. TB rib   *(AIIMS Dec 1998)*
    C. TB pelvis   D. TB pleura
Ans. is 'A' TB spine

34. Tuberculosis of the spine starts in: *(BHU 98)*
    A. Vertebral body   B. Nucleus pulposus
    C. Annulus fibrosis D. Paravertebral fascia
Ans. is 'A' Vertebral body

35. The most common type of spinal tuberculosis is:
    (BHU 98, Bihar 1988) (Kerala 88) (JIPMER 88)
    A. Anterior   B. Posterior
    C. Central   D. Paradiscal
Ans. is 'D' Paradiscal
    - The initial focus of tubercular infection usually begins in the cancellous bone of vertebral body near the disk (in most common paradiscal type)

35. Commonest site for tuberculous spondylitis: *(AI 1998)*
    A. T12/L1   B. C6-7
    C. L4-5   D. S1-2
Ans. is 'A' T12/L1
    - Order of involvement of Pott's spine is dorsal >lumbar> dorsolumbar junction

36. The most common cause of kyphosis in a male is:
    (National Board 97)
    A. Congenital   B. Tuberculosis
    C. Trauma   D. Secondaries
Ans. is 'B' Tuberculosis
    - Tuberculosis is the most common cause of kyphosis in males. The deformity being maximum in dorsal spine > lumbar spine > cervical spine.

37. The commonest infective lesion of the spine in India is:
    A. Pyogenic infection   B. Fungal   *(AIIMS 96)*
    C. TB   D. Typhoid
Ans. is 'C' TB
    - One fifth of TB population is in India.
    - Three percent are suffering from skeletal tuberculosis, of which spinal TB is the most common.

38. The ideal surgical treatment for Pott's paraplegia is:
    (UPSC 1997, 88 Tamil Nadu 1994)
    A. Laminectomy and decompression
    B. Anterior decompression and bone grafting
    C. Anterolateral decompression
    D. Costotransversectomy
Ans. is 'B' Anterior decompression and bone grafting
    - Surgical options for most of the cases are—anterior decompression + bone grafting or anterolateral decompression + bone grafting are 2 procedures with similar success rates. Here option B is preferred because it also has bone grafting with it.

39. The most common cause of paraplegia of early onset of Tuberculosis of spine is: *(Karnataka 1992)*
    A. Spinal artery thrombosis
    B. Sudden collapse of vertebra
    C. Sequestrum pressing on cord
    D. Cold abscess pressing on the cord
Ans. is 'D' Cold abscess pressing on the cord

- Early onset paresis is due to inflammatory edema, granulation tissue, an abscess, caseous material. It has good prognosis. Late onset paresis is due to increasing deformity or reactivation of disease, or bony sequestrum, stenosis of the vertebral canal, fibrosis or vascular insufficiency and has poor prognosis.

40. Surgical treatment in Pott's spine is indicated if there is: *(PGI 1991)*
   A. Progressive loss of function in spite of medical treatment
   B. No improvement in motor power in spite of 3 months of treatment
   C. There is no improvement in fever in 3 months of treatment
   D. Patient who is an adult or middle age

Ans. is 'A' Progressive loss of function in spite of medical treatment; and 'B' No improvement in motor power in spite of 3 months of treatment.

41. Short long bones of hand and foot are commonly infected by the following organism: *(Tamil Nadu 88, Bihar 88)*
   A. Pyogenic
   B. Tuberculous
   C. Fungal
   D. All of the above

Ans. is 'B' Tuberculous
   - Spina ventosa is the name given to tuberculosis of the phalanges of hand.

42. In bony ankylosis, there is: *(UP 98)*
   A. Painless, no movement
   B. Painful complete movement
   C. Painless complete movement
   D. Painful incomplete movement

Ans. is 'A' Painless, no movement

43. A 25-year-old male complaints of pain in lower back region for three months. Has history of slipping of bathroom slippers. Mild weakness of both lower limbs but can walk without support. There is 30% sensory loss and has bladder symptoms. D12-L1 is tender. X-ray shows paradiscal destruction of vertebrae and MRI shows destruction with indentation of thecal sac. Management is:
   A. Wait and watch
   B. Domiciliary ATT
   C. Admit and ATT
   D. ATT and Decompression

Ans. is 'D' ATT and Decompression as bladder symptoms are present.

Indications of surgery in any disease of spine
   - Deterioration in neural or clinical status on treatment
   - No improvement in neural or clinical status after conservative trial of 3–4 weeks or
   - Bowel bladder involvement

44. Anterolateral decompression (ALD) and anterior decompression (AD) for Pott's spine all are true except:
   A. ALD and AD results are the same
   B. ALD position of patient is right lateral
   C. ALD laminectomy is always a part
   D. ALD part of ribs is removed and spinal nerves exposed.

Ans. is 'C' ALD laminectomy is always a part
   - Surgical options for most of the cases are anterior decompression + bone grafting or anterolateral decompression + bone grafting and both have similar success rates.
   - Structures removed in Anterolateral decompression are part of rib, intercostal nerves, one side transverse process, one pedicle and small part of vertebral body.
   - These surgeries are carried out in right lateral position (right side down and left side up) approaching the spine from left side as the vessel handled is aorta on left side which is thick muscular vessel with more resilience to handling pressure as compared to vena cava which is friable to handle
   - Posterior structures like lamina are never removed because disease destroys anteriorly and if surgeon destroys posteriorly then there will be instability.

Table 3.1: Staging of tuberculosis of the joints and its outcome in general.

	Stages	Clinical	Radiology	Usual effective treatment	Expectation
I.	Synovitis (FABER) Apparent lengthening	Movements present >75%	Soft tissue swelling, osteoporosis	Chemotherapy and rarely synovectomy	Retention of near full, mobility
II.	Early arthritis (FADIR +<1 cm shortening)	Movements present 50–75%	In addition to I, moderate diminution of joint space and marginal erosions	Chemotherapy and rarely synovectomy or debridement	Restoration of 50–75% of mobility
III.	Advanced arthritis (FADIR +>1 cm shortening)	Loss of movements of >75% in all directions	In addition to II, marked diminution of joint space and destruction of joint surfaces	Chemotherapy and surgery. Generally arthrodesis,* arthroplasty/excision arthroplasty in lower limbs	Ankylosis
IV.	Advanced arthritis with subluxation/dislocation-wandering acetabulum/ pestle and mortar appearance	Loss of movements of >75% in all directions	In addition to III, joint is disorganized with subluxation/dislocation	Chemotherapy and surgery. Generally arthrodesis* arthroplasty/excision arthroplasty in lower limbs	Ankylosis*
V.	Aftermath/terminal or gross arthritis	Gross deformity and ankylosis	In addition to IV, grossly deformed articular margins ± degenerative osteoarthrosis	Chemotherapy and surgery. Generally arthrodesis* arthroplasty/excision arthroplasty in lower limbs	Ankylosis*

* Arthrodesis: Surgical fusion of joint. Ankylosis: Pathological fusion of joint.

TUBERCULOSIS OF HIP: INITIAL FOCUS IN ACETABULUM (MOST COMMON SITE) AND FEMUR (BABCOCK'S TRIANGLE)

- **Stage 1:** Stage of synovitis - **FABER** (Flexion, Abduction and External rotation). Lengthening.
- **Stage 2:** Stage of early arthritis - FADIR + <1 cm shortening (Flexion, Adduction and Internal rotation).
- **Stage 3:** Stage of advanced arthritis - FADIR +>1 cm shortening (Flexion, Adduction and Internal rotation).
- **Stage 4:** Stage of subluxation/dislocation—wandering acetabulum or pestle and mortar appearance.
- **Stage 5:** Stage of sequelae, ankylosis or severe arthritis.

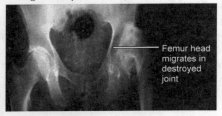

Fig. 3.6: Wandering acetabulum (actually wandering femur head)

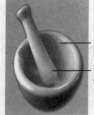

Fig. 3.7: Pestle and Mortar

Note: FABER at Hip seen in synovitis/infection/anterior dislocation/iliotibial band contracture (polio) FADIR at hip seen in arthritis/posterior dislocation

Treatment of Tuberculosis of Hip

A. **Remove:** Excision arthroplasty of hip (problems of instability and shortening)
   - Girdlestone excision arthroplasty. Head and neck of femur are removed.
B. **Fuse: Arthrodesis** causes increased damage to one joint above and one joint below
C. **Replace**, e.g. total hip replacement

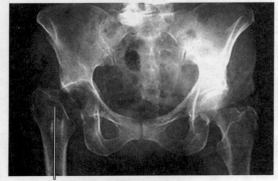

Fig. 3.8: Excision arthroplasty

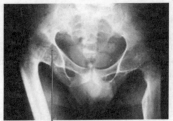

Fig. 3.9: Arthrodesed hip joints (Cobra plate is used for hip arthrodesis)

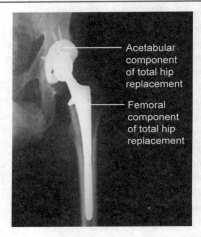

Fig. 3.10: Total hip replacement

Stage 1 and 2 ATT and traction and if required joint debridement or synovectomy.

Stage 3, 4 and 5 ATT and joint replacement/arthrodesis/osteotomy/excision arthroplasty.

MULTIPLE CHOICE QUESTIONS

1. First radiological sign for active tubercular arthritis is: *(NEET DEC 2016)*
   A. Localized osteoporosis B. Sclerosis
   C. Joint space reduction D. Osteophytes
   Ans. is 'A' Localized osteoporosis

2. Deformity of hip joint in case of tubercular synovitis of hip joint is: *(NEET 2015)*
   A. Flexion abduction external rotation
   B. Flexion adduction external rotation
   C. Flexion abduction internal rotation
   D. Flexion adduction internal rotation
   Ans. is 'A' Flexion abduction external rotation

3. Wandering acetabulum is seen in: *(JIPMER 2014)*
   A. Fracture of acetabulum B. Hip dislocation
   C. Rheumatoid arthritis D. TB of hip
   Ans. 'D' TB of hip
   - Wandering acetabulum is seen in tuberculosis of hip, stage 4 when destroyed head dislocates from the acetabulum.

4. Apparent lengthening of limb is seen in which TB hip stage of? *(NEET Pattern 2013)*
   A. 1 B. 2
   C. 3 D. 4
   Ans. is 'A' 1

Tuberculosis of Bone and Joints

5. Girdlestone arthroplasty is carried out for: *(NEET Pattern 2012)*
   A. Chronic elbow infections B. Acute elbow infections
   C. Chronic hip infections D. Acute hip infections

   Ans. is 'C' Chronic hip infections

6. TB Sicca involves: *(NEET Pattern 2012)*
   A. Shoulder B. Elbow
   C. Hip D. Knee

   Ans. is 'A' Shoulder

7. A 30-year-old male HIV positive on antiretroviral therapy has pain in right hip region. Flexion, abduction and external rotation deformity of right hip for 2 months, what is the most likely diagnosis? *(AIPG-2008)*
   A. Avascular necrosis B. TB hip
   C. Transient synovitis D. Septic arthritis

   Ans. is 'B' TB Hip

	TB hip in HIV	AVN hip in HIV
Incidence	More Common	Less Common
Deformity	FABER-stage of synovitis may be prolonged on treatment, then subsequently with onset of arthritis – FADIR	Limitation of abduction and internal rotation so initially position is adduction and external rotation (opposite to movements limited) and than subsequently with onset of arthritis FADIR
	Unilateral (usually)	Bilateral (usually)

TUBERCULOSIS OF KNEE: INITIAL FOCUS IS IN SYNOVIUM!

- Tubercular arthritis is insidious in onset and often monoarticular in involvement. It **is the most common cause of monoarticular arthritis in children.**
- Tubercular arthritis is a **synovial disease**, so peripheral destruction of joint occurs earlier than the central part and movements are lost gradually.
- At times with tubercular arthritis both sides of joint are involved and two foci of tuberculosis will be directly opposite each other **(kissing arthritis).**
- Affected joint will be stiff and soon the night cries develop, because irritation from the process is low grade, muscle spasm protects the part quite satisfactorily during the day, but when the child is asleep, the protective action of muscle is lost and on motion pain is produced.
- **Synovial fluid shows elevated (TLC) lowered sugar level and poor mucin.**
- Tuberculosis of the knee is the classical cause of triple deformity, which includes *posterior subluxation of tibia, external (lateral) rotation of tibia and flexion of knee (PERF).*
- It can be treated by ATT and joint replacement/arthrodesis (Charnley's method). **Wilkinson joint debridement procedure** is done for tuberculosis of knee early stages.

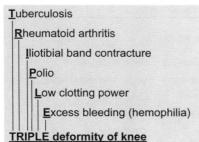

Note: Triple deformity can also be seen in rheumatoid arthritis, Iliotibial band contracture, poliomyelitis and hemophilic arthropathy.

MULTIPLE CHOICE QUESTIONS

1. Triple deformity true statements are: *(PGI Nov 2018)*
   A. TB Knee
   B. Post subluxation of tibia, External rotation of Leg, Flexion of knee
   C. Post subluxation of femur, External rotation of Leg, Flexion of knee
   D. Post subluxation of tibia, External rotation of Leg, Extension of knee
   E. Iliotibial tract is important for mechanism

   Ans. is 'A' TB Knee; 'B' Post subluxation of tibia, External rotation of Leg, Flexion of knee; & 'E' Iliotibial tract is important for mechanism

2. A 20-year-old male presents with history of gradual onset pain and swelling in left knee since 6 months. Now since last 1 month patient has started limping while walking and also has flexion deformity of knee. Ultrasonography shows presence of synovial thickening. What is the most probable diagnosis? *(NEET DEC 2016)*
   A. Tuberculosis of knee
   B. Pigmented villonodular synovitis
   C. Synovial sarcoma D. Hemarthrosis

   Ans. is 'A' Tuberculosis of knee

3. Which of the following is a feature of triple deformity of the knee joint? *(CET July 16)*
   A. Posterior subluxation of tibia
   B. Internal rotation of tibia
   C. Medial angulation of tibia
   D. Recurvatum

   Ans. is 'A' Posterior subluxation of tibia

4. Complication of joint TB: *(NEET Pattern 2012)*
   A. Fibrous ankylosis B. Bony ankylosis
   C. Normal healing D. None

   Ans. is 'A' Fibrous ankylosis

5. Treatment of triple deformity is: *(AMU 95)*
   A. ATT B. ATT + Immobilization
   C. ATT + Immobilization + Debridement
   D. ATT + Replacement

   Ans. is 'D' ATT + Replacement

   – Treatment of triple deformity is replacement/arthrodesis

6. Triple deformity of knee is classically seen in: *(AIIMS Dec 1994)*
   A. Fracture patella B. Tuberculosis
   C. Rheumatic arthritis D. Rheumatoid arthritis

   Ans. is 'B' Tuberculosis

7. The most common cause of monoarthritis in children is: *(Andhra 1989)*
   A. Septic arthritis B. Tuberculous arthritis
   C. Osteoarthritis D. Rheumatoid arthritis
   E. Any of the above

   Ans. is 'B' Tuberculous arthritis

   Tubercular arthritis is insidious in onset and often monoarticular in involvement. It is the most common cause of monoarticular arthritis in children.

Chapter 4: Orthopedics Oncology

DIFFERENTIAL DIAGNOSIS OF BONE TUMORS

- Osteomyelitis has same clinical presentation as Ewing's sarcoma and osteosarcoma
- Myositis ossificans mimics osteosarcoma
- Stress fracture
- Bone infarct mimics enchondroma
- Bone islands mimics osteoid osteoma
- Fibrous dysplasia mimics Giant cell tumor
- Post-traumatic osteolysis
- Brown tumor (seen in Hyperparathyroidism)
- Paget's disease.

POLYOSTOTIC BONE LESIONS

- Fibrous dysplasia
- Enchondroma
- Osteochondroma
- Ewing's sarcoma
- Giant cell tumor (Goltz syndrome)
- Metastasis
- Multiple myeloma
- Bone infarction
- Osteomyelitis.

MULTIPLE CHOICE QUESTIONS

1. In which of the following multiple lesions are not seen? *(JIPMER May 2016)*
   A. Enchondroma
   B. Osteoid osteoma
   C. Fibrous dysplasia
   D. GCT

   Ans. is 'B' Osteoid osteoma

2. Background lesions simulating bone tumors are all except: *(AIIMS MAY 2011)*
   A. Fibrous dysplasia
   B. Bone island
   C. Hurler's syndrome
   D. Bone infarct

   Ans. is 'C' Hurler's syndrome

MOST COMMON SITE OF PRIMARY BONE TUMORS

Epiphyseal

- **Chondroblastoma (before physeal closure)**-purely epiphyseal
- Osteoclastoma/Giant cell tumor (after physeal closure in adults)
- Articular osteochondroma
- Clear cell chondrosarcoma

Metaphyseal (Most Common Site for Bone Tumors)

Chondrosarcoma Enchondroma
Osteochondroma Osteoblastoma
Bone cyst **Osteosarcoma**
Osteoclastoma (in children)

Note: Osteomyelitis also starts in metaphysis.

Diaphyseal

1. Round cell lesions—**Ewing's sarcoma**
2. Lymphoma
3. Multiple myeloma
4. **Adamantinoma**
5. **Osteoid osteoma**

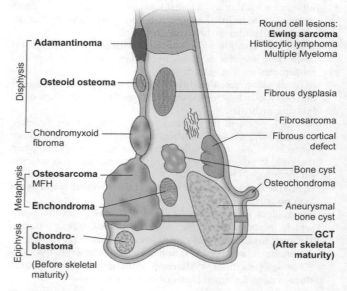

Fig. 4.1: Sites of bone tumors

Most Common Sites

Unicameral bone cyst	Upper end Humerus
Aneurysmal bone cyst	**Lower limb metaphysis (Tibia and femur)**
Osteochondroma	Distal femur
Osteoid osteoma	**Femur >Tibia**
Osteoblastoma	Vertebrae
Osteoma (Ivory or Compact or Eburnated)	Skull and facial bones
Enchondroma	Short bones of **hand**

Orthopedics Oncology

Chordoma	**Sacrum** (most common) > sphenooccipital region (clivus)> anterior vertebral body, i.e. involves only axial skeleton
Adamantinoma (Long bone)	Tibia
Ameloblastoma	Mandible
Osteoclastoma (GCT)	Lower end of Femur
Fibrous dysplasia	**Upper femur monostotic (commoner)** **Craniofacial region – Polyostotic**
Multiple myeloma	Lumbar vertebrae
Osteosarcoma	Lower end of femur
Ewing's sarcoma	Femur
Chondrosarcoma	Pelvis
Secondary tumors	**Dorsal vertebrae** (Secondaries in bone are commonest from **Breast** > prostate > lung > kidney)

Note: Most common tumor of **mandible** is **squamous cell carcinoma**.

MULTIPLE CHOICE QUESTIONS

1. Which among the following is/are metaphyseal tumor? *(PGI May 2017)*
   A. Chondrosarcoma B. Enchondroma
   C. Giant cell tumor D. Ameloblastoma
   E. Osteosarcoma
Ans. is 'A' Chondrosarcoma; 'B' Enchondroma; 'E' Osteosarcoma

2. Epiphysis involved in which bone tumor? *(NEET 2015)*
   A. Osteosarcoma B. Multiple myeloma
   C. Giant cell tumor D. Ewing's sarcoma
Ans. is 'C' Giant cell tumor

3. Epiphyseal tumor before fusion of epiphysis: *(NEET Pattern 2014, 2012)*
   A. Chondroblastoma B. Chondrosarcoma
   C. Ewing's sarcoma D. Giant cell tumor
Ans. is 'A' Chondroblastoma

4. Tumor in Diaphysis: *(NEET Pattern 2012)*
   A. Osteogenic sarcoma B. Ewing's sarcoma
   C. Osteoclastoma D. Osteochondroma
Ans. is 'B' Ewing's sarcoma

5. GCT is: *(NEET Pattern 2012)*
   A. Epiphyseal B. Epiphyseometaphyseal
   C. Metaphyseal D. Metaphyseodiaphyseal
Ans. is 'B' Epiphyseometaphyseal > 'A' Epiphyseal

6. Most common tumor of hand: *(NEET Pattern 2012)*
   A. Enchondroma B. Squamous cell carcinoma
   C. Chondroblastoma D. Melanoma
Ans. is 'B' Squamous cell carcinoma—is the most common tumor of hand most common tumor involving bones of hand is enchondroma.

Note: Always beware of first choice, please read carefully before answering. Most students get this one wrong! And mark enchondroma.

7. Solitary bone cyst is most common in the: *(AI 2004)*
   A. Upper end of humerus B. Lower end of humerus
   C. Upper end of fibula D. Lower end of femur
Ans. is 'A' Upper end of humerus

8. The following lesions are classically seen in metaphysis: *(PGI June 2002)*
   A. Osteomyelitis B. Osteosarcoma
   C. Chondrosarcoma D. Osteoclastoma
   E. Ewing's sarcoma
Ans. is 'A' Osteomyelitis; 'B' Osteosarcoma; and 'C' Chondrosarcoma
   – Osteoclastoma is epiphyseal
   – Ewing's sarcoma is diaphyseal

9. Most common site of Osteogenic sarcoma is: *(AI 2001)*
   A. Femur, upper end B. Femur, lower end
   C. Tibia, upper D. Tibia, lower end
Ans. is 'B' Femur lower end
   – Osteosarcoma and GCT involves lower end of femur commonly

10. Bone tumors seen in diaphysis: *(PGI Dec 2K)*
    A. Chondrosarcoma B. Ewing's tumor
    C. Osteoclastoma D. Chondroblastoma
    E. Osteoid osteoma
Ans. is 'B' Ewing's tumor; 'E' Osteoid osteoma
   – Diaphyseal lesions: Ewing sarcoma, Lymphomas, Myeloma, Adamantinoma, Osteoid osteoma.

11. Chordoma can occur over all the following sites, *except*:
    A. Rib B. Clivus *(AI 2000)*
    C. Sacrum D. Vertebral body
Ans. is 'A' Rib
   – Chordoma occurs only in vertebrae and clivus

AGE PREDILECTION

Important Ages as per the Questions Asked

1st decade usually **Ewing's sarcoma** (Can be 5–20 years), Unicameral Bone Cyst other tumors that can be seen at this age are Retinoblastoma, Rhabdomyosarcoma and Metastasis from Neuroblastoma.

2nd decade usually osteosarcoma (Can affect all ages), Aneurysmal Bone Cyst.

After skeletal maturity **Giant cell tumor** (20–40 years — classical **is 30 years**), Adamantinoma, enchondroma.

After 40 metastases > multiple myeloma, Chondrosarcoma.

Note: Ewing's sarcoma is commonest bone tumor of 1st decade but its peak incidence is 2nd decade.

MULTIPLE CHOICE QUESTIONS

1. Not a common tumor of 1st decade of life: *(NEET Pattern 2012)*
   A. Ameloblastoma B. Neuroblastoma
   C. Retinoblastoma D. Rhabdomyosarcoma
Ans. is 'A' Ameloblastoma

2. True about bone tumor is: *(AIIMS Nov 1999)*
   A. Multiple myeloma is seen in more than 55 years age and above
   B. Osteogenic sarcoma fourth decade
   C. Chondrosarcoma first decade
   D. Osteoclastoma fifth decade
Ans. is 'A' Multiple myeloma—more than 55 years age and above

3. A 10-year-old boy, LEAST common cause of proximal lytic lesion of head of femur is: *(AIIMS June 1997)*
   A. Plasmacytoma   B. Metastasis
   C. Histiocytosis   D. Bone tumor

Ans. is 'A' Plasmacytoma
- If multiple myeloma occurs as a solitary lesion it is known as Plasmacytoma
- Rare before 40 years of age

Imaging of Bone Tumors

Questions to ask when looking at an X-ray: (Watt 1985).
- Solitary or Multiple.
- What type of bone involved.
- **Where is the lesion in bone Middle (diaphysis) or Ends (Epiphysis or metaphysis).**
- **Well or ill defined-Ill defined malignant lesion, well defined benign lesion.**
- Cortical destruction-malignant lesion.
- **Bony reaction – Narrow zone – benign lesion and wide zone – malignant lesion.**
- Center Calcified Cartilaginous Tumors

Classical Radiological Features*

Sunray appearance*/ Codman's triangle	**Osteosarcoma** but can be seen in any malignant lesion
Onion peel appearance*	**Ewing sarcoma** but can be seen in any malignant lesion or chronic osteomyelitis
Soap bubble appearance*	**Osteoclastoma (GCT)**, adamantinoma
Ground glass appearance	Fibrous Dysplasia
Patchy calcification*	Chondrogenic tumors (Chondrosarcoma > Chondroblastoma)
Homogeneous calcification	Osteogenic tumors (Osteosarcoma)

Note: *While marking answers on calcifications choose cartilaginous tumors before osteogenic and amongst cartilaginous prefer malignant more than benign*

Winking Owl Sign vs Blind Bat Sign

CT is most helpful in assessing ossification and calcification and in evaluating the integrity of the cortex. It is also the best imaging study to localize the nidus of an osteoid osteoma, to detect a thin rim of reactive bone around an aneurysmal bone cyst, to evaluate calcification in a suspected cartilaginous lesion, and to evaluate endosteal cortical erosion in a suspected chondrosarcoma. CT of the lungs also is the most effective study to detect pulmonary metastases.

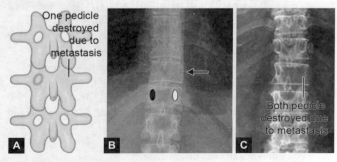

Figs 4.2A to C: (A and B) Winking owl sign (One pedicle destroyed due to metastasis), (C) Blind bat sign (Both pedicle destroyed due to metastasis)

Technetium bone scans are used to determine the activity of a lesion and to determine the presence of multiple lesions or skeletal metastases. Bone scans frequently are falsely negative in multiple myeloma and some cases of renal cell carcinoma. Excluding these exceptions, however, most other malignant neoplasms of bone show increased uptake on technetium bone scans. A normal bone scan is reassuring; however, the converse statement is not true because benign active lesions of bone also show increased uptake.

MRI has replaced CT as the study of choice to determine the size, extent, and anatomical relationships of bone and soft-tissue tumors. **It is the most accurate technique for determining the limits of disease within and outside bone.** With regard to most neoplasms, however, the MRI appearance requires biopsy to diagnose.

Angiography, which previously was used to determine the relationship of a neoplasm to the vessels, has been supplanted by MRI.

Positron emission tomography, although considered investigational in the field of musculoskeletal oncology, is proving to be useful in staging, planning the biopsy, evaluating the response to chemotherapy, and helping to direct subsequent treatment. It is considered better than Bone Scan for metastasis.

Tumors that metastasize from bone to bone:
BONE: Osteosarcoma/Neuroblastoma/Ewing's Sarcoma (Maximum incidence of a particular tumor type).

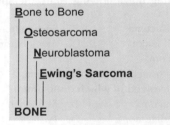

Neuroblastoma is the Most Common Tumor to have Bone Metastasis in Children

Important Notes

In a patient older than age 40 with a new, painful bone lesion, metastatic carcinoma > multiple myeloma are the most likely diagnoses even if the patient has no known history of carcinoma.

Breast cancer and Prostate cancer are the two most common primary sources for bone metastases.

If a patient has no known primary tumor, however, the most likely sources are lung cancer and renal cell carcinoma.

Biopsy: It is the gold standard for any tumor.

MULTIPLE CHOICE QUESTIONS

1. Soap bubble appearance in X-ray suggests: *(JIPMER Nov 2017)*
   A. Osteogenic sarcoma   B. Ewing's sarcoma
   C. Osteoclastoma   D. Chondrosarcoma

Ans. is 'C' Osteoclastoma

2. Which of the following is not a type of geographic lesion of bone? *(DNB June 2017)*
   A. Fibrous dysplasia   B. Brodie's abscess
   C. Giant cell tumor   D. Ewing's sarcoma

Ans. 'D' Ewing's sarcoma
   I Geographic lesions:
      IA: Well defined with sclerotic margins: Simple Bone Cyst (SBC), Fibrous dysplasia

IB: Well defined without sclerotic rim: Aneurysmal Bone Cyst (ABC) Giant Cell Tumor (GCT)

IC: Ill defined margins: Chondrosarcoma

II Moth Eaten: Multiple Lytic lesions: Myeloma metastasis

III Permeative: Poorly demarcated, numerous lytic lesions: Ewings sarcoma, Myeloma, metastasis.

3. Dense calcification is found in all except: *(NEET Dec 2016)*
   A. Osteosarcoma
   B. Chondroblastoma
   C. Synovial sarcoma
   D. Osteoblastoma

Ans. 'C' Synovial sarcoma

4. Which of the following is wrongly matched? *(TN 2014)*
   A. Osteosarcoma — Sunray appearance
   B. Chondroblastoma — Soap bubble appearance
   C. Ewing's sarcoma — Onion peel appearance
   D. Secondaries of spine — winking owl sign

Ans. 'B' Chondroblastoma — Soap bubble appearance

5. Which of the following childhood tumors most frequently metastasizes to the bone? *(NEET Pattern 2012)*
   A. Neuroblastoma   B. Ganglioneuroma
   C. Wilms' tumor   D. Ewing's sarcoma

Ans. is 'A' Neuroblastoma

CLASSIFICATION

Enneking's

Classification system for staging benign and malignant musculoskeletal tumors (i.e. tumor of bone and soft tissue).

Benign

1. Latent
2. Active
3. Aggressive

Benign = Arabic numbers

- **Stage 1.** *Latent:* lesions are **intracapsular**, usually **asymptomatic**, and frequently incidental findings. Radiographic features include a well-defined margin with a thick rim of reactive bone. There is no cortical destruction or expansion. These lesions do not require treatment because they do not compromise the strength of the bone and usually resolve spontaneously. An example is a small asymptomatic non-ossifying fibroma discovered incidentally on radiographs taken to evaluate an unrelated injury.
- **Stage 2.** *Active:* lesions also are **intracapsular**, but are **actively growing** and can cause symptoms or lead to pathological fracture. They have **well-defined margins** on radiographs but may expand and thin the cortex. Usually they have only a thin rim of reactive bone and narrow zone of activity. An example is Aneurysmal bone cyst. Treatment usually consists of extended curettage.
- **Stage 3.** *Aggressive:* lesions are **extracapsular**. Their aggressive nature is apparent clinically and radiographically. They usually have broken through the reactive bone and possibly the cortex. MRI may show a soft-tissue mass, and metastases may be present in 5% of patients with these lesions. An example is Giant cell tumor. Treatment consists of extended curettage and marginal or even wide resection, and local recurrences are common.

Malignant = Roman Numerals

I   =   Low grade
II =   High grade
III =   Metastases
A   =   Intracompartmental
B   =   Extracompartmental

Anatomical compartments are determined by the natural anatomical barriers to tumor growth, such as cortical bone, articular cartilage, fascial septa, or joint capsules.

Low-grade lesions are designated as stage I. These lesions are well-differentiated, have few mitoses, and exhibit only moderate cytological atypia. The risk for metastases is low (<25%).

IA Low grade, intracompartmental G 1 T 1 M 0

Stage IA: Wide excision and are usually amenable to limb salvage procedures.

IB Low grade, extracompartmental G 1 T 2 M 0

Stage IB: Such tumors may be treated with wide excision, but the choice between amputation and limb salvage depends on the estimated amount of residual tumor left behind after a limb salvage procedure.

High-grade lesions are designated as stage II. They are poorly differentiated with a high mitotic rate and a high cell-to-matrix ratio. The risk for metastases is >25%

IIa High grade, intracompartmental G 2 T 1 M 0

IIb High grade, extracompartmental G 2 T 2 M 0

Stage II: These tumors are high grade, are usually extracompartmental, and have a significant risk for skip metastases. They usually are not amenable to limb salvage operations and require radical amputation or disarticulation in most patients. However, bone tumors responsive to chemotherapy may be treated successfully using wide excision and adjuvant therapy.

Stage III: Refers to any lesion that has metastasized regardless of the size or grade of the primary tumor. No distinction is made between lymph node metastases or distant metastases because both circumstances are associated with an equally poor prognosis.

IIIa Low or High grade, intracompartmental G 1-2 T 1 M 1 with metastases.

IIIb Low or High grade, extracompartmental G 1-2 T 2 M 1 with metastases.

Stage III: Tumors at this stage responsive to chemotherapy may be treated with aggressive resection. Those that are not responsive to chemotherapy should be treated with palliative resection.

> **Note:** Benign bone tumor has well defined margin and uniform consistency on feel. Malignant tumor has ill defined margins and variable consistency on feel.

Consistencies of tissues in human body

1. *Hard—Bone (feel of forehead)*
2. *Firm—cartilage (feel of the tip of the nose)*
3. *Soft—soft tissues (feel of lips)*

Treatment

The goal of treatment in a patient with a primary malignancy of the musculoskeletal system is to make the patient disease free. The goal of treatment of a patient with metastatic carcinoma to bone is to minimize pain and to preserve function. The optimal treatment of the tumor often requires a combination of radiation therapy, chemotherapy, and surgery.

Radiation Therapy

Most primary bone malignancies are relatively radio-resistant. Exceptions are the **marrow cell tumors, including multiple myeloma, lymphoma, and Ewing sarcoma, which are each exquisitely sensitive. Carcinomas metastatic to bone, with the exception of renal cell carcinoma, also frequently are sensitive to radiation treatment. Most radiation treatment protocols deliver 150 to 200 cGy/d until the target dose is achieved. This dose ranges from 30 to 40 Gy for myeloma to 60 Gy for treatment of a soft-tissue sarcoma. Radiotherapy is rarely used for benign conditions. (Possible exceptions include an extensive pigmented villonodular synovitis that cannot be controlled by surgery or a large spinal giant cell tumor).**

Radiation therapy is associated with significant acute and long-term complications. Acutely, the most common complication is skin irritation. Other common acute side effects include gastrointestinal upset, urinary frequency, fatigue, anorexia, and extremity edema. Late effects include chronic edema, fibrosis, osteonecrosis, and pathological fracture. Malignant transformation of irradiated tissues (i.e. radiation sarcoma) is being reported with increasing frequency in survivors of childhood and adolescent cancers. These secondary sarcomas occur with a mean lag time of approximately 10 years and often are associated with a poor prognosis. **Most common type is osteosarcoma.**

Radio-Resistant Bone Tumor

- Metastatic renal cell carcinoma
- Synovial cell sarcoma
- Malignant fibrous histiocytoma
- Rhabdomyosarcoma
- Fibrosarcoma
- Liposarcoma
- Osteosarcoma
- Fibrosarcoma of bone
- Chondrosarcoma
- Malignant GCT

Chemotherapy

Adjuvant chemotherapy refers to chemotherapy administered postoperatively to treat presumed micrometastases. Neoadjuvant chemotherapy refers to chemotherapy administered before surgical resection of the primary tumor. Preoperative chemotherapy frequently causes regression of the primary tumor, making a successful limb salvage operation easier. **Neoadjuvant chemotherapy followed by surgical resection allows for histological evaluation of the effectiveness of treatment. This is one of the most valuable prognostic indicators of successful long-term outcome.** In addition, histological evaluation may lead to alteration of further chemotherapy in poor responders. Preoperative chemotherapy theoretically may decrease the spread of tumor cells at the time of surgery. **On the same approach there is improvement in survival of osteosarcoma and the current 5-year survival rate for osteosarcoma is approximately 70%.** The role of chemotherapy is less well defined for adult soft-tissue malignancies, with most investigations showing modest improvements in outcome. In general, chemotherapy is not useful for cartilaginous lesions and most other low-grade malignancies.

Surgical Therapy

In orthopedic oncology, the surgical margin is described by one of four terms—intralesional, marginal, wide, or radical. Amputations and limb-sparing resections may be associated with any of the four types of margins, and the margin must be specifically defined with each procedure.

Intralesional: Enters tumor leaving gross residual tumor within the bed.

Marginal: Plane through reactive zone around tumor.

Wide local excision (Most commonly used) cuff of normal tissue completely encircling, the tumor is taken out. (Usual cuff of normal tissue is **3 cm**).

Radical or amputation: Tissue from joint to joint and muscle from origin to insertion is excised.

Curettage is removing or curetting or scooping out the contents of the lesion, e.g. for simple bone cyst. If to it additional chemical (Phenol/Poly Methy/Methacrylate/Liquid Nitrogen/hydrogen peroxide/Argon beam laser) is added to kill the residual cells to decrease the rate for recurrence it is called as extended curettage. Extended curettage is used for GCT, Enchondroma and Aneurysmal bone cyst. **Least rate of recurrence in extended curettage is seen with Liquid Nitrogen.**

> Note: Most of the benign tumors and cartilaginous tumors are treated by surgery. **Osteosarcoma** and cartilaginous tumors are **radio-resistant**.

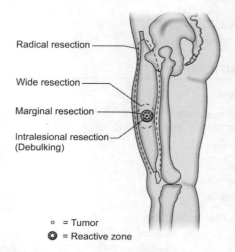

Fig. 4.3: Enneking's margins for tumor excision

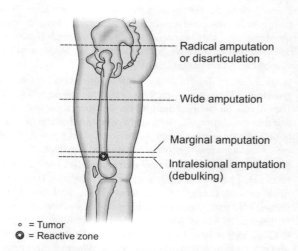

Fig. 4.4: Enneking's margins for amputation

MULTIPLE CHOICE QUESTIONS

1. Most radio-resistant tumor: (JIPMER MAY 2017)
   A. Osteosarcoma
   B. Malignant fibrous histiocytoma
   C. Ewing's sarcoma
   D. Multiple myeloma

   Ans. is 'A' Osteosarcoma

2. Radio-resistant bone tumor among the following: (PGI Nov 2016)
   A. Ewing's
   B. Osteosarcoma
   C. Multiple myeloma
   D. Chondrosarcoma
   E. Lymphoma

   Ans. is 'B' Osteosarcoma and 'D' Chondrosarcoma

3. Active benign tumor (Enneking) all are true *except*:
   A. Intracapsular (AIIMS May 2011)
   B. Well defined margins
   C. Wide area of activity (> 5 cm)
   D. Treated by extended curettage

   Ans. is 'C' Wide area of activity (> 5 cm)
   – Benign lesions have narrow zone of activity. Zone of activity refers to area of destruction and periosteal reaction around the lesion.

4. Classification system of bone tumors is: (AIIMS Nov 07)
   A. Enneking   B. Manchester
   C. Edward   D. TNM

   Ans. is 'A' Enneking

5. All of the following tumors are benign tumor *except*: (PGI Dec 06) (PGI Dec 03) (AI 1998)
   A. Chondroma   B. Chordoma
   C. Osteochondroma D. Enchondroma

   Ans. is 'B' Chordoma
   – Chordoma is a malignant tumor arising from notochordal remnants.

6. According to a newer hypothesis Ewing's sarcoma arises from: (AI 1999)
   A. Epiphysis   B. Diaphysis
   C. Medullary cavity D. Cortex

   Ans. is 'C' Medullary cavity
   – Marrow tumors (medullary cavity tumors)—Ewing's sarcoma, Plasma cell tumor, multiple myeloma, Lymphoma.

CYSTIC LESIONS OF BONE

Unicameral Bone Cyst: True Cyst!

Unicameral bone cysts are most common in the proximal humerus and femur. The lesions are most active during skeletal growth and **usually heal spontaneously at maturity.** Unicameral bone cysts **often are asymptomatic**, unless a pathological fracture has occurred. Plain radiographs reveal a **centrally located, purely lytic lesion with a well-marginated outline.** Occasionally (20%), a thinned cortical fragment fractures and falls into the base of the lesion confirming its empty cystic nature. This **"fallen fragment" sign is pathognomonic of a unicameral bone cyst, bone fragment, may also hinge around and move with fluid called as trap door sign.** Unicameral bone cysts are classified as active when they are within 1 cm of the physis and latent when they are closer to the diaphysis. Small, asymptomatic lesions in the upper extremities can be treated with observation with serial plain radiographs. Larger lesions (lesions at risk for pathological fracture), symptomatic lesions, and lesions in the lower extremities usually are treated with curettage (with or without bone grafting or internal fixation) or aspiration and injection (often using steroids, bone marrow aspirate, demineralized bone matrix, or sclerosant).

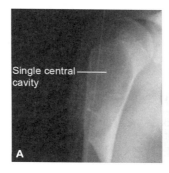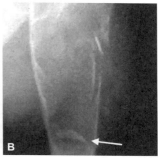

Figs. 4.5A and B: (A) Unicameral or simple bone cyst (B) Fallen fragment (leaf) sign

Aneurysmal Bone Cyst (ABC)—Pseudocyst!

Aneurysmal bone cysts are locally destructive, blood-filled reactive lesions of bone and are not considered to be true neoplasms. Most commonly involves the lower limbs. Vertebral lesions, accounting for 15–20% of these entities, are located in the posterior elements.

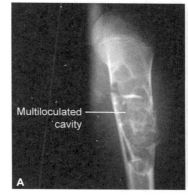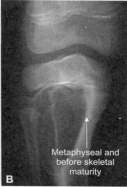

Figs. 4.6A and B: Aneurysmal bone cyst

Radiographs reveal an expansile lytic lesion that elevates the periosteum, but remains contained by a thin shell of cortical bone. An aneurysmal bone cyst can have well-defined margins or a permeative appearance that mimics a malignancy. It is most often eccentrically located in the metaphysis. When differentiating between a unicameral and aneurysmal bone cyst using MRI, the presence of a **double-density fluid level and intralesional septations** usually indicates an aneurysmal bone cyst.

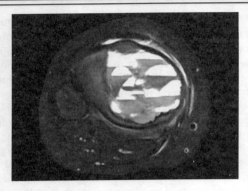

Fig. 4.7: Double-Density fluid level on MRI

An aneurysmal bone cyst can arise de novo, but areas similar to an aneurysmal bone cyst are found in various other lesions, **such as Giant cell tumor, chondroblastoma, osteoblastoma, fibrous dysplasia, non-ossifying fibroma, and chondromyxoid fibroma.**

Aneurysmal bone cysts are treated with extended curettage and grafting with a bone graft substitute. Lesions in the spine or pelvis can be treated with **preoperative embolization to minimize surgical blood loss.** Low-dose irradiation has been reported to be an effective method of treatment, often associated with rapid ossification; however, it is not used routinely because of the potential for malignant transformation.

	Unicameral bone cyst	Aneurysmal bone cyst
Age	1st decade	2nd decade
Site	**Proximal humerus, femur**	Lower limb (however can occur anywhere)
Location	**Central (concentric)**	Eccentric
Expansile	Expansile	More expansile
Symptoms	Asymptomatic	Pain is present
Cavity	Single, Straw colored fluid	Multiloculated, Hemorrhagic fluid
Treatment	Curettage	Extended curettage

Radiolucent Bone Lesion with Well Defined Borders

Eccentric and Expansile (NAG – EXPANDS)

1. Non-ossifying fibroma
2. Aneurysmal bone cyst
3. Giant cell tumor

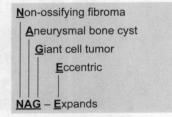

Centric Nonexpansile (or minimally expansile) with Marginal Sclerosis (BEECH - CYST)

Brodie's abscess
Brown tumor of hyperparathyroidism
Eosinophilic granuloma
Enchondroma
Chondroblastoma
Hemophilia – Pseudotumor
Simple bony cyst

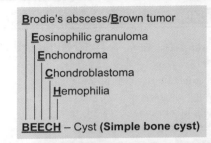

MULTIPLE CHOICE QUESTIONS

1. Fallen fragment sign is a feature of: *(NEET Pattern 2018, 2013)*
   A. Simple bone cyst   B. Aneurysmal bone cyst
   C. Giant cell tumor   D. Fibrous dysplasia
   Ans. is 'A' Simple bone cyst

2. Which of the following is/are true about simple bone cyst? *(PGI MAY 2016)*
   A. Most commonly occur in adult
   B. Commonest site is the upper end of the humerus
   C. Cortex may be thin
   D. Cause pathological fracture
   E. No risk of recurrence after removal
   Ans. is 'B' Commonest site is the upper end of the humerus; 'C' Cortex may be thin; 'D' Cause pathological fracture

3. X-ray upper end humerus, diagnosis is: *(AI 2016)*

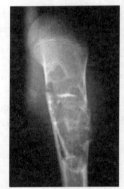

   A. Giant cell tumor   B. Simple bone cyst
   C. Aneurysmal bone cyst   D. Osteosarcoma
   Ans. is 'C' Aneurysmal bone cyst

4. All are true about aneurysmal bone cyst *except*: *(NEET Pattern 2013)*
   A. Eccentric
   B. Expansile and lytic
   C. Treated by simple curettage
   D. Metaphysis of long bones
   Ans. is 'C' Treated by simple curettage
   – Treatment is extended curettage

5. Pediatric patient with upper humerus lytic lesion with cortical thinning which is not a treatment modality:
   A. Sclerosant   *(AIIMS Nov 2012)*
   B. Radiotherapy
   C. Curettage and bone grafting
   D. Steroids
   Ans. is 'B' Radiotherapy

6. **Secondary aneurysmal bone cyst arises in:** *(PGI June 07)*
   A. Osteoclastoma   B. Chondroblastoma
   C. Fibrous dysplasia   D. GCT
   E. All of the above

Ans. is 'E' All of the above

7. **True about simple bone cyst:** *(PGI Dec 2005)*
   A. Seen in children
   B. Present as well demarcated radiolucent lesions
   C. Pathological fracture seen
   D. Commonest site is diaphysis

Ans. is 'A' Seen in children; 'B' Present as well demarcated radiolucent lesions; 'C' Pathological fracture seen
   Cysts are metaphyseal

8. **A classical expansile lytic lesion in the transverse process of a vertebra is seen in:** *(PGI Dec 2004, AI 2003)*
   A. Osteosarcoma
   B. Aneurysmal bone cyst
   C. Osteoblastoma
   D. Metastasis

Ans. is 'B' Aneurysmal bone cyst
   Lytic Lesion in Posterior Element of Vertebrae (i.e. spinous process, transverse process, and pedicle) Expansile and Purely lytic, Aneurysmal Bone Cyst, Non-expansile and partly or extensively ossified, Osteoblastoma
   Body of vertebra is involved in GCT

9. **An 8-year-old male has expansile lytic cavity in upper end of humerus. Cavity in centre has a cortical fragment. What is the diagnosis?** *(AIIMS May 2002, Nov 89, AI 2001; AIIMS Dec 1995)*
   A. UBC   B. ABC
   C. GCT   D. Enchondroma

Ans. is 'A' UBC, Expansile Cyst in upper end humerus goes towards UBC > ABC. Also cortical fragment in center means Fallen Fragment Sign.

OSTEOCHONDROMA

Osteochondromas are **developmental malformations** rather than true neoplasms and are thought to originate within the periosteum as small cartilaginous nodules.

The lesions consist of a bony mass, often in the form of a stalk, produced by progressive endochondral ossification of a growing cartilaginous cap. In contrast to true neoplasms, their growth usually parallels that of the patient and usually ceases when skeletal maturity is reached. Most lesions are found during the period of rapid skeletal growth. About 90% of patients have only a single lesion. Osteochondromas are found on the metaphysis of a long bone near the physis they are seen most often on the distal femur, the proximal tibia, and the proximal humerus.

Many of these lesions cause no symptoms and are discovered incidentally. Some cause pain by Bursitis of overlying bursa **(most common cause of pain)**, fracture through stalk or pedunculated (narrow based) lesion, sarcomatous change and Impingement of neighboring structure, e.g. nerve, vessel, etc. The physical finding usually is a palpable mass.

Multiple hereditary exostoses **(diaphyseal aclasia)** constitute an autosomal dominant (Chromosome 8, 11, 19 involved) condition with variable penetrance, **disturbances in growth also occur,** such as bowing of the radius and shortening of the ulna, producing ulnar deviation of the hand (Madelung deformity).

Osteochondromas are of two types: Pedunculated and broad-based or sessile. Pedunculated tumors are more common, and any definite stalk is directed away from the physis adjacent to which it takes its origin. The projecting part of the lesion has cortical and cancellous components, both of which are continuous with corresponding components of the parent bone.

The lesion is covered by a cartilaginous cap that often is irregular and usually cannot be seen on radiographs; occasionally, calcification within the cap may be seen. They usually angle away from the growth plate.

Typically, the cap is only a few millimeters thick in adults, although it may be 2 cm thick in a child. Plain radiographs usually are sufficient to make a diagnosis. **It looks smaller than it feels because the cartilage cap is not seen on X-ray.** CT or MRI sometimes is needed to confirm the diagnosis.

The incidence of malignant degeneration is approximately **1% for patients with a solitary osteochondroma and 6%** for patients with **multiple hereditary exostoses**. Malignant transformation should be suspected when a previously quiescent lesion in an adult grows rapidly; any further enlargement after skeletal maturity takes place, loss of corticomedullary differentiation takes place it usually takes the form of a low-grade **chondrosarcoma**. In these cases, the **cartilage cap usually is more than 2 cm thick.** (Best evaluated by MRI).

Surgery (en bloc resection-extraperiosteal resection) is indicated for lesion that causes—pain, symptomatic impingement on neurovascular structure, compromise of joint function, cosmetic deformity, painful bursa formation and rapid increase in size of lesion or when imaging features suggest malignancy.

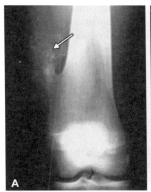 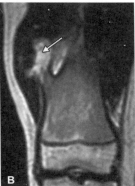

Figs. 4.8A and B: Exostosis/osteochondroma

Patients with multiple hereditary exostoses may require osteotomies to correct deformity.

Trevor's disease is osteochondroma on epiphyseal side of growth plate.

MULTIPLE CHOICE QUESTIONS

1. **Diaphyseal aclasia is etiologically:** *(PGM-CET 2015)*
   A. Congenital   B. Developmental
   C. Metabolic   D. Inflammatory

Ans. is 'B' Developmental

2. **Factors indicating malignant degeneration in Osteochondroma:** *(AIIMS May 2014)*
   A. Size   B. Pain
   C. Weight loss   D. Thickness of cartilage

Ans. is 'D' Thickness of cartilage

3. All of the following are the causes of sudden increase in pain in osteochondroma, except: *(AIIMS May 2006)*
   A. Sarcomatous change B. Fracture
   C. Bursitis D. Degenerative changes

Ans. is 'D' Degenerative changes

4. All the statements are true about exostosis, except: *(AI 06)*
   A. It occurs at the growing end of bone
   B. Growth continues after skeletal maturity
   C. It is covered by cartilaginous cap
   D. Malignant transformation may occur

Ans. is 'B' Growth continues after skeletal maturity
   – Growth of osteochondroma stops with skeletal maturity. If it continues to grow after skeletal maturity it indicates malignant transformation.

5. Which of the following statements is true about osteo-chondromatosis? *(PGI Dec 01)*
   A. Usually affects long bones, but can also occur in skull and pelvis
   B. Usual site is metaphyseal region
   C. Also known as multiple exostoses, diaphyseal aclasia
   D. It does not interfere with general body stature
   E. Autosomal dominant in inheritance

Ans. is 'A' Usually affects long bones, but can also occur in skull and pelvis; 'B' Usual site is metaphyseal region; 'C' Also known as multiple exostoses, diaphyseal aclasia; 'E' Autosomal dominant in inheritance
   – Remember the fact that using the suffix tosis' means **multiple** lesions, e.g. osteochondromatosis means multiple osteochondromas. Osteochondromas can cause growth disturbances.

6. Most common benign tumor of the bone is: *(AIIMS Dec 1995)*
   A. Giant cell tumor B. Simple bone cyst
   C. Osteochondrorna D. Enchondroma

Ans. is 'C' Osteochondroma

Note:
   – **Commonest benign bone lesion is fibrous cortical defect > osteochondroma**
   – **Commonest true benign bone tumor is osteoid osteoma** as above two conditions are not true tumors.

OSTEOID OSTEOMA

Osteoid Osteoma—MC Femur Diaphysis

- It is commonest **benign true bone tumor**, exceeded in incidence only by osteochondroma and non-ossifying fibroma.
- The typical patient with an osteoid osteoma has **pain that is worse at night and is relieved by aspirin or other non-steroidal antiinflammatory medications**. When the lesion is in a vertebra, scoliosis may occur.

Osteoid Osteoma: Both Osteoblastic & Osteoclastic cells are seen

- The lesion has central lysis with surrounding sclerosis. Growing center is called as Nidus (Seed).
- **CT is the best study to identify the nidus** and confirm the diagnosis.
- D/D of osteoid osteoma is bone island.
- Radiofrequency ablation is used for osteoid osteoma.

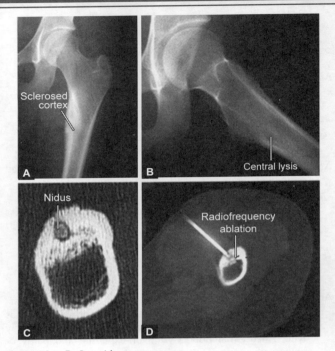

Figs. 4.9A to D: Osteoid osteoma

- Surgical management involves removal of the entire nidus done by burr-down technique.

Note: The literature now supports that osteoid osteoma is showing higher incidence in metaphysis. Even than the clinical scenario given is such that it is mentioned as diaphyseal.

MULTIPLE CHOICE QUESTIONS

1. Which of the following is true regarding osteoid osteoma? *(DNB Pattern 2018)*
   A. The femur and tibia are the commonest bones involved
   B. Radiologically appears as a radiolucent lesion surrounded by dense bone
   C. It is a benign bone tumor, presents with severe pain that is typically relieved by aspirin
   D. All of the above

Ans. is 'D' All of the above

2. Which of the following is not true about osteoid osteoma? *(DNB June 2017)*
   A. Most common true benign tumor of bone
   B. Occurs between 10–30 years of age
   C. Lesion appears ill defined on X-ray with permeative margins
   D. Bone scan shows increased uptakes in the lesion

Ans. is 'C' Lesion appears ill defined on X-ray with permeative margins

3. Osteoid osteoma consists of: *(NEET 2015)*
   A. Osteoblasts B. Osteoclasts
   C. Both of the above D. None of the above

Ans. is 'C' Both of the above

4. Which is the commonest true benign bone tumor?
   A. Osteoid osteoma B. Hemangioma *(NEET 2015)*
   C. Osteochondroma D. Enchondroma

Ans. is 'A' Osteoid osteoma

5. A 10-year-old child has a lesion in the diaphysis of bone in the cortex with central lysis and surrounding sclerosis: *(AIIMS Nov 2014)*
   A. Osteoid osteoma
   B. Eosinophilic granuloma
   C. Fibrous cortical defect
   D. Fibrous dysplasia

Ans. is 'A' Osteoid osteoma

6. Tumor with maximum bone matrix: *(NEET Pattern 2012)*
   A. Osteoid osteoma
   B. Chondrosarcoma
   C. Enchondroma
   D. None

Ans. is 'A' Osteoid osteoma

Osteosarcoma > Osteoid Osteoma for bone tumor with Bone matrix.

7. A patient presents with pain in the thigh, relieved by aspirin. X-ray shows a radiolucent mass surrounded by sclerosis. Diagnosis is: *(NEET Pattern 2012)*
   A. Osteoma
   B. Osteoid osteoma
   C. Osteoblastoma
   D. Osteoclastoma

Ans. is 'B' Osteoid osteoma

8. Nidus is seen in: *(NEET Pattern 2012)*
   A. Osteoid osteoma
   B. Osteosarcoma
   C. Ewing's sarcoma
   D. Chondroblastoma

Ans. is 'A' Osteoid osteoma

9. Pain in osteoid osteoma is specifically relieved by: *(NEET Pattern 2012)*
   A. Salicylates
   B. Narcotic analgesics
   C. Radiation
   D. Splinting

Ans. is 'A' Salicylates

10. Babu a 19-year-old male has a small circumscribed sclerotic swelling over diaphysis of femur; likely diagnosis is: *(AIIMS Nov 2001)*
    A. Osteoclastoma
    B. Osteosarcoma
    C. Ewing's sarcoma
    D. Osteoid osteoma

Ans. is 'D' Osteoid osteoma
   – Well circumscribed sclerotic swelling over diaphysis of a long bone (femur) in a 19 years old suggests the diagnosis of osteoid osteoma.

FIBROUS CORTICAL DEFECT (NON-OSSIFYING FIBROMA)

These are common **developmental abnormalities** and are believed to occur in 35% of children. Usually they are found incidentally. Generally, these lesions occur in the metaphyseal region of long bones in individuals 2–20 years old.

Although any bone may be involved, femur is the commonest. On plain radiographs, a non-ossifying fibroma appears as a well-defined lobulated lesion located eccentrically in the metaphysis.

Histologically, Giant cells and foam cells are almost always apparent.

Most non-ossifying fibromas are asymptomatic and regress spontaneously in adulthood. Recurrence after curettage is rare.

MULTIPLE CHOICE QUESTION

1. True about non-ossifying fibroma of bone: *(PGI June 03); (PGI Dec 02)*
   A. Present until 3rd and 4th decade
   B. Eccentric
   C. Sclerotic margin
   D. Histologically Giant cell with foam cell
   E. Metaphyseal lesion

Ans. is 'B' Eccentric; 'C' Sclerotic margin; 'D' Histologically Giant cell with foam cell and 'E' Metaphyseal lesion.

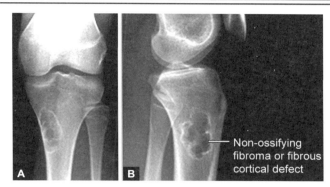

Figs. 4.10A and B: Non-ossifying fibroma (Closely Mimics GCT)

CHONDROMA

Chondromas are benign lesions of **hyaline cartilage**. They are the most common tumor of the small bones of the hands and feet. They usually arise in the medullary canal, where they are referred to as "enchondromas".

Enchondroma: D/D is bone infarct

- Enchondroma—most common tumor of bones of hand.
- Multiple enchondromatosis is also known as Ollier disease.
- Maffucci's syndrome is Enchondroma, subcutaneous hemangioma and phlebolith.

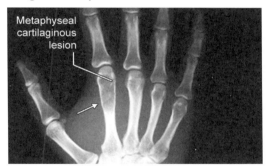

Fig. 4.11: Enchondroma

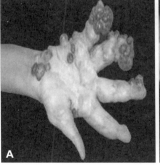 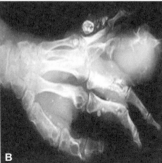

Figs. 4.12A and B: Mafucci syndrome: (A) Hemangiomas (B) Phleboliths and Enchondromas

- Malignant transformation to chondrosarcoma may occur in <2% in solitary cases, 30% in Ollier's disease and 100% in Maffucci's syndrome.
- Treatment is extended curettage.

MULTIPLE CHOICE QUESTIONS

1. Development of Chondrosarcomas is related with:
   (NEET 2015)
   A. Maffucci syndrome
   B. Felty syndrome
   C. Ollier's disease
   D. None of the above

   Ans. is 'A' Maffucci syndrome

2. Maffucci syndrome:
   (DNB June 2017, NEET Pattern 2012)
   A. Multiple enchondromatosis with hemangiomas
   B. Multiple osteochondromatosis with hemangiomas
   C. Multiple osteochondromas
   D. Multiple Giant cell tumor

   Ans. is 'A' Multiple enchondromatosis with hemangiomas.

3. Most common tumor in bones of hand:
   (NEET 2018, AIIMS June 1997)
   A. Exostosis
   B. Giant cell tumor
   C. Enchondroma
   D. Synovial sarcoma

   Ans. is 'C' Enchondroma

   Enchondromas are most common type of hand bone tumor".
   – Phalanges of hand are involved most commonly and *the proximal phalanx is the most common site*.

CHONDROBLASTOMA/CODMAN'S TUMOR— EPIPHYSEAL BEFORE SKELETAL MATURITY

Chondroblastoma is well-circumscribed lesion usually centered in an epiphysis of a long bone. Often it has a surrounding rim of reactive bone, and 30–50% exhibit calcification on plain radiographs.

In chondroblastomas, Calcification is present and may surround individual cells, giving the classic "chicken wire" appearance.

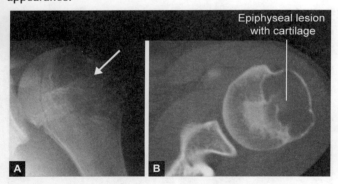

Figs. 4.13A and B: Chondroblastoma (Codman's tumor)

In contrast to chondroblastomas, however, giant cell tumors usually do not have a rim of sclerotic bone or intralesional calcification; and may have a soft-tissue component are not as aggressive as giant cell tumors. Treatment consists of extended curettage and bone grafting or placement of bone cement.

MULTIPLE CHOICE QUESTIONS

1. Identify the lesion in the X-ray: (AI 2016)

   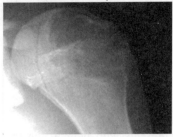

   A. Chondroblastoma   B. Osteoclastoma
   C. ABC   D. Eosinophilic granuloma

   Ans. is 'A' Chondroblastoma

2. A 15-year-old boy presented with painful swelling over the left shoulder. Radiograph of the shoulder showed an osteolytic area with stippled calcification over the proximal humeral epiphysis. Biopsy of the lesion revealed an immature fibrous matrix with scattered giant cells. Which of the following is the most likely diagnosis?
   (AIIMS May 2013, Nov 2004)
   A. Giant cell tumor   B. Chondroblastoma
   C. Osteosarcoma   D. Chondromyxoid fibroma

   Ans. is 'B' Chondroblastoma
   – Painful swelling over the left shoulder, osteolytic area and stippled calcification over proximal humeral epiphysis in a 15 years old suggest the diagnosis of chondroblastoma

3. Dense calcification is found in: (AIIMS May 2002)
   A. Osteosarcoma   B. Chondroblastoma
   C. Synovial sarcoma   D. Osteoblastoma

   Ans. is 'B' Chondroblastoma
   – *You can simply solve this question by knowing very simple fact that punctate calcification is seen in cartilaginous tumors and amongst the given options. Only Chondroblastoma is cartilaginous.*

CHONDROMYXOID FIBROMA

Chondromyxoid fibroma is a rare lesion of cartilaginous origin, Although chondromyxoid fibromas may occur at any age, most occur in patients 10–30 years old. Any bone may be involved, but the proximal tibia is the most common location.

In contrast to other cartilaginous lesions, radiographic evidence of intralesional calcification usually is absent.

Treatment consists of resection or extended curettage.

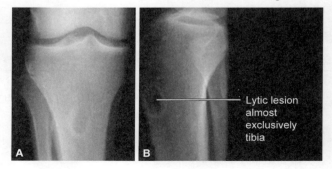

Figs. 4.14A and B: Chondromyxoid fibroma

LANGERHANS CELL HISTIOCYTOSIS (LCH): DESTRUCTION DUE TO HISTIOCYTES, IDIOPATHIC

1. Letterer-Siwe disease: a fulminant systemic disease, age group < 3 years, fatal.
2. Hand-Schuller-Christian disease: Triad of skull lesions (lytic lesion), Exophthalmos and diabetes insipidus.
3. Eosinophilic Granuloma: Solitary lesion of bone or lung (Pulmonary histiocytosis X) 1st decade of life. Skull is the most common site in skeletal system – Bevelled edge lytic lesion is seen in skull (double contour).

Biopsy: Gold standard (cells with Birbeck's granules (tennis racket appearance) under election microscopy)

Treatment

Spontaneous resolution. Highly radiosensitive and Excision + Curettage for resistant cases.

GIANT CELL TUMOR (OSTEOCLASTOMA)

They typically occur in patients **20–40 years old**, and there is a slight **female predominance**. The most common location for this tumor is the distal femur, followed closely by the proximal tibia.

Tumor of lower end radius is GCT till proved otherwise.

Multiple giant cell like bone tumors—Goltz syndrome. GCT has egg shell crackling on palpation.

Although these tumors typically are benign, pulmonary metastases occur in approximately 3% of patients.

Malignant giant cell tumors represent less than 5% of total GCT. **Malignancy in GCT-Osteosarcoma or Malignant Fibrous Histiocytoma or Fibrosarcoma.**

Radiographic findings often are diagnostic. The lesions are eccentrically located in the epiphyses of long bones and usually about the subchondral bone. Although rare in skeletally immature patients, giant cell tumors arise in the metaphysis in this age group. Radiographically, the lesions are purely lytic. The lesion frequently expands or breaks through the cortex; however, intraarticular extension is rare because the subchondral bone usually remains intact.

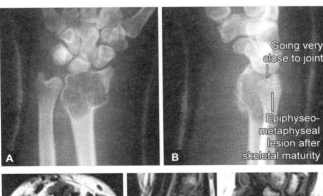
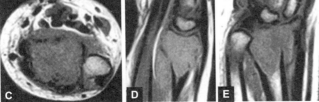

Figs. 4.15A to E

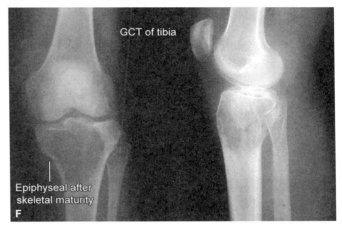

Figs. 4.15A to F: (A to E) Giant cell tumor of lower end radius; (F) Giant cell tumor of upper end tibia

Microscopically, giant cell tumors are composed of many multinucleated giant cells (typically 40–60 nuclei per cell) in a sea of mononuclear stromal cells (malignant cells). **The nuclei of the mononuclear cells are identical to the nuclei of the giant cells, a feature that helps to distinguish giant cell tumors from other tumors that may contain many giant cells.**

Giant cell variants (Tumor with giant cells)

- Brown tumor of hyperparathyroidism
- **Aneurysmal bone cyst (closest)** and unicameral bone cyst
- **Non-ossifying fibroma (commonest)** and Fibrous dysplasia
- Osteoblastoma and Osteosarcoma
- Metastatic carcinoma with giant cells
- Chondromyxoid fibroma and Chondroblastoma
- Pigmented villonodular synovitis (mostly occurrning in knee)
- Benign fibrous histiocytoma
- *Malignant fibrous histiocytoma*
- *Fibrosarcoma*
- *Clear cell chondrosarcoma.*

Treatment of Osteoclastoma (GCT)

1. Extended Curettage by PMMA or phenol or liquid nitrogen and bone grafting
   It is procedure of choice for most lesions.
2. Excision
   Lower end of ulna
   Upper end of fibula
3. Excision and replacement by vascularized bone graft
   Lower end of radius where upper end of fibula is grafted
4. Excision and arthrodesis or prosthetic replacement or Turn – O – Plasty (Bone ends are cut and rotated)
   Lower end femur and upper end tibia
5. **Treatment of recurrent lesions is the same as for primary lesions.** After biopsy shows that the tumor is still benign, repeat curettage or resection should be performed.
6. Amputation
   Malignant recurrent GCT of extremity
7. Radiotherapy
   Spine (RT may cause malignant transformation of GCT).

Orthopedics Quick Review

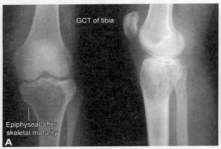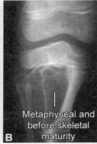

Figs. 4.16A and B: (A) GCT upper end tibia (B) ABC upper end tibia

	Giant Cell Tumor	Aneurysmal Bone Cyst
Category of tumor	Aggressive tumor	Active tumor
Age	After skeletal maturity	Before skeletal maturity
Region	**Epiphyseal tumor** (next to the joint surface) and extending to the metaphyseal region	**Metaphyseal tumor** rarely goes to the epiphyseal region (if after skeletal maturity)
Radiological appearance	Soap bubble appearance- free septations	Air fluid levels—irregular septations separating blood filled sinusoids (seen on MRI)
Bones affected	1. Lower end femur 2. Upper end tibia 3. Lower end radius (characteristic site)	Lower limbs (tibia)

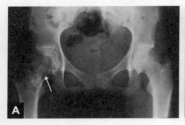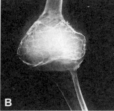

Figs. 4.17A and B: GCT upper end femur, GCT lower end femur

MULTIPLE CHOICE QUESTIONS

1. A patient with GCT which of the following is false: *(NEET Pattern 2019)*
   A. Epiphyseometaphyseal location
   B. Eccentric
   C. Defined margins
   D. Chemotherapy is the mainstay of treatment

   Ans. is 'D' Chemotherapy is the mainstay of treatment
   Chemotherapy is not used in GCT.

2. The most likely diagnosis for the tumor at upper end of tibia is: *(NEET Pattern 2019, AIIMS Nov 2015)*

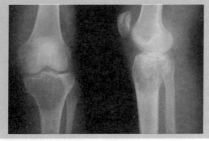

   A. GCT   B. UBC
   C. ABC   D. CB

   Ans. is 'A' GCT

3. What is the diagnosis: *(AIIMS Nov 2018)*

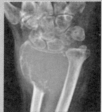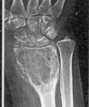

   A. Aneurysmal Bone Cyst   B. Giant Cell Tumor
   C. Osteosarcoma   D. Osteoclastoma

   Ans. is 'B' Giant Cell Tumor

4. X-ray of Tibia of an adolescent boy is shown. Probable diagnosis: *(JIPMER May 2018)*

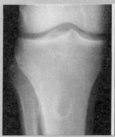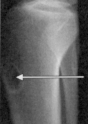

   A. Chondromyxoid fibroma B. Osteosarcoma
   C. Bone cyst with fracture D. Fibrosis cystica

   Ans. is 'A' Chondromyxoid fibroma

5. True statement regarding GCT is/are: *(PGI May 2016)*
   A. Malignant tumor
   B. Most commonly seen around knee
   C. Seen before puberty
   D. Local radiation is the treatment
   E. Egg shell crackling is seen

   Ans. is 'B' Most commonly seen around knee; and 'E' Egg shell crackling is seen

6. True about giant cell tumor (GCT): *(PGI May 2017)*
   A. Most commonly seen in 20–40 year age group
   B. Proximal femur is affected most commonly
   C. May involve sacrum
   D. Occur as multiple lesions
   E. Pulmonary metastasis occur rarely

   Ans. is 'A' Most commonly seen in 20–40 year age group; 'C' May involve sacrum; and 'E' Pulmonary metastasis occur rarely

Another variety of question.

7. Regarding GCT Bone true is: *(PGI Nov 2016)*
   A. Common in 20–40 years age group
   B. Proximal femur involvement may be seen
   C. Best managed by extended curettage followed by bone grafting
   D. Closest differential is ABC
   E. 3% cases have metastasis to lungs

   Ans. is 'A' Common in 20–40 years age group; 'B' Proximal femur involvement may be seen; 'C' Best managed by extended curettage followed by bone grafting; 'D' Closest differential is ABC; and 'E' 3% cases have metastasis to lungs

Orthopedics Oncology

8. About Giant cell tumor, all are true *except*:
   (AIIMS May 2016)
   A. Commonly presents in the 20-40 year age group
   B. Matrix consists of proliferating mononuclear cells
   C. Osteoclast giant cells constitute the proliferative component of the tumor
   D. It is a benign tumor which may have lung metastasis.

Ans. is 'C' Osteoclast Giant cells constitute the proliferative component of the tumor

9. A 30-year-old male presented with hip pain for last 6 months. Hip X-ray is as shown below. What is the likely diagnosis? (AIIMS May 2016)

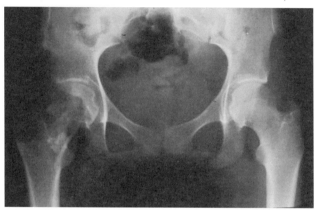

   A. Giant cell tumor   B. Simple Bone Cyst
   C. Adamantinoma   D. Ewing's sarcoma

Ans. is 'A' Giant cell tumor

10. What is the most likely diagnosis of the X-ray depicted below? (APPG 2015)

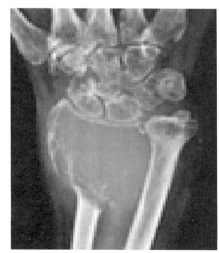

   A. Chondrosarcoma   B. Osteoclastoma
   C. Osteogenic sarcoma   D. Osteoid sarcoma

Ans. is 'B' Osteoclastoma

11. Soap bubble appearance on X-ray is seen in which bone tumor? (NEET Pattern 2013)
   A. Osteogenic sarcoma   B. Giant cell tumor
   C. Multiple myeloma   D. Chondroblastoma

Ans. is 'B' Giant cell tumor

12. Which of the following is epiphyseal tumor?
    (NEET Pattern 2012)
    A. Giant cell tumor   B. Osteogenic Sarcoma
    C. Ewing sarcoma   D. Osteoid osteoma

Ans. is 'A' Giant cell tumor

13. GCT malignant component is: (NEET Pattern 2012)
    A. Giant cells   B. Mononuclear cells
    C. Both   D. None

Ans. is 'B' Mononuclear cells

14. Which of the following is a variant of giant cell tumor?
    (AIIMS May 2011)
    A. Ossifying fibroma   B. Non-ossifying fibroma
    C. Osteogenic sarcoma   D. Chondroblastoma

Ans. is 'B' Non-ossifying fibroma
   – Eccentric lytic lesion with no calcification is the commonest differential.
   – Ossifying fibroma, chondroblastoma and osteosarcoma will have calcification hence non-ossifying fibroma is a preferred answer here.

Note: Closest differential is ABC.

15. The differential diagnosis of lesion, histologically resembling giant cell tumor in the small bones of the hands or feet, includes all of the following *except*: (AIIMS May 06)
    A. Aneurysmal bone cyst
    B. Fibrosarcoma
    C. Osteosarcoma
    D. Hyperparathyroidism

Ans. is 'C' Osteosarcoma
   – All mentioned tumor contain giant cells but osteosarcoma is extremely rare in short bones of hand and feet.

16. Osteoclastoma is treated with:
    (PGI Dec 2K, PGI June 2001)
    A. Joint replacement   B. Excision
    C. Curettage   D. Arthrodesis
    E. Chemotherapy

Ans. is 'A' Joint replacement; 'B' Excision; 'C' Curettage; 'D' Arthrodesis.
   – Chemotherapy has no role in GCT.

17. Soap bubble appearance at lower end of radius, the treatment of choice is: (AIIMS June 1998)
    A. Local excision
    B. Excision and bone grafting
    C. Amputation
    D. Radiotherapy

Ans. is 'B' Excision and bone grafting

ADAMANTINOMA—TIBIA

- Adamantinoma is seen in second or third decade of life.
- It is almost exclusively found in **tibial diaphysis**.
- **Pain** is the most common symptom a palpable mass may be present.
- The most common radiographic appearance is that of multiple, sharply demarcated radiolucent lesions in the tibial diaphysis.
  – Soap Bubble appearance.

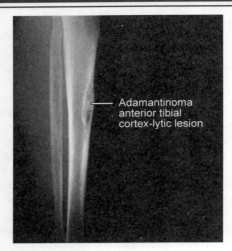

Fig. 4.18: X-ray both bone leg

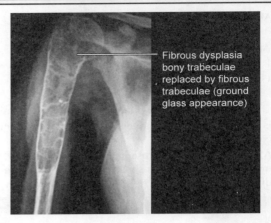

Fig. 4.19: X-ray upper end humerus

- Late metastases to inguinal nodes and lung can rarely occur.
- The optimal treatment of adamantinoma is wide resection or amputation.

AMELOBLASTOMA

Ameloblastoma is an epithelial tumor arising from ameloblast (enamel forming cell). The most common site is posterior mandible in the **area of molar teeth**. It is a slow growing, locally invasive cystic benign tumor that causes expansion of outer table more than inner table of mandible. Cystic degeneration may cause softening and egg shell crackling on palpation, it rarely metastasizes and has honey comb/soap bubble appearance on X-ray.

Treatment is wide local Excision.

Please note that most common tumor of mandible is squamous cell carcinoma.

FIBROUS DYSPLASIA

Fibrous dysplasia is a **developmental anomaly** of bone formation that may exist in a monostotic or polyostotic form. The hallmark is replacement of normal bone and marrow by fibrous tissue and small woven spicules of bone. Fibrous dysplasia can occur in the epiphysis, metaphysis, or diaphysis. It may affect one bone (monostotic form) or several bones (polyostotic form).

The monostotic form is the most common and is usually diagnosed in patients between 20 and 30 years of age. The polyostotic form typically manifests in children <10 years of age and may progress with age.

Monostotic fibrous dysplasia most commonly affects the **femur**.

Polyostotic fibrous dysplasia most commonly affects the maxilla and other craniofacial bones.

McCune-Albright syndrome refers to polyostotic fibrous dysplasia, cutaneous pigmentation (café au lait spots), and endocrine abnormalities (Precoceous puberty). The cafe au lait spots seen in Albright-McCune syndrome have characteristically irregular ragged borders (commonly called "coast of Maine" borders), as opposed to the smoothly marginated borders ("coast of California") of the spots seen in neurofibromatosis.

Mazabraud syndrome is polyostotic fibrous dysplasia with intramuscular myxomas. Other less common endocrine disorders include thyrotoxicosis, Cushing syndrome, acromegaly, hyperparathyroidism, hyperprolactinemia, and pseudo-precocious puberty in boys.

"Fibrous dysplasia of proximal femur has shepherd crook deformity".

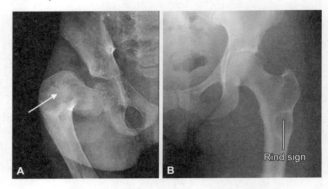

Figs. 4.20A and B: (A) Shepherd crook deformity (B) Rind sign

Malignant change has been reported occasionally with and without prior radiotherapy.

Radiographic Findings

In long bones, the fibrous dysplastic lesions have **ground-glass appearance.**
- The multiloculated translucent lesion may be surrounded by a sclerotic rim the so called **'Rind sign'**.

Involvement of facial bones may create a leonine appearance (leontiasis ossea).

On biopsy: Chinese Letter Pattern is recognised

Surgical treatment (Curettage + bone grafting) is indicated when significant deformity or pathological fracture occurs or when significant pain exists.

OSTEOFIBROUS DYSPLASIA: CAMPANACCI DISEASE! OR OSSIFYING FIBROMA!

Osteofibrous dysplasia (ossifying fibroma of long bones, also known as **Campanacci disease**) is a rare lesion usually affecting the tibia and fibula.

Orthopedics Oncology

Patients usually are in the first two decades of life.

The middle third of the tibia is the most frequently affected is enlarged and often bowed anterolaterally.

Pain usually is absent, unless pathological fracture has occurred. The radiographs show eccentric intracortical osteolysis with expansion of the cortex.

Histological studies reveal zonal architecture with loose fibrous tissue in the center of the lesion and a band of bony trabeculae rimmed by active osteoblasts at the periphery. Recurrence rates are high after curettage or marginal resection in children. Conversely, recurrence rates are low after surgery in skeletally mature patients. Pathological fractures can be treated nonoperatively. Surgical management is aimed at preventing or correcting deformity.

Osteofibrous Dysplasia (Female)	Adamantinoma (Male)	Fibrous Dysplasia (Female)
Tibial Diaphysis + Fibula	Tibia (MC Long Bone)	Femur, Craniofacial area
Swelling + Deformity	Swelling	Deformity
Trabecular Bone with Fibrous Stroma with osteoblasts	Epithelial Cells	Trabecular Bone with Fibrous Stroma
Soap Bubble ± ground glass	Soap Bubble	Ground glass

MULTIPLE CHOICE QUESTIONS

1. McCune-Albright syndrome features are: *(PGI May 2016)*
   A. High calcium
   B. Presents around puberty
   C. Cysts in long bones
   D. Precocious puberty
   E. High ACTH levels

Ans. is 'B' Presents around puberty; 'C' Cysts in long bones; and 'D' Precocious puberty

2. Fibrous dysplasia, true is: *(AI 2016)*
   A. X-ray shows increase bone density
   B. More common in females as compared to males
   C. Rare in < 40 yrs age
   D. Monostotic fibrous is seen in McCure Albright syndrome

Ans. is 'B' More common in females as compared to males

3. X-ray proximal femur in a patient with pain hip. The deformity shown is: *(AI 2016)*

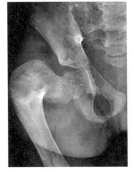

   A. Blade of grass deformity B. Shepherd crook deformity
   C. Chicken wire appearance   D. Corduroy appearance

Ans. is 'B' Shepherd crook deformity

4. Mandible most common tumor: *(NEET Pattern 2012)*
   A. Ameloblastoma
   B. Squamous cell carcinoma
   C. Osteoid osteoma
   D. Metastasis

Ans. is 'B' Squamous cell carcinoma

5. Characteristic radiological feature of fibrous dysplasia is: *(AIIMS May 2010)*
   A. Cortical thickening
   B. Cortical calcification
   C. Ground glass appearance
   D. Bone enlargement

Ans. is 'C' Ground glass appearance

6. True about Ameloblastoma: *(PGI Dec 2006)*
   A. Cystic lesion
   B. Rapidly growing
   C. Malignant disease
   D. MC site is tibia

Ans. is 'A' Cystic lesion
   - Most common site of ameloblastoma is mandible.
   - Most common site of ameloblastoma of long bones (i.e. adamantinoma) is Tibial diaphysis.
   - Adamantinoma is a slow growing benign locally aggressive tumor with late metastasis
   - Well demarcated lytic (cystic) or mixed lytic/sclerotic lesion involving the cortex.

7. A 33-year-old man presented with a slowly progressive swelling in the middle 1/3rd of his right tibia. X-rays examination revealed multiple sharply demarcated radiolucent lesions separated by areas of dense and sclerotic bone. Microscopic examination of a biopsy specimen revealed island of epithelial cells in a fibrous stroma. Which of the following is the most probable diagnosis? *(AIIMS May 2004)*
   A. Adamantinoma
   B. Osteofibrous dysplasia
   C. Osteosarcoma
   D. Fibrous cortical defect

Ans. is 'A' Adamantinoma

8. Most common site of admantinoma of the long bones is: *(AIIMS May 2002)*
   A. Femur
   B. Ulna
   C. Tibia
   D. Fibula

Ans. is 'C' Tibia
   - Ameloblastoma—Most common site mandible.
   - Ameloblastoma of long bones—Called adamantinoma and is most common in tibial diaphysis.

9. Most common site of origin of amelobastoma is: *(AIIMS Nov 2001)*
   A. Mandible near molar tooth
   B. Middle alveolar margins
   C. Hard palate
   D. Mandible near symphysis menti

Ans. is 'A' Mandible near molar tooth

OSTEOSARCOMA: CANCER OF YOUNG

Osteosarcoma is a tumor **characterized by the production of osteoid matrix by malignant cells.** It is the second most common primary malignancy of bone behind multiple myeloma. Onset can occur at any age; however, primary high-grade osteosarcoma occurs most commonly in the **second decade of life. Osteosarcoma may be more common in patients with the hereditary form of retinoblastoma and Li-Fraumeni syndrome.** All skeletal locations can be affected; however, most primary osteosarcomas occur at the sites of the most rapid bone growth, including the distal femur, the proximal tibia, and the proximal humerus.

Almost all patients with high-grade osteosarcoma report progressive **pain.** Night pain may be an important clue to the true diagnosis; however, only about 25% of patients experience this phenomenon.

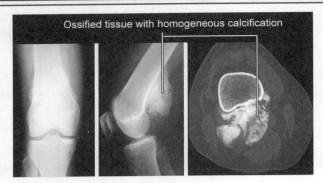

Fig. 4.21: X-ray knee

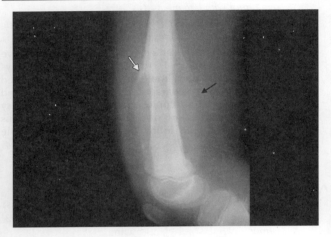

Fig. 4.22: Codman's triangle

Periosteal reaction may take the form of **"Codman's triangle"**, or it may have a **"sunburst"** or **"hair on end"** appearance. MRI is the best test to measure the extent of the tumor within the bone and in the soft tissue and to determine the relationship of the tumor to nearby anatomical structures. A bone scan should be obtained to look for skeletal metastases, and radiographs and CT scans of the chest should be done to search for pulmonary metastases; **the lungs are the most common sites of metastases.**

Histologically osteoid production from the tumor cells must be shown.

This osteoid matrix presents as calcification.

Periosteal osteosarcoma is an intermediate-grade malignancy that arises on the surface of the bone.

Pulsatile bone tumors in following order answer must be preferred.

Osteosarcoma>ABC>Angioendothelioma of bone >GCT.

Amongst metastasis renal and thyroid have pulsatile metastasis.

CT scan may be helpful in differentiating osteosarcoma from myositis ossificans or an osteochondroma. The ossification in myositis ossificans is more mature at the periphery of the lesion, whereas the center of osteosarcoma is more heavily ossified.

Secondary osteosarcomas occur at the site of another disease process. They rarely occur in young patients, but constitute almost half of the osteosarcomas in patients older than age 50 years. The most common factors associated with secondary osteosarcomas include Paget disease and previous radiation treatment. The incidence of osteosarcoma in Paget disease is approximately 1%. Paget osteosarcoma most commonly occurs in patients in the sixth to eighth decades of life, and the pelvis is the most common location. Radiation-induced osteosarcoma occurs in approximately 1% of patients who have been treated with greater than 2500 cGy and can occur in unusual locations, such as the skull, spine, clavicle, ribs, scapula, and pelvis. Although osteosarcoma is the most common radiation-induced sarcoma, fibrosarcoma and malignant fibrous histiocytoma also are relatively common in this setting. The time to onset of the secondary osteosarcoma averages approximately **10–15 years after radiation exposure.**

Other conditions that have been reported to be associated with secondary osteosarcomas include fibrous dysplasia, bone infarcts, osteochondromas, chronic osteomyelitis, dedifferentiated chondrosarcomas, melorheostosis, osteogenesis imperfecta and Paget's disease (osteitis deformans).

With today's multiagent chemotherapy regimens and appropriate surgical treatment, most series report long-term survival of 60–75% for patients with high-grade osteosarcoma without metastases at initial presentation and 90% for low-grade lesions.

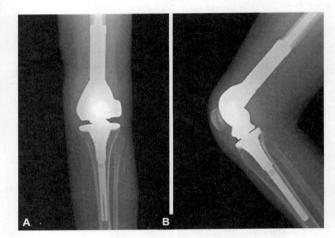

Figs. 4.23A and B: Osteosarcoma excised and replacement done

The most important prognostic factor at the time of diagnosis is the **extent of the disease (staging).** Approximately 15% of patients with osteosarcoma have detectable **pulmonary metastases** at the time of diagnosis. As a group, these patients continue to have a poor prognosis with less than 20% long-term survival. Patients with **non-pulmonary metastases (e.g. bone metastases) have an even worse prognosis.** Patients with "skip" metastases (i.e. a metastasis within the same bone as the primary tumor or across the joint from the primary tumor) have the same poor prognosis as patients with distant metastases.

The next most important prognostic feature is the grade of the lesion. Paget osteosarcomas and radiation-induced osteosarcoma have a poor prognosis.

It is highly radio-resistant and ideally treated by chemotherapy followed by limb salvage surgery/amputation followed by chemotherapy.

Rosens T-10 Protocol for osteosarcoma: Patients were treated with high-dose methotrexate (HDMTX) and citrovorum factor rescue (CFR), Adriamycin, and the combination of bleomycin, cyclophosphamide and dactinomycin (BCD) given for 4-6 weeks prior to definitive surgery. Histologic examination of the resected primary tumor determined the effect of preoperative chemotherapy with many primary tumors showing greater than 90% tumor necrosis attributable to preoperative chemotherapy. All patients having this favorable effect of chemotherapy on the primary tumor were continued on the same chemotherapy regimen postoperatively. However, in those patients not having a good effect of preoperative chemotherapy on the primary tumor, HDMTX with CFR was subsequently deleted from their postoperative chemotherapy and they were placed on a regimen containing cisplatinum at the dose of 120 mg/m^2 with mannitol diuresis combined with Vincristine or Adriamycin in addition to BCD.

This individualized chemotherapeutic strategy has yielded the highest disease-free survival rate (70%) reported to date for osteogenic sarcoma.

Note: Etoposide is not included in the 'T-10' protocol for osteosarcoma.

MULTIPLE CHOICE QUESTIONS

1. A 12-year-old boy presents with chronic knee pain for 2 years. Knee X-ray is shown. Probable diagnosis?
   (JIPMER May 2018)

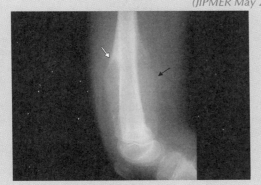

   A. Chronic osteomyelitis   B. Osteosarcoma
   C. Rickets   D. Hyperparathyroidism

Ans. is 'B' Osteosarcoma (Codman's Triangle is shown)

2. Peak incidence of osteosarcoma occurs at:
   (JIPMER May 2018)
   A. 2nd decade   B. 3rd decade
   C. 5th decade   D. 6th decade

Ans. is 'A' 2nd decade

3. Most common site of metastases in case of osteosarcoma is:
   (DNB June 2017)
   A. Brain   B. Lungs
   C. Liver   D. Bladder

Ans. is 'B' Lungs

4. Which of the following is bone forming malignant tumor?
   (DNB JULY 2016)
   A. Osteoid osteoma   B. Osteosarcoma
   C. Chondrosarcoma   D. Giant cell tumor

Ans. is 'B' Osteosarcoma

5. Which is intramedullary tumor among carcinoma of bone:
   (NEET Dec 2016)
   A. Classical osteosarcoma   B. Parosteal osteosarcoma
   C. Periosteal osteosarcoma   D. None of the above

Ans. is 'A' Classical osteosarcoma

6. 33 year old female presents with a slow growing bony mass along the distal femur cortex in the metaphyseal region with an appreciable gap between the cortex and tumor without any cortical invasion. What is the usual treatment for the same?
   (NEET Dec 2016)
   A. Local resection   B. Amputation
   C. Chemotherapy   D. Radiotherapy

Ans. is 'A' Local resection

7. 22 year old male present with bony mass in the metaphyseal region of right. knee with typical sun ray appearance and CT Scan of the chest reveals osteoblastic metastases. What is the most probable diagnosis?
   (NEET Dec 2016)
   A. Osteosarcoma   B. Chondrosarcoma
   C. Ewing's sarcoma   D. Osteochondroma

Ans. is 'A' Osteosarcoma

8. Age group affected by osteosarcoma: *(NEET Dec 2016)*
   A. Up to 10 years   B. 10-20 years
   C. 30-40 years   D. Older than 45 years

Ans. is 'B' 10-20 years

9. The following reaction is associated with which tumor:
   (AI 2016)

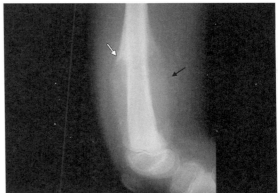

   A. Osteosarcoma   B. Chondroblastoma
   C. Ewing's sarcoma   D. Codman's tumor

Ans. is 'A' Osteosarcoma

10. Calcification in osteosarcoma is due to presence:
    (NEET 2015)
    A. Osteoid matrix   B. Osteoblasts
    C. High calcium levels in serum
    D. High calcitonin

Ans. is 'A' Osteoid matrix

11. Osteosarcoma occurs in: *(DNB July 2016, TN 2015)*
    A. Osteoma   B. Osteoporosis
    C. Osteomalacia   D. Osteitis deformans

Ans. 'D' Osteitis deformans

12. In young person most common cancer among following is:
    (PGI May 2015)
    A. Giant cell   B. Osteosarcoma
    C. Chondrosarcoma   D. Ewing sarcoma
    E. Multiple myeloma

Ans. is 'B' Osteosarcoma

13. Characteristic histopathological feature of osteosarcoma is:
    A. Codman's triangle   *(JIPMER 2014)*
    B. Matrix new bone formation with Codman's triangle
    C. Malignant cells with osteoid formation
    D. Spindle cells

Ans. 'C' Malignant cells with osteoid formation

14. True about Osteosarcoma: *(PGI Nov 2014)*
    A. Primary osteosarcoma most commonly occurs in age group of less than 20 years
    B. Periosteal reaction is present
    C. Present as elevated soft tissue mass
    D. Commonly associated with osteoid osteoma
    E. Formation of bone by the tumor cells is characteristic

Ans. is 'A' Primary osteosarcoma most commonly occurs in age group of less than 20 years; 'B' Periosteal reaction is present; 'C' Present as elevated soft tissue mass; and 'E' Formation of bone by the tumor cells is characteristic.

15. In osteogenic sarcoma predominant histological finding is:
    A. Giant cells *(NEET 2015)*
    B. Osteoid forming tumor cells
    C. Fibroblastic proliferation
    D. Chondroblasts

Ans. is 'B' Osteoid forming tumor cells

16. Children with germline retinoblastoma are more likely to develop other primary malignancies in their later lifetime course. Which of the following can occur in such patients? *(AIIMS Nov 2013)*
    A. Osteosarcoma of lower limbs and soft tissue sarcoma
    B. Thyroid carcinoma   C. Seminoma
    D. Squamous cell carcinoma

Ans. is 'A' Osteosarcoma of lower limbs and soft tissue sarcoma

17. X-ray appearance of osteosarcoma are all *except*: *(NEET Pattern 2012)*
    A. Periosteal reaction   B. Codman's triangle
    C. Soap-bubble   D. Sunray appearance

Ans. is 'C' Soap-bubble

18. Codman's triangle and onion peel appearance are most commonly seen in: *(NEET Pattern 2012)*
    A. Benign bone tumors   B. Malignant bone tumors
    C. Traumatic conditions   D. Paget's disease

Ans. is 'B' Malignant bone tumors

19. Matrix forming tumor is: *(NEET Pattern 2012)*
    A. Osteosarcoma   B. Chondrosarcoma
    C. Fibrosarcoma   D. Ewing's sarcoma

Ans. is 'A' Osteosarcoma

20. Osteosarcoma most commonly affects: *(NEET Pattern 2012)*
    A. Femur   B. Humerus
    C. Tibia   D. Vertebrae

Ans. is 'A' Femur

21. Radiation induced tumor: *(NEET Pattern 2012)*
    A. Osteosarcoma   B. Ewing's sarcoma
    C. Multiple myeloma   D. Chondrosarcoma

Ans. is 'A' Osteosarcoma

22. Which of the following malignant tumors is radio-resistant? *(NEET Pattern 2012)*
    A. Ewing's sarcoma   B. Retinoblastoma
    C. Osteosarcoma   D. Neuroblastoma

Ans. is 'C' Osteosarcoma

23. Which of the following is a pulsatile tumor? *(AIIMS May 2010)*
    A. Osteosarcoma   B. Chondrosarcoma
    C. Osteoclastoma   D. Ewing's sarcoma

Ans. is 'A' Osteosarcoma

24. True about osteosarcoma: *(PGI Nov 2009)*
    A. Involves epiphysis of long bones
    B. Most commonly involve knee and distal femur
    C. Spread to lung through hematogenous route
    D. Exclusively found in adolescent and early adult life
    E. X-ray has sunray appearance

Ans. is 'B' Most commonly involve knee and distal femur; 'C' Spread to lung through hematogenous route; 'E' X-ray: sunray appearance.

25. An 8-year-male progressive swelling upper end tibia – irregular, local temperature raised, variable consistency and ill defined margins: *(DPG 2009)*
    A. Giant cell tumor   B. Ewing's sarcoma
    C. Osteogenic sarcoma   D. Secondary metastasis

Ans. is 'C' Osteogenic sarcoma
    – The clinical presentation in question can occur both in Ewing's sarcoma and osteosarcoma.
        - History of trivial trauma
        - Progressive swelling
        - Raised local temperature
        - Variable consistency
        - Ill defined margins.
    – However, swelling is around the knee joint at upper end of tibia, which favors the diagnosis of osteosarcoma (metaphyseal lesion).
    – Ewing's sarcoma usually occurs in the diaphysis of the bone (middle of the shaft).

26. 'T'-10 Protocol' for treatment of osteosarcoma includes all of the following, *except*: *(AI 2009)*
    A. High dose methotrexate
    B. Bleomycin, Cyclophosphamide Doxorubicin (BCD)
    C. Vincristine   D. Etoposide

Ans. is 'D' Etoposide

27. All of the following investigations are needed for the diagnosis of osteosarcoma, *except*: *(All India 2007)*
    A. MRI of femur   B. Bone marrow biopsy
    C. Bone scan   D. CT chest

Ans. is 'B' Bone marrow biopsy
    – **A biopsy of the lesion** (not bone marrow biopsy) should always be carried out before commencing treatment.
        - Bone scan, MRI and CT chest are used.

28. Management plan for osteogenic sarcoma of the lower end of femur must include? *(AI 2004)*
    A. Radiotherapy, amputation, chemotherapy
    B. Surgery alone
    C. Chemotherapy + Limb Salvage Surgery + Chemotherapy
    D. Chemotherapy + Radiotherapy

Ans. is 'C' Chemotherapy + Limb Salvage Surgery + Chemotherapy

29. Which of the following bone tumor present secondaries in lung with pneumothorax: *(AIIMS Sept 1996, AIIMS Dec 1995)*
    A. Osteosarcoma   B. Ewing's sarcoma
    C. Osteoclastoma   D. Chondroblastoma

Ans. is 'A' Osteosarcoma
    – Both osteogenic sarcoma and Ewing's sarcoma may have metastasis to lung.
    – However, it is much more common in osteogenic sarcoma and about 10% of patients have pulmonary metastasis by the time they are first seen. Incidence of pneumothorax is higher in osteosarcoma metastasis.

Orthopedics Oncology

EWING SARCOMA

Ewing sarcoma is the fourth most common primary malignancy of bone, but it is the second most common (after osteosarcoma) in patients younger than 30 years of age and the most common in patients younger than 10 years of age. **Its maximum incidence is seen in 2nd decade of life.**

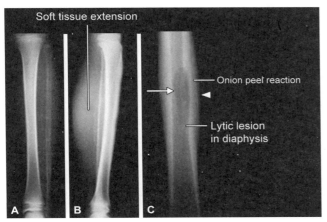

Figs. 4.24A to C: Ewing's sarcoma

Pain is an almost universal complaint of patients with Ewing sarcoma.

In addition to pain, patients also may have fever, erythema, and swelling suggesting osteomyelitis. Laboratory studies may reveal an increased white blood cell count, an elevated erythrocyte sedimentation rate, and an elevated C-reactive protein. To complicate matters further, a needle aspirate of Ewing sarcoma may grossly resemble pus, and the tissue may be sent in its entirety to microbiology and none to pathology. (As a general rule, most biopsy specimens should be sent for culture and pathological analysis.)

Classically, Ewing sarcoma appears radiographically as a *destructive lesion in the diaphysis* of a long bone with an "onion skin" periosteal reaction. In reality, Ewing sarcoma more often originates in the metaphysis of a long bone, but frequently extends for a considerable distance into the diaphysis.

MRI of the entire bone should be ordered to evaluate the full extent of the lesion, which typically extends beyond the abnormality apparent on plain films.

MRI also is useful to evaluate the extent of the soft-tissue mass, which often is very large. All patients should have a baseline radiograph and a CT scan of the chest because the **lung is the most common site of metastases.**

A bone scan should be performed because bone is the second most common site of metastases. In contrast to other bone sarcomas, a bone marrow aspirate should be obtained as a routine part of the staging of Ewing sarcoma to rule out diffuse systemic disease.

Ewing's sarcoma is part of a family of peripheral neuroectodermal tumors (PNET) that share a common cytogenetic translocation of chromosomes 11 and 22, **t(11:22.)**, differing only in their degree of neural differentiation, **Ewing's sarcoma is poorly differentiated whereas PNET exhibits definite neural differentiation. (N myc positive).**

The t(11; 22) (q24; q12) is the most common translocation diagnostic of Ewing sarcoma and is present in greater than 90% of cases. Other diagnostic translocations, including t(21; 22) (q22; q12), t(7; 22) (p22; q12), trisomy 8 and trisomy 12.

MIC2(CD99) is a specific marker for Ewing's sarcoma and peripheral primitive neuroectodermal tumors and is expressed on short-arm of chromosome x and y. In addition, Ewing sarcomas usually are periodic acid–Schiff positive (owing to intracellular glycogen) and reticulin negative. This is in contrast to lymphomas, which are periodic acid–Schiff negative and reticulin positive.

The worst prognostic factor is the presence of distant metastases. Even with aggressive treatment, patients with metastases have only a 20% chance of long-term survival.

The size of the primary lesion has been shown consistently to be of prognostic significance, although specific parameters have not been firmly established. Location also has been reported to be of prognostic significance, but it is difficult to differentiate the effects of location and size because most proximally located tumors are larger at presentation than distally located tumors.

Histological grade is of no prognostic significance because all Ewing sarcomas are considered high grade.

Fever, anemia, and elevation of laboratory values (white blood cell count, erythrocyte sedimentation rate, lactate dehydrogenase) have been reported to indicate more extensive disease and a worse prognosis.

Older age at presentation (with a cut off around 12–15 years old) and **male gender** also have been reported to be associated with a worse prognosis.

The specific translocation, t(11;22) versus t(21;22), does not seem to affect the clinical course; however, secondary genetic alterations, such as aberrant p53 expression, may prove to be important. As with osteosarcoma, histological response to neoadjuvant chemotherapy has been shown to be prognostically important.

The treatment of Ewing sarcoma must include neoadjuvant or adjuvant chemotherapy, or both, to treat distant metastases that may or may not be readily apparent at the initial staging. Before the use of multiagent chemotherapy, long-term survival was less than 10%. Today, most centers report long-term survival rates of 60–75%.

- Chemotherapy is much more effective and include vincristine, actinomycin D, cyclophosphamide, bleomycin, adriamycin, ifosfamide and etoposide.

    ABCD: Actinomycin D/**B**leomycin/**C**yclophosphamide/ **D**oxorubicin

- Best results are achieved by Preoperative chemotherapy; then wide excision (or amputation) if tumor is in favorable site and further chemotherapy for 1 year. Subsequently Radiotherapy may be given.

MULTIPLE CHOICE QUESTIONS

1. What is true regarding Ewing's Sarcoma?
   (PGI Nov 2018)
   A. Common in Elderly
   B. It mimics Osteomyelitis
   C. Onion peel reaction is seen
   D. CD99 marker is positive
   E. Originates from marrow

   Ans. is 'B' It mimics Osteomyelitis; 'C' Onion peel reaction is seen; 'D' CD99 marker is positive; 'E' Originates from marrow

2. Which of the following is/are true about Ewing sarcoma?
   (PGI NOV 2016)
   A. Vascular origin
   B. Ewing's sarcoma is second most common primary malignant bone tumor in children and adolescent after Osteosarcoma
   C. Metaphysis of long bone is most common site
   D. Fever and weight loss may be present
   E. Surgery is very useful in management
Ans. is 'B' Ewing's sarcoma is second most common primary malignant bone tumor in children and adolescent after Osteosarcoma; 'D' Fever and weight loss may be present; 'E' Surgery is very useful in management

3. Characteristic translocation seen in Ewing's sarcoma:
   (AI 2016)
   A. t(2;8)   B. t(11;22)
   C. t(x;18)   D. t(14;18)
Ans. is 'B' t(11;22)

4. A 5-year child with pain and swelling over tibia, X-ray done most probable diagnosis based on periosteal reaction seen on X-ray: (AI 2016)

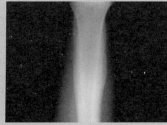

   A. Osteosarcoma   B. GCT
   C. Ewing's sarcoma D. Chondrosarcoma
Ans. is 'C' Ewing's sarcoma

5. 'Ewing's sarcoma is characterized by all except:
   (Maharashtra PG 2016)
   A. Diaphysis in location
   B. Locally malignant
   C. Soap bubble appearance
   D. Onion peel appearance on X-ray
Ans. is 'C' Soap bubble appearance

6. A 7-year-old boy presents with swelling and pain over tibia. On X-ray there is periosteal reaction in diaphysis. Probable diagnosis is: (AIIMS May 2014)
   A. Osteomyelitis   B. Chondroblastoma
   C. Ewing's sarcoma D. Osteosarcoma
Ans. is 'C' Ewing's sarcoma
Diaphysis + Periosteal reaction = Ewing's sarcoma

7. Most common site of Ewing's sarcoma:
   (NEET Pattern 2013)
   A. Upper end of tibia   B. Shaft of tibia
   C. Lower end of femur   D. Shaft of femur
Ans. is 'D' Shaft of femur

8. Maximum incidence of Ewing's occurs in:
   (NEET Pattern 2012)
   A. 1st decade   B. 2nd decade
   C. 3rd decade   D. 4th decade
Ans. is 'B' 2nd decade

9. Small round cell tumor among the following:
   (NEET Pattern 2012)
   A. Ewing's sarcoma B. Chondrosarcoms
   C. Metastasis   D. Rhabdomyosarcoma
Ans. is 'A' Ewing's sarcoma

10. Glycogen Positive cells are seen in: (NEET Pattern 2012)
    A. Ewing's sarcoma B. Osteosarcoma
    C. Fibrosarcoma   D. Osteoid osteoma
Ans. is 'A' Ewing's sarcoma

11. Mass in anterior aspect of thigh fixed to bone the procedure to be carried out: (NEET Pattern 2012)
    A. Incisional biopsy   B. Excisional biopsy
    C. FNAC   D. Radiotherapy
Ans. is 'B' Excisional biopsy

12. 1st decade most common bone tumor:
    (NEET Pattern 2012)
    A. Ewing's sarcoma B. Osteosarcoma
    C. Multiple myeloma D. Metastasis
Ans. is 'A' Ewing's sarcoma

13. PAS positive cells are seen in: (NEET Pattern 2012)
    A. Ewing's sarcoma B. Osteosarcoma
    C. Chondrosarcoma   D. Multiple myeloma
Ans. is 'A' Ewing's sarcoma

14. Mic 2 positive cells are seen in: (NEET Pattern 2012)
    A. Ewing's sarcoma B. Osteosarcoma
    C. Chondrosarcoma   D. Multiple myeloma
Ans. is 'A' Ewing's sarcoma

15. CD 99 is marker of: (NEET Pattern 2012)
    A. Dermatofibrosarcoma protuberans
    B. Ewing's sarcoma
    C. Osteosarcoma   D. Metastasis
Ans. is 'B' Ewing's sarcoma

16. Ewing's Sarcoma is associated with which genetic defect?
    A. 13q14   B. c-myc   (AI 2012)
    C. Trisomy 8   D. t(22,11)
Ans. is 'C' Trisomy 8

17. Poor prognostic sign for Ewing's sarcoma is:
    (AIIMS Non 2010)
    A. Fever   B. Age <12 years
    C. Grade   D. Females
Ans. is 'A' Fever

18. A 7-year-old boy with h/o trauma 2 months back now presents with fever and acute pain over thigh. On X-ray femoral shaft shows lesions with multiple laminated periosteal reaction next line of management: (AIIMS Nov 09)
    A. CRP measurement B. Core biopsy
    C. Tc99 MDP scan   D. MRI
Ans. is 'D; MRI
  – Information in this question are: 1st Decade, diaphyseal lesion with onion peel reaction goes towards Ewing's sarcoma. Next best investigation is MRI for soft tissue involvement, marrow involvement and micrometastasis. Overall the best investigation is Biopsy to confirm the diagnosis but MRI is done before the biopsy, to localize the best site for biopsy.

Orthopedics Oncology

19. A 15-year-old boy is injured while playing cricket. X-rays of the leg rule out a possible fracture. The radiologist reports the boy has an evidence of aggressive bone tumor with both bone destruction and soft tissue mass. The bone biopsy reveals a bone cancer with neural differentiation. Which of the following is the most likely diagnosis?

(AIIMS May 2006)

A. Chondroablastoma B. Ewing's sarcoma
C. Neuroblastoma D. Osteosarcoma

Ans. is 'B' Ewing's sarcoma

- **Ewing's sarcoma is part of a family of peripheral neuroectodermal tumors** *(PNET)* *that share a coimnon cytogenetic translocation of chromosomes 11 and 22, t(11:22.) and round cells, differing only in their degree of neural differentiation, Ewing's sarcoma is poorly differentiated whereas PNET exhibits definite neural differentiation.*

CHORDOMA

Chordoma is a rare malignant neoplasm that arises from notochord remnants. Chordoma is the second most common primary malignancy in the spine (behind myeloma) and is the most common primary malignancy of the **sacrum**. Greater than 50% of chordomas arise in the sacrococcygeal area, and more than 30% arise at the base of the skull. The remainder are dispersed throughout the rest of the spine.

- *On Biopsy*: **Physaliferous cells** are seen.

Treatment is surgical resection with wide margins. Radiation may be beneficial for patients in whom resection is not feasible.

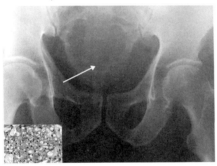

Fig. 4.25: Chordoma (Sacrum) & Physaliferous cells (Cells with small nuclei and vacuoles in cytoplasm)

MULTIPLE CHOICE QUESTIONS

1. Physaliferous cells are seen in: *(PGM-CET 2015)*
   A. Phyllodes tumor B. Chordoma
   C. Meningioma D. Pheochromocytoma

Ans. is 'B' Chordoma

2. Chordoma commonly involves: *(PGI June 02)*
   A. Dorsal spine B. Clivus
   C. Lumbar spine D. Sacrum

Ans. is 'B' Clivus; 'D' Sacrum

3. Which of the following is not a benign bone tumor?
   A. Osteoid osteoma B. Chondroma *(AI 1996)*
   C. Enchondroma D. Chordoma

Ans. is 'D' Chordoma

- Chordoma is a malignant tumor arising from notochordal remnants.

CHONDROSARCOMA

It occurs over a broad age range, with peaks between 40 and 60 years for primary chondrosarcoma and between 25 and 45 years for secondary chondrosarcoma. Chondrosarcoma can occur in any location; however, most are located in a proximal location such as the **pelvis (most common site)**, proximal femur, and proximal humerus. **Although chondrosarcomas rarely occur in the hand, they are the most common malignant tumor of bone in this location.**

Secondary chondrosarcomas arise at the site of a preexisting benign cartilage lesion. They occur most frequently in the setting of **multiple enchondromas and multiple hereditary exostoses**. Other conditions that have been reported to be associated with secondary chondrosarcoma include synovial chondromatosis, chondromyxoid fibroma, periosteal chondroma, chondroblastoma, previous radiation treatment, and fibrous dysplasia.

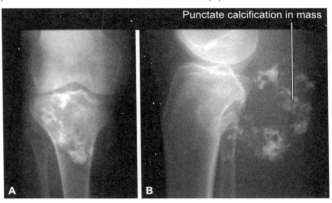

Figs. 4.26A and B: Chondrosarcoma

The radiographic appearance of chondrosarcoma frequently is similar to enchondroma, it is a lesion arising in the medullary cavity with irregular matrix calcification. The pattern of calcification has been described as "punctate", "popcorn", or "comma-shaped". Compared with enchondroma, however, chondrosarcoma has a more aggressive appearance with bone destruction, cortical erosions, periosteal reaction, and rarely a soft-tissue mass. A CT scan can be helpful to show endosteal erosions or other evidence of a destructive lesion and to differentiate benign from malignant cartilage lesions.

Chondrosarcoma can produce hyperglycemia in 85% cases. metastasis from Chondrosarcoma most commonly goes to lungs (hematogenous).

Treatment is wide local excision/Radical excision.

MULTIPLE CHOICE QUESTIONS

1. Commonest site of occurrence of chondrosarcoma is:
   A. Pelvis B. Femur *(AI Dec 15)*
   C. Ribs D. Proximal tibia

Ans. is 'A' Pelvis

2. Tumor with calcification is seen in: *(NEET Pattern 2012)*
   A. Unicameral bone cyst B. Chondroblastoma
   C. Osteoclastoma D. Chondrosarcoma

Ans. is 'D' Chondrosarcoma

- Malignant are preferred over Benign lesions.

3. Which of the following tumor is associated with hyperglycemia? *(AI 2010)*
   A. Ewing's sarcoma B. Osteosarcoma
   C. Multiple myeloma D. Chondrosarcoma

Ans. is 'D' Chondrosarcoma

4. A 45 years male presented with an expansile lesion in the centre of femoral metaphysis. The lesion shows endosteal scalloping and punctuate calcifications. Most likely diagnosis is: *(AI 2002)*
   A. Osteosarcoma
   B. Chondrosarcoma
   C. Simple bone cyst
   D. Fibrous dysplasia

Ans. is 'B' Chondrosarcoma

So,

Dense homogeneous calcification	Osteoid tumors
Dense punctate calcification	Chondroid matrix

HEMANGIOMA OF BONE

Hemangioma is a common benign bone lesion. It is estimated that 10% of the population has asymptomatic hemangioma of the vertebral bodies. Hemangiomas also are common in the skull. They usually are discovered as incidental findings.

The radiographic appearance in the spine usually is characteristic, with thickened, vertically oriented trabeculae giving the classic **"jailhouse" (Corduroy) appearance**. In cross-section, these thickened trabeculae have a "polka dot" pattern on CT scan.

Treatment usually is not necessary.

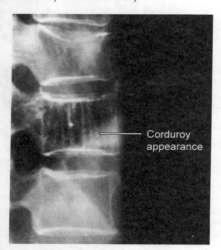

Fig. 4.27: Hemangioma

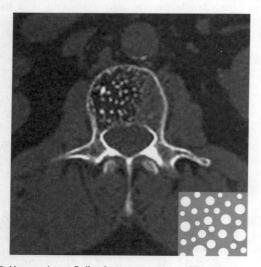

Fig. 4.28: Hemangioma: Polka dot appearance on CT Scan

Selective arterial embolization also can be used as definitive treatment for symptomatic lesions in surgically inaccessible locations.

Low-dose radiation also is an option for inoperable lesions but carries the risk of malignant degeneration.

Vertebroplasty is also performed for painful hemangioma.

MULTIPLE CHOICE QUESTIONS

1. Striated Vertebra are seen in: *(NEET Pattern 2012)*
   A. Metastasis
   B. Tuberculosis
   C. Hemangioma
   D. Osteoblastoma

Ans. is 'C' Hemangioma

2. Which of the following statements is true regarding hemangioma of the bone? *(PGI Dec 01)*
   A. Occurs commonly in skull bones
   B. Requires observation as it is premalignant
   C. Hamartomatous in origin
   D. Forms 10–12% of the bone tumors
   E. Local gigantism occurs when it occurs in an extremity

Ans. is 'A' Occurs commonly in skull bones; 'C' Hamartomatous in origin; 'E' Local gigantism occurs when it occurs in an extremity.

MULTIPLE MYELOMA AND PLASMACYTOMA

Elderly with bone pains, increased ESR and hypercalcemia is multiple myeloma till proved otherwise.

Multiple myeloma is the most common primary malignancy of bone, representing more than 40% of primary bone cancers. Its peak incidence is in the fifth to seventh decades with a 2:1 male predominance. Multiple myeloma and metastatic carcinoma should be included in the differential diagnosis for any patient older than age 40 with a new bone tumor.

Bone pain is the most common complaint for patients with multiple myeloma or with a solitary plasmacytoma. In contrast to most bone tumors, however, other systemic problems, such as weakness, weight loss, anemia, thrombocytopenia, peripheral neuropathy (especially with the osteosclerotic type of multiple myeloma), hypercalcemia, or renal failure, frequently are present at the time of diagnosis of multiple myeloma. Symptoms usually are of short duration because of the aggressive nature of the disease. Pathological fractures are relatively common. The spine is the most common location followed by the ribs and pelvis.

Radiographically, multiple myeloma appears as multiple, **"punched-out"**, sharply demarcated, purely lytic lesions without any surrounding reactive sclerosis. The lack of reactive bone formation also is shown by the fact that most lesions are **negative on bone scan**. Occasionally, myeloma is characterized by marked bone expansion, giving rise to a "ballooned" appearance. The osteoclast activating factor (OAF) released by plasma cells cause lytic bone lesions with almost no osteoblastic activity. Therefore, bone scan is less useful than plain X-ray and serum alkaline phosphatase level is normal.

The diagnosis usually can be confirmed by serum immunoelectrophoresis, which shows a monoclonal gammopathy. In addition to a complete blood count and serum chemistries, staging studies include a skeletal survey and a bone marrow biopsy. Occasionally, biopsy of the bone lesion is required to establish the diagnosis.

Histologically, multiple myeloma appears as sheets of plasma cells. These are small, round blue cells with "clock face" nuclei and abundant cytoplasm with a perinuclear clearing or "halo". Amyloid production can be abundant. **(With the exception of patients on long-term hemodialysis, the presence of amyloid in bone usually means a diagnosis of multiple myeloma.)** In patients with a solitary plasmacytoma, the pathological differential diagnosis may include chronic osteomyelitis with abundant plasma cells. In this situation, immunohistochemistry can be helpful.

Plasmacytoma exhibits monoclonal k or l light chains, whereas the plasma cells of chronic osteomyelitis are polyclonal. Also, myeloma cells usually stain positive for the natural killer antigen CD56, whereas reactive plasma cells usually do not.

Immunohistochemistry also can be helpful in poorly differentiated cases when lymphoma could be in the differential diagnosis. Lymphoma cells usually stain positive for CD45 (leukocyte common antigen) and CD20 (a B-cell marker), whereas myeloma cells usually are negative.

Diagnosis of MM is made if plasmacytosis (>10%) is present with either:
- Lytic bone lesion
- Serum or urine M component
- Progressive increase in M component over time or
- Extramedullary mass lesion develop.

The primary treatment of multiple myeloma is chemotherapy includes - alkylating agents, e.g. Melphalan (L-PAM = L-phenylalanine mustured), cyclophosphamide or chlorambucil and prednisolone in intermittent pulses followed by IFN - maintenance therapy. Symptomatic bone lesions usually respond rapidly to radiation treatment. The orthopedic surgeon most commonly is consulted to treat impending or actual pathological fractures of the spine, acetabulum, proximal femur, or proximal humerus. Because most of these patients have a short life expectancy, every effort should be made to perform the operation that would allow the earliest resumption of full activity. This may include debulking the tumor and using internal fixation augmented with methacrylate. If this method would not allow immediate full weight bearing, cemented total joint arthroplasty or hemiarthroplasty should be considered. In most patients, local radiation treatment should be instituted approximately 3 weeks after surgery or when the wound appears to be healed.

Despite aggressive treatment, the prognosis for multiple myeloma continues to be poor. Most patients die as a result of their disease within 3 years after diagnosis. Long-term survival is exceedingly rare. Patients who present with a solitary plasmacytoma without evidence of systemic involvement (i.e. negative bone marrow biopsy and negative skeletal survey) have a better prognosis. Although more than half of patients who present with a solitary plasmacytoma eventually go on to develop multiple myeloma, some patients have a considerable disease-free interval, and a few remain continuously disease-free.

MULTIPLE CHOICE QUESTIONS

1. Most common primary bone tumor is: *(TN 2015)*
   A. Multiple myeloma B. Osteosarcoma
   C. Chondrosarcoma   D. Metastasis
   Ans. 'A' Multiple myeloma

2. Lytic punched out lesions in the skull X-ray, most likely diagnosis: *(TN 2014, 2000)*
   A. Osteosarcoma   B. Multiple myeloma
   C. Metastasis   D. Eosinophilic granuloma
   Ans. 'B' Multiple myeloma

3. Moth eaten bone is: *(NEET Pattern 2013)*
   A. Osteoid osteoma   B. Multiple myeloma
   C. Eosinophilic granuloma D. Chondromyxoid fibroma
   Ans. is 'B' Multiple myeloma

4. A 70-year-old male complains of multiple bone pains, on evaluation he has high ESR, high Calcium values, lytic lesion in multiple bones >20% plasma cells in peripheral smear. Most likely diagnosis is: *(AIIMS May 2013)*
   A. Multiple myeloma   B. Hairy cell leukemia
   C. Plasma cell leukemia D. Metastasis periosteal
   Ans. is 'C' Plasma cell leukemia
   - More than 20% plasma cells in PS—Plasma cell leukemia

5. All are true for multiple myeloma *except*: *(PGI Nov 09)*
   A. Hypercalcemia
   B. Increased Serum Alkaline phosphatase
   C. Monoclonal M Band
   D. Bone marrow plasma cells <5%
   Ans. is 'B' Increase Serum Alkaline phosphatase; 'D' Bone marrow plasma cells <5%
   - ALP is usually not raised in Multiple myeloma until fracture occurs
   - Bone marrow plasma cells are >10% in Multiple Myeloma

6. A patient with pain in back. Lab investigation shows elevated ESR. X-ray skull shows multiple punched out lytic lesions. Most important Investigation to be done is: *(AIIMS June 2000)*
   A. Serum acid phosphatase
   B. CT head with contrast
   C. Whole body scan
   D. Serum electrophoresis
   Ans. is 'D' Serum electrophoresis
   - This patient has:
     - Multiple punched out lytic lesions of skull.
     - Elevated ESR
     - Back pain
   - Diagnosis is multiple myeloma.
   - Multiple myeloma is diagnosed by M bands on serum electrophoresis.
   - Punched out lesions of skull are seen both in Eosinophilic granuloma and multiple myeloma. However, bevelled edges (double contour) is characteristic of eosinophilic granuloma due to uneven destruction of the inner and outer table of the skull.
     - Punched out lesions of skull—Multiple myeloma
     - Punched out lesions with bevelled edges—Eosinophilic granuloma.

METASTATIC CARCINOMA

Metastatic Bone Disease

- Most common primary is Breast > Prostate overall
- **Most common sites of primary for bone metastasis.**
  - In males – Prostate > Lung
  - In Female – Breast > Lung
  - In Children – Neuroblastoma

- Skeletal sites most frequently involved
  - Spine (Dorsal)
- Lytic expansile metastasis seen in
  - Renal cancer
  - Thyroid carcinomas
- Purely Osteoblastic secondaries
  - Prostate/Carcinoid/Medulloblastoma
- Metastasis distal to knee and elbow is rare and usually arises from a primary tumors of the
  - Bronchus, Bladder and Colon (BBC)

"BBC Can Go Anywhere even distal to Elbow and Knee"

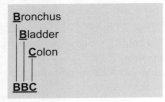

Bronchus
Bladder
Colon
BBC

Metastasis from Bone to Bone—'BONE'

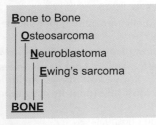

Bone to Bone
Osteosarcoma
Neuroblastoma
Ewing's sarcoma
BONE

Sarcomas of soft tissue origin do not frequently involve bone, the ones involving are 'SARLA'

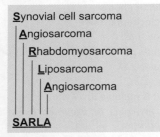

Synovial cell sarcoma
Angiosarcoma
Rhabdomyosarcoma
Liposarcoma
Angiosarcoma
SARLA

Rhabdomyosarcoma is the most common soft tissue tumor in child.
Liposarcoma is the most common soft tissue tumor in adult.
Sarcomas metastasizing through lymphatic and causing lymph node involvement are:

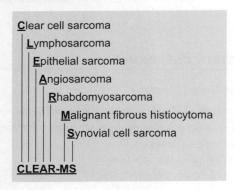

Clear cell sarcoma
Lymphosarcoma
Epithelial sarcoma
Angiosarcoma
Rhabdomyosarcoma
Malignant fibrous histiocytoma
Synovial cell sarcoma
CLEAR-MS

Causes of Lytic Lesions in Skull

- Metastasis
- Eosinophilic granuloma and Epidermoid
- Lymphoma/Langerhans Cell histiocytosis
- Tuberculosis
- Hyperparathyroidism
- Osteomyelitis
- Radiation
- Multiple myeloma

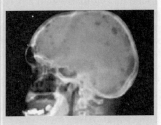

Pigmented Villo Nodular Synovitis

Idiopathic proliferation of synovial tissue in joint, tendon sheath or bursa. May arise from intra-articular or extra-articular synovial tissue. Locally aggressive lesion destroys soft tissues and bones.

- Involvement order is **knee** > hip > shoulder
- Chromosome 5, 7 associated

Insidious onset, slow progressive course, mild pain and decreased range of movement is seen. There can be episodes of mechanical locking/giving way.

- Soft tissue calcification is unusual
- X-ray bony changes - marginal erosions and cysts
- Knee - brown fluid or hemarthrosis is seen.
- Treatment - Synovectomy (open/arthroscopic)
- External beam radiotherapy is used in some cases
- Advanced cases - arthrodesis/arthroplasty

Synovial Cell Sarcoma

Synovial cell sarcoma (previously called 'synovioma') is an uncommon malignant mesenchymal neoplasm comprising 8–10% of soft tissue sarcomas.

The term 'synovial cell sarcoma' is however a misnomer as synovial cell sarcomas do not arise from synovium the term was designated because the histological appearance of cells from synovial sarcoma resemble normal synovial tissue.

Etiology

- Most synovial sarcomas are associated with a characteristic translocation involving chromosome X and chromosome 18: t (X; 18) giving rise to SYT – SSX fusion genes.

Origin/Site of Predilection

- Synovial cell sarcomas usually arise from deep soft tissues in the vicinity of joint capsules, tendon sheath and bursae.
- Most synovial sarcomas are extraarticular and only less than 10% are intra-articular.
- Most common site of synovial sarcomas is around the extremities (83%) although uncommonly tumors may also develop in the head and neck or different viscera.
- The most common site is the lower extremity especially around the knee and foot.

Age at Presentation

- Tumor most frequently occurs in young adults between 15 and 35 years of age and rarely appears in individuals over 50 years of age.

Sex
- There is no sex predilection although recently slight male predominance has been suggested.

Presentation
- Most common presenting symptom is a deep seated mass/swelling that has been present for be a long time.
- Usually slow growing with an indolent course (but aggressive in late stages).
- **Synovial sarcomas are morphologically biphasic as they have dual lines of differentiation (Epithelial and Mesenchymal).**

Treatment is excision and chemotherapy has been advocated by some.

Oncogenic Osteomalacia

Hypophosphatemic Vitamin D resistant rickets or osteomalacia can be associated with
- Hemangiopericytomas
- **Fibrosarcoma**
- GCT
- Osteosarcoma
- Pigmented Villo Nodular synovitis

The mediator is phosphatonin; FGF-23

It is a reversible condition along with malignancy.

MULTIPLE CHOICE QUESTIONS

1. Which metabolic condition has phosphaturia and osteomalacia: *(AIIMS Nov 2018)*
   A. Fibrosarcoma
   B. Osteosarcoma
   C. Undifferentiated sarcoma
   D. Malignant peripheral nerve sheath tumor

   Ans. is 'A' Fibrosarcoma

2. A 55-year-old male complains of bone pain since 2 yrs. The skull radiograph of the patient is suggestive of: *(NEET 2018)*

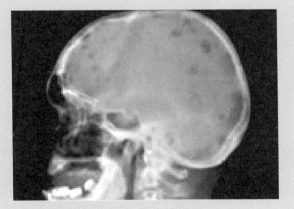

   A. Multiple myeloma
   B. Hyperparathyroidism
   C. Eosinophilic granuloma
   D. Paget's disease

   Ans. is 'A' Multiple myeloma

3. Oncogenic osteomalacia is mediated by: *(NEET Dec 2016)*
   A. Phosphatonin
   B. Calcitonin
   C. Interleukin 2
   D. Interleukin 6

   Ans. is 'A' Phosphatonin

4. Most common primary cancer for metastatic bone tumor: *(AI 2016)*
   A. Ca stomach
   B. Ca breast
   C. Ca rectum
   D. Ca color

   Ans. is 'B' Ca Breast

5. Osteosclerotic metastases is/are common in cancer of:
   A. Prostate *(PGI May 2015)*
   B. Breast
   C. Lung
   D. Malignant melanoma
   E. Renal cell carcinoma

   Ans. is 'A' Prostate; and 'B' Breast

6. Most common site of metastasis in skeleton: *(NEET 2015)*
   A. Femur
   B. Tibia
   C. Vertebrae
   D. Skull

   Ans. is 'C' Vertebrae

7. Most common malignancy that metastasizes to the spine is: *(APPG 2015)*
   A. Thyroid
   B. Prostate
   C. Lung
   D. Breast

   Ans. is 'D' Breast

8. Which of the following is not a cause of these lesions in skull? *(APPG 2015)*

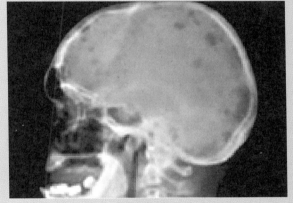

   A. Paget's disease
   B. Hyperparathyroidism
   C. Histiocytosis X
   D. Multiple myeloma

   Ans. is 'A' Paget's disease

9. Osteoblastic secondaries are seen in: *(AIIMS May 2013, NEET Pattern 2013)*
   A. Prostate metastasis
   B. Lung metastasis
   C. Bladder metastasis
   D. Stomach metastasis

   Ans. is 'A' Prostate metastasis

10. Most common cause of metastasis to orbit:
    A. Breast *(AIIMS Nov 2013)*
    B. Ovary
    C. Endometrial carcinoma
    D. Wilms'

    Ans. is 'A' Breast

11. All are common sites of primary for bone metastasis except: *(NEET Pattern Dec 2016, 2013)*
    A. Breast
    B. Prostate
    C. Brain
    D. Kidney

    Ans. is 'C' Brain

12. Most common bone tumor: *(NEET Pattern 2016, 2013)*
    A. Osteoid osteoma
    B. Metastasis
    C. Multiple myeloma
    D. Osteosarcoma
Ans. is 'B' Metastasis

13. Metastasis not found in: *(NEET Pattern 2012)*
    A. Femur
    B. Humerus
    C. Fibula
    D. Spine
Ans. is 'C' Fibula

14. In carcinoma prostate with bone metastasis which is raised? *(NEET Pattern 2012)*
    A. ESR
    B. Alkaline phosphatase
    C. Acid phosphatase
    D. Bilirubin
Ans. is 'B' Alkaline phosphatase

15. Pigmented Villo Nodular Synovitis is seen at most commonly: *(NEET Pattern 2012)*
    A. Knee
    B. Hip
    C. Shoulder
    D. Elbow
Ans. is 'A' Knee

16. Synovial sarcoma gene affected is: *(NEET Pattern 2012)*
    A. SYT-SSX
    B. MIC 2
    C. RAS
    D. P53
Ans. is 'A' SYT-SSX

17. Involvement of regional lymph nodes is seen in: *(NEET Pattern 2012)*
    A. Osteogenic sarcoma
    B. Synovial sarcoma
    C. Osteoclastoma
    D. Fibrosarcoma
Ans. is 'B' Synovial sarcoma

18. Phelps sign is seen in: *(NEET Pattern 2012)*
    A. Glomus tumor
    B. Osteoblastoma
    C. Osteoid osteoma
    D. Unicameral bone cyst
Ans. is 'A' Glomus tumor

19. All of the following statements about synovial cell sarcoma, are true, except: *(AI 2010)*
    A. Originate from synovial lining
    B. Occur more often at extra-articular sites
    C. Usually seen in patients less than 50 years of age
    D. Knee and foot are common sites involved
Ans. is 'A' Originate from synovial lining
    – The term 'synovial cell sarcoma' is however a misnomer as synovial cell sarcomas do not arise from synovium.
    – Most synovial sarcomas are extra-articular and only less than 10% are intraarticular.

Synovial cell sarcoma does not arise from synovial lining
The term synovial sarcoma is a misnomer. The term originates from the histological appearance of cells which can resemble synovial cells. These tumors, however, do not arise from synovial tissue.

20. True about Bone metastasis: *(PGI Nov 2009)*
    A. 5% bone metastasis are symptomatic
    B. Higher serum levels of alkaline phosphatase
    C. Most common secondary in female is breast
    D. Prostate produce osteosclerotic lesion
    E. Commonly involves hand and feet bones

Ans. is 'B' Higher serum levels of alkaline phosphatase; 'C' Most common secondary in female is breast; 'D' Prostate produce osteosclerotic lesion
    – Most common tumor producing bone metastasis in females is breast carcinoma and in males is prostatic carcinoma.
    – Prostatic carcinoma produces osteoblastic (osteosclerotic) lesions.
    – Osteoblastic lesions are associated with higher serum levels of alkaline phosphatase (reflecting high activity of osteoblasts).
    – Metastases below elbow and knee are rare.

21. Metastases least common in: *(PGI June 09, Dec 07, June 04)*
    A. Skull
    B. Pelvis
    C. Vertebrae
    D. Proximal part of long bones of the upper limb
    E. Small bones of the hand
Ans. is 'E' Small bones of the hand
    – The commonest site for bone metastases are the VERTEBRAE
    – Extremities distal to elbow and knee are least commonly involved sites.

22. Most common soft tissue tumor in a child: *(PGI June 2K)*
    A. Rhabdomyosarcoma
    B. Histiocytoma
    C. Fibrosarcoma
    D. Liposarcoma
Ans. is 'A' Rhabdomyosarcoma
    – Rhabdomyosarcoma, the most common childhood soft-tissue sarcoma, is often located in the head and neck (40%) and in the trunk and extremities (25%).

23. Expansile lytic osseous metastases are characteristics of primary malignancy of: *(JIPMER May 2017)*
    A. Kidney
    B. Bronchus
    C. Breast
    D. Prostate
Ans. is 'A' Kidney
    – Renal (kidney) carcinoma and thyroid carcinoma—expansile osteolytic bone metastasis.

24. A 60-year-old male has bone pain, vertebral collapse, fracture pelvis, the probable diagnosis is: *(AIIMS Sept 1996)*
    A. Multiple myeloma
    B. Secondaries
    C. TB
    D. Hemangioma of bone
Ans. is 'B> A' Secondaries > Multiple myeloma
    – The information in this question are
      i. Age — 60 years;
      ii. Bone pain;
      iii. Vertebral collapse;
      iv. Pathological fracture pelvis
    – All these clinical features can occur both in multiple myeloma and metastatic bone disease, metastasis will be preferred over multiple Myeloma. In > 40 years of age.

Orthopedics Oncology

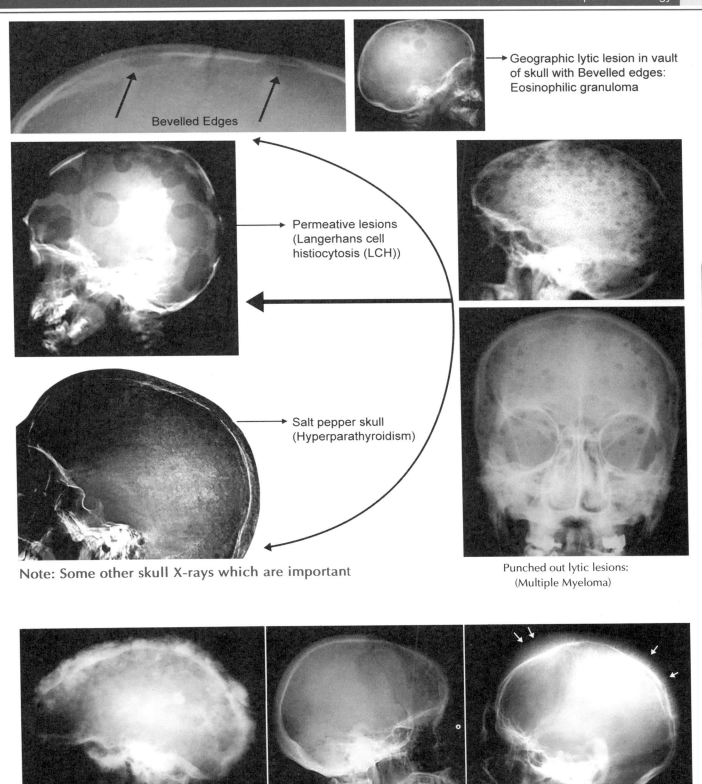

Note: Some other skull X-rays which are important

CHAPTER 5: Fracture and Fracture Healing

ANATOMY OF BONE

In children, a typical long bone has two ends or epiphyses an intermediate portion diaphysis connecting part between the two metaphysis. There is a thin plate of growth cartilage one at each end, separating the epiphysis from the metaphysis. This is called the physeal plate. At maturity, the epiphysis fuses with the metaphysis and the physeal plate is replaced by bone. The articular ends of the epiphyses are covered with articular cartilage. The rest of the bone is covered with periosteum which provides attachment to tendons, muscles, ligaments, etc. **The strands of fibrous tissue connecting the bone to the periosteum are called Sharpey's fibers.**

Microscopically, bone can be classified as either woven or lamellar.

Woven bone or immature bone is characterized by random arrangement of cells and collagen it is associated with periods of rapid bone formation, such as in the initial stages of fracture healing.

Lamellar bone or mature bone has an orderly cellular distribution and properly oriented collagen fibres. The basic structural unit of lamellar bone is the **osteon**. It consists of a series of concentric laminations or lamellae surrounding a central canal, the Haversian canal. These canals run longitudinally and connect freely with each other and with Volkmann's canals. Which run horizontally from endosteal to periosteal surfaces. The lamellae may be arranged densely to form the cortical bone, or loosely to form the cancellous bone. The shaft of a bone is made up of cortical bone; the ends mainly of cancellous bone. The junction between the two known as corticocancellous junction is a common site of fractures.

Flowchart 5.1: Classification of bone components

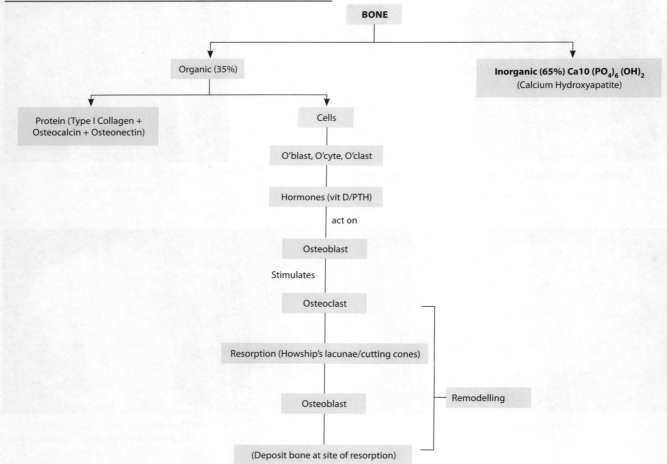

Fracture and Fracture Healing

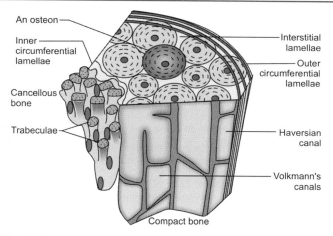

Fig. 5.1: Bone

GROWTH OF A LONG BONE

Limbs appear at the end of 1st month of intrauterine life. All long bones, with the exception of the clavicle, develop from cartilaginous primordia (endochondral ossification). This type of ossification commences in the middle of the shaft (primary center of ossification) before birth usually beginning by the **end of 2nd month of intrauterine life**.

Muscles and joints appear in 3rd month. The secondary ossification centers (the epiphyses) appear at the ends of the bone, mostly around and after birth.

Endochondral Ossification

- When bone formation takes pace in pre-existing cartilage.
- The cartilage model formed from mesenchymal tissue acts as a scaffold for ossification but does not itself become bone.
- Long bones, vertebrae, pelvis, and bones of the base of skull.

Intramembranous Ossification

- When bone formation occurs directly in primitive connective tissue by proliferation, hypertrophy and transformation of cells into osteoblasts.
- Progressive bone formation results in the fusion of adjacent bony areas within the membrane to form spongy bone
- Skull vault, maxilla, majority of mandible and **clavicle**.

The bone grows in length by a continuous growth at the Epiphyseal plate. The increase in the girth of the bone is by subperiosteal new bone deposition. The secondary centers of ossification, not contributing to the length of a bone, are termed the apophysis (e.g. apophysis of the greater trochanter). At the end of the growth period, the epiphysis fuses with the metaphysis and the growth stops. The time and sequence of appearance and fusion of epiphysis has great clinical relevance in deciding the true age (bone age) of a person, and in differentiating an Epiphyseal plate from a fracture.

Milking position to remember age of ossification or skeletal maturity—**joints that face towards sky or god like shoulder/ wrist/knee usually ossify around 18 and joints that face towards ground like elbow/hip and ankle fuse around 16.**

CELLS OF BONE

Osteoblast

- Mononuclear cells derived from marrow stromal cells by differentiation of preosteoblasts. The single nucleus is eccentrically placed and the abundant rough endoplasmic reticulum (RER) is characteristic of a cell engaged in protein synthesis. **They are rich in alkaline phosphatase.**
- It is responsible for the synthesis of major protein of bone including type I collagen and non-collagen proteins such as—**osteocalcin (bone Gla protein) and osteonectin.** It plays a central role in osteoclastic function (i.e. involved in initiation and control of osteoclastic activity) **Osteoblasts have specific surface receptors for 1,25-Dihydroxy vitamin D3 and Parathyroid hormone.**

Osteocytes

- By the end of bone remodelling cycle, the osteoblast either remains on newly formed surface as quiescent lining cell or become enveloped in the matrix as resting osteocytes. So these are spent osteoblasts.
- *Their function is obscure*: They may under the influence of PTH, participate in **bone resorption (osteocytic osteolysis) and calcium ion transport.**

Osteoclast

- It is multinucleated giant cell
- It is the principal mediator of bone resorption and is formed by fusion of mononuclear cells.
- The characteristic feature is the area of in folded plasma membrane **ruffled border** which is the site of bone resorption.
- In order to create this enclosed space, the osteoclast attaches to the bone through special attachment proteins called integrins.
- It contains characteristic enzymes Tartrate resistant acid phosphatase (TRAP) and carbonic anhydrase.

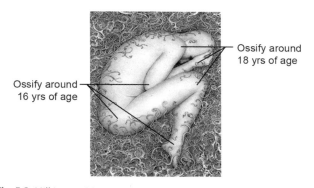

Fig. 5.2: Milking position

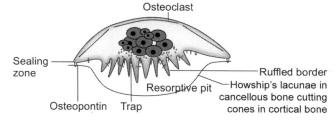

Fig. 5.3: Osteoclast

- With resorption of organic matrix, the osteoclasts are left in shallow excavations—**Howship's lacunae** in cancellous bone and cutting cones in cortical bones. By identifying these excavations one can distinguish 'resorption surface' from the smooth 'formation surface' or 'resting surface'.

BONE HISTOLOGY

1. Name the joints that ossify around 16: *(PGI Nov 2018)*
- A. Ankle
- B. Knee
- C. Hip
- D. Elbow
- E. Wrist

Ans. is 'A' Ankle 'C' Hip 'D' Elbow

2. The tensile strength of a bone is due to: *(DNB JULY 2016)*
- A. Strands of collagen
- B. Hydroxyapatite crystals
- C. Periosteum
- D. Metaphysis

Ans. is 'A' Strands of collagen

Compressile strength of bone is due to proteoglycans.

3. Proximal tibial epiphysis fuses at. *(NEET DEC 2016)*
- A. 12-14 years
- B. 14-16 years
- C. 16-18 years
- D. 18-20 years

Ans. is 'C' 16-18 years

4. Which of the following is the most metabolically active part of long bone? *(NEET DEC 2016)*
- A. Epiphysis
- B. Metaphysis
- C. Diaphysis
- D. Physis

Ans. is 'D' Physis

Physis or growth plate has highest turnover and metabolic activity in the bone

5. Osteoclasts have all of the following except: *(AI Dec 15)*
- A. Bone resorption
- B. Receptor for parathormone
- C. Ruffled border
- D. Rank ligand

Ans. is 'B' Receptor for parathormone

6. Most vascular zone of the bone is: *(AI Dec 15)*
- A. Metaphysis
- B. Diaphysis
- C. Epiphysis
- D. Medullary Cavity

Ans. is 'A' Metaphysis

7. PTH acts directly on which cells? *(AI Dec 15)*
- A. Osteoclasts
- B. Osteocytes
- C. Osteoblasts
- D. Macrophages

Ans. is 'C' Osteoblasts

8. Intramembranous ossification is seen in which bones:
- A. Pelvis
- B. Long bones
- C. Maxilla
- D. None *(NEET Pattern 2013)*

Ans. is 'C' Maxilla

9. Major Mineral of the bone is: *(NEET Pattern 2013; AIIMS May 2010)*
- A. Calcium chloride
- B. Hydroxyapatite
- C. Calcium oxide
- D. Calcium carbonate

Ans. is 'B' Hydroxyapatite

- Inorganic component of bone is consists of *mineral phase* which is principally composed of calcium and phosphate, mostly in the form of *hydroxyapatite* $[Ca_{10}(PO_4)_6(OH)_2]$.

10. True about Osteoclast is all except: *(PGI June 2K)*
- A. Derived from monocytes
- B. Stimulated by PTH
- C. Phagocytosis of foreign bodies
- D. Resorption of bone

Ans. is 'C > B' Phagocytosis of foreign bodies > Stimulated by PTH

- Osteoblasts have specific surface receptors for agent, such as 1,25-dihydroxy vitamin D3 and parathyroid hormone. These receptors are not present on osteoclast.

FRACTURE HEALING

1. Stage of hematoma
2. Stage of granulation tissue
3. Stage of callus **(Earliest at 3 weeks)**
4. Stage of consolidation—woven bone is seen **(Clinically bone is united)**
5. Stage of remodelling

Note: In open fractures hematoma is lost so there are problems of fracture healing.

Callus in initial stage is soft and doesn't restrict movements in all planes; but the woven bone does.

Note: Callus is earliest seen at 3 weeks and is earliest Radiological indicator for fracture healing.

High oxygen tension, high pH (aiding alkaline phosphate activity) and stability (micromovement) predispose to osteoblasts hence enhances rate of union.

STAGE OF REMODELLING

Bone biologists call it 'modelling' and describe it a process of readaptation of the skeleton to the loads which will be applied to it. It involves replacement of woven bone by lamellar bone. By 3–4 weeks the fracture is consolidated enough to allow penetration and bridging of the area by bone remodelling unit—i.e. osteoclast cutting cones/Howship's lacunae followed by osteoblast closing cones. Remodelling activity peaks around 8 week following fracture. Thicker lamellar bone is laid down where stresses are high; unwanted buttresses are curved away and medullary cavity is reformed. **So there is osteoclastic activity at tension site and osteoblastic activity at the compression site.**

Bone Apposition after Skeletal Maturity!

- Since bone itself is a hard and unyielding structure, it can only increase in size by the relatively slow process of appositional growth that is bone deposition on bone surface increasing width of bone.

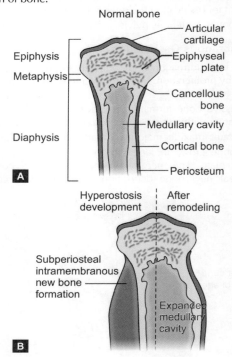

Figs. 5.4A and B: Bone apposition—sequential increase in width of bone with age

- Bone remodelling requires a raw surface for bone deposition which can only take place by resorption of bone by osteoclast (Howship's lacuna in trabecular bone or cutting cones in cortical bone are formed as a result of bone resorption carried out by osteoclasts).
- Once this resorption surface is formed than osteoblast will accumulate to form new bone on surface which is called as bone apposition or bone deposition and these cells form the closing cones.
- Thus in adult, skeleton after cessation of skeleton growth, new lamellar bone formation occurs only after an episode of bone resorption. This constraint applies with in the cortex, where the physical lack of space for new bone necessitates preceding resorption, and it also seems to apply to periosteal and endosteal surfaces.
- There are two, pathological exceptions to this rule. One is during the production of callus in a healing fracture where woven bone will form without resorption and after cancellous autograft, where new bone will form directly on to the cancellous graft not requiring resorption.

So Bone Apposition is Seen in

Howship's lacunae or cutting cones in normal adults (after resorption).

Subperiosteal cambium layer in fractured bones (best example of bone apposition) and after cancellous bone grafting (both these conditions resorption is not required).

BONE TURNOVER

Bone is constantly renewed, with a turnover rate of ~10% per year (4% in cortical bone and 25% in trabecular bone). Modelling and remodelling are both expression of bone turnover, in which bone is serially removed by osteoclasts and laid down by osteoblasts in a closely coupled fashion.

Thus remodelling = Resorption + Bone apposition (Formation)

Bone Remodelling: Renews Bone and Maintains Bone Homeostasis!

- It is divided into four discrete phases: quiescence, activation, resorption, reversal and formation.

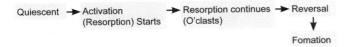

BONE MODELLING—TERM BY BONE PATHOLOGIST!

It refers to over all consequences for the whole bone of the sum of all the units of remodelling activity which are occurring throughout the bone it has usually predominant osteoclastic activity at tension site and osteoblastic activity at compression site. By progressive bone deposition on to one surface (to compression site) and resorption from other (tension site), it is responsible for the gross changes in the shape of bones which occur during development and adaptation of bone to applied loads which is illustrated by Wolff's law.

Majority of modelling activity ceases with skeletal maturity, progressive modelling throughout adult life in responsible for the gradual widening of bones with age.

Thus bone remodelling has both osteoclastic and osteoblastic activity at compression or tension side but the forces on bone decide where remodelling takes place with compressile forces at compression site and with tensile forces tension site and in bone modelling there is osteoclastic activity at tension site and osteoblastic activity at compression site.

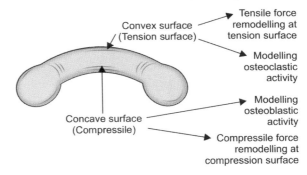

Fig. 5.5: Overall osteoclastic activity at tension surface and osteoblastic activity at compression surface

Markers of Bone Formation

1. Serum bone specific alkaline phosphatase
2. **Serum osteocalcin (very important marker)**
3. Serum peptide of type I procollagen
4. Type 1 collagen extension peptide*

*Are product of type I collagen degradation and are more specific.

Osteocalcin or bone Gla protein (BGP) is raised in diseases with increased bone turnover, e.g. Paget's disease, renal osteodystrophy and primary hyperparathyroidism.

Markers of Bone Resorption

Urine and serum cross linked N telopeptide
- Urine and serum cross linked C telopeptide
- Urine total free deoxypyridinoline
- **Urine hydroxyproline (very important marker)**
- Urine hydroxylysine glycosides
- Serum tartrate resistant acid phosphatase (TRAP)
- Serum bone sialoprotein

TRAP/TRAF (tumor necrosis factor receptor associated factor) regulates osteoclast formation.

Tetracycline administered in vivo becomes fixed in new forming mineralizing bone and exhibit a characteristic fluorescence when viewed by ultraviolet light. When two doses of tetracycline are given a number of days apart, two bands of fluorescence will be separated by an interval of unlabelled new bone that has formed during the period between doses. **Thus rate of mineralization of newly formed osteoid is estimated by tetracycline labelling.**

MULTIPLE CHOICE QUESTIONS

1. True about fracture healing is/are: *(PGI May 2017)*
   A. Micromovement promotes healing
   B. In primary healing, cartilage involvement is there
   C. Woven bone is formed in primary fractures
   D. In secondary healing, cartilage involvement is there
   E. Immobilization is golden rule for all fractures

Ans. is 'A' Micromovement promotes healing; and 'D' In secondary healing, cartilage involvement is there

2. Which of these is not a marker of bone formation?
   (JIPMER Nov 2017)
   A. Serum Bone specific alkaline phosphatase
   B. Serum cross linked N-telopeptide
   C. Serum Osteocalcin   D. Type 1 procollagen peptide
Ans. is 'B' Serum cross linked N-telopeptide

3. Which among the following is indicative of bone resorption?
   (JIPMER Nov 2017)
   A. Osteocalcin   B. Urine hydroxyproline
   C. Bone specific alkaline phosphatase
   D. Type 1 procollagen
Ans. is 'B' Urine hydroxyproline

4. Increase Callus or Cartilage formation is seen in:
   (AIIMS Nov 16)
   A. Rigid immobilization B. Necrosis of bone ends
   C. Increase mobilization D. Compression plating
Ans. is 'C' Increase mobilization

5. Wolff's law states that: (CET Nov 15)
   A. If a bone is continuously subjected to a particular stress it will adapt to become stronger to resist that loading
   B. Only Diaphysis allows longitudinal growth in childhood
   C. Any infection not showing periosteal reaction within 1 week of symptoms can be ruled out to be osteomyelitis
   D. Angular deformities will progress till the closure of physis
Ans. is 'A' If a bone is continuously subjected to a particular stress it will adapt to become stronger to resist that loading

6. The tensile strength of a bone is due to: (CET July 16)
   A. Strands of collagen   B. Hydroxyapatite crystals
   C. Periosteum   D. Metaphysis
Ans. is 'A' Strands of collagen

7. Callus formation is seen between what duration of fracture healing: (NEET 2015)
   A. 0–2 weeks   B. 2–4 weeks
   C. 4–12 weeks   D. 12–16 weeks
Ans. is 'C' 4–12 weeks

8. Bone resorption is inhibited by: (PGM-CET 2015)
   A. Parathyroid hormone   B. Thyroid hormones
   C. Cortisol   D. Estrogen
Ans. is 'D' Estrogen

9. The first center of primary ossification appears at:
   A. At the end of 2 months in intrauterine life
   B. Beginning of 3rd month   (AIIMS Nov 2011)
   C. End of 3rd month
   D. End of 4th month
Ans. is 'A' At the end of 2 months in intrauterine life

10. Rate of mineralization of newly formed osteoid can be estimated by the following: (AI 09)
    A. Von Kossa staining for calcium
    B. Alzarin red stain   C. Labelled tetracycline
    D. Immunofluorescence
Ans. is 'C' Labelled tetracycline

11. Indicators of bone formation and resorption which of the following is false: (AIIMS MAY 2008)
    A. Osteocalcin is marker of bone formation
    B. Hydroxyproline is marker of bone resorption
    C. N and C terminal procollagen for bone formation
    D. N and C terminal telopeptide for bone formation
Ans. is 'D' N and C terminal telopeptide for bone formation

12. Marker for bone formation is:
    (All India 2007, PGI Dec 07, AIIMS June 1987)
    A. Tartrate resistant acid phosphate
    B. Osteocalcin   C. Urinary calcium
    D. Serum nucleotidase
Ans. is 'B' Osteocalcin
   – During bone growth and development, bone formation, i.e. osteoblastic activity predominates Osteocalcin is used as sensitive and specific serum marker for osteoblastic activity.

13. Bone apposition is best in: (AIIMS Nov 01)
    A. Osteoblastic activity at the area of stress
    B. Endochondral ossification
    C. Subperiosteal cambium layer
    D. Osteoblastic activity in Howship's lacunae
Ans. is 'C' Subperiosteal cambium layer

14. Regarding bone remodelling, all are true except:
    (AIIMS May 01)
    A. Osteoclastic activity at the compression site
    B. Osteoclastic activity at the tension site
    C. Osteoclastic activity and osteoblastic activity are both needed for bone remodelling in cortical and cancellous bones
    D. Osteoblasts transforms into osteocytes
Ans. is 'A' Osteoclastic activity at the compression site
   Thus bone remodelling has both osteoclastic and osteoblastic activity at compression or tension side but the forces on bone decide where remodelling takes place compressile forces compression site and tensile forces tension site and in bone modelling there is osteoclastic activity at tension site and osteoblastic activity at compression site. Thus the best answer here will be (a) but this is with respect to modelling not remodelling.

FRACTURE: DIAGNOSIS AND PATTERN

Radiological Feature

Partial or complete **loss of continuity of cortex.**

Clinical Features

Tenderness is the commonest (consistent) sign of fracture.

Abnormal mobility and loss of transmitted movements is surest sign of fracture.

*Crepitus occurs because of rubbing of both fracture ends together and gives sense of friction between fractured ends, it should not be elicited as it may cause neurogenic shock **or may cause comminution at fracture ends due to rubbing of bone ends.** Crepitus may also be positive in bursitis or subcutaneous emphysema. Thus crepitus is not a very reliable sign of fracture as the above two, but if abnormal mobility and loss of transmitted movements are not mentioned than crepitus has to be chosen as the answer.

Fracture

Pathological	The broken bone has an underlying disease most common cause in India is nutritional disorder.
Comminuted	Fracture in multiple pieces and intermediate fragment has only one cortex.
Segmental	Fracture at two levels in the same bone with intermediate segment having two cortices.
Avulsion	Bone piece pulled-off by attached muscle or ligament.
Burst	Vertebral body fracture where fragments burst out in different directions - Compression injury.

- Fractures can be Classified on basis of **Pattern of injury**
- **Transverse fractures (fracture forms an angle of less than 30 degrees with horizontal)** – Tension/direct trauma

Fracture and Fracture Healing

- Oblique fractures (fracture forms an angle of more than 30 degrees with horizontal) – Compression injury.
- Spiral fractures – Twisting injury and it has maximum chances of union.
- Bending – Butterfly (Comminuted) fracture.
- Direct – Comminuted fracture.
- Direct trauma – Transverse > Comminuted fracture.

- Most consistent symptom of fracture—*Pain*
- Most consistent sign of fracture—*Tenderness*

FRACTURE CLASSIFICATION ON THE BASIS OF RELATIONSHIP WITH EXTERNAL ENVIRONMENT

Closed Fracture

A fracture hematoma not communicating with external environment, i.e. overlying skin and soft tissue are intact.

Open Fracture

A fracture hematoma communicating with external environment, i.e. overlying skin (and soft tissue) is breached.

Gustilo and Anderson classification is used for open fracture

Grade	Characteristic Feature
I	Clean wound of < 1 cm length
II	Wound > 1 cm in length without extensive soft tissue damage, skin flap or avulsion
III	Wound associated with extensive soft tissue damage, comminution, contamination or segmental fractures
IIIA	Adequate periosteal coverage is there
IIIB	**Significant periosteal stripping and it requires secondary bone coverage procedure like skin grafting or flap**
IIIC	Open fracture with vascular injury that requires vascular repair

Tscherne Classification is used for Skin Lesions in Closed Fractures

Management Plan of Open Fractures:

- Tscherne described four eras of open fracture treatment: life preservation (1st era), limb preservation (2nd era), infection avoidance (3rd era) and function preservation (4th era).

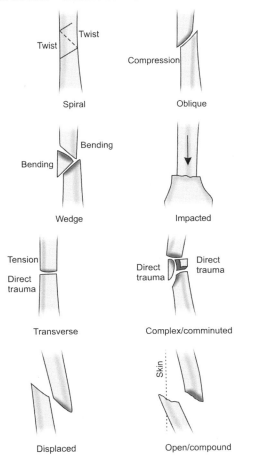

Fig. 5.6: Fracture pattern and mode of injury

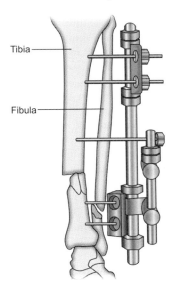

Fig. 5.7: External fixator—usual treatment of open fracture

- We are in fourth era of functional preservation which includes the following principles:
  1. All open fractures are emergencies.
  2. Begin appropriate antibiotic therapy in emergency room.

MULTIPLE CHOICE QUESTIONS

1. Diagnostic sign of a fracture: *(NEET Pattern 2013)*
   - A. Abnormal mobility at fracture site
   - B. Pain at the fracture site
   - C. Tenderness
   - D. Swelling

   Ans. is 'A' Abnormal mobility at fracture site

2. Direct impact on the bone will produce a: *(AIIMS May 2003)*
   - A. Transverse fracture
   - B. Oblique fracture
   - C. Spiral fracture
   - D. Comminuted fracture

   Ans. is 'A > D' Transverse fracture > Comminuted fracture

3. The most common sign of fresh fracture is: *(Andhara 99, JIPMER 98, PGI 97)*
   - A. Crepitus
   - B. Bony tenderness
   - C. Deformity
   - D. Abnormal mobility
   - E. Shortening of bone

   Ans. is 'B' Bony tenderness

3. Immediately debride the wound of contaminated and devitalized tissue, copiously irrigate, and repeat debridement within 24–72 hours (Delayed wound closure is preferable).
4. Stabilize the fracture and Perform early autogenous cancellous bone grafting if required.
5. Rehabititate the involved extremity aggressively.

Type and Method of fixation:

Grade I	Technique that is suitable for closed fracture management, i.e. Debridement and internal fixation by intramedullary nail and plate.
Grades II, IIIA	Within 6 hours of injury same as Grade I. After 6 hours same as grades IIIB and IIIc.
Grades III B, III C	Debridement and external fixation

Note: Remember usual treatment for open fractures is debridement (more important) and external fixator.

MULTIPLE CHOICE QUESTIONS

1. A patient with open wound with fracture of both bones of right lower limb came to the emergency. The doctor labelled the injury as 3B according to Gustillo Anderson Classification. Which of the following would represent the injury? *(AIIMS Nov 2017)*
   A. Open wound with fracture with wound <1 cm
   B. Open wound with fracture, 1 to 10 cm wound size, but mild soft tissue injury
   C. Open wound >10 cm, though soft tissue coverage not required
   D. Open wound > 10 cm, with extensive injury requiring soft tissue coverage

Ans. 'D' Open wound > 10 cm, with extensive injury requiring soft tissue coverage

2. Which of the following injuries can be classified as Gustilo-Anderson Grade III injuries? *(CET Nov 15)*
   A. Open fracture with clean wounds less than 1 cm long
   B. Open fractures with a laceration more than 1 cm long usually up to 10 cm, with extension tissue damage, flaps or avulsions
   C. Open segmental fractures, open fracture with extensive soft tissue damage
   D. Compartment syndrome with an open fracture

Ans. is 'C' Open segmental fractures, open fracture with extensive soft tissue damage

3. Open fracture in children is managed by: *(JIPMER 2014)*
   A. Debridement
   B. External fixation
   C. Open reduction and Internal fixation
   D. Intramedullary nail

Ans. 'A' Debridement

4. A patient with gun shot wound in tibia presents with comminuted fracture tibia with 2 cm wound. This belongs to what grade of Gustilo-Anderson classification of open fractures: *(AIIMS May 2013)*
   A. Grade I
   B. Grade II
   C. Grade IIIA
   D. Grade IIIB

Ans. is 'C' Grade IIIA (Comminuted fracture)

5. Vascular repair to be done in which Gustilo-Anderson type:
   A. IIIC
   B. I   *(NEET Pattern 2013)*
   C. II
   D. IIIb

Ans. is 'A' IIIC

6. A patient presents with Open fracture of Tibia with 1.5 cm opening in skin. Which grade it belongs?
   (JIMPER 2003, AMU 2003 JIMPER 2000, 1993)
   A. Grade I
   B. Grade II
   C. Grade III A
   D. Grade III B

Ans. is 'B' Grade II

7. Internal Fixation is primarily used in all except:
   (Manipal 1999) (Rohtak 98) (UP 1998, Delhi 97)
   A. Compound fractures
   B. Multiple fractures
   C. Fractures in elderly patient
   D. Fracture neck of femur

Ans. is 'A' Compound fracture

CRUSH SYNDROME

It is seen when a limb is compressed for many hours, resulting in massive crushing of muscles and **release of large amounts of myohemoglobin.**

Pathophysiology

- Due to ischemia, tissues die and accumulate toxic metabolites. When limb is freed, reperfusion injury occurs due to reactive oxygen metabolites. The ion pumps in the capillary and muscle cells fail, leading to fluid shifts which cause swelling leading to compartment syndrome and further ischemia.
  Toxic metabolites (myohemoglobin) are released into circulation resulting.
  Myohemoglobinuria can cause **acute tubular necrosis** and **renal failure**. So the features are:
  1. Rhabdomyolysis
  2. **Hypocalcemia**
  3. Hyperuricemia
  4. Hyperphosphatemia
  5. **Hyperkalemia** ~ Cardiac arrest
  6. Cardiomyopathy
  7. Myoglobinemia and myoglobinuria
  8. Metabolic acidosis
  9. Acute tubular necrosis and ARF
  10. DIC.

Management

Most important measure is prevention, which is achieved by maintaining high urine output by giving large volumes of intravenous crystalloid. Forced mannitol alkaline diuresis is maintained until myoglobin is no longer detected in urine. If oliguria persists, renal dialysis will be needed.

MULTIPLE CHOICE QUESTIONS

1. Crush syndrome: *(PGI Nov 2015)*
   A. Most common in earthquakes and bombings
   B. Causes acute glomerulonephritis
   C. Release of myoglobin in blood
   D. Occurs due to massive crushing of muscles
   E. Causes acute tubular necrosis

Ans. is 'A' Most common in earthquakes and bombings; 'B' Causes acute glomerulonephritis; 'C' Release of myoglobin in blood;

'D' Occurs due to massive crushing of muscles; 'E' Causes acute tubular necrosis

2. Which of the following is not a component of the crush syndrome: *(AIIMS May 02)*
   A. Myohemoglobinuria B. Massive crushing of muscles
   C. Acute tubular necrosis D. Bleeding diathesis

Ans. is 'D' Bleeding diathesis

3. Crush syndrome is managed by: *(AIIMS Nov 1993)*
   A. 20% Dextrose B. Hydrocortisone
   C. Maintaining high urine output
   D. Acidification of urine

Ans. is 'C' Maintaining high urine output

PATHOLOGICAL FRACTURE

A fracture in an abnormal bone is referred to as pathological fracture. Vertebral bodies (thoracic and lumbar) are the most often affected bones followed by neck femur and lower end radius (Colle's fracture). **Most common cause is osteoporosis followed by metastasis. In India most common cause is nutritional.**

Important Points to be Remember

- Commonest local cause of pathological fractures is secondary to malignant lesion, most common site is **thoracic vertebrae**.
- Commonest generalized cause is osteoporosis site is again vertebral column.
- Pathological fracture in generalized disease usually heal in time.
- Pathological fracture in benign lesion usually heal but take longer time.
- Pathological fracture in infected/malignant lesion may not unite at all.

Mirel's Criteria for Risk of Pathological Fracture

- Mirel's developed a scoring system based on, the presence or absence of pain, and the size, location, and radiographic appearance of the lesion to quantify the risk of impending pathological fracture in **malignant lesion**.

	Number Assigned		
Variable	1	2	3
Site	Upper limb	Lower limb	Peritrochanteric
Pain	Mild	Moderate	Severe
Lesion	Blastic	Mixed	Lytic
Size	<1/3 diameter of bone	1/3–2/3	>2/3 diameter of bone

- So patients with maximum risk of pathological fracture are having lytic peritrochanteric lesion involving >2/3 diameter with severe pain.
- Patients with < 7 score are observed, but those with score > 8 should have prophylactic internal fixation.

Treatment

- When patient has sustained a true pathological fracture surgical stabilization with internal fixation is usually indicated.
- Because of poor bone quality, augmentation of fixation with bone grafting/bone cement may be necessary.
- Radiation therapy is also given for metastatic or malignant lesions.

MULTIPLE CHOICE QUESTIONS

1. Pathological fracture not found in: *(PGI Nov 2014)*
   A. Bone cyst B. Osteoporosis
   C. Chronic osteoyelitis D. Osteochondroma
   E. Osteogenesis imperfecta

Ans. is None

2. Most common cause of pathological fracture in India is:
   A. Paget's B. Sarcoidosis *(AI 2012)*
   C. Nutritional D. Steroids

Ans. is 'C' Nutritional

3. Mirel's criteria is developed for the evaluation of:
   A. Risk of fatigue fracture *(Jipmer 2000, AIIMS 92)*
   B. Severity of osteoporosis
   C. Risk of pathological fracture after metastasis
   D. Severity of neurological defect

Ans. is 'C' Risk of pathological fracture after metastasis

4. The commonest cause of pathological fracture is generalized affection is: *(UP 99, Jipmer 97, Bihar 90)*
   A. Carcinoma B. Osteoporosis
   C. Cyst D. All of the above

Ans. is 'B' Osteoporosis

6. The treatment of choice in pathological fractures is: *(Bihar 88)*
   A. Internal Fixation B. Plaster of Paris casts
   C. Skin traction D. External skeletal fixation

Ans. is 'A' Internal Fixation

STRESS/FATIGUE FRACTURE

Stress fracture is due to imbalance between load and resistance of bone. It is of 2 types:

1. **Fatigue Fracture:** caused by application of abnormal stress on normal bone.
2. **Insufficiency Fracture:** caused by normal activity on weak bone.

Sites of Stress Fractures

Lower Extremity

- **March fracture is a** stress fatigue fracture of second metatarsal neck > 3rd metatarsal neck.
- The most common site is metatarsal neck followed by tibia (proximal third in children, middle third in athlete and lower third in elderly).
- Femoral neck (inferomedial compression side in young and superior tension side in older patients).
- Rarely fibula lower end **(runners fracture).**

Upper Extremity

- Olecranon is most common site of upper limb stress fractures.

Pelvis and Spine

- Pars inter articularis of 5th lumbar vertebral (causing spondylolysis) is commonest in spine.

Clinical Presentation

- Load related pain often bilateral
- The hallmark physical finding is tenderness with palpation and stress.

Investigation

MRI provide excellent sensitivity and superior specificity compared to bone scan in differentiating from infections or tumors.

Bone scan is preferable for bilateral cases due to feasibility, also bilateral cases go in favor of stress fracture as compared to Infection or tumor and also can scan the whole body.

- Treatment is symptomatic with cast and cessation of activity.

Orthopedics Quick Review

MULTIPLE CHOICE QUESTIONS

1. Which part of 2nd metatarsal is involved in the march fracture? *(AIIMS May 2017)*
   - A. Head
   - B. Neck
   - C. Shaft
   - D. Base

   Ans. is 'B' Neck

2. Most common site of stress fracture. *(AIIMS May 2017, NEET DEC 2016)*
   - A. 2nd metacarpal
   - B. 2nd metatarsal
   - C. Fibula
   - D. Ribs

   Ans. is 'B' 2nd metatarsal

3. Investigation of choice in stress fracture:
   - A. MRI
   - B. CT   *(AIIMS May 2015)*
   - C. Bone scan
   - D. X-ray

   Ans. is 'A' MRI

4. Differential diagnosis of stress fracture: *(PGI 2006)*
   - A. Infection
   - B. Tumor
   - C. Neuropathic joints
   - D. Osteochondritis

   Ans. is 'A' Infection; 'B' Tumor

5. An army recruit, smoker and 6 months into training started complaining of pain at posteromedial aspect of both legs. There was acute point tenderness and the pain was aggravated on physical activity. The most likely diagnosis is: *(AI 2004)*
   - A. Buerger's disease
   - B. Gout
   - C. Lumbar canal stenosis
   - D. Stress fracture

   Ans. is 'D' Stress fracture

   - The hallmark physical finding is focal bone pain (tenderness) with palpation and stress. Also bilateral goes in favor of stress fracture.

6. What is March fracture? *(PGI June 2K, 99 Tamil Nadu 1993, Bihar 1989, NEET 2015, JIPMER 2014, 2010)*
   - A. Fracture of 2nd metatarsal
   - B. Fracture of 4th metatarsal
   - C. Fracture of cuboids
   - D. Fracture of tibia

   Ans. is 'A' Fracture of 2nd metatarsal

   - Most common site for march fracture is 2nd **metatarsal followed by 3rd metatarsal.**

7. Stress fracture is treated by: *(Delhi 1990)*
   - A. Rest
   - B. Cast immobilization
   - C. Closed reduction
   - D. Internal fixation

   Ans. is 'B' Cast immobilization

NON-UNION

- **Fracture not united at end of 9 months** and there is no progress in fracture healing in last 3 months is Non-union.
- Non-unions may be of two types—hypertrophic non-union (have viable ends and exuberant callus formation) and atrophic non-union (non-viable bone ends and no callus formation). As a generalization, those non-unions with better blood supply and some degree of micromotion at fracture site develop more callus, while those with either no motion, excess motion, or distraction and a less rich blood supply produce less callus.

Hypertrophic Non-union

1. Elephant's foot: Insecure fixation causing abundant callus
2. Horse's hoof: Les abundant Callus (as compared to Elephant's foot): Moderately unstable fracture
3. Oligotrophic: Minimal or no Callus but vascularized bone ends.

Atrophic non-union: Absence of Callus

- Torsion/wedge: Avascular intermediate fragment
- Comminuted: One or more avascular fragments
- Gap non-union: Loss of bone between the fracture ends.

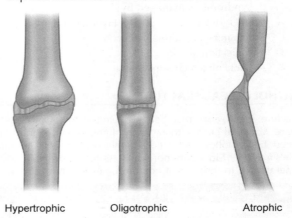

Hypertrophic   Oligotrophic   Atrophic

Fig. 5.8: Types of non-union

- Head injury, High Oxygen tension, high pH, stability, compression and intermittent shear force, micro-movements at fracture site and released from platelets favor callus formation. Hence enhance union.

Bone Union Depends on:

1. Age: Younger better
2. Type of bone: Cancellous better
3. Fracture type: **Spiral better than oblique which is better than transverse. Comminuted heal slowest.**
4. Soft tissue interposition or disturbed vascularity is inhibitory
5. Reduction
6. Immobilization helps union (Micromovements enhance union)
7. Closed fractures heal better
8. Compression at fracture site enhances union

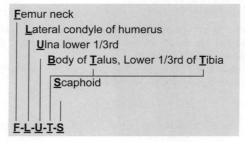

Fractures known for non-union: "FLUTS"

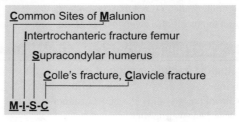

Fractures known for malunion: "MISC"

NON-UNION OR DELAYED UNION—5 PRINCIPLES OF TREATMENT

A.
1. Open Reduction
2. Freshen Margins of fracture ends
3. Bone graft
4. Stable fixation
5. Postoperative splint

B. **Infected non-unions**
1. If no gap – External fixator + Bone graft
2. If gap then ilizarov fixator + bone grafting
3. For infected non-union of tibia with very big gap
   i. Tibialization of fibula: Huntingtons procedure (Fibula fills the gap in tibia)
   ii. Non-vascularized fibular graft
   iii. Vascularized fibular transfer

C. **Recent advances:** Bone Morphogenic proteins are Growth factors in transforming growth factor B (TGF-B). They cause osteoinduction which is dose dependent. In fractures they enhance fracture healing and they are also used for spinal fusion.

Note: Hypertrophic Non-union is treated by stabilization of fracture ends.

Complications of Fracture

Immediate Complications	Early Complications	Delayed Complications
1. Hypovolemic shock	1. Hypovolemic shock	1 **Problems of union**
2. Injury to major vessels and nerves	2. ARDS	– Delayed union
3. Injury to muscles and tendons	3. Fat embolism syndrome	– Non-union
4. Injury to joints	4. DVT and Pulmonary embolism	– Malunion
5. Injury to viscera	5. Aseptic traumatic fever	2. Avascular necrosis
6. Gas gangrene	6. Septicemia (in open fracture)	3. Shortening
	7. Crush syndrome	4. **Joint stiffness**
	8. **Infection**	5. Sudeck's dystrophy (Reflex Sympathetic Dystrophy)
	9. **Compartment syndrome**	6. Osteomyelitis
		7. Ischemic contracture
		8. Myositis ossificans
		9. Osteoarthritis

MULTIPLE CHOICE QUESTIONS

1. Hypertrophic non-union following a fracture, most appropriate treatment would be: *(AI 2016)*
   A. Stabilization
   B. Bone grafting
   C. Stabilization and bone grafting
   D. None of the above

   Ans. is 'A' Stabilization

2. Following are immediate complications of fracture: *(PGI May 2015)*
   A. Vascular ischemia   B. Neuronal injury
   C. Malunion   D. Compartment syndrome
   E. Avascular necrosis

   Ans. is 'A' Vascular ischemia and 'B' Neuronal injury

3. Which of the following cause malunion except? *(PGI May 2015)*
   A. Open fracture   B. Infection
   C. Bone grafting   D. Soft tissue interposition
   E. Proper alignment of fracture

   Ans. is 'C' Bone grafting and 'E' Proper alignment of fracture

4. True about fracture healing except: *(NEET Pattern 2012)*
   A. Nutrition affects healing
   B. Stable fixation promotes healing
   C. Compression at fracture site causes non-union
   D. Hormonal status may affect healing

   Ans. is 'C' Compression at fracture site causes non-union
   – Compression at fracture site increases union

5. Fracture healing is affected by all except: *(NEET Pattern 2012)*
   A. Osteoporosis   B. Infection
   C. Poor blood supply   D. Soft tissue interposition

   Ans. is 'A' Osteoporosis

6. Factors affecting bone healing are all except: *(NEET Pattern 2012)*
   A. Age   B. Sex
   C. Vascularity   D. Comminution

   Ans. is 'B' Sex

7. The time necessary for healing of fracture depends on the following factors: *(UP 98, NB 1989, Rohtak 89)*
   A. Age of the patient   B. Location of the fracture
   C. Type of the fracture
   D. Degree of damage to soft tissues
   E. All of the above

   Ans. is 'E' All of the above

8. All of the following factors facilitate non-union except: *(AI 1997, Bihar 1990)*
   A. Hematoma formation
   B. Periosteal injuries
   C. Absence of nerve supply   D. Chronic infection

   Ans. is 'A' Hematoma formation
   – A hematoma enhances fracture healing it is the first stage of fracture healing

9. Delayed union of fracture of a bone following a surgical treatment may be due to: *(NB 1990)*
   A. Infection   B. Inadequate circulation
   C. Inadequate mobilization   D. All of the above

   Ans. is 'D' All of the above

Chapter 6: Advanced Trauma Life Support

SEQUENCE OF EVENTS ACCORDING TO ATLS (ADVANCED TRAUMA LIFE SUPPORT)

Management of Polytrauma Patients/Life Threatening Conditions

- The assessment of severely injured patient consists of four overlapping phases:
    1. Rapid primary evaluation
    2. Restoration of vital functions
    3. Detailed secondary evaluation and
    4. Definitive care

Prehospital phase:
 − Airway maintenance
 − Control of external bleeding and shock
 − Immobilization of the patient
 − Immediate transport to closest appropriate facility

Hospital phase:
 − Triage
 − Primary survey (ABCDEF)

A. **Airway maintenance with cervical spine protection:**
    1. The finding of non-purposeful motor responses strongly suggests the need for definitive airway management.
    2. Assume a cervical spine injury in any patient with multisystem trauma, especially those with altered level of consciousness or blunt injury above the clavicle.
    3. Open the airway by Chin lift or Jaw thrust maneuver.

B. **Breathing and ventilation:**
    Tension pneumothorax, flail chest with pulmonary contusion, massive hemothorax and open pneumothorax must be detected in primary survey.

C. **Circulation with hemorrhage control:**
    Major areas of occult blood loss are the chest, abdomen, retroperitoneum, pelvis and long bones. They should be carefully handled.

D. **Disability: Neurological status (GCS especially the best motor response)**

E. **Exposure/Environmental control: Prevent Hypothermia**

F. **Fracture splintage-Rule of splintage:** The joints above and below the fracture should be immobilized.

 − Consider need for patient transfer
 − Secondary survey (head to toe evaluation and patient history): only after vital functions are normalized
 − Continued postresuscitation monitoring and re-evaluation
 − Definitive care.

SOME SALIENT POINTS REGARDING CERVICAL SPINE INJURY

- Patients with maxillofacial or head trauma should be presumed to have an unstable cervical spine injury and the neck should be immobilized until an injury has been excluded. The absence of neurological deficit does not exclude injury to cervical spine.
- Patients who are wearing helmet and require airway management: one person provides manual in line stabilization (MILS) from below, while the second person expands the helmet laterally and removes it.
- A normal lateral cervical spine film does not exclude the possibility of cervical-spine injury.
- Cervical spine stabilization should be done and then airway maintenance should be carried out.

```
Airway maintenance with cervical spine stabilization
                    │
                Breathing
                    │
               Circulation
```

Please note that order of resuscitation according to ATLS is A–B–C and according to ACLS is C–A–B.

MULTIPLE CHOICE QUESTIONS

1. While attending to a victim of RTA, who is otherwise conscious, all the following can be done except?
    (AIIMS Nov 2017)
    A. Roll the patient making sure there is no movement of the spine on to a hard board
    B. Strap the patients head thorax & pelvis to a flat hard board in supine position
    C. Turn the patient to one side
    D. Assess the patient by asking his name

Ans. is 'C' Turn the patient to one side

All resuscitations of a polytraumatized patient should be performed using Advanced trauma life support (ATLS) guidelines. Assessment of the patient is performed using a stepwise longitudinal approach. Spine must be immobilized appropriately before starting the resuscitation protocol.

Primary survey: Airway (with cervical spine protection first), Breathing, Circulation are assessed.

The goal is to immediately provide the patent airway while maintaining a manual in line stabilization of spinal cord.

Airway
- Ask the patient any question, e.g. Ask his name, ask how he/she is feeling. If the patient responds verbally, means he/she has an intact airway, is breathing, is thinking. Also the patient's level of consciousness can be briefly assessed (OPTION D CORRECT).

- If the patient is unresponsive, check airway patency by looking at patients chest. Look for chest expansion, listen and feel for air movement. If doubtful airway patency can be maintained using jaw thrust (head tilt/chin lift maneuver only if cervical spine injury has been ruled out). Because the most common cause of airway obstruction is base of tongue falling backward into the posterior pharynx. Jaw thrust will uplift the tongue and relieve the obstruction.
- Definitive Airway management achieves 3 Ps: Airway patency, aspiration protection and positive pressure ventilation.
- Intubation is the criterion standard of airway management: Orotracheal/Nasotracheal intubation.
- Surgical airway: Circothyrodotomy is usually a last resort when intubation is unsuccessful.

The spine should be protected immediately at all times during the management of the multiply injured patient. This may be achieved manually (Manual in line stabilization) or with a combination of semi-rigid cervical collar, side head supports for head immobilization and strapping and using a spine board. Strapping for stabilization should be applied to the shoulders/Thorax and pelvis as well as the Head to prevent the neck becoming the centre of rotation of the body (OPTION B CORRECT)

The ideal position is with the spine immobilized in a neutral position on a firm surface/hard board. If the neck is not in the neutral position, proper immobilization is achieved with the patient in neutral position, such that no rotation/bending of spinal column should be allowed. If the patient is awake and conscious/cooperative/neurologically normal, as mentioned in the question, they should actively move their neck into line, because these are unlikely to have acute cervical spine injury. If unconscious, this is done passively.

Patient should be LOG ROLLED, when moving to and fro from the hard board. The Four person log roll is the standard maneuver to allow examination of the back and transfer on and off back boards. Neutral anatomic alignment of the entire vertebral column must be maintained while rolling and lifting the patient. (OPTION A CORRECT).

Hence option C becomes an incorrect choice... Considering, the patient can be a suspected spine injury patient hence should be least mobilized.

Imaging

When available, all such patients should undergo Multi-detector axial CT. CT is the most sensitive imaging modality to evaluate spine injury/fractures.

2. A female child with abuse has fracture pelvis, multiple injuries and is bleeding the immediate step on presentation to the hospital is: *(AIIMS Nov 2014)*
   A. Blood transfusion   B. Airway assessment
   C. Inform the police   D. Splint

Ans. is 'B' Airway assessment

3. A victim of road traffic accident with fracture shaft femur first line of management: *(AIIMS May 2014)*
   A. Splint   B. IV fluids
   C. Airway maintenance D. Breathing

Ans. is 'C' Airway maintenance

4. The correct order of priorities in the initial management of road traffic accident patient is: *(AI 99, 92)*
   A. Airway, Breathing, Circulation, treatment of extracranial injuries
   B. Treatment of extracranial injuries Airway, Breathing, Circulation
   C. Circulation, Airway, Breathing, treatment of extracranial injuries
   D. Airway, circulation, breathing treatment of extracranial injuries

Ans. is 'A' Airway, Breathing, Circulation, treatment of extracranial injuries

5. In an injury with multiple fractures, most important is: *(JIPMER 99, DELHI 1998, PGI 94, PGI 86)*
   A. Airway maintenance
   B. Blood transfusion
   C. Intravenous fluids
   D. Open reduction of fractures

Ans. is 'A' Airway maintenance
   – Airway management is the first priority in trauma patients.

6. Severely injured patient with Cervical spinal fracture and unconsciousness first thing to be done is: *(AIIMS 95)*
   A. GCS scoring
   B. Cervical spine stabilization
   C. Mannitol drip to decrease ICT
   D. Airway maintenance

Ans. is 'B' Cervical spine stabilization
   – Cervical spine stabilization is very important while maintaining airway and if we have to choose one than cervical spine stabilization is done first then only airway has to be secured.

CHAPTER 7: Upper Limb Traumatology

SHOULDER ANATOMY

Normal function of the shoulder is a balance between mobility and stability. The bony anatomy contributes little to stability and has been compared with a golf ball on a tee. The bony anatomy of the shoulder joint does not provide inherent stability. The glenoid fossa is a flattened, dishlike structure. **Only one fourth of the large humeral head articulates with the glenoid at any given time.** The glenoid is encircled by the labrum, a dense fibrocartilaginous tissue, which increases the depth of the socket by 50% around the humeral head and increases stability.

Humeral head is rotated 15–20° posteriorly in relation to the shaft. (Retroversion)

Integral to the glenoid labrum is the insertion of the tendon of the long head of the biceps, which inserts on the superior aspect of the joint and blends to become indistinguishable from the posterior glenoid labrum.

Four rotator cuff muscles are—supraspinatus, infraspinatus, subscapularis and teres minor.

They are dynamic stabilisers of shoulder. Their impingement causes painful arc syndrome.

> **S**upraspinatus (Most commonly damaged)
> **I**nfraspinatus
> **T**eres minor
> **S**ubscapularis (Forgotten tendon)
> **SITS**

The tendon of rotator cuff muscles blend with the joint capsule and form a musculotendinous collar that surrounds the posterior, superior, and anterior aspect of gleno-humeral joint. **The inferior part of shoulder joint capsule is the weakest area.**

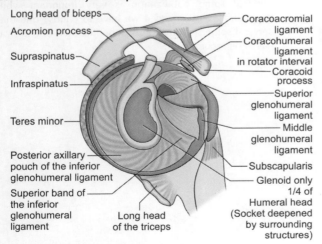

Fig. 7.1: Anatomy of shoulder

The tendon of the **long head of biceps brachii muscle passes superiorly through the joint** and restricts upward movement of humeral head on glenoid cavity.

Rotator interval is interval between leading edge of supraspinatus and superior edge of subscapularis. Coracohumeral ligament passes within rotator interval.

The **Quadrangular space (Quadrilateral space, foramen of Velpeau) contains axillary nerve and posterior circumflex humeral artery and vein.**

2 triangular spaces
- Upper: Circumflex scapular vessels
- Lower: Radial nerve and profunda brachii artery.

Lift Off Test (Gerber's test)

Lift off test is done to assess the strength of **subscapularis muscle** and detect a rupture of the subscapularis tendon. Subscapularis functions primarily as an internal rotator of the shoulder. The test is performed with the arm extended and internally rotated such that the dorsum of the hand rests against the lower back. Subscapularis is maximally active in this position. Patient is then instructed to lift his/her hand off the back (Lift-off) (Attempting further internal rotation). If the patient is able to lift the dorsum of the hand off the back the subscapularis tendon is intact and the test is considered negative.

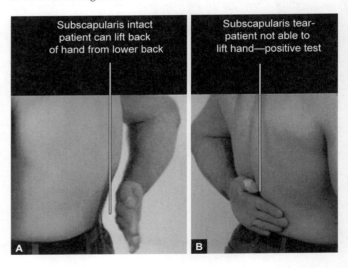

Figs. 7.2A and B: Lift off test

If the patient is not able to lift the dorsum of the hand off the back the subscapularis tendon is torn and the test is considered positive.

Flowchart 7.1: Rotator cuff tear

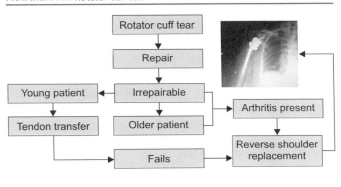

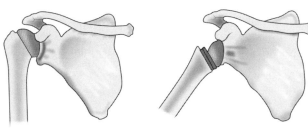

Fig. 7.3: Types of shoulder replacement

Shoulder replacement is carried out for shoulder arthritis and reverse shoulder replacement is carried out in patients with deltoid dysfunction or rotator cuff arthropathy.

Lesions Associated with Recurrent Dislocation

In 1938, Bankart published his classic paper in which he recognized two types of acute dislocations. In the first type, the humeral head is forced through the capsule where it is the weakest, generally anteriorly and inferiorly in the interval between the lower border of the subscapularis and the long head of the triceps muscle. In the second type, the humeral head is forced anteriorly out of the glenoid cavity and tears not only the fibrocartilaginous labrum from almost the entire anterior half of the rim of the glenoid cavity, but also the capsule and periosteum from the **anterior surface of the neck** of the scapula. This traumatic detachment of the glenoid labrum has been called the Bankart lesion. Most authors agree that the Bankart lesion is the most commonly observed pathological lesion in recurrent subluxation or dislocation of the shoulder.

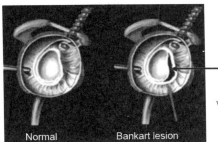

Fig. 7.4: Bankart lesion

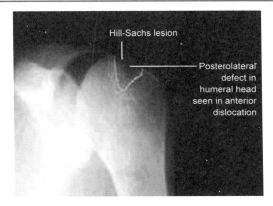

Fig. 7.5: Hill-Sachs lesion

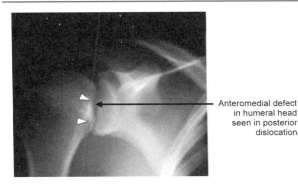

Fig. 7.6: Reverse Hill-Sachs lesion

A humeral head impaction fracture can be produced as the shoulder is dislocated anteriorly, and the humeral head is impacted against the rim of the glenoid at the time of dislocation. **This Hill-Sachs lesion is a defect in the posterolateral aspect of the humeral head.** If these lesions involve more than 20% of the glenoid, they can result in recurrent instability despite having an excellent soft-tissue repair. They are also called as impression fractures.

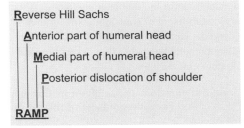

MULTIPLE CHOICE QUESTIONS

1. Shoulder flexion is done by: *(DNB JUNE 2017)*
   A. Posterior fibres of deltoid B. Pectoralis major
   C. Pectoralis minor D. Latissimus dorsi

Ans. is 'B' Pectoralis major

2. Bankart's lesion is seen in: *(AI 2016)*
   A. Recurrent anterior shoulder dislocation
   B. Posterior shoulder dislocation
   C. Rotator cuff tear
   D. Interior shoulder dislocation

Ans. is 'A' Recurrent anterior shoulder dislocation

3. What is the normal orientation of humeral head?
(CET July 16)
   A. Retroversion of 80 degrees
   B. Retroversion of 30 degrees
   C. Anteversion of 15 degrees
   D. Anteversion of 50 degrees

Ans. is 'B' Retroversion of 30 degrees

4. Which of the following structure passes through the quadrangular space? (AI Dec 15)
   A. Axillary nerve
   B. Radial nerve
   C. Median nerve
   D. Brachial artery

Ans. is 'A' Axillary nerve

5. The posterolateral lesion in the head of humerus in cases of recurrent anterior shoulder dislocation is:
   A. Bankart's lesion (DNB July 2017, JIPMER 2014)
   B. Hill-Sachs lesion
   C. Reverse Hill-Sachs lesion
   D. Greater tuberosity avulsion fracture

Ans. 'B' Hill-Sachs lesion

6. A 42-year-old man is diagnosed to have irreparable tear of the rotator cuff. Treatment of choice will be:
   A. Tendon transfer (AIIMS May 2015)
   B. Total Shoulder replacement
   C. Reverse shoulder replacement
   D. Acromioplasty

Ans is 'A' Tendon transfer

7. Bankart's lesion involves the—of the glenoid labrum:
(AIIMS May 2014) (AIIMS Nov 2006, 2K, May 1993, UP 2K)
   A. Anterior lip
   B. Superior lip
   C. Antero-superior lip
   D. Antero-inferior lip

Ans. is 'A' Anterior lip

8. Avulsion of capsulolabral complex is seen from which part of glenoid in bankarts lesion? (DNB JUNE 2017)
   A. Anteroinferior
   B. Posteroinferior
   C. Anterosuperior
   D. Posterosuperior

Ans. is 'A' Anteroinferior
Please note Anterior lip is a better answer.

9. Dynamic stabilisers of shoulder joint: (AIIMS Nov 2013)
   A. Glenoidal labrum
   B. Rotator cuff muscles
   C. Glenohumeral ligament
   D. Coracohumeral ligament

Ans. is 'B' Rotator cuff muscles

10. For long the muscle was not given its due importance and was called Forgotten muscle of rotator cuff which one is it? (AIIMS May 2013)
    A. Subscapularis
    B. Supraspinatus
    C. Infraspinatus
    D. Teres minor

Ans. is 'A' Subscapularis

11. Most common muscle damaged in rotator cuff:
(NEET Pattern 2016, 2012)
    A. Supraspinatus
    B. Infraspinatus
    C. Subscapularis
    D. Teres minor

Ans. is 'A' Supraspinatus

12. Painful arc syndrome is caused by impingement of:
(NEET Pattern 2013)
    A. Subacromial bursa
    B. Subdeltoid bursa
    C. Rotator cuff tendon
    D. Biceps tendon

Ans. is 'C' Rotator cuff tendon

13. Rotator cuff muscle all are true except:
    A. Supraspinatus
    B. Subscapularis
    C. Infraspinatus
    D. Teres major

Ans. is 'D' Teres major

14. Lift off test is done for: (AIIMS May 2012, AIPG 2010)
    A. Supraspinatus
    B. Infraspinatus
    C. Teres minor
    D. Subscapularis

Ans. is 'D' Subscapularis

15. Rotator interval is between:
(MAHE 2005, AIIMS 06, JIPMER 02)
    A. Supraspinatus and teres minor
    B. Teres major and teres minor
    C. Supraspinatus and subscapularis
    D. Subscapularis and infraspinatus

Ans. is 'C' Supraspinatus and subcapsularis
   – Rotator interval is a triangular portion of shoulder capsule which lies between **supraspinatus and subscapularis tendon and coracohumeral ligament passes through it.**

16. Muscle crossing through the shoulder joint is:
(NIMHANS 98, PGI 95)
    A. Biceps short head
    B. Biceps long head
    C. Triceps long head
    D. Coracobrachialis

Ans. is 'B' Biceps long head
   – Long head of biceps goes through the shoulder joint

17. Weakest portion of shoulder joint capsule is:
(PGI 93, AI 92, AIIMS 90)
    A. Anterior
    B. Posterior
    C. Inferior
    D. Superior

Ans. is 'C' Inferior
Shoulder is weakest inferiorly but dislocates anteriorly because it is the direction of force that decides the dislocation but never the anatomical weakness for a particular joint, e.g. the force that causes anterior dislocation (Abduction and external rotation) is much more common as in throwing objects like ball or javelin as compared to force that causes inferior dislocation.

18. Hill-Sachs lesion in recurrent shoulder dislocation is:
(NEET 2016, AIIMS 1992) (JIPMER 1992)
    A. Injury to humeral head
    B. Rupture of tendon of supraspinatus muscle
    C. Avulsion of glenoid labrum
    D. None of the above

Ans. is 'A' Injury to humeral head

MODE OF INJURY CAUSING SHOULDER DISLOCATION

- *Anterior dislocation:* **Abduction and External rotation force**
- *Posterior dislocation:* Indirect force producing marked internal rotation and adduction
- *Inferior dislocation:* Severe hyperabduction force
  Position of arm in shoulder dislocation
  1. Anterior Dislocation (**Subcoracoid** > Preglenoid > Subclavicular type)
     Slight abduction and external rotation
  2. Posterior Dislocation
     Difficult to diagnose because the patient may have normal contour of shoulder. Holds injured shoulder in internal rotation and examiner cannot externally rotate it
  3. Inferior Dislocation (Luxatio erecta/Subglenoid)
     Locked in full abduction, fixed by the side of head.

Anterior Dislocation of Shoulder—Most Common Type of Shoulder Dislocation

Mechanism of Injury: Abduction and External rotation force.

Types: Subcoracoid > Preglenoid > Subclavicular

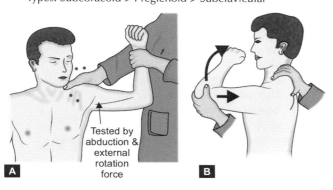

Figs. 7.7A and B: (A) Anterior instability; (B) Posterior instability

Clinical Features

- Patient keeps his arm slightly abducted.
- Normal round contour of shoulder is lost and it becomes flat.
- **Bryant's test:** Anterior axillary fold is at lower level.
- **Dugas test:** It is not possible for the patient to bring the elbow close to the body and touch the tip of opposite shoulder.
- **Callaway's test:** Vertical circumference of axilla is increased as compared to the normal side.
- **Hamilton ruler test:** Because of flattening of shoulder, it is possible to place a ruler on the lateral side of arm and it touches acromion and lateral condyle of humerus simultaneously (in normal it would not due to shoulder contour).

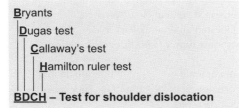

BDCH – Test for shoulder dislocation

- A-P X-ray show overlapping shadow of humeral head and glenoid fossa; and lateral view show humeral head out of line with the socket.

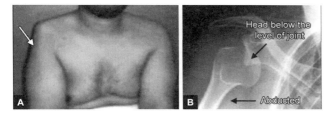

Figs. 7.8A and B: Shoulder dislocation (A) Lost contour of shoulder; (B) Abducted arm in anterior shoulder dislocation

Management

- Commonly used reduction techniques are Stimson's gravity method, Hippocratic method and Kocher's method.

Kocher's method
Stimson's gravity method
Hippocratic method

KSH – Maneuver for reduction of anterior dislocation

- Kochers method is done by traction in slight abduction and external rotation to increase deformity required to unlock the surfaces followed by adduction and internal rotation. Post reduction there is positioning of the limb in adduction and internal rotation called as chest arm bandage x 3 weeks.

"Most common early complication of anterior dislocation of shoulder is nerve injury"

Most commonly injured nerve in anterior dislocation of shoulder is circumflex branch of axillary nerve. The injury to nerve is usually neuropraxia.

Inferior dislocation also axillary nerve involvement is the commonest.

Other Nerves Rarely Involved:
- Musculocutaneous nerve
- Radial nerve
- Avulsion of brachial plexus

Recurrent dislocation is most common in shoulder joint, accounting for nearly 50% of all dislocations. Most commonly it is subcoracoid type. Second common joint for recurrent dislocation is patella and rarest joint to dislocate is ankle:

- Matsen's classification system is useful to differentiate recurrent and non-recurrent dislocations.

Differences between recurrent and non-recurrent anterior dislocation

Feature	Recurrent	Non-recurrent (Post-traumatic-acute)
Bankarts lesion	Common	Uncommon
Hill-Sachs lesion	Common	Uncommon
Lax capsule	Common	Uncommon
Rupture of anterior capsule	Uncommon	Common
Associated Injuries (Nerve injury Rotator cuff injury/Fractures)	Rare	Common

TUBS VS AMBRII

Matsen's classification for recurrent instability of shoulder.

TUBS	AMBRII
T: Traumatic	A: Atraumatic
U: Unidirectional	M: Multidirectional
B: Bankart's	B: Bilateral
S: Surgery	R: Rehabilitation
	I: Inferior capsular shift procedure
	I: Internal closure

Surgeries for recurrent dislocation of shoulder:

1. *Bankart's operation:* Detached anterior structures are attached to the rim of the-glenoid cavity with suture.

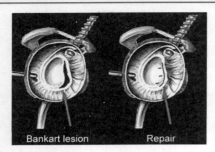

Fig. 7.9: Bankart's repair

2. *Putti Platt's operations:* Subscapularis tendon and capsule is overlapped and tightened.

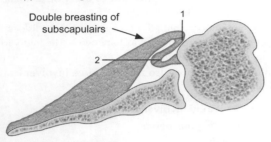

Fig. 7.10: Putti Platt's operation

3. *Laterjet Bristow's operation:* Transplantation of coracoid process with its attachments to the anterior rim of glenoid.
4. Neers capsular shift for multidirectional instability.
5. In failed reconstructions, glenoid deficiency may be treated with the Laterjet procedure or iliac crest bone graft.
6. Neglected shoulder dislocation—surgically managed.

MULTIPLE CHOICE QUESTIONS

1. Kocher manoeuver is used for: (NEET DEC 2016)
   A. Shoulder reduction   B. Elbow reduction
   C. Ankle dislocation   D. Knee dislocation
Ans. is 'A' Shoulder reduction

2. Most common joint to be dislocated in the body is:
   A. Shoulder   B. Hip (NEET DEC 2016)
   C. Elbow   D. Knee
Ans. is 'A' Shoulder

3. What is the most common sequelae of traumatic shoulder dislocation in young adults? (AIIMS Nov 2017)
   A. Frozen shoulder
   B. Recurrent shoulder dislocation
   C. Normal shoulder healing and movements
   D. Subscapular tendinitis
Ans. is 'B' Recurrent shoulder dislocation

4. Shoulder dislocation false is: (AI 2016)
   A. Most common early complication of anterior dislocation shoulder is nerve injury
   B. Hill Sachs is seen in recurrent anterior shoulder dislocation
   C. Rotator cuff injury is a common cause of recurrent dislocation
   D. Posterior dislocation presents with difficulty in external rotation of shoulder
Ans. is 'C' Rotator cuff injury is a common cause of recurrent dislocation

5. Putti Platt's operation involves tightening of which muscle? (AI 2016)
   A. Supraspinatus   B. Subscapularis
   C. Infraspinatus   D. Deltoid
Ans. is 'B' Subscapularis

6. Which of the following is true about anterior shoulder dislocation? (CET July 16)
   A. It is most common type of shoulder dislocation
   B. It is most commonly subclavicular
   C. Patient keeps his arm in saluting position
   D. Injury to brachial plexus may occur
Ans. is 'A' It is most common type of shoulder dislocation

7. Hamilton Ruler test sign is positive in which of the above mentioned conditions? (AI Dec 15)
   A. Anterior dislocation of shoulder
   B. Acromioclavivular joint dislocation
   C. Posterior dislocation of shoulder
   D. Luxatio erecta
Ans. is 'A' Anterior dislocation of shoulder

8. Following Defect (lesion) is NOT responsible for recurrent anterior dislocation of shoulder: (Maharashtra PG 2016)
   A. Bankart's lesion
   B. Hill-Sachs lesion
   C. Bristow's lesion
   D. A defect in the anterior-inferior capsule
Ans. is 'C' Bristow's lesion

9. All are seen in anterior shoulder dislocation except:
   A. Elevated anterior axillary fold (TN 2014)
   B. Duga's positive
   C. Hamilton Ruler positive
   D. Increased vertical circumference
Ans. is 'A' Elevated anterior axillary fold

10. Commonest type of shoulder dislocation: (NEET Pattern 2013 PGI 87)
    A. Subcoracoid   B. Subglenoid
    C. Posterior   D. Subclavicular
Ans. is 'A' Subcoracoid

11. Uncomplicated shoulder dislocation most commonly occurs in the following direction: (NEET Pattern 2012)
    A. Anterior   B. Posterior
    C. Superior   D. Medially
Ans. is 'A' Anterior

12. Nerve injured in anterior dislocation of shoulder: (NEET Pattern Dec 2016, 2012)
    A. Radial   B. Axillary
    C. Long thoracic   D. Median
Ans. is 'B' Axillary

13. Neglected shoulder dislocation in a young labourer is: (NEET Pattern 2012)
    A. Medically managed   B. Surgically managed
    C. Neglected   D. Counselled
Ans. is 'B' Surgically managed

14. In Recurrent Anterior dislocation of shoulder, the movements that causes dislocation is:
    (AIIMS Nov 2011, Andhra 99,94, KA 97, AI 1989)

A. Flexion and internal rotation
B. Abduction and external rotation
C. Abduction and internal rotation
D. Extension

Ans. is 'B' Abduction and external rotation

15. Recurrent dislocations are least commonly seen in:
    A. Ankle   B. Hip   (AI 2009, Delhi 94)
    C. Shoulder   D. Patella

Ans. is 'A' Ankle

16. All are related to recurrent shoulder dislocation except:
    (AIIMS May 2006, TN 2000, KA 98, UP 02, Karnataka 89)
    A. Hill sachs defect   B. Bankart lesion
    C. Lax capsule   D. Rotator cuff injury

Ans. is 'D' Rotator cuff injury

17. Traumatic glenohumeral instability in one direction with Bankarts lesion are treated by: (NIMHANS 2003)
    A. Conservative methods   B. Surgery
    C. Rehabilitation   D. Inferior capsule shift

Ans. is 'B' Surgery

– Treatment of traumatic unidirectional instability— Surgery.
– Treatment of non-traumatic multidirectional instability —* Rehabilitation.

18. Following anterior dislocation of the shoulder, a patient develops weakness of flexion at elbow and lack of sensation over the lateral aspect forearm; nerve injured is: (AI 2001)
    A. Radial nerve   B. Musculocutaneous nerve
    C. Axillary nerve   D. Ulnar nerve

Ans. is 'B' Musculocutaneous nerve

– The most common complication of anterior dislocation of shoulder is axillary (circumflex) nerve injury.
– There is consequent paralysis of the deltoid muscle, with a *small area of anaesthesia at the lateral aspect of the upper arm.*
– However, in this question the sensation are lost on lateral aspect of forearm (not arm). Lateral side of forearm has sensory supply from lateral cutaneous nerve of forearm, a branch of *musculocutaneous nerve.* Musculocutaneous nerve also supplies the biceps brachii (a flexor of elbow joint).
– Therefore, musculocutaneous nerve injury will cause sensory loss over lateral aspect of the forearm with weakness of flexion at elbow.

INFERIOR DISLOCATION OF SHOULDER

Inferior (Downward/subglenoid) dislocation of shoulder is known as luxatio erecta. It is caused by severe hyper abduction force. With the humerus as the lever and acromian as fulcrum, the humeral head is lifted across the inferior rim of glenoid socket and pokes into axilla (subglenoid position). The patient comes with his forearm resting on head. Potentially serious consequences, e.g. neurovascular damage is quite common. (Axillary nerve injured).

• Reduced by pulling upwards in the line of abducted arm with counter traction downwards.

It is usually indicative of hyperlaxity syndrome and usually such patients have multidirectional instability.

MULTIPLE CHOICE QUESTIONS

1. Nerve injured inferior dislocation of shoulder:
   A. Radial nerve   (NEET Pattern 2012)
   B. Axillary nerve
   C. Posterior cord of brachial plexus
   D. Ulnar nerve

Ans. is 'B' Axillary nerve

2. Luxatio erecta: (NEET 2016, TN 98)
   A. Tear of the glenoid labrum
   B. Inferior dislocation of shoulder
   C. Anterior dislocation of shoulder
   D. Defect in the humeral head

Ans. is 'B' Inferior dislocation of shoulder

POSTERIOR DISLOCATION OF SHOULDER—OFTEN MISSED CLINICALLY

Mechanism of Injury Indirect force producing marked internal rotation and adduction, <u>most commonly during a fit, convulsion or an electric shock.</u>

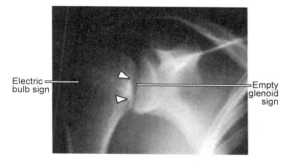

Fig. 7.11: X-ray: posterior dislocation

Clinical presentation often missed clinically. The classical clinical feature is **arm is held in medial rotation** and is locked in that position, and an examiner cannot externally rotate it.

Investigation Reliance is placed on a single A-P X-ray which may look almost normal. In A-P X-ray because of medial rotation head looks abnormal **(electric bulb sign)** and it stands away some what from glenoid fossa **(empty glenoid sign)**. Reverse Hill Sach's Lesion may be seen.

McLaughlin procedure is done for recurrent posterior shoulder dislocation with reverse Hill Sachs lesion.

MULTIPLE CHOICE QUESTIONS

1. Light bulb sign is seen in: (JIPMER 2014)
   A. Anterior dislocation of shoulder
   B. Posterior dislocation of shoulder
   C. Fracture acromion
   D. Clavicular fracture

Ans. 'B' Posterior dislocation of shoulder

2. 40-year-old male who was unconscious and presented with Bilateral Adduction and internal rotation of shoulder: (AIIMS Nov 2012)
   A. Anterior dislocation   B. Posterior dislocation
   C. Cleidocranial dislocation   D. Brachial plexus injury

Ans. is 'B' Posterior dislocation

3. In posterior dislocation of shoulder Hill Sach lesion is seen in: *(AI 2012)*
   A. Anterior
   B. Anteromedial
   C. Posterior
   D. Posteromedial

Ans. is 'B' Anteromedial

4. Which is true about shoulder dislocation? *(MAHE 2003, TN 98)*
   A. Anterior dislocation is more common than posterior
   B. Fixed medial rotation in posterior dislocation
   C. Kocher's maneuver is effective in anterior dislocation
   D. All of the above

Ans. is 'D' All of the above

5. Which is true regarding shoulder dislocation? *(SGPGI 2002, NIMHANS 99)*
   A. Posterior dislocation is often over-looked
   B. Pain is severe in anterior dislocation
   C. Radiography may be misleading in posterior dislocation
   D. All of the above

Ans. is 'D' All of the above

TEST FOR EVALUATION OF GLENOHUMERAL JOINT INSTABILITY IN RECURRENT DISLOCATION

Anterior Instability

1. **Anterior Apprehension Tests**
   In general these maneuver mimics the positioning of subluxation or dislocation, application of anterior directed force to the humeral head from the back or abduction and external rotation of arm results in patients apprehension that the joint will dislocate. And the patient does not allow the test to be performed.

   Variations include:
   - Fulcrum test
   - Crank test
   - Surprise test (most accurate)
   - Jobe relocation test

2. **Posterior Instability (Adduction and internal rotation force)**
   - Jerk (provocative) test
   - Posterior apprehension test
   - Posterior clunk test
   - Push-Pull test

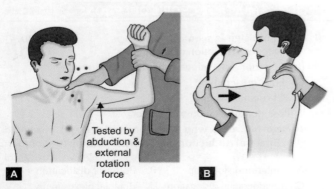

Figs. 7.12A and B: (A) Anterior instability; (B) Jerk test (Posterior instability)

3. Inferior Instability Test and Sign (Indicative of Multidirectional instability)-Sulcus Test

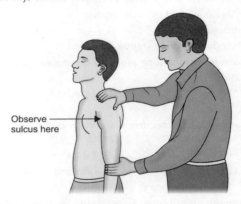

Fig. 7.13: Sulcus test (Multidirectional instability) or inferior instability

MULTIPLE CHOICE QUESTIONS

1. Which of the following is test of posterior glenohumeral instability? *(JIPMER May 2016, AIIMS May 10, 09)*
   A. Fulcrum
   B. Sulcus test
   C. Jerk test
   D. Crank test

Ans. is 'C' Jerk test

2. A 6-year-old boy has a history of recurrent dislocation of the right shoulder. On examination, the orthopedician puts the patient in the supine position and abducts his arm to 90° with the bed as the fulcrum and then externally rotates it but the boy does not allow the test to be performed. The test done by the orthopedician is: *(AIIMS May 2001)*
   A. Apprehension test
   B. Sulcus test
   C. Dugas test
   D. McMurray's test

Ans. is 'A' Apprehension test

FRACTURE AROUND SHOULDER AND ARM

Clavicle Fracture

1. Mechanism of Injury. Fall on shoulder or outstretched hand
2. The weakest point of midclavicle is the junction of middle and outer third (i.e. medial 2/3rd and lateral 1/3rd).
3. Clavicle fractures are classified by the location of the fracture in the proximal, central, or distal third of the bone. **Eighty percent of clavicle fractures occur in the middle third**, and most of these are amenable to closed management.
4. Clavicle is the most common fractured bone (over all) in adults and during birth.
5. Clavicle is the 4th common fractured bone in children after distal radius and ulna; hand injuries; elbow injuries in order of priority.
6. Sling immobilization/Figure of eight bandage is adequate nonoperative treatment for most isolated clavicle fractures.
7. Malunion is the most common complication.
8. Surgical treatment of clavicle fractures is generally reserved for fractures of the lateral clavicle, middle third fractures with >2 cm of shortening, open fractures, symptomatic nonunions, or fractures with associated neurovascular injury, in patients with a floating shoulder or other complex injuries to the

shoulder girdle where addressing the clavicle may improve overall stability of the upper extremity. Surgical option are plating and K-wire fixation.

Floating Shoulder

The term floating shoulder is used to describe a glenoid neck fracture with an associated clavicle fracture. This combination of injuries leaves the glenohumeral joint with no intact bony contact to the rest of the skeleton. Surgery is often considered in these injuries.

MULTIPLE CHOICE QUESTIONS

1. Most common bone to fracture in body: *(NEET Pattern 2012)*
   A. Clavicle B. Humerus
   C. Tibia D. Femur

Ans. is 'A' Clavicle

2. Shoulder X-ray highest bony landmark is: *(NEET Pattern 2012)*
   A. Greater tuberosity B. Lesser tuberosity
   C. Head D. Acromion

Ans. is 'D' Acromion

3. The most common bone fractured during birth: *(CMC 2002, MP 1998)*
   A. Clavicle B. Scapula
   C. Radius D. Humerus

Ans. is 'A' Clavicle

4. Clavicular fracture is usually treated by: *(UP 2001, Tamil Nadu 1999, Andhra 99, JIPMER 87)*
   A. Traction
   B. Open Reduction and Internal fixation
   C. Figure of eight bandage
   D. Plate and Screw fixation

Ans. is 'C' Figure of eight bandage

ACROMIOCLAVICULAR DISLOCATION

Acromioclavicular (AC) joint injury typically occurs due to a fall onto the acromion. Stability of the AC joint is dependent upon both the AC and coracoclavicular (CC) ligaments.

It is classified into type 1 to 6 by Rockwood classification

Treatment

Type 1 to 3 conservative

Velpeau bandage (dressing) is used in acromioclavicular dislocation, fracture clavicle and shoulder dislocation but it is most effective in acromioclavicular dislocation as it pushes lateral end of shoulder downwards and arm upwards, and thus helps maintaining reduction.

Type 4 to 6 open reduction and internal fixation

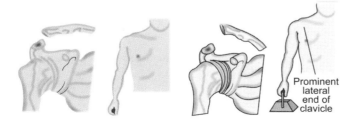

Fig. 7.14: Acromioclavicular dislocation

MULTIPLE CHOICE QUESTION

1. Velpeau bandage and Sling and Swathe splint are used in? *(AIIMS Nov 08)*
   A. Shoulder dislocation
   B. Fracture scapula
   C. Acromioclavicular dislocation
   D. Fracture clavicle

Ans. is 'C' Acromioclavicular dislocation

FRACTURES OF SURGICAL NECK HUMERUS

Proximal humeral fractures are relatively common and occur most often as the result of falls or motor vehicle trauma.

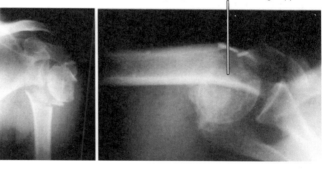

Fig. 7.15: Fracture proximal humerus

The incidence increases with age and in the elderly the cause is typically a low-energy injury. Elderly osteoporotic females are usually involved. In such cases it is usually impacted.

Displaced injuries are best classified by the system developed by Neer and are labeled two, three, or four part fractures. The four potential parts are the humeral head, the greater tuberosity, the lesser tuberosity, and the shaft.

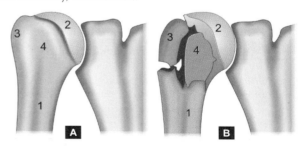

Figs. 7.16A and B: Fractures of the proximal humerus. Diagram of (A) the normal and (B) a fractured proximal humerus, showing the four main fragments, showing the four main fragments, two or more of which are seen in almost all proximal humeral fractures 1-shaft of humerus; 2-head of humerus; 3-greater tuberosity; 4-lesser tuberosity.

When considering treatment options it is important to consider the age and functional expectations of the patient. Most nondisplaced fractures can be treated with a short period of sling immobilization. Early range of motion has been shown to improve functional outcomes. **(This is the case with elderly patients with impacted fractures).**

Two-part fractures with a displaced head fragment may be amenable to closed reduction and percutaneous fixation.

Two-part fractures of the greater tuberosity are best treated with open reduction and internal fixation if displaced more than 3–5 mm because there is increased risk of disability in patients who require overhead function especially abduction and external rotation. (Supraspinatus Assists deltoid in abduction and Infraspinatus/Teres minor - Laterally (externally) rotates arm and all these are attached on greater tuberosity).

Open reduction and internal fixation, is indicated for most three-part fractures of the proximal humerus.

Four-part fractures are at very high risk for development of complete osteonecrosis of the humeral head, resulting in functional limitation. For this reason, hemiarthroplasty of the shoulder is usually considered.

Note: If the question does not mention about age or classification than treatment of choice will be sling and analgesics as this is very commonly seen in osteoporotic females and it is very often impacted in them.

Note: The most common nerve involved in neck humerus fracture is axillary nerve (supplies deltoid and teres minor). The next common nerve involved is suprascapular nerve (supplies supraspinatus—abductor and infraspinatus—external rotator)

Injury	Common Nerve Involvement
Anterior or inferior shoulder dislocation	Axillary, (circumflex humeral) nerve
Fracture surgical neck humerus	Axillary nerve
Fracture shaft humerus	Radial nerve
Fracture supracondylar humerus	AIN > Median > Radial > Ulnar (AMRU)
Medial condyle humerus	Ulnar nerve
Elbow dislocation	Ulnar nerve
Monteggia fracture dislocation	Posterior interosseous nerve
Volkman's ischemic contracture	Anterior Interosseous nerve
Lunate dislocation	Median nerve
Hip dislocation	Sciatic nerve
Knee dislocation	C. Peroneal nerve

MULTIPLE CHOICE QUESTIONS

1. What is the type of fracture shown in the X-ray of left shoulder? *(AIIMS Nov 2017)*

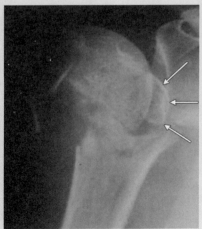

   A. Neer classification grade 4
   B. Ideberg classification grade 4
   C. Garden classification grade 3
   D. Schatzker classification grade 5

Ans. is 'A' Neer classification grade 4

2. A patient had met with an accident and he can not abduct his right arm and can not lift it. On examination tenderness felt near right upper arm. X-ray showed fracture surgical neck of humerus. Muscle that was paralysed was: *(JIPMER May 2016)*
   A. Subscapularis   B. Supraspinatus
   C. Infraspinatus   D. Teres major

Ans. is 'B' Supraspinatus

   The best answer here is deltoid (axillary nerve) since it is not mentioned, so we choose supraspinatus (suprascapular nerve).

3. In fracture of surgical neck of humerus which nerve is involved? *(NEET 2015)*
   A. Axillary   B. Median
   C. Ulnar   D. Radial

Ans. is 'A' Axillary

4. Most common complication of mid shaft humerus fracture is: *(NEET 2015)*
   A. Radial nerve palsy   B. Median nerve palsy
   C. Nonunion   D. Malunion

Ans. is 'A' Radial nerve palsy

5. Which of the following is least likely associated with vascular injury? *(NEET Pattern 2013)*
   A. Fracture supracondylar femur
   B. Fracture supracondylar humerus
   C. Fracture shaft of femur   D. Fracture shaft humerus

Ans. is 'D' Fracture shaft humerus

6. Nerve injured in fracture of medial epicondyle of humerus: *(NEET Pattern 2013)*
   A. Anterior interosseous   B. Median
   C. Ulnar   D. Radial

Ans. is 'C' Ulnar

7. Proximal humerus fracture which has maximum chances of avascular necrosis: *(NEET Pattern 2012)*
   A. One part   B. Two part
   C. Three part   D. Four part

Ans. is 'D' Four part

8. Trauma to neck of humerus, nerve damaged: *(NEET Pattern 2012)*
   A. Radial   B. Ulnar
   C. Median   D. Axillary

Ans. is 'D' Axillary

9. Posterior Elbow dislocation most common nerve involved is: *(NEET Pattern 2012)*
   A. Ulnar   B. Median
   C. Radial   D. Musculocutaneous

Ans. is 'A' Ulnar

10. Treatment of choice for fracture neck of humerus in a 70-year-old male:
    (PGI 2000, UP 2K, AIIMS June 1999, PGI 94, MAHE 96)
    A. Analgesic with triangular sling
    B. U-slab   C. Arthroplasty
    D. Open reduction - Internal fixation

Ans. is 'A' Analgesic with triangular sling

11. Which of the following movements will be affected if the greater tubercle of the humerus is lost? *(AIIMS Nov 2000)*
    A. Abduction and lateral rotation
    B. Adduction and flexion
    C. Adduction and medial rotation
    D. Flexion and medial rotation

Ans. is 'A' Abduction and lateral rotation

12. Fracture neck humerus is common in: *(TN 97)*
    A. Elderly woman   B. Young lady
    C. Children   D. All of these

Ans. is 'A' Elderly woman

HUMERAL SHAFT FRACTURE

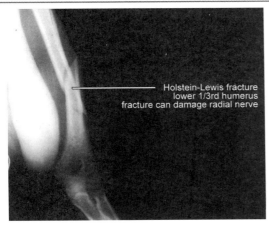

Fig. 7.17: Fracture humerus involving radial nerve

Incidence

- Upper 1/3rd 15%
- Mid 1/3rd 35%
- Lower 1/3rd 50% Holstein Lewis Sign. Radial nerve gets entrapped at fracture site.

Humerus shaft fracture: The most common cause of delayed union or non-union is distraction at fracture site due to gravity and weight of plaster. A spiral fracture of the distal third of the humerus is called a Holstein-Lewis fracture. It is frequently associated with radial nerve palsy. Coaptation splint/Hanging cast is used for non-operative management. Plating for treatment (usually) if surgery indicated.

MULTIPLE CHOICE QUESTIONS

1. Which of the following is/are indication of surgical management of fracture shaft humerus? *(PGI NOV 2016)*
   A. Fracture in elderly
   B. Radial nerve involvement after manipulation
   C. Pathological fractures
   D. Vascular injury   E. Multiple fractures

Ans. is 'B' Radial nerve involvement after manipulation; 'C' Pathological fractures; 'D' Vascular injury; 'E' Multiple fractures

2. Nerve commonly damaged in fracture shaft humerus is: *(NEET DEC 2016)*
   A. Axillary nerve   B. Radial nerve
   C. Ulnar nerve   D. Median nerve

Ans. is 'B' Radial nerve

3. Hanging cast is used in: *(NEET Pattern 2012 AIIMS Dec 1995)*
   A. Fracture Femur   B. Fracture Radius
   C. Fracture Tibia   D. Fracture humerus

Ans. is 'D' Fracture humerus

4. The most important cause of non-union of fracture of humeral shaft is: *(Orissa 1990)*
   A. Comminuted fracture
   B. Compound (Open) fracture
   C. Overriding of fracture ends
   D. Distraction at fracture site
   E. Operative reduction

Ans. is 'D' Distraction at fracture site

INJURIES AROUND ELBOW

Elbow Anatomy

- Capitellum is the first ossification centre about the elbow to appear. It appears around 2 years of age.
- The mnemonic "CRITOE" is helpful in remembering the progression of the radiographic appearance of ossification centre about the elbow in children:
  - C : Capitellum – 2 years
  - R : Radius head – 4 years
  - I : Internal (medial) epicondyle – 6 years
  - T : Trochlea – 8 years
  - O : Olecranon – 10 years
  - E : External (Lateral) epicondyle – 12 years

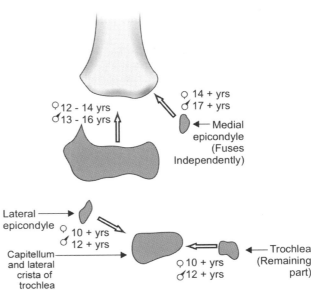

Fig. 7.18: Order of fusion with humerus

Carrying angle: Angle between long axis of arm and forearm angle is more in females because of lower level of trochlea in female. Normal value is 5–15°. Cubitus Varus is reduced carrying angle and cubitus valgus is increased carrying angle. Varus-distal part towards midline and valgus is distal part away from midline.

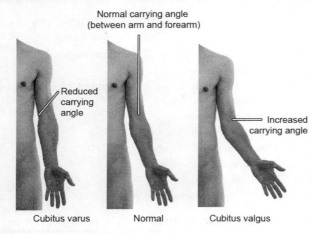

Fig. 7.19: Carrying angle

Note: Malunion around elbow causes Varus = cubitus (elbow) varus. Non-union around elbow causes valgus = cubitus valgus

Supracondylar fracture humerus—causes malunion hence cubitus varus and this fracture is above the growth plate hence static cubitus varus.

Non-union is unknown in supracondylar fracture humerus hence cubitus valgus is not seen as a complication of this fracture.

Lateral condyle fracture humerus is known for non-union and it involves growth plate hence it causes cubitus valgus that can be progressive.

Lateral condyle fracture humerus very rarely undergoes malunion in such cases it can cause progressive cubitus varus.

But in lateral condyle humerus cubitus valgus is much more common than varus.

Note: Jupiter classification is for fractures of lower end humerus. Lateral Column fractures cause Cubitus valgus and medial column fractures can cause cubitus varus in case of complications.

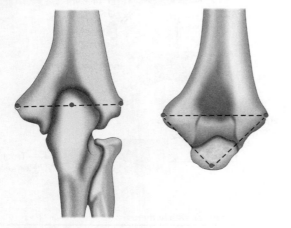

Fig. 7.20: Three point relationship

Three Point Bony Landmarks In Elbow

- The tips of medial and lateral epicondyles and the olecranon.
- Form Isosceles triangle—In Elbow flexion of 90 degree.
- Lie transversely in straight line—Elbow Extension.

- *Three point bony relationship is not disturbed in fracture supracondylar humerus as the fracture occurs above the level of these bony landmarks.*
    - A. With disturbed (increased) intercondylar distance:
        1. Fracture lateral epicondyle and condyle
        2. Fracture medial epicondyle and condyle
        3. Fracture intercondylar humerus.
    - B. With maintained intercondylar distance:
        1. Fracture olecranon (i.e. upper end ulna)
        2. Elbow dislocation (classical example)
- Weak posterior capsule may disrupt three point bony relation by promoting subluxation or dislocations of elbow.

Radial head, lateral epicondyle and tip of olecranon form a triangle over the posterolateral aspect of elbow joint. This space is occupied by anconeus muscle and so known as **anconeus triangle**.

MULTIPLE CHOICE QUESTIONS

1. Deformity with decreased carrying angle is:
   (DNB JUNE 2017)
   - A. Cubitus varus
   - B. Mannus varus
   - C. Cubitus valgus
   - D. Mannus valgus

   Ans. is 'A' Cubitus varus

2. Cubitus valgus develops as complication of:
   (NEET DEC 2016)
   - A. Jupiter fracture
   - B. Smiths fracture
   - C. Malgaigne fracture
   - D. Staddle fracture

   Ans. is 'A' Jupiter fracture

3. First to appear amongst the ossification centres about the elbow is:
   (UP 2003, PGI 96, Assam 99)
   - A. Radial head
   - B. Olecranon
   - C. Lateral epicondyle
   - D. Capitellum

   Ans. is 'D' Capitellum

4. Three bony point relationship is maintained in:
   (NEET 2016, CET Dec 2015, AIIMS June 2000, Dec 1995, Nov 93, May 93, 91)
   - A. Supracondylar Fracture humerus
   - B. Dislocation of elbow
   - C. Fracture Lateral condyle
   - D. Intercondylar Fracture

   Ans. is 'A' Supracondylar fracture humerus

5. Posterolateral anconeus triangle is formed by:
   (Jipmer 2000, KA 2001)
   - A. Head of radius, lateral epicondyle, medial epicondyle
   - B. Head of radius, lateral epicondyle, olecranon
   - C. Olecranon, medial epicondyle, neck of radius
   - D. Neck of radius, head of radius, lateral epicondyle

   Ans. is 'B' Head of radius, lateral epicondyle, olecranon

AGE GROUPS OF FRACTURES AROUND ELBOW

1. Lower humeral epiphyseal slip: 1–3 years
2. Supracondylar humerus fracture: 5–8 years
3. Lateral condyle humerus fracture: 5–15 years

FRACTURE SUPRACONDYLAR HUMERUS

Supracondylar humeral fractures in children are most common elbow injuries, especially in children aged 5–8 years. They account for 50–70% of all elbow fractures.

Mechanism

- Most common type of supracondylar fracture—Extension type (~98% of all supracondylar fracture).
- Most common type of distal fragment displacement in extension type fracture supracondylar humerus.
  "Posteromedial displacement with internal rotation".

Characteristic Displacements

Medial (Internal) rotation/Medial tilt/Medial or lateral shift
 |**I**mpaction (proximal shift)
 |**D**orsal displacement/Dorsal tilt
MID

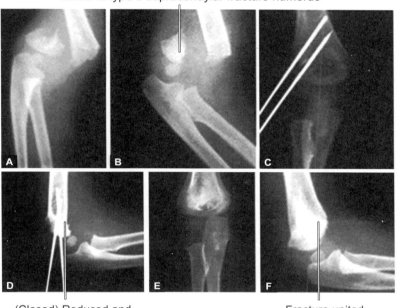

Gartland type 3 supracondylar fracture humerus

Figs. 7.21A to F: Displaced supracondylar fracture humerus

Most common type of displacement in flexion type (2%) fracture supracondylar humerus Anterior displacement.

Gartland Classification is used for Supracondylar Fractures

- Treatment is closed reduction and cast if it fails or if fracture is displaced than closed reduction and K-wire fixation.

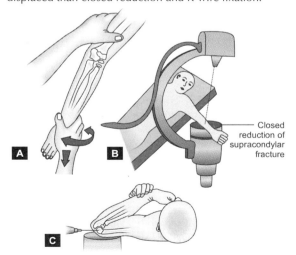

Figs. 7.22A to C: Closed reduction and fixation

- **Admission to hospital is essential following reduction:**
  Potential problem with close reduction and cast management of fracture supracondylar humerus is increased swelling and potential development of compartment syndrome, hence they require observation.

Complications of Fracture Supracondylar Humerus

1. Malunion Most Common Complication
   Posteromedially displaced fracture tend to develop Cubitus varus (gun stock deformity).
   - Cubitus varus deformity in fracture supracondylar humerus is managed by French/modified French osteotomy (lateral closing wedge osteotomy).
   - **Baumans Angle**-angle between the physis and long axis of humerus normal value **75–90 degrees** it is increased in cubitus varus

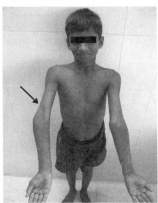

Fig. 7.23: Cubitus varus

2. Vascular (brachial artery) injury
3. Nerve injury (anterior interosseous n.> median n. >radial n>ulnar. n): These are usually neuropraxia, hence transient.

Anterior interosseous nerve (Supplies FPL, Pronator Quadratus + Lat. 1/2 FDP)
Median nerve
Radial nerve
Ulnar nerve
AMRU
Note: AIN controls thumb flexion (FPL = Flexor Pollicis Longus)

4. Volkmann's ischemia and compartment syndrome
5. Elbow stiffness
6. Myositis ossificans
7. Avascular necrosis of trochlea. (rare)
8. Tardy ulnar nerve palsy

Fracture supracondylar humerus is:
- **Most common fracture associated with vascular injury.**
- Most common fracture to involve brachial artery. (10% cases).
- Most common cause of volkmann's ischemia and compartment syndrome in children.
- Most common cause of volkmann's ischemic contracture.
- Non-union is unknown.

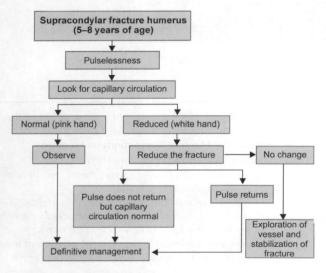

ELBOW DISLOCATION

The most common dislocation is **posterior** or **posterolateral** and is usually the result of a fall with forearm supinated and the elbow either extended or partially flexed.

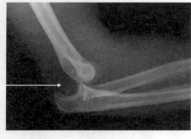

Fig. 7.24: Elbow dislocation

Simple dislocations of the elbow result in injuries of the medial and lateral collateral ligament complexes without bony injury. Complex dislocations are those associated with fractures about the elbow. Associated soft tissue injuries may involve the brachial artery, *ulnar nerve (most commonly)*, median and radial nerve.

Elbow dislocation:
- **Most common joint to dislocate in children**
- Coronoid process is posterior to humerus
- Most prominent part is olecranon in dislocated elbow
- Myositis ossificans is late complication

Urgent closed reduction is recommended. Difficulty obtaining stable closed reduction should increase suspicion of complex dislocation or other associated injuries. Radiographs should be repeated after reduction and carefully scrutinized to confirm concentric reduction and identify any associated fractures that may not have been visible with the joint displaced. Simple dislocations rarely require surgical treatment.

Any complex dislocation of the elbow should be definitively addressed within a few days or as soon as the patient's overall condition allows.

Note: A notoriously unstable injury is the elbow dislocation with associated fractures of the radial head and coronoid process of the ulna. This pattern has been termed the terrible triad of the elbow. Surgical treatment is required to restore stability to the elbow.

Side swipe injury-open fracture dislocation of elbow seen due to accidents involving side swipe over elbow, it has high rates of complications like:
1. Vascular injury
2. Nerve injury
3. Stiffness
4. Myositis ossificans
5. Recurrent dislocation

MULTIPLE CHOICE QUESTIONS

1. A patient of supracondylar humerus fracture is unable to flex interphalangeal joint of the thumb. Which nerve is most likely injured? *(AIIMS May 2018)*
   A. Median nerve
   B. Superficial branch of ulnar nerve
   C. AIN
   D. PIN
   Ans. is 'C' AIN

2. An 8-year-old fall on outstretched elbow leading to a supracondylar fracture (type II). The late complication would be: *(PGI Nov 2017)*
   A. Volkmann ischemia   B. Malunion
   C. No union   D. Ulnar nerve palsy
   E. Brachial nerve palsy
   Ans. is 'A' Volkmann ischemia 'B' Malunion and 'D' Ulnar nerve palsy

3. Preferred treatment of cubitus varus is: *(DNB JULY 2016)*
   A. Medial closing wedge osteotomy
   B. Lateral closing wedge osteotomy
   C. Medial opening wedge osteotomy
   D. Lateral opening wedge osteotomy
   Ans. is 'B' Lateral closing wedge osteotomy

4. A patient presents to you with musculoskeletal complaints. The main concern is to differentiate articular versus non articular origin of pain. Which of the following feature is suggestive of non articular origin of pain? (NEET 2018)
   A. Pain or decrease range of motion on active and passive movement both
   B. Swelling
   C. Crepitation
   D. Pain on active movement but not on passive movement

Ans. is 'D' Pain on active movement but not on passive movement
Differentiation between articular and extraarticular joint disorders
Articular disorders are characterized by internal/deep joint pain that is exacerbated by active and passive motion and by reduced range of motion; Extraarticular disorders are associated with joint pain with active motion rather than passive motion in addition, range of motion often is preserved.

5. Most common deformity after malunited supracondylar humerus fracture is: (NEET DEC 2016)
   A. Flexion deformity   B. Extension deformity
   C. Cubitus varus   D. Cubitus valgus

Ans. is 'D' Cubitus varus

6. You are an intern in a busy casualty. A patient comes with upper limb fracture. According to priority to be given, which of these should be reviewed urgently by an Orthopedic resident? (NBE Pattern 2018)
   A. Patient with delayed capillary refill time in fingers of the involved limb
   B. Having Intra-articular extension of the fracture
   C. With Abrasion over the fracture of more than 10 cm
   D. Having Weakness of wrist extensors

Ans. is 'A' Patient with delayed capillary refill time in fingers of the involved limb

7. In the fracture seen in the X-ray below, what is the most commonly expected vascular injury?

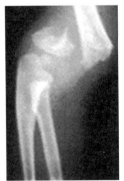

   A. Brachial artery   B. Radial artery
   C. Ulnar artery   D. Cubital vein

Ans. is 'A' Brachial artery

8. Supracondylar fracture humerus, true is: (AI 2016)
   A. Flexion type is the most common type
   B. Malunion causing gunstock deformity is the MC complication
   C. Definitive management requires open reduction
   D. Radial nerve injury is commonly seen

Ans. is 'B' Malunion causing gunstock deformity is the MC complication

9. A child presents with the following deformity. Most common etiology is: (AIIMS Nov 18)

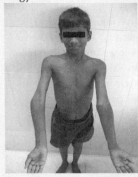

   A. Supracondylar humerus fracture
   B. Lateral condyle humerus fracture
   C. Radial head dislocation
   D. Monteggia fracture dislocation

Ans. is 'A' Supracondylar humerus fracture

10. Preferred treatment of cubitus varus is: (CET July 16)
    A. Medial closing wedge osteotomy
    B. Lateral closing wedge osteotomy
    C. Medial opening wedge osteotomy
    D. Lateral opening wedge osteotomy

Ans. is 'B' Lateral closing wedge osteotomy

11. All are true regarding supracondylar humerus fracture in children except: (PGI May 2016)
    A. Extension type is more common than flexion type
    B. Gartland classification is used for flexion type injury
    C. Gartland III fracture shows 'fat pad sign'
    D. Median nerve is most commonly injured nerve
    E. Cubitus valgus is most common complication

Ans. is 'B' Gartland classification is used for flexion type injury; 'C' Gartland III fracture shows 'fat pad sign'; 'D' Median nerve is most commonly injured nerve; and 'E' Cubitus valgus is most common complication

12. In Supracondylar fracture of humerus in children if the radial pulse is absent, what is next line of management?
    A. Emergency brachial artery exploration (JIPMER 2015)
    B. Closed reduction of fracture and look of reappearance of pulse
    C. Closed reduction, above elbow slab plaster and observe
    D. Open reduction and internal fixation of fracture

Ans. 'B' Closed reduction of fracture and look of reappearance of pulse

13. Most common type of supracondylar fracture in children: (NEET 2015)
    A. Posteromedial extension   B. Posterolateral extension
    C. Anteromedial flexion   D. Anterolateral flexion

Ans. is 'A' Posteromedial extension

14. True about supracondylar fracture: (PGI Nov 2015)
    A. Most common fracture in adults
    B. Posterior medial displacement of posterior fragment
    C. Bauman angle is used during correction
    D. Ulnar Nerve most commonly injured
    E. Brachial artery is least commonly injured

Ans. is 'B' Posterior medial displacement of posterior fragment; 'C' Bauman angle is used during correction

15. The most common complication after supracondylar fracture humerus is: *(NEET 2016, PGM-CET 2015)*
    A. Cubitus varus B. Cubitus valgus
    C. Median nerve injury D. Ulnar nerve injury
Ans. is 'A' Cubitus varus

16. Pointing index is a complication seen in: *(JIPMER 2014)*
    A. Lateral humeral condyle fracture
    B. Supracondylar fracture of humerus
    C. Shoulder dislocation
    D. Fracture of shaft of humerus
Ans. 'B' Supracondylar fracture of humerus

17. The most common type of elbow dislocation is: *(NEET 2016, TN 2014)*
    A. Posterior B. Posteromedial
    C. Posterolateral D. Lateral
Ans. 'A' Posterior

18. All of the following are complications of supracondylar fracture of humerus in children, except: *(AIIMS May 2014)*
    A. Compartment syndrome B. Myositis ossificans
    C. Malunion D. Non-union
Ans. is 'D' Non-union

19. Supracondylar fracture true: *(AIIMS Nov, May 2013)*
    A. Distal segment displaced anterior is more common
    B. Cubitus valgus malunion more common than varus
    C. Nerve injury transitory
    D. Elbow flexion weakness
Ans. is 'C' Nerve injury transitory

20. Late complication of elbow dislocation: *(NEET Pattern 2013)*
    A. Median nerve injury B. Brachial artery injury
    C. Myositis ossificans D. All of the above
Ans. is 'C' Myositis ossificans

21. True about supracondylar fracture of humerus: *(NEET Pattern 2012)*
    A. Common in adults
    B. Extension type most common
    C. Flexion type is most common
    D. None
Ans. is 'B' Extension type most common

22. In extension type of supracondylar fracture, the usual displacement is: *(NEET Pattern 2013)*
    A. Anteromedial B. Anterolateral
    C. Posteromedial D. Posterolateral
Ans. is 'C' Posteromedial

23. Deformity in posterior elbow dislocation: *(NEET Pattern 2012)*
    A. Flexion B. Extension
    C. Both D. None
Ans. is 'A' Flexion

24. What is seen on X-ray with posterior elbow dislocation: *(NEET Pattern 2012)*
    A. Coronoid process posterior to humerus
    B. Coronoid process anterior to humerus
    C. Coronoid process below humerus
    D. None
Ans. is 'A' Coronoid process posterior to humerus

25. In posterior dislocation of elbow, most prominent part: *(NEET Pattern 2012)*
    A. Coronoid B. Radial head
    C. Olecranon D. None
Ans. is 'C' Olecranon

26. Early complication of elbow dislocation are all except: *(NEET Pattern 2012)*
    A. Myositis ossificans B. Median nerve injury
    C. Brachial artery injury D. Radial nerve injury
Ans. is 'A' Myositis ossificans

27. Supracondylar fracture humerus treatment is:
    A. Open reduction and K-wire fixation *(NEET Pattern 2012)*
    B. Closed reduction and K-wire fixation
    C. Excision
    D. Below elbow slab
Ans. is 'B' Closed reduction and K-wire fixation

28. Elbow dislocation going into most commonly: *(NEET Pattern 2012)*
    A. Posterolateral B. Posteromedial
    C. Anterior D. Lateral
Ans. is 'A' Posterolateral

29. Microcirculation blockade is a feature of: *(NEET Pattern 2012)*
    A. Sudecks dystrophy B. Myositis ossificans
    C. Compartment syndrome D. Crush syndrome
Ans. is 'C' Compartment syndrome

30. The malunion of supracondylar fracture of the humerus most commonly leads to: *(AIIMS May 2006, 97, KA 98, PGI 97, TN 97 AI 94)*
    A. Flexion deformity B. Cubitus varus
    C. Cubitus valgus D. Extension deformity
Ans. is 'B' Cubitus varus
    – Cubitus varus, also known as a "gunstock deformity" is the most common complication of supracondylar fracture humerus, due to malunion. It is static.

31. The following fractures are known for Non-union except: *(AIIMS May 2006, PGI Dec 2005, 95 UP 02, AI 02, BHU 99, AMU 98, TN 96, DNB 1990)*
    A. Fracture of lower half of tibia
    B. Fracture of neck of femur
    C. Fracture of scaphoid
    D. Supracondylar fracture of humerus
Ans. is 'D' Supracondylar fracture of humerus

32. A 10-year-old boy presenting with a cubitus varus deformity and a history of trauma 3 months back on clinical examination, has the preserved 3 bony point relationship of the elbow. The most probable diagnosis is: *(AIIMS May 2004, 94, AI 94)*
    A. Old unreduced dislocation of elbow
    B. Non-union lateral condylar humerus
    C. Malunited intercondylar fracture of humerus
    D. Malunited supracondylar fracture of humerus
Ans. is 'D' Malunited supracondylar fracture of humerus
    – Cubitus varus deformity with maintained three bony point relationship after 3 months of injury suggests the diagnosis of malunited supracondylar fracture humerus.

33. **Supracondylar fracture is usually caused by:**
    (MAHE 2002, SGPGI 2001) (AIIMS Nov 2000)
    A. Hyperflexion injury   B. Axial rotation
    C. Extension injury   D. Hyperextension injury

Ans. is 'D' Hyperextension injury
- Supracondylar fracture (most common extension type) occurs due to hyperextension injury, usually due to fall on outstretched hand.
- Flexion type of supracondylar fracture occurs due to fall directly on elbow.

34. **Most common elbow injury in adolescents is:**
    (UP 2001, AMU 97, AI 90)
    A. Dislocation   B. Physeal injury
    C. Supracondylar fracture D. Olecranon fracture

Ans. is 'B' Physeal injury
- During adolescent growth spurts, physeal plate is weaker than the surrounding bone, therefore it is the most common site of injury.

FRACTURE LATERAL CONDYLE HUMERUS

- This is a transphyseal **intraarticular** injury usually involving immature skeleton of children and adolescent.
- The lateral condylar (or capitellar) epiphysis begins to ossify during the first year of life and fuses with shaft at 12–16 years. Between these ages it may be sheared off or avulsed by forceful traction. The maximum chances of injury is between 5–15 years.
They are the **most common distal humeral epiphyseal fractures**

Mechanism of Fracture Lateral Condyle Humerus Fall on outstretched arm with Varus stress (mostly) that "Pulls off" (avulses) lateral condyle or Valgus force (rarely) in which radial head directly pushes off the lateral condyle.

Milch described two basic types of lateral condylar fractures.

In the type I fracture, the fracture line courses medially to the trochlea through and into the capitellar-trochlear groove. This type I fracture is rare; it is a **true Salter-Harris type IV** fracture but is frequently **stable**.

In the type II fracture described by Milch, which is more common, the fracture line extends into the area of the trochlea and produces inherent instability of the elbow. It is Salter-Harris type II fracture.

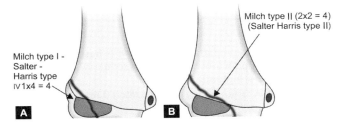

Figs. 7.25A and B: Fracture lateral condyle humerus

Remember Multiplication:
- **Milch type I is Salter Harris type IV 1 x 4 = 4**
- **Milch type II is Salter Harris type II 2 x 2 = 4**

Results are unsatisfactory after closed treatment so open reduction and internal fixation with K-wires/screws is necessary—hence the term fracture of necessity.

Fractures of necessity (requiring surgery)
- *Galeazzi fracture dislocation* (Classical Example)
- *Lateral condyle fracture humerus*
- *Displaced fracture olecranon and patella*
- *Fracture neck femur*
- *Monteggia fracture in adults*
- *Articular fractures*

1. **Non-union is most frequent problematic complication.**
   - **The most common sequela of non-union with displacement is the development of progressive cubitus valgus deformity.**
   - Treatment of cubitus valgus—Milch Osteotomy.
2. **Cubitus varus/lateral spur formation is the reported complication following lateral condyle fracture subsequent to malunion of fractures** after surgical intervention
   - **Treatment of cubitus varus-Modified French Osteotomy.**
   - Remember that cubitus valgus is much more common than true cubitus varus in fracture lateral condyle humerus, because non-union is more common than malunion in fracture lateral body humerus.
3. **Tardy ulnar nerve palsy** is a late complication of progressive **cubitus valgus > cubitus varus** deformity occuring in lateral condylar fractures.
4. Growth (physeal) arrest, avascular necrosis and fishtail deformity are other rare complications.

Tardy Ulnar Nerve Palsy

Tardy ulnar nerve palsy as a late complication of fracture lateral condyle physis is well known, especially after the development of cubitus valgus and less commonly after cubitus varus.

The symptoms are usually gradual in onset and may appear years after injury. Motor loss occur first, with sensory changes developing later.

Anterior transposition of ulnar nerve is most commonly used procedure.

MULTIPLE CHOICE QUESTIONS

1. All of the following are true regarding fractures of lateral condyle of humerus except: *(NEET DEC 2016)*
   A. Usually seen at 6-10 years of age
   B. Results in Gun stock deformity
   C. Cubitus valgus occurs
   D. Tardy ulnar nerve palsy is seen

Ans. is 'B' Results in Gun stock deformity

2. A child following fall on outstretched arm, presented with tenderness and crepitus over lateral condyle humerus alongwith instability of elbow. The condition of the child can cause following complications: *(PGI Nov 2017)*
   A. Malunion
   B. Nonunion
   C. Ulnar Nerve Palsy
   D. Volkmann's Ischaemic Contracture
   E. Recurrent dislocation of elbow

Ans. is 'A' Malunion; 'B' Nonunion; and 'C' Ulnar Nerve Palsy

3. A six-year-old child presented with a valgus deformity at his right elbow since 3 years that is gradually progressive. He has a history of cast applied for 6 weeks after fall on outstretched hand 3 years back. The probable fracture was: *(CET Nov 15)*
   A. Lateral Condylar fracture of Humerus
   B. Supracondylar Fracture of Humerus
   C. Posterior dislocation of elbow
   D. Fracture medial condyle of humerus

Ans. is 'A' Lateral Condyle fracture of Humerus

4. Identify the cause of Deformity in the image below: *(AIIMS Nov 2015)*

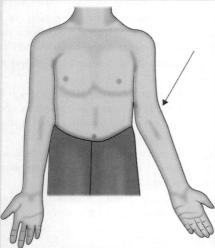

   A. Humerus lateral condylar fracture
   B. Supracondylar fracture humerus
   C. Fracture shaft humerus
   D. Medial Condyle fracture of humerus

Ans. is 'A' Humerus lateral condylar fracture

Cubitus valgus is seen which is caused by Non-union of fracture lateral condyle Humerus

5. The most common complication of lateral humeral condyle fracture in children is: *(JIPMER 2014)*
   A. Valgus deformity   B. Varus deformity
   C. Malunion   D. Hyperextension

Ans. 'A' Valgus deformity

6. Most common complication of lateral condyle humerus fracture: *(NEET Pattern 2012)*
   A. Malunion   B. Non-union
   C. VIC   D. Median nerve injury

Ans. is 'B' Non-union

7. Which fracture requires open reduction in children? *(AI 2001, 91, AIIMS 1992, 91)*
   A. Fracture of both bones of forearm
   B. Epiphyseal separation of tibia
   C. Intercondylar fracture of femur
   D. Lateral condyle fracture of humerus

Ans. is 'D' Lateral condyle fracture of humerus

8. A 6-year-old child has an accident and had fracture elbow, after 4 years presented with tingling and numbness in the ulnar side of finger, fracture is: *(AIIMS June 1999)*
   A. Supracondylar fracture humerus
   B. Lateral condylar fracture humerus
   C. Olecranon fracture
   D. Dislocation of elbow

Ans. is 'B' Lateral condylar fracture humerus
   – Fracture elbow with tingling subsequently after few years—"Tardy ulnar nerve palsy". Most common cause is fracture lateral condyle humerus.

9. Tardy ulnar nerve palsy seen in: *(AIIMS Dec 1998, 91, PGI 92, Bihar 90)*
   A. Medial condyle fracture humerus
   B. Lateral condyle fracture humerus
   C. Supracondylar fracture humerus
   D. Fracture shaft humerus

Ans. is 'B' Lateral condyle fracture humerus; >'C' Supracondylar fracture humerus

10. Fracture lateral condyle of the humerus is a common injury in children. Which one of the following is the most ideal treatment for a displaced fracture lateral condyle of the humerus in a 7-year-old child? *(Karnataka 89)*
    A. Open reduction and plaster immobilization
    B. Closed reduction and plaster immobilization
    C. Open reduction and internal fixation
    D. Excision of the fractured fragment

Ans. is 'C' Open reduction and internal fixation

COMPARTMENT SYNDROME-TIGHT CAST THINK OF COMPARTMENT SYNDROME

In acute compartment syndromes increased pressure in a close fascial space causes loss of microcirculation.

Most commonly compartment syndrome involves deep posterior compartment of leg>deep flexor compartment of forearm (commonest in children).

It is most commonly seen following fractures of tibia and supracondylar humerus.

Most common cause is fractures and dislocations: Other Causes of compartment syndrome
1. **Crush injury/Burn/Infection/Surgical procedure/Tight circumferential dressing**
2. **Exercise**—Exercise may increase intracompartmental pressure and muscle edema, so it is avoided in cases of acute compartmental syndrome.

Clinical Features

The diagnosis of compartment syndrome is based on dramatically increasing pain (out of proportion to injury) after fracture/any injury (1st symptom).

Pain and resistance on passive stretch (Distal most joint of extremity) (1st sign).

In compartment syndrome the order of compression of vascular structures with increase of intracompartmental pressure is: capillary compression, venous compression, arterial compression. Pulselessness is a late feature and it is not a reliable indicator of compartment syndrome. **The presence of pulse does not exclude the diagnosis.**

Pressures in the deep volar compartment are significantly elevated compared with pressures in other compartments. **Deep flexor muscles are involved particularly flexor digitorum profundus>Flexor Pollicis Longus.**

Treatment

- **The limb should be kept at the level of heart rather than elevated.**
- **Removal of all circumferential dressing reduce pressure upto 85%.**
- Fasciotomy is recommended in the presence of clinical signs of compartment syndrome, such as undue pain and a palpable firmness in the forearm. The morbidity caused by fasciotomy is minimal, whereas that caused by an untreated compartment syndrome is much greater. The general indications for fasciotomy are Impending tissue ischemia or it may be considered when the tissue pressure reaches 30 mm Hg or the difference between diastolic blood pressure and compartment pressure is less than 30 mm of Hg. (normal compartment pressure is 8–10 mm of Hg and pressure at calf during walking is 200–300 mm of Hg).

A higher pressure is a strong indication that fasciotomy should be recommended. In a hypotensive patient, the acceptable pressure is lower. Mubarak recommended that fasciotomy be performed in (1) normotensive patients with positive clinical findings, compartment pressures of greater than 30 mm Hg, and when the duration of the increased pressure is unknown or thought to be longer than 8 hours; (2) uncooperative or unconscious patients with a compartment pressure greater than 30 mm Hg; (3) patients with low blood pressure and a compartment pressure greater than 20 mm Hg; (4) clinical signs such as demonstrable motor or sensory loss, and (5) interrupted arterial circulation to the extremity for more than 4 hours.

Fasciotomy must release skin, superficial fascia and deep fascia.

Note: Pallor, Paresthesias and pulselessness are late signs of compartment syndrome.

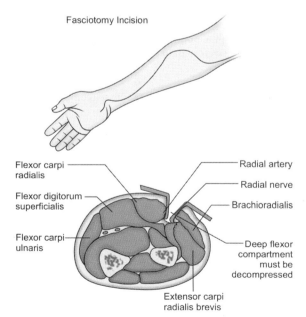

Fig. 7.26: Forearm fasciotomy

Volkmann's Ischaemic Contracture (VIC)

Volkmann's Ischaemic Contracture (VIC): Most commonly in upper limbs (After supracondylar fracture).

If a compartment syndrome is untreated or inadequately treated, compartment pressures continue to increase until irreversible tissue ischemia occurs. In Volkmann ischemic contracture earliest changes usually involve the **flexor digitorum profundus muscles** in the middle third of the forearm followed by **flexor pollicis longus**. The typical clinical picture of established Volkmann contracture includes elbow flexion, forearm pronation, wrist flexion, thumb adduction, metacarpophalangeal joint extension, and finger flexion.

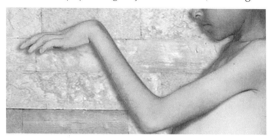

Fig. 7.27: Volkmann's Ischemic Contracture (VIC)

The earliest nerve involved is **Anterior interosseous** > median > ulnar.

During the early stages of a mild contracture, dynamic splinting (Turn Buckle splint) to prevent wrist contracture, functional training, and active use of the muscles may be helpful. After 3 months, the involved muscle-tendon units can be released and lengthened.

Muscle Sliding Operation of Flexors for Established Volkmann Contracture.

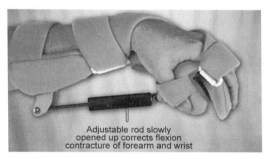

Fig. 7.28: Turn buckle splint—VIC

The muscle sliding operation was first described by Page in 1923. It has been used for Volkmann and other contractures caused by conditions such as brain damage and burns. In the case of Volkmann contracture, usually the muscle is fibrotic and noncontractile, and its release may decrease the degree of deformity and contractures.

If Median and ulnar nerve sensory changes are present with progression of VIC a careful neurolysis (release of nerve adhesions) and the excision of any fibrotic muscle mass encountered may be done.

Osteotomies and tendon releases and transfers can be carried out in late stages.

MULTIPLE CHOICE QUESTIONS

1. Earliest sign of compartment syndrome of leg is:
   (AIIMS Nov 2018)
   A. Tingling or numbness
   B. Skin mottling
   C. Pulselessness
   D. Pain on Passive stretch

Ans. is 'D' Pain on Passive stretch

2. Signs of compartment syndrome include: *(PGI MAY 2018)*
   A. Pain on passive flexion
   B. Pain on active flexion
   C. Swelling of fingers
   D. Pallor
   E. Paresthesias

Ans. is 'B' Pain on active flexion 'C' Swelling of fingers 'D' Pallor and 'E' Paresthesias

3. In fasciotomy done for compartment syndrome, you incise: *(NEET 2018)*
   A. Skin
   B. Skin and subcutaneous fat
   C. Skin, superficial fascia subcutaneous fat and deep fascia
   D. Skin and superficial fascia

Ans. is 'C' Skin, superficial fascia subcutaneous fat and deep fascia

4. Earliest way to detect development of compartment syndrome by a nurse in a patient with cast is: *(AIIMS Nov 2017)*
   A. Check radial pulse by displacing the cast
   B. Decreased response to analgesia
   C. Change in color of fingers
   D. Change in odor

Ans. is 'B' Decreased response to analgesia

5. Compartment syndrome is commonly seen in: *(DNB JUNE 2017)*
   A. Fracture of proximal tibia
   B. Fracture shaft humerus
   C. Fracture of femur shaft
   D. Fracture distal end radius

Ans. is 'A' Fracture of proximal tibia

6. Fasciotomy -all of the following are cut except: *(DNB JUNE 2017)*
   A. Skin
   B. Superficial fascia
   C. Deep fascia
   D. Muscles

Ans. is 'D' Muscles

7. Which is the earliest reliable sign of compartment syndrome? *(CET July 16)*
   A. Stretch pain
   B. Pulselessness
   C. Paraesthesia
   D. Pallor

Ans. is 'A' Stretch pain

8. The typical clinical picture of established Volkmann's ischemic contracture includes: *(PGI May 2016)*
   A. Elbow flexion
   B. Forearm pronation
   C. Wrist flexion
   D. Thumb abduction
   E. MCP Joint flexion

Ans. is 'A' Elbow flexion; 'B' Forearm pronation; and 'C' Wrist flexion

9. In Supracondylar fracture of humerus in children if the radial pulse is absent, what is next line of management?
   A. Emergency brachial artery exploration *(JIPMER 2015)*
   B. Closed reduction of fracture and look for reappearance of pulse
   C. Closed reduction, above elbow slab plaster and observe
   D. Open reduction and internal fixation of fracture

Ans. is 'B' Closed reduction of fracture and look for reappearance of pulse

10. A case of comminuted fracture of tibia presenting with severe pain in the calf on dorsiflexion of the foot. There is also numbness on the sole of foot. Distal pulses are present. What is the probable diagnosis? *(JIPMER 2015)*
    A. Rupture of Achilles tendon
    B. Gastroenemius and Soleus muscle tear
    C. Compartment syndrome
    D. Tarsal tunnel syndrome

Ans. 'C' Compartment Syndrome

11. Most common cause of acute compartment syndrome in children is: *(NEET 2015)*
    A. Fracture supracondylar humerus
    B. Transphyseal humerus fracture
    C. Fracture radius/ulna
    D. Fracture shaft humerus

Ans. is 'A' Fracture supracondylar humerus

12. Volksmann ishcaemic contracture *(PGI Nov 2015)*
    A. Due to injury of nerves
    B. Flexor Digitalis superficialis usually involved
    C. Treated when more than 30 degrees deformity
    D. Treated by releasing flexor pulleys
    E. Anterior interossei nerve is involved

Ans. is 'C' Treated when more than 30 degrees deformity and 'E' Anterior interossei nerve is involved

13. 'Volkmann's Ischaemic Contracture" mostly involves which muscle in Upper Limb. *(Maharashtra PG 2016)*
    A. Flexor digitorum superficialis
    B. Pronator teres
    C. Flexor digitorum profundus
    D. Flexor carpi radialis longus

Ans. is 'C' Flexor digitorum profundus > Flexor pollicis longus

14. Volkmann's contracture, which artery is involved: *(NEET Pattern 2012)*
    A. Radial
    B. Brachial
    C. Ulnar
    D. Interosseus

Ans. is 'B' Brachial

15. Calf pressure during walking is: *(NEET Pattern 2012)*
    A. 200–300 mm Hg
    B. 200–300 cm of H_2O
    C. 20–30 mm Hg
    D. 20–30 cm of H_2O

Ans. is 'A' 200–300 mm Hg

16. Dye is injected in one of the extremities in a child and is followed by pain and swelling of upper limb, paraesthesias of fingers, stretch pain and normal peripheral pulses, management is: *(May AIIMS 2012)*
    A. Aspiration
    B. Anti-Inflammatory
    C. Observation
    D. Fasciotomy

Ans. is 'D' Fasciotomy
   – As patient is clinically a case of compartment syndrome -pain on passive stretch and he has paraesthesias so fasciotomy is indicated.
   – Remember Pulses can be normal in compartment syndrome.

17. In posterior compartment syndrome which passive movement causes pain? *(AIIMS Nov 2008)*
    A. Dorsiflexion of foot
    B. Foot inversion
    C. Toe dorsiflexion
    D. Toe Plantar flexion

Ans. is 'C' Toe dorsiflexion
   – Toe dorsiflexion as passive stretch should be performed at distal most joint of the extremity.

18. All are correct regarding compartment syndrome except:
    A. Pulse is a reliable indicator *(PGI Dec 2005, 05)*
    B. Pain on passive stretching
    C. Interstitial pressure> capillary pressure
    D. Paraesthesia are seen late

Ans. is 'A' Pulse is a reliable indicator
   – Peripheral pulses can be normal in compartment syndrome

19. The most common cause of Volkmann's ischaemic contracture (VIC) in a child is: (AIIMS 1999)
    A. Intercondylar fracture of humerus
    B. Fracture both bone of forearm
    C. Fracture lateral condyle of humerus
    D. Supracondylar fracture of humerus

Ans. is 'D' Supracondylar fracture of humerus
    – VIC develops most commonly after supracondylar humerus fracture in children.

20. The most common nerve involved in Volkmann's Ischemic contracture: (AI 1999)
    A. Radial   B. Ulnar
    C. Median   D. Posterior interosseous

Ans. is 'C' Median
    – AIN>Median>ulnar nerve

MYOSITIS OSSIFICANS/HETEROTOPIC OSSIFICATION-HISTORY OF MASSAGE THINK OF IT

It is heterotopic calcification and ossification in muscle tissue. The name is **misnomer as there is no myositis** (inflammation of muscle) and rarely ossification in the muscle (because the mineral phase differs from that in bone and no true bone matrix is formed). Myositis is usually seen in 2nd to 3rd decade of life.

Causes

- Injury (trauma) is an important factor when associated with massage. Myositis Ossificans is seen in **Elbow (MC) followed by hip joint.**
- In elbow Myositis is seen more commonly anteriorly than posteriorly.
- **Massage to the elbow and vigorous passive stretching to restore movements is aggravating factor.** It occurs in muscles which are vulnerable to heavy loads, such as **brachialis (commonest)**, biceps. Surgical trauma specially total hip replacement, is precipitating factor.
- MO not associated with traumatic injury is termed as Pseudomalignant myositis ossificans and it is seen in—Neurological disorders, e.g. GB syndrome, AIDS encephalopathy, closed head injury, hypoxic brain injury, Polio, Hemophilia and burns.

Pathogenesis: Bone formation in muscle represents metaplasia of fibroblast at the site of injury

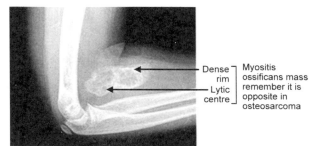

Fig. 7.29: X-ray: elbow- myositis ossificans

4 Zonal Pattern (CT best demonstrates) was described by -Ackerman

X-ray evidence by 3–6 wks of development

There is peripheral ossification and central lucency of the mass (opposite in osteosarcoma).

The mass is usually separated from underlying bone by at least a thin line and lesion are usually located in the diaphysis. If the lesion is in continuity with the bone it is not myositis ossificans and the possibility of tumor or infection arises.

It is distinguished from **Tumor calcinosis**, which is a metabolic disorder, often associated with collagen diseases scleroderma and dermatomyositis. This disorder is associated with hyperphosphatemia is often **bilateral seen around knee** or hip. Phosphate binders may have a role in treatment but surgery may be required in symptomatic case.

Parameter	Myositis Ossificans	Tumor Calcinosis
Etiology	Traumatic	Idiopathic/Familial
Side/Site	Unilateral-Elbow	Bilateral-Knee
Symptom	Painful	Painless
Marker	ALP Levels Increased	PO4 Levels Increased

It is distinguished from ectopic calcification, which occurs in the capsule of joints, commonly the shoulder and is caused by inflammatory reaction around deposits of hydroxy appetite crystals and it is seen in CRF, hypo/hyper parathyroidism, TB and supraspinatous tendinitis.

Treatment of Myositis Ossificans

30% of cases resolves spontaneously

Treatment is normally by 'watchful inactivity'. Relative rest of the affected extremity is helpful, with motion and activity gradually resumed as the acute phase subsides. **In acute phase the treatment consist of limiting motion x 3 weeks. Followed by only active exercises upto 12 months.** Surgical excision in toto is after 1 year if progress is not satisfactory.

Low dose irradiation, bisphosphonates and indomethacin may prevent heterotopic ossification, but the radiation should be avoided in children.

MYOSITIS OSSIFICANS PROGRESSIVA

It is a rare autosomal dominant (AD) disorder of connective tissue differentiation. **Main pathogenic mechanism is defective regulation of the induction of endochondral ossification.** The proliferating loose myxoid fibrous tissue infiltrates and replaces normally formed fibrous connective tissue and striated muscle.

Endochondral ossification is a feature of maturing lesion. Only the absence of normal anatomical orientation differentiates this heterotopic bone from normal.

Bone morphogenetic protein 4 is over expressed and Basic fibroblast growth factor which is an extremely potent stimulator of angiogenesis (in vivo) is elevated in urine during acute flare up stage.

Clinical Features

Seen in 1st decade of life.

Begins as painful erythematous subfascial nodule mostly located on posterior aspect of neck and back which gradually calcify and eventually ossify (heterotopic ossification).

The heterotopic ossification progress in axial to appendicular, cranial to caudal and proximal to distal direction. So the most commonly involved site is neck followed by spine and shoulder girdle and same is the order for limitation of motion.

The ossification is irreversible, unlike other forms of heterotopic ossification.

Diaphragm, extraocular muscles and smooth muscles are characteristically spared.

Primary congenital skeletal abnormality is deformity of great toe.

Limitations of jaw mobility, extremely limited chest expansion, reduced lung volumes (~ 44% of normal) but relatively preserved flow rates and scoliosis/hypokyphosis are other feature.

Life expectancy is decreased and premature death usually result from **respiratory failure due to restrictive lung disease** and their complications.

MULTIPLE CHOICE QUESTIONS

1. All of the following are features of myositis ossificans except: *(CET Nov 15)*
   A. Commonly occurs around the elbow
   B. It matures from inside out
   C. Massage is a known associated factor
   D. Can be post-traumatic
Ans. is 'B' It matures from inside out

2. Most common site of myositis ossificans:
   A. Knee   B. Elbow *(NEET Pattern 2013)*
   C. Shoulder   D. Wrist
Ans. is 'B' Elbow > Hip

3. False about myositis ossificans progressiva (child with heterotopic ossifications) is: *(AI 08)*
   A. Pneumonia is common
   B. Life longevity is normal
   C. Most common site involved is the spine
   D. Onset is before 6 year
Ans. is 'B' Life longevity is normal

4. In myositis ossificans mature bone is seen:
   (MAHE 2004, AMU 2003, NIMHANS 03 SGPGI 99) (KA 2002, TN 99)
   A. At periphery   B. In center
   C. Whole muscle mass D. In the joint capsule
Ans. is 'A' At periphery

5. A person of 60 years age is suffering from myositis ossificans progressiva. The usual cause of death:
   A. Nutritional deficiency B. Bed sore *(AIIMS 2000)*
   C. Lung disease   D. Septicemia
Ans. is 'C' Lung disease
   – Severe restrictive chest wall disease is the cause of death in myositis ossificans progressiva

6. Treatment of Acute Myositis Ossificans is:
   (NEET 2016, AIIMS 91, TN 91)
   A. Active mobilization   B. Passive mobilization
   C. Infra Red Therapy   D. Immobilization
Ans. is 'D' Immobilization

7. Myositis ossificans is due to: *(Bihar 1990)*
   A. Migration osteoblasts to haematoma
   B. New bone formation
   C. Ossification of subperiosteal haematoma
   D. All of the above
Ans. is 'D' All of the above

PULLED ELBOW/NURSE MAID'S ELBOW

It is **subluxation of radial head** or more accurately subluxation of the annular (orbicular) ligament which slips up over the head of radius into the radiocapitellar joint.

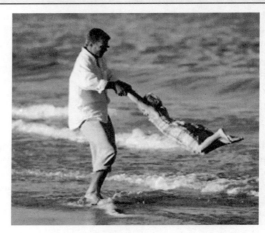

Fig. 7.30: Violent force to elbow – pulled elbow!

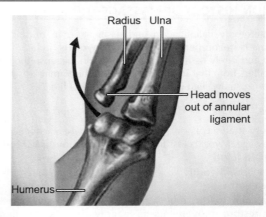

Fig. 7.31: Pulled elbow

Mechanism of Injury

Traction to elbow.

Clinical Features

- Maximum incidence in 1–4 years age group.
- The child holds the elbow in slight flexion with the forearm pronated.

X-rays are normal

Treatment

- Reduced by flexing the elbow to 90 degrees and rapidly and firmly rotating the forearm into full supination **on outdoor basis without anaesthesia** Immobilization is not necessary.
- Supination is a gravity assisted movement and pulled elbow may be reduced spontaneously by gravity, but this may take time.

MULTIPLE CHOICE QUESTIONS

1. What is not true about pulled elbow? *(NEET 2015)*
   A. Occurs due to sudden axial pull on extended elbow
   B. Forearm is held in pronation and extension
   C. Most commonly occurs between 2–5 years of age
   D. Treatment is quick pronation and flexion of elbow
Ans. is 'D' Treatment is quick pronation and flexion of elbow

2. A mother catches her 3-year-old child by wrist and lifts her. The child does not move her elbow and cries most likely cause is: *(AIIMS Nov 2014, TN 02, AIIMS May 01)*
   A. Shoulder dislocation
   B. Elbow dislocation
   C. Pulled elbow
   D. Colles fracture

Ans. is 'C' Pulled elbow

3. Pulled elbow means: *(NEET Pattern 2012)*
   A. Fracture of head of radius
   B. Subluxation of head of radius
   C. Fracture dislocation of elbow
   D. Fracture ulna

Ans. is 'B' Subluxation of head of radius

4. A one-and-a-half-year-old child holding her father's hand slipped and fell but did not let go of her father's hand. After that she continued to cry and hold the forearm in pronated position and refused to move the affected extremity. Which of the following management at this stage is most appropriate?
   (AIIMS Nov 2004, 93, JIPMER 01, AMU 99)
   A. Supinate the forearm
   B. Examine the child under GA
   C. Elevate the limb and observe
   D. Investigate for osteomyelitis

Ans. is 'A' Supinate the forearm
   – This is a case of pulled elbow.
   – *Treatment is simple*. The child's attention is diverted, the elbow is quickly supinated and then slightly flexed.

RADIAL HEAD FRACTURES

Radial head fractures are common injuries and may occur in association with dislocation of the elbow.

A radial head fracture with an associated injury to the interosseous membrane is termed an *Essex-Lopresti* fracture-dislocation. Causes (wrist pain displacement at the distal radio-ulnar joint, and/or proximal migration of the radius evident on X-ray). If signs of instability in any plane are present, every attempt should be made to preserve the radial head or perform arthroplasty with a metallic radial head implant.

Remember in children radial neck fractures are more common than radial head fractures.

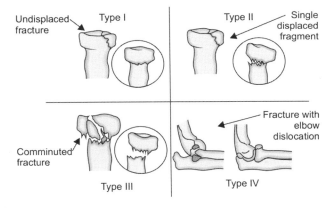

Fig. 7.32: Radial head fracture

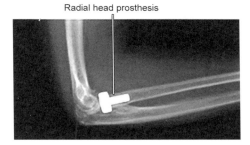

Fig. 7.33: Prosthetic replacement of radial head

Classically the head of radius should not be excised in children because. It will interfere with the synchronous growth of radius and ulnar producing wrist and elbow deformity. **It leads to proximal radial migration and subluxation of inferior radio-ulnar joint.** It causes weakness of extremity and discomfort in distal radio-ulnar joint with heavy activities. **May produce cubitus valgus deformity and instability.**

The Floating Elbow

The floating elbow occurs when there are ipsilateral fractures of the humerus and forearm. The elbow segment is unsupported proximally and distally, requiring stabilization of both injuries.

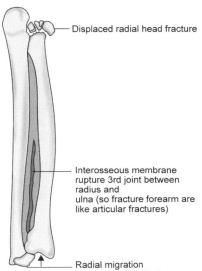

Fig. 7.34: Essex lopresti: radial head fracture can cause wrist pain

MULTIPLE CHOICE QUESTIONS

1. X-ray of a 10-year-old child is shown. Which of the following is incorrect? *(JIPMER May 2018)*

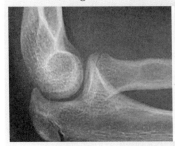 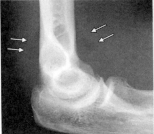

A. Anterior pad of fat sign present
B. Fracture of radius head
C. Radius head articulation is seen
D. Supracondylar humerus fracture can raise anterior fat pad.

Ans. is 'B' Fracture of radius head

In children radial neck fracture is seen. Undisplaced supracondylar fracture humerus can raise the fat pad due to hematoma this is called as fat pad sign.

Fat pad sign

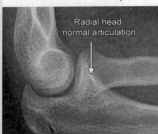
Normal anterior fat pad

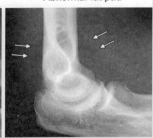
Abnormal fat pad

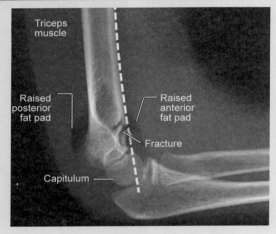

2. Essex lopresti lesion in upper limb: *(NEET Pattern 2014, 2013)*
   A. Injury to interosseous membrane
   B. Radial head fracture
   C. Radial shaft fracture
   D. Radial shaft and radio-ulnar joint fracture

Ans. is 'A' Injury to interosseous membrane

3. Excision of head of radius in a child should not be done because: *(JIPMER 2001)*
   A. It produces instability of elbow joint
   B. It leads to secondary Osteoarthritis of elbow
   C. It causes subluxation of inferior radio-ulnar joint
   D. It causes myositis ossificans

Ans. is 'C' It causes subluxation of inferior radio-ulnar joint

4. Open Reduction is not required in which fracture:
   A. Patella *(AIIMS May 1995)*
   B. Outer 1/3 of radius head   C. Condyle of humerus
   D. Olecranon displaced fracture

Ans. is 'B' Outer 1/3 of radius head
   – Involvement of outer 1/3rd of head is an indication for excision of the fragment (not open reduction).

5. If head of the radius is removed, it will result in: *(PGI 1991)*
   A. Lengthening of limb   B. Valgus deformity
   C. Varus deformity   D. No deformity

Ans. is 'B' Valgus deformity
   – Classically the head of radius should not be excised in children because. It will interfere with the synchronous growth of radius and ulnar producing wrist and elbow deformity.
   – It leads to proximal radial migration and subluxation of inferior radio-ulnar joint. It causes weakness of extremity and discomfort in distal radio-ulnar joint with heavy activities. May produce cubitus valgus deformity and instability.

FRACTURES OF THE OLECRANON

Fractures of the olecranon can be caused either by direct trauma, such as falling on the tip of the elbow, or by indirect trauma, such as falling on a partially flexed elbow with indirect forces generated by the triceps muscle avulsing the olecranon.

In fractures of the olecranon in adults, when the fragments are separated, open reduction and internal fixation are necessary **(Tension Band Wiring)**.

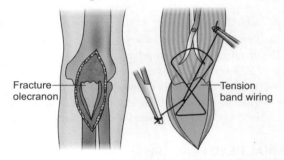

Fig. 7.35: Tension band wiring for fracture olecranon

Excision of a proximal fragment can be used only if enough of the olecranon is left to form a stable base for the trochlea. It is not indicated if a comminuted fracture extends as far distally as the coronoid process for fear of producing elbow instability.

Advantages of excision are that

It is an easy and rapid procedure and It eliminates the possibility of delayed union, non-union and post-traumatic arthritis.

Disadvantages include:

Triceps weakness, Elbow instability and Loss of elbow motion.

MULTIPLE CHOICE QUESTIONS

1. In fracture of the olecranon, excision of the proximal fragment is indicated in all of the following situations except: *(AI 2004)*
   A. Old ununited fractures   B. Non-articular fractures
   C. Fracture extending to coronoid process
   D. Elderly patient

Ans. is 'C' Fracture extending to coronoid process

2. An oblique fracture of olecranon. If displaced proximally. The treatment is: *(AIIMS Sp 96)*
   A. Excision and resuturing   B. Tension band wiring
   C. Elbow is immobilized by cast
   D. Open reduction and external fixation

Ans. is 'B' Tension band wiring

MONTEGGIA FRACTURE DISLOCATION

- Fractures between the **proximal third of the ulna** and the base of olecranon combined with **dislocation of the proximal radioulnar joint**. Direction of dislocation of radial head is used for classification.

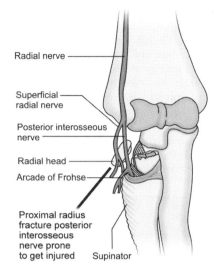

Fig. 7.36: Elbow anatomy

Bado's Classification

Type	Direction of radial head dislocation	Direction of apex of ulnar shaft fracture angulation
I (most common)	Anterior	Anterior (also called as extension type)
II	Posterior	Posterior
III	Lateral	Lateral
IV	Anterior	Fracture of both radius and ulnar-Radius is fractured in proximal third below the bicipital groove

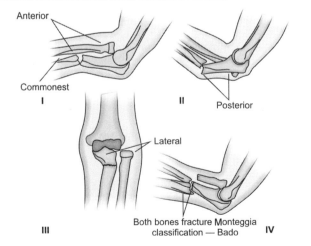

Fig. 7.37: Monteggia fracture—Bado classification

Treatment

The clue to successful treatment is to restore the length of the fractured ulna; only then can the dislocated joint be fully reduced and remain stable.

In adults treatment is reduction and fixation.

In children treatment is reduction and cast application

Posterior interosseous nerve has been most commonly injured nerve in association with Monteggia fracture dislocation because it takes a turn around radial head and is injured with its dislocation. This causes paralysis of thumb and finger extensors.

MULTIPLE CHOICE QUESTIONS

1. In a patient with history of trauma and X-ray showing fracture of proximal part of medial bone of forearm with dislocation. The muscles which may get paralysed:
   (DNB JULY 2016)
   A. Flexor carpi ulnaris
   B. Adductor pollicis
   C. Extensor pollicis longus
   D. Opponens pollicis

Ans. is 'C' Extensor pollicis longus

2. Which of the following is not true about monteggia fracture dislocation? *(NEET DEC 2016)*
   A. Fracture of proximal third of ulna with dislocation of radial head
   B. Extension type is a commoner type
   C. Ulna angulates posteriorly in the extension type
   D. Malunion occurs commonly in conservatively managed patients

Ans. is 'C' Ulna angulates posteriorly in the extention type

3. What is the diagnosis of this fracture?
   (AIIMS May 2016, APPG 2015)

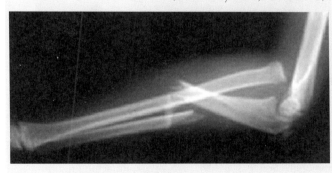

   A. Monteggia fracture type I
   B. Side swipe fracture
   C. Galeazzi fracture
   D. Monteggia fracture type II

Ans. is 'A' Monteggia fracture type I

4. Monteggia fracture is a: *(JIPMER 2014, 2012)*
   A. Fracture of atlas
   B. Fracture of radial styloid
   C. Fracture of proximal 1/3 of ulna with dislocation of proximal radioulnar joint
   D. Fracture of distal 1/3 of radius with dislocation of distal radioulnar joint

Ans. 'C' Fracture of proximal 1/3 of ulna with dislocation of proximal radioulnar joint.

5. In Monteggia fracture, which is true about ulnar fracture and head of radius most commonly?
   A. Both ulnar fracture and head of radius is displaced posteriorly. *(AIIMS Nov 2006, JIPMER 1992)*
   B. Both ulnar fracture and head of radius is displaced anteriorly.
   C. Ulnar fractures is posteriorly and head of radius is displaced anteriorly.
   D. Ulnar fracture is anteriorly and head of radius is displaced posteriorly.

Ans. is 'B' Both ulnar fracture and head of radius is displaced anteriorly

6. Posterior interosseous nerve is injured in: *(Andhra 1999)*
   A. Posterior dislocation of elbow
   B. Monteggia fracture dislocation
   C. Reversed Monteggia fracture dislocation
   D. Supracondylar fracture of humerus

Ans. is 'B' Monteggia fracture dislocation

FRACTURES OF THE DISTAL THIRD OF THE RADIUS WITH DISLOCATION OF THE DISTAL RADIOULNAR JOINT (GALEAZZI FRACTURE-DISLOCATION)

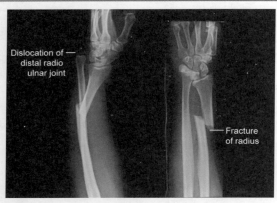

Fig. 7.38: Galeazzi fracture-dislocation

The combination of **fracture of the distal third of the shaft of the radius and dislocation of the distal radioulnar joint** (along with damage to interosseous membrane and Triangular Fibro Cartilage complex) is called Galeazzi Fracture dislocation **(the fracture of necessity)**. A treatment regimen of closed reduction and cast immobilization has a high rate of unsatisfactory results. Open reduction and internal fixation with plate is the treatment of choice in adult.

MULTIPLE CHOICE QUESTIONS

1. Which of the following is not true about Galeazzi fracture dislocation? *(NEET DEC 2016)*
   A. Fracture of distal third of radius and dislocation of distal radio-ulnar joint
   B. Results from fall on outstretched hand
   C. The distal end of ulna dislocates volarly after disruption of distal radio-ulnar joint
   D. Radius is angulated medially and anteriorly

Ans. is 'C' The distal end of ulna dislocates volarly after disruption of distal radio-ulnar joint

2. Which of the following statements correctly define Galeazzi fracture dislocation? *(AIIMS May 2017)*
   A. Radial fracture with disruption of triangular fibrocartilage complex and lower radio-ulnar joint
   B. Ulnar fracture with disruption of triangular fibrocartilage complex and lower radio-ulnar joint
   C. Ulnar shaft fracture and disruption of superior radio-ulnar joint
   D. Radial collateral ligament tear with interosseous membrane tear and radial shaft fracture

Ans. is 'A' Radial fracture with disruption of triangular fibrocartilage complex and lower radio-ulnar joint

3. Fracture of necessity is used to describe: *(NEET DEC 2016)*
   A. Cottons fracture
   B. Galeazzi fracture
   C. Monteggia fracture
   D. Rolando fracture

Ans. is 'B' Galeazzi fracture

4. AP & Lat. View of wrist is given. What is your diagnosis? *(AIIMS Nov 2015)*

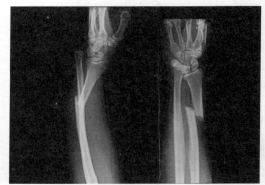

   A. Galeazzi
   B. Monteggia
   C. Smith
   D. Colles

Ans. is 'A' Galeazzi

5. Galeazzi fracture is: *(Andhra 98, Karnataka 97)*
   A. Supracondylar fracture of the humerus
   B. Fracture of the distal radius with inferior radioulnar joint dislocation
   C. Fracture of radius in the proximal site and dislocation of the elbow
   D. Fracture of the radial head

Ans. is 'B' Fracture of the distal radius with inferior radioulnar joint dislocation

FRACTURE BOTH BONES FOREARM

Mechanism of Injury

A twisting force (usually fall on hand) produce spiral fracture with both bones broken at different level (radius usually at higher level). A direct blow or angulating force causes a transverse fracture of both bones at the same level.

Treatment Rationale

A fracture of shaft of radius at the junction of upper and middle thirds proximal to pronator teres is therefore situated between two groups of muscles. The proximal fragment has only supinators inserted into it and the distal fragment has only pronators. Thus causing supination of proximal fragment and pronation of distal fragment. **Fractures of upper third of radius, therefore, should usually be immobilized with the hand and forearm supinated,** so that the distal fragment is rotated into the same axis as the proximal fragment.

If the fracture is at, or below, **the middle third** (distal to pronator teres) of the bone, the proximal fragment has both supinators and pronators muscles attached to it. It therefore takes up the mid position half way between full supination and full pronation, and this forearm fracture should usually be immobilized with the hand and **forearm in the mid (neutral) position.**

Open reduction and internal fixation by plating for displaced diaphyseal fractures in the adult are generally accepted as the best method of treatment and in children they are managed by Cast.

Night stick fracture is isolated fracture of ulna caused by blow on Ulna causing transverse fracture that is usually non-displaced or minimally displaced and can be managed by cast displaced fractures are usually treated with compression plating.

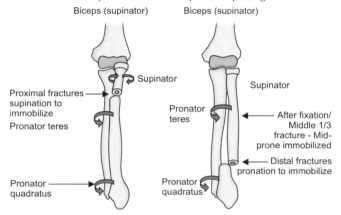

Fig. 7.39: Forces in different region of forearm

MULTIPLE CHOICE QUESTIONS

1. Fracture of proximal forearm cast position is:
   (NEET Pattern 2013)
   A. Pronated flexion   B. Neutral position
   C. Supinated position   D. Position does not matter
   Ans. is 'C' Supinated position

2. Fracture of both bone forearm at same level, position of the arm in plaster is: *(AIIMS June 1999)*
   A. Full supination   B. 10 degree supination
   C. Full pronation   D. Mid-prone
   Ans. is 'D' Mid-prone
   - In children, and sometimes also in adults, it is worth-while first to attempt manipulative reduction under anaesthesia. If this is successful a full-length arm plaster is applied with *elbow at a right angle and the forearm in a position midway between pronation and supination (mid-prone position).*

3. The treatment of choice of fracture of radius and ulna in an adult is: *(Delhi 1992)*
   A. Plaster for 4 weeks
   B. Closed reduction and calipers
   C. Reduction and stabilization with plating
   D. Kuntscher nails
   Ans. is 'C' Reduction and stabilization with plating

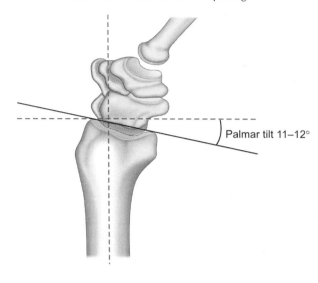

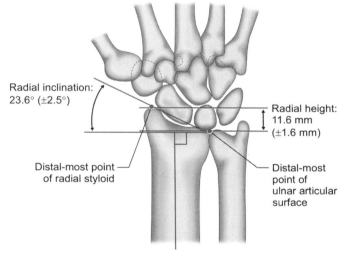

Fig. 7.40: Normal anatomy distal radius

COLLES FRACTURE

Colles fracture is **fracture of lower end of radius at its corticocancellous junction** mostly occurring in post-menopausal osteoporotic elderly women; as a result of fall on outstretched hand, with wrist in extension. It is one of the **most common fractures in elderly.**

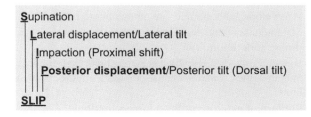

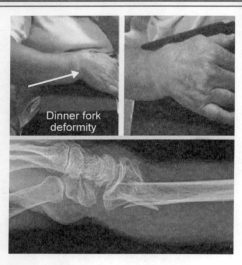

Fig. 7.41: Colles fracture

Most Colles fractures can be successfully treated nonoperatively and cast is applied on opposite forces to displacement. **That's why position of immobilization in Colles fracture is:**

P ronation
| P almar angulation
| | U lnar deviation
Pro-Pag-Unda—Called as Hand shaking cast

In younger patients, near-normal function and clinical and radiographic appearance are expected. If maintenance of reduction of Colles or Smith fractures requires prolonged immobilization in extreme positions, or reduction is lost early in treatment, closed reduction followed by percutaneous K-wire fixation is done.

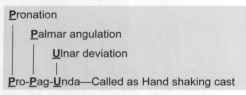
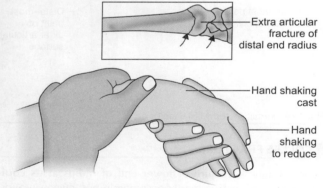

Fig. 7.42: Reduction of Colles fracture

Complications of Colles Fracture:

- *Joint Stiffness:* **Finger stiffness is most common complication.** Wrist, elbow, and shoulder are other joints to become stiff.
- Malunion is the 2nd most common complication and it leads to **dinner fork deformity.**
- Sudeck's osteodystrophy/Reflex sympathetic dystrophy. Colles fracture is the commonest cause of Sudeck's dystrophy in upper limb.
- **Rupture of extensor pollicis longus tendon.**

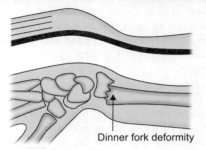

Fig. 7.43: Malunited colles

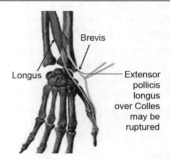

Fig. 7.44: EPL injury

- Carpal tunnel syndrome causing median nerve compression.
- Carpal instability.
- Triangular-fibrocartilage complex (TFCC) injury and subluxation of inferior radioulnar joint.
- Delayed union and nonunion are extremely rare.

TFCC

Triangular fibro cartilage complex: It connects ulnar styloid process to carpals and distal radius. It includes dorsal radioulnar ligaments, ulnotriquetral and ulnolunate ligaments, ulnar collateral ligament, articular disc and Extensor Carpi Ulnaris (ECU) sheath. It stabilizes Distal Radio Ulnar Joint (DRUJ). TFCC injury causes DRUJ instability and wrist pain

MULTIPLE CHOICE QUESTIONS

1. All of the following are displacements of Colle's fracture except: *(DNB JULY 2016)*
   A. Dorsal tilt
   B. Impaction
   C. Supination
   D. Medial displacement
Ans. is 'D' Medial displacement

2. Which of the following is true about Colles Fracture? *(NEET 2016, CET Nov 15)*
   A. Volar angulation with Radial deviation occurs
   B. It is an intra articular fracture
   C. It may lead to gunstock deformity due to malunion
   D. It is associated with dorsal angulation
Ans. is 'D' It is associated with dorsal angulation

3. Colles fracture: *(PGI May 2016)*
   A. Fracture line is at radioulnar joint
   B. Fracture line extends to the carpal joint
   C. 2 cm proximal to the radiocarpal joint
   D. Distal fragment is ulnar deviated
   E. Distal fragment is palmar fixed
Ans. is 'C' 2 cm proximal to the radiocarpal joint

4. All are true about colles fracture except: *(NEET 2015)*
   A. In old age
   B. Dorsal shift
   C. At cortico-cancellous junction
   D. Garden spade deformity

Ans. is 'D' Garden spade deformity

5. Colles fracture which of the following is not true?
   (AIIMS Nov 2014)
   A. Dorsal tilt
   B. Volar tilt
   C. Lateral displacement
   D. Supination

Ans. is 'B' Volar tilt

6. Commonest fracture in elderly with fall on outstretched hand is: *(NEET Pattern 2013)*
   A. Colles fracture
   B. Bennetts fracture
   C. Galeazzi fracture
   D. Monteggia fracture

Ans. is 'A' Colles fracture

7. Modified Allen's test is for proper arterial supply at the:
   (AIIMS Nov 2012)
   A. Arm
   B. Forearm
   C. Wrist
   D. Elbow

Ans. is 'C' Wrist

8. Dinner fork deformity is seen in: *(NEET Pattern 2012)*
   A. Colles fracture
   B. March fracture
   C. Lateral condyle fracture
   D. Supracondylar fracture

Ans. is 'A' Colles fracture

9. Most common complication of Colles:
   (Neet Pattern 2012, Karnataka 2K, NB 2K, AI 97, 95, AIIMS May 1995)
   A. Malunion
   B. Avascular necrosis
   C. Finger stiffness
   D. Rupture of EPL tendon

Ans. is 'C' Finger stiffness

10. Position of wrist in cast of Colles fracture is: *(JIPMER 98)*
    A. Palmar deviation and pronation
    B. Palmar deviation and supination
    C. Dorsal deviation and pronation
    D. Dorsal deviation and supination

Ans. is 'A' Palmar deviation and pronation

11. Colles fracture is: *(WB 93, AMU 92, DNB 1990)*
    A. Common in adolescence
    B. A fracture about the ankle joint
    C. Common in elderly women
    D. A fracture of head of the radius

Ans. is 'C' Common in elderly women
    Colles is seen in osteoporotic elderly female

12. All of the following can be the complications of a malunited Colles fracture except: *(AI 2004, 96)*
    A. Rupture of flexor pollicis longus tendon
    B. Reflex sympathetic dystrophy (RSD)
    C. Carpal tunnel syndrome
    D. Carpal instability

Ans. is 'A' Rupture of flexor pollicis longus tendon

SUDECK'S OSTEONEURO DYSTROPHY

Sudeck's osteoneurodystrophy/reflex sympathetic dystrophy/algodystrophy/complex regional pain syndrome

Complex regional pain syndrome (CRPS) type I is a regional pain syndrome that usually develops after tissue trauma. The symptoms are unrelated to the severity of the initial trauma and are not confined to the distribution of a single peripheral nerve. **CRPS type II (causalgia) is a regional pain syndrome that develops after injury to a peripheral nerve, usually a major nerve trunk.** Spontaneous pain initially develops within the territory of the affected nerve but eventually may spread outside the nerve distribution. Median > Sciatic (Tibial trunk) are the most common nerves involved.

Pain is the primary clinical feature of CRPS. Vasomotor dysfunction, sudomotor abnormalities, or focal edema may occur alone or in combination but must be present for diagnosis. In CRPS, localized sweating (increased resting sweat output) and changes in blood flow may produce temperature differences between affected and unaffected limbs.

The most characteristic symptom is **pain out of proportion to the inciting event in both severity and duration.** It is often burning in character. Hence the term 'Causalgia' which means burning pain.

Swelling is the most consistent physical finding. It often begins in area of injury and is soft initially as the process continues, oedema gradually becomes firm and involves much broader area.

Stiffness and discolouration of skin (red, blue and/or pallor) are other classic signs.

Trophic skin changes i.e. skin is shiny, thin with loss of normal wrinkles and creases are characteristically seen late. The most common radiographic finding is **localized osteopenia**-increased blood flow to the bone. Prognosis is directly related to the time to diagnosis and initiation of therapy. **The goal is to break abnormal sympathetic Reflex and to restore motion.**

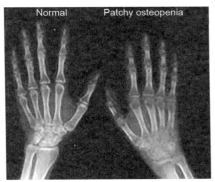

Fig. 7.45: Patchy osteopenia

The natural history of typical CRPS may be more benign than Reflected in the literature. A variety of surgical and medical treatments have been developed, with conflicting reports of efficacy. Clinical trials suggest that early mobilization with physical therapy or a brief course of glucocorticoids may be helpful for CRPS type I. Other medical treatments include the use of adrenergic blockers, nonsteroidal anti-inflammatory drugs, calcium channel blockers, phenytoin, opioids, and calcitonin. Stellate ganglion blockade is a commonly used invasive therapeutic technique that often provides temporary pain relief, but the efficacy of repetitive blocks is uncertain.

Recovery is prolonged **and** painful both for patient and surgeon. 3 years usually elapse before the bones are remineralized and it is rare that full range of movements returns.

Note: Reflex Sympathetic Dystrophy-**Patchy** Osteopenia
Hyperparathyroidism- **Generalised** Osteopenia
Tuberculosis- **Disuse** Osteopenia

MULTIPLE CHOICE QUESTIONS

1. CRPS: *(PGI Nov 2015)*
   A. Type 1 due to nerve injury
   B. Type 2 due to fracture complication
   C. Tissue necrosis and gangrene are common feature
   D. Burning pain is seen
   E. Patchy osteopenia is seen

Ans. is 'D' Burning pain is seen; 'E' Patchy osteopenia is seen

2. A lady with Colles fracture. The fracture healed but after few days patient develops pain and swelling over wrist and forearm, red hot and shiny skin and on X-ray-patchy osteopenia. Diagnosis is: *(AIIMS May 2013)*
   A. Sudeck's osteodystrophy
   B. Causalgia
   C. Non-union
   D. Nerve injury

Ans. is 'A' Sudeck's osteodystrophy

3. Sudeck's dystrophy symptoms are all except: *(NEET Pattern 2012)*
   A. Pain
   B. Increased bone density
   C. Sweating
   D. Stiffness

Ans. is 'B' Increased bone density

4. Regarding Sudeck's osteodystrophy all are true except: *(AIIMS Nov 2000, PGI 93)*
   A. Burning pain
   B. Stiffness and swelling
   C. Erythematous and cyanotic discolouration
   D. Self limiting and good prognosis

Ans. is 'D' Self limiting and good prognosis
   – Recovery is prolonged and painful both for patient and surgeon. 3 years usually elapse before the bones are remineralized and it is rare that full range of movements returns.

5. Sudeck's atrophy is associated with: *(Delhi 1999)*
   A. Osteopetrosis
   B. Osteophyte formation
   C. Osteopenia
   D. Osteochondritis

Ans. is 'C' Osteopenia

6. Stellate ganglion block is useful in: *(AIIMS Nov 1999)*
   A. Sudeck's osteodystrophy
   B. Compound palmar ganglion
   C. Tenosynovitis
   D. Osteoarthritis of first CMC joint

Ans. is 'A' Sudeck's osteodystrophy

7. A 40-year-old female presented to the clinic after 3 months of traumatic tibial fracture with history of pain and swelling of right leg since 8–10 days. Her skin of that was shiny, cold and edematous. There was no history of hypertension and diabetes. What is the diagnosis?
   A. Complex regional pain syndrome I
   B. Complex regional pain syndrome II
   C. Fibromyalgia
   D. Peripheral neuropathy

Ans. is 'A' Complex regional pain syndrome Type I (CRPS I)

SMITH'S FRACTURE: REVERSE COLLES!

Smith fracture is treated by close reduction and immobilization in long arm (above elbow) cast with forearm in supination and wrist in extension (dorsiflexion).

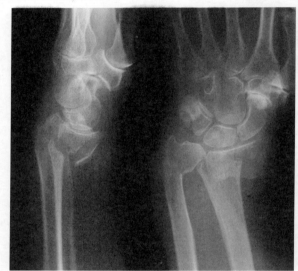

Fig. 7.46: Smith fracture = Reverse Colles fracture

Definition	Colles Fracture/Pouteau's fracture	Smith Fracture/Reverse Colles Fracture
Displacement	**S**upination 　**L**ateral displacement/Lateral tilt angulation 　　**I**mpaction (Proximal shift) 　　　**P**osterior displacement/Posterior tilt/angulation **SLIP**	**P**ronation 　**P**almar angulation 　　**U**lnar deviation **Pro-Pag-Unda**
Position of Cast	**P**ronation 　**P**almar angulation 　　**U**lnar deviation **Pro-Pag-Unda**	**S**upination 　**L**ateral displacement/Lateral tilt angulation 　　**I**mpaction (Proximal shift) 　　　**P**osterior displacement/Posterior tilt/angulation **SLIP**
Extent of Cast	Below elbow	Above elbow

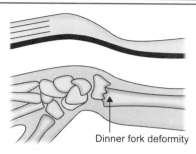

Fig. 7.47: Malunited Colles

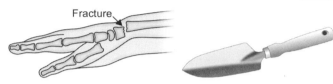

Fig. 7.48: Smith fracture – reverse Colles! "Garden Spade Deformity"

MULTIPLE CHOICE QUESTIONS

1. Garden spade deformity is seen in: *(NEET Pattern 2013)*
   A. Barton's fracture   B. Colles fracture
   C. Smith's fracture   D. Bennet's fracture

Ans. is 'C' Smith's fracture

2. Smith's fracture involves which bone? *(NEET Pattern 2012)*
   A. Distal radius   B. Proximal ulna
   C. Metatarsal   D. Patella

Ans. is 'A' Distal radius

3. Management of Smith's fracture is: *(AI 94)*
   A. Open reduction and fixation
   B. Plaster cast with forearm in pronation
   C. Closed reduction with below-elbow cast
   D. Above-elbow cast with forearm in supination

Ans. is 'D' Above-elbow cast with forearm in supination
   – Treatment is closed reduction and immobilization in cast with forearm in supination and wrist in extension.
   – Percutaneous pinning may be done in unstable fractures.

BARTON'S FRACTURE

A fracture dislocation in which the carpus and a rim of distal radius are displaced together.

They usually require open reduction and internal fixation. These fractures are almost impossible to treat by closed means although few advocate an attempt of non-operative management Plate fixation of volar Barton fractures is carried out.

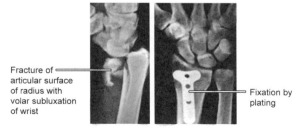

Fig. 7.49: Barton fracture

Chauffeur's Fracture is Intra-articular radial styloid fracture.

MULTIPLE CHOICE QUESTIONS

1. Barton's fracture is: *(NEET Pattern 2013; 2012)*
   A. Fracture distal end humerus
   B. Extra-articular fracture distal end radius
   C. Intra-articular fracture distal end radius
   D. Intra-articular fracture distal end radius with carpal bone subluxation

Ans. is 'D' Intra-articular fracture distal end radius with carpal bone subluxation

2. All are injuries of lower end of radius except: *(TN 98, PGI 95)*
   A. Smith's fracture   B. Colles fracture
   C. Night stick fracture D. Barton's fracture

Ans. is 'C' Night stick fracture
   – Night stick fracture: Isolated fracture of ulna.

3. Barton's fracture of the wrist: *(TN 92)*
   A. Involves radiocarpal subluxation
   B. Is a severe form of a Colles' fracture
   C. Is often treated by cast   D. All of the above

Ans. is 'A' Involves radiocarpal subluxation
   – *Colles fracture and Smith's fracture:* Extra-articular fracture of distal end radius.
   – *Barton's fracture:* Intra-articular fracture of distal end radius with carpus dislocation.

CARPAL INJURIES

Relative Incidence of Carpal Bone Fractures

Scaphoid > Triquetral > Trapezium

Fracture Scaphoid—Tenderness in anatomical snuff box!

Scaphoid is the most commonly fractured bone in the carpus, in adult as well as children. Scaphoid fracture is seen most commonly in males between the ages of 15 and 30. Middle third **(Waist)** fractures are most common accounting for 70% of scaphoid fractures > proximal pole fracture (20%) > distal pole fracture (10%), in adults and adolescents. **Distal pole avulsion type fracture is most common fracture type in children.**

- Most of the **blood supply to the scaphoid enters distally**, so blood supply of scaphoid diminishes proximally. This accounts for the fact that 1% of distal third, 20% of middle third, 40% of proximal third and 100% of proximal pole fractures result in avascular necrosis or non-union of the proximal fragment.

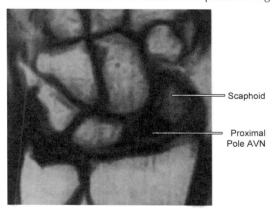

Fig. 7.50: AVN scaphoid

- A delay in diagnosis and treatment of this fracture may alter the prognosis for union.
- A wrist sprain that is sufficiently severe to require radiographic examination initially should be treated as a possible fracture of the scaphoid, and radiographs should be repeated in 2 weeks even though initial radiographs may be negative.
- **Fullness and tenderness in anatomical snuff box.** Proximal pressure along the axis of the thumb may be painful.
- Recent fracture shows only in the oblique view.
- MRI can diagnose occult fractures.
- MRI, especially with gadolinium enhancement, also is useful in assessing the vascularity of a fractured scaphoid.

Nondisplaced, Stable Scaphoid Fractures: Scaphoid Glass Holding Cast

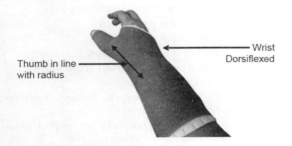

Fig. 7.51: Glass holding cast—scaphoid

Displaced, Unstable Scaphoid Fractures: Headless Screw (Herbert) is used

- Complication Nonunion > Avascular Necrosis.

MULTIPLE CHOICE QUESTIONS

1. Scaphoid fracture which area has maximum chances of Avascular Necrosis? *(NEET Pattern 2019)*
   A. Proximal 1/3　　B. Middle 1/3
   C. Distal 1/3
   D. Scaphoid Tubercle Fracture

Ans. is 'A' Proximal 1/3

- Most of the **blood supply to the scaphoid enters distally**, so blood supply of scaphoid diminishes proximally. This accounts for the fact that 1% of distal third, 20% of middle third, 40% of proximal third and 100% of proximal pole fractures result in avascular necrosis or non-union of the proximal fragment.

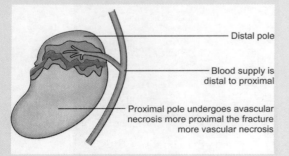

Fig. 7.52: Scaphoid blood supply

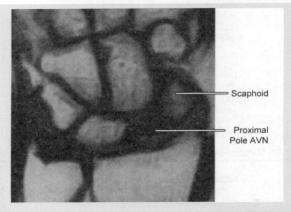

Fig. 7.50: AVN scaphoid

2. A young man had a fall on his outstretched hand, presented to the hospital with pain on the radial side of wrist and swelling in the anatomical snuff box. X-ray showed the following findings. What is the diagnosis? *(AIIMS Nov 2017)*

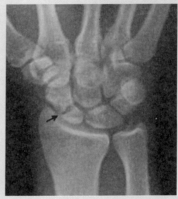 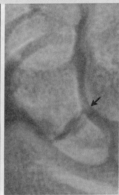

   A. Scaphoid fracture
   B. Trans scaphoidperilunate disruption fracture
   C. Hook of hamate fracture
   D. Distal radius fracture

Ans. 'A' Scaphoid fracture

3. 1st Carpal bone to ossify: *(AIIMS Nov 2017)*
   A. Trapezoid　　B. Capitate
   C. Lunate　　D. Pisiform

Ans. B. Capitate

Ossification of the Carpal Bones

Ossification of the carpal bones occurs in a predictable sequence, starting with the capitates and ending with the pisiform.

At birth, there is no calcification in the carpal bones. Although there is great individual variability, approximate ossification times are as follows:

- *Capitate:* 1-3 months
- *Hamate:* 2-4 months
- *Triquetrum:* 2-3 years
- *Lunate:* 2-4 years
- *Scaphoid:* 4-6 years
- *Trapezium:* 4-6 years
- *Trapezoid:* 4-6 years
- *Pisiform:* 8-12 years

4. Treatment of scaphoid fracture: *(NEET DEC 2016)*
   A. Conservative
   B. Compression Screws
   C. Compression Plating
   D. Traction

Ans. is 'A' Conservative

5. Ossification center of scaphoid appears at: *(CET Nov 15)*
   A. 1–6 months
   B. 1 to 2 years
   C. 2 to 4 years
   D. 4 to 6 years

Ans. is 'D' 4 to 6 years (~5 years)

6. Axis of upper limb passes through: *(NEET Pattern 2013)*
   A. Capitulum
   B. Trochlea
   C. Olecranon
   D. Radial styloid

Ans. is 'A' Capitulum

7. Most common complication of scaphoid fracture:
   (NEET Pattern 2013)
   A. Malunion
   B. Avascular necrosis
   C. Wrist stiffness
   D. Arthritis

Ans. is 'B' Avascular necrosis
   – Nonunion > Avascular necrosis

8. Which one of the following statements is not correct regarding fracture of the scaphoid: *(UPSC 01)*
   A. It is the most commonly fractured carpal bone
   B. Persistent tenderness in the anatomical snuffbox is highly suggestive of fracture
   C. Immediate X-ray of hand may not reveal fracture line
   D. Malunion is a frequent complication

Ans. is 'D' Malunion is a frequent complication
   – The problem of union in scaphoid fracture are delayed union or non-union (not malunion).

9. A patient reported with a history of fall on an outstretched hand, complains of pain in the anatomical snuffbox and clinically no deformities visible. The diagnosis is:
   (DNB June 2017, Andhra 99, NIMS 98) (AI 92, AIIMS 90)
   A. Colles' fracture
   B. Lunate dislocation
   C. Barton's fracture
   D. Scaphoid fracture

Ans. is 'D' Scaphoid fracture
   – Tenderness in anatomical snuffbox think of fracture scaphoid

10. In children fracture scaphoid is through rare but usually involves: *(JIPMER 98, AIIMS 92)*
    A. Waist
    B. Proximal pole
    C. Neck
    D. Distal pole

Ans. is 'D' Distal pole

"Although uncommon, fractures of the scaphoid in children tend to be avulsions of the distal pole accounting for 75%, with 20% of the waist and 5% of the proximal pole".

11. Most common site of scaphoid fracture is:
    (NEET 2016, AI 1997)
    A. Waist
    B. Proximal fragment
    C. Distal fragment
    D. Tilting of the lunate

Ans. is 'A' Waist

12. The best radiological view for fracture scaphoid is:
    (Assam 95, PGI 91, AI 89)
    A. AP
    B. PA
    C. Lateral
    D. Oblique

Ans. is 'D' Oblique

13. In non-union of scaphoid vascularized muscle pedicle graft is taken from: *(PGI 93, AIIMS 90)*
    A. Pronator teres
    B. Brachioradialis
    C. Pronator quadratus
    D. Extensor pollicis longus

Ans. is 'C' Pronator quadratus

WRIST DISLOCATION

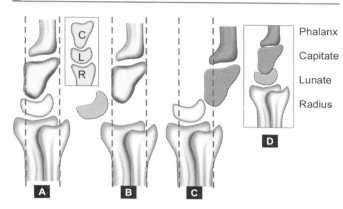

Figs. 7.53A to D: (A) Normal; (B) Lunate dislocation; (C) Perilunate dislocation; (D) Normal

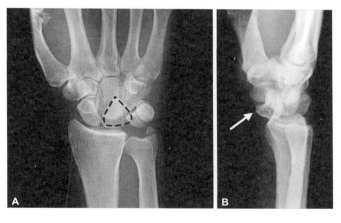

Figs. 7.54A and B: (A) Pie Sign (Lunate dislocation); (B) Spilled tea pot sign (Lunate dislocation)

1. Lunate dislocation
   – Lunate dislocate anteriorly but the rest of the carpals remain in position.
2. Perilunate dislocation
   – The lunate remains in position and the rest of the carpals dislocate dorsally.
   – **Perilunate is more common.**
   – Complications may be AVN, osteoarthritis and median nerve injury.
   – The most common type of perilunate instability is transscaphoid perilunate fracture dislocation.
   – **Median nerve is most commonly involved** nerve.
   – The most commonly used method of closed reduction is **Tavernier's maneuver.**

Note: Scapholunate dissociation has Terry Thomas Sign.

Orthopedics Quick Review

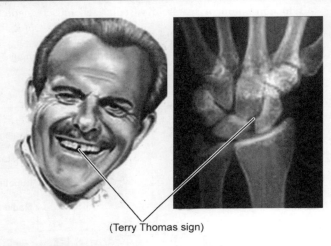

Fig. 7.55: Terry Thomas Sign

Note: Scapholunate ligament is commonly injured at wrist.

MULTIPLE CHOICE QUESTIONS

1. Perilunate dislocation is: *(NEET 2018)*
   A. Lunate and carpal bones dislocate anteriorly
   B. Lunate stays in place and carpal bones dislocate
   C. Lunate and carpal bones dislocate posteriorly
   D. Lunate dislocates anteriorly, but carpal bones stay in place

   Ans. is 'B' Lunate stays in place and carpal bones dislocate

2. A patient presents with wrist trauma. On investigations patient is diagnosed to have a sprained wrist without any evidence of fracture. there is tenderness in anatomical snuffbox. Which ligament is commonly involved?
   (NEET DEC 2016)
   A. Scapholunate ligament   B. Radial collateral ligament
   C. Lunotriquetral ligament   D. Ulnar collateral ligament

   Ans. is 'A' Scapholunate ligament

3. The most common nerve involvement in dislocation of Lunate is: *(NIMS 2000) (UP 1998)*
   A. Median nerve   B. Anterior interosseus
   C. Posterior interosseus   D. Median nerve

   Ans. is 'A' Median nerve

HAND INJURIES

Thumb-Carpometacarpal (CMC) Fracture Dislocations

The majority of thumb CMC joint injuries are fracture dislocation rather than pure dislocations. The majority of thumb metacarpal base fractures are intra-articular. These intra-articular fractures are of two types.

Bennet's Fracture

In 1882, Bennett, an Irish surgeon, described an **intra articular** fracture through the **base of the first metacarpal** in which the shaft is laterally dislocated by the unopposed **pull of the abductor pollicis longus**. The medial projection of the thumb metacarpal base on which the volar oblique ligament attaches remains in place. The technique of closed pinning described by Wagner is preferred, but should reduction be unsatisfactory, open reduction is indicated.

Note: Bennet's fractures is common in Boxers but Boxers fractuers is eponym for 5th metacarpal neck fracture.

Rolando Fracture (Comminuted First Metacarpal Base)

In 1910, Rolando described a T- or Y-shaped **intra-articular fracture involving the base of 1st metacarpal** that usually does not result in diaphyseal displacement as in a Bennet' fracture. Because of the likelihood of posttraumatic arthritis after these fractures accurate reduction is important.

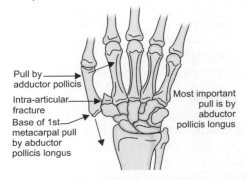

Fig. 7.56: Bennett's fracture (common fracture in boxer's)

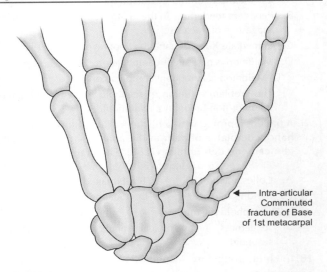

Fig. 7.57: Rolando fracture

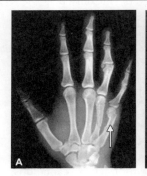 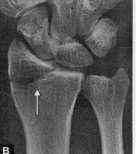

Fig. 7.58: (A) Boxer's Fracture (fracture neck of 5th metacarpal) (B) Chauffeur's fracture (Fracture of radial styloid)

Note: In boxers— Boxer's fracture is more common than Bennett's fracture

Upper Limb Traumatology

MULTIPLE CHOICE QUESTIONS

1. Which Bone does not form the Wrist joint:
   (AIIMS Nov 2018)
   A. Radius
   B. Triquetrum
   C. Scaphoid
   D. Ulna

   Ans. is 'D' Ulna
   Wrist is radio-carpal joint. Ulna is not part of wrist point.

2. Mc bone to get fractured in fall on outstretched hand is:
   (NEET 2018)

   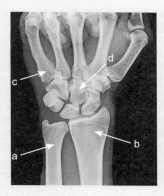

   A. Lower End Ulna
   B. Lower End Radius (Colles fracture)
   C. 5th Metacarpal
   D. Capitate

   Ans. is 'B' Lower End Radius (Colles fracture)

   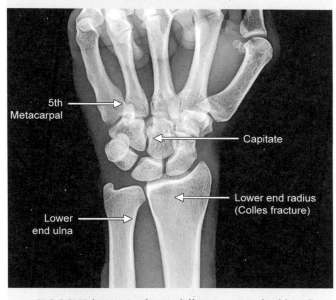

   "FOOSH" (Fracture due to fall on outstretched hand)
   – Fracture clavicle
   – Surgical neck of humerus fracture
   – Supracondylar fracture humerus and lateral condyle fracture humerus
   – Head and neck fracture of radius
   – Galeazzi fracture dislocation
   – Colle's fracture (Most common)
   – Radial styloid fracture
   – Fracture scaphoid

3. Bennett's fracture is an:
   (DNB June 2017, TN 2015, 2004, 2003)
   A. Extra-articular fracture of the 1st metacarpal
   B. Extra-articular fracture of 2nd metatarsal
   C. Intra-articular fracture of the 1st metacarpal
   D. Intra-articular fracture of the 2nd metacarpal

   Ans. is 'C' Intra-articular fracture of the 1st metacarpal

4. One of the common fractures that occur during boxing by hitting with a closed fist is: (NEET 2015)
   A. Monteggia fracture dislocation
   B. Galeazzi fracture dislocation
   C. Bennett's fracture dislocation
   D. Smith's fracture

   Ans. is 'C' Bennett's fracture dislocation

5. Boxer's fracture is: (DNB June 2017, NEET Pattern 2013)
   A. Radial styloid fracture
   B. Reverse colle's fracture
   C. 5th metacarpal fracture
   D. 1st metacarpal fracture

   Ans. is 'C' 5th metacarpal fracture

6. Rolando Fracture involves base of: (NEET Pattern 2012)
   A. 1st metacarpal
   B. 2nd metacarpal
   C. 3rd metacarpal
   D. 4th metacarpel

   Ans. is 'A' 1st metacarpal

7. A Bennett's fracture is difficult to maintain in a reduced position mainly because of the pull of the:
   (Karnataka 99, AIIMS May 94, PGI 92)
   A. Flexor pollicis longus
   B. Flexor pollicis brevis
   C. Extensor pollicis brevis
   D. Abductor pollicis longus
   E. Adductor pollicis

   Ans. is 'D' Abductor pollicis longus

8. The term Bennett's fracture is used to describe:
   (Karnataka 1989)
   A. Fracture-dislocation of metacarpophalangeal joint of thumb
   B. Interphalangeal fracture dislocation of thumb
   C. Anterior marginal fracture of distal end of radius
   D. Fracture dislocation of trapeziometacarpal joint

   Ans. is 'D' Fracture dislocation of trapeziometacarpal joint

CHAPTER 8: Spinal Injury

COMMONEST MODE OF SPINAL INJURY

- In developing country, e.g. **India—Fall from height**
- In **developed countries—Road traffic accident**

MULTIPLE CHOICE QUESTIONS

1. **The commonest cause of spinal cord injuries in our country is:** *(SGPGI 2003, AMU 2002)*
   A. Road traffic accident
   B. Fall from a height
   C. Fall into well
   D. House collapse

   Ans. is 'B' Fall from a height

SPINAL SHOCK

Sometimes physical energy of the injury mechanism causes immediate depolarization of axonal membranes in the neural tissue. This results in functional neurological deficit that exceeds the actual tissue disruption. This condition is referred to as spinal shock. The presence of spinal shock causes the absence of all reflexes. And it typically lasts up to 24–48 hours after the injury. **The bulbocavernosus reflex is the reflex that returns first, thus marking the end of spinal shock.**

When a spinal cord injury is suspected methyl prednisolone (steroid) should be started. Most benefit occurs in the first 8 hours, and additional effect occurs with in first 24 hours.

Reflex	Location of lesion (Root value)	Normal response	Abnormal response	Significance
Cremasteric	T12-L1	Stroking the medial thigh proximal to distal produce upward motion of scrotum^Q	No motion of scrotum	Return of normal response of bulbocavernosus, anal and cremasteric reflex indicate that the spinal shock is over
Anal wink	S2-S4	Stroking perianal skin cause anal sphincter contraction	No anal sphincter contraction	
Bulbocavernosus	S3-S4	Squeezing the glans penis in males, applying pressure to clitoris in females, or tugging (pulling) the bladder catheter in either cause anal sphincter contraction^Q	No anal sphincter contraction	

The dose of methyl prednisolone is 30 mg/kg loading dose + 5.4 mg/kg/hour **maintenance dose** for 24 hours **and if patient presents after 3 hours of injury for 48 hours.**

Areflexic bladder bower and lower limbs
- With symmetrical involvement conus medullaris syndrome
- Asymmetrical involvement cauda equina syndrome

MULTIPLE CHOICE QUESTIONS

1. **Earliest reflex to reappear after spinal shock:** *(AIIMS Nov 2018, NEET Pattern 2013)*
   A. Knee jerk
   B. Ankle jerk
   C. Bulbocavernous reflex
   D. Abdominal reflex

   Ans. is 'C' Bulbocavernous reflex

2. **A patient presents with normal Babinsky reflex with ankle areflexia with presence of saddle anesthesia and difficulty in micturition. What is the most probable diagnosis?** *(DNB JUNE 2017)*
   A. Cauda equina syndrome
   B. Brown Sequard syndrome
   C. Leriche syndrome
   D. Williams syndrome

   Ans. is 'A' Cauda equina syndrome

3. **Acute flaccid complete paralysis with areflexia and loss of perianal reflexes, below the level of spinal cord injury is due to:** *(DNB JUNE 2017)*
   A. Spinal shock
   B. Denervation
   C. Malingering
   D. UMN paralysis

   Ans. is 'A' Spinal shock

4. **Not true for atlanto-axial joint:** *(PGI May 2016)*
   A. Vertebral artery passes posterior to foramen magnum
   B. Atlanto-axial joint with have ellipsoid joint
   C. Atlanto-occipital joint will have flexion and extension movement
   D. Atlanto-occipital joint is pivot joint
   E. Post-longitudinal ligaments passes through the spinal canal

   Ans. is 'A' Vertebral artery passes posterior to foramen magnum; 'B' Atlanto-axial joint with have ellipsoid joint; and 'D' Atlanto-occipital joint is pivot joint

- Vertebral arteries travel through foramen magnum
- Atlanto-occipital joint is condyloid joint allowing flexion and extension
- Atlanto-axial: Pivot joint
- Post-longitudinal ligaments is on posterior part of vertebral body and are in spinal canal.

5. **Spinal injury with no radiological finding is commonly seen in:** *(AIIMS Nov 2013)*
   A. Children   B. Older men
   C. Older woman   D. In middle aged

Ans. is 'A' Children

SCIWORA:
- **S**pinal **C**ord **I**njury **W**ithout **O**bvious **R**adiological **A**bnormality is seen in children due to flexibility of spine.

6. **Denis gave how many columns theory to define stability of spine:** *(DNB June 2017, AIIMS Nov 2012)*
   A. 1   B. 2
   C. 3   D. 4

Ans. is 'C' 3

Explanation
Denis' Three-Column Theory
- Proposed by Francis Denis, three-column concept divides a spinal segment into three parts: Anterior, middle, and posterior colums.
- The anterior column comprises the anterior longitudinal ligament and the anterior half of the vertebral body; the middle column comprises the posterior half of the vertebral body and the posterior longitudinal ligament; the posterior column comprises the pedicles, the facet joints and the supraspinous ligaments.
- **Significance:** If 2 out of 3 columns are involved it is labelled as unstable spinal injury.

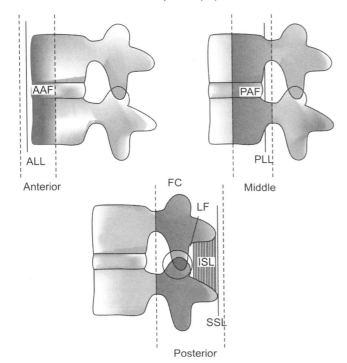

Fig. 8.1: Denis 3 columns

7. **Which is not a feature of cervical syringomyelia:** *(AIIMS Nov 2012)*
   A. Hypertrophy of abductor pollicis brevis
   B. Burning sensation in arm
   D. Biceps reflex absent
   D. Extensor plantar

Ans. is 'A' Hypertrophy of abductor pollicis brevis

Explanation
- Syringomyelia is a generic term referring to a disorder in which a cyst or cavity forms within the spinal cord. This cyst, called a syrinx, can expand and elongate over time, destroying the spinal cord. Cervical Syringomyelia has variable clinical presentations which include asymmetric weakness and atrophy of hands, lower limb spasticity, areflexia of upper extremity, dissociated sensory loss in the neck and arms (classic cape like distribution) and increased tone and hyperreflexia of lower limb. Thus there is wasting of hand and not hypertrophy.

Diagnostic modality is MRI

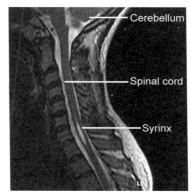

- Treatment is surgical

8. **In spinal shock:** *(NIMHANS 99)*
   A. Knee jerk is the first reflex to return
   B. High thoracic lesions are commonly associated with more severe neurological deficits
   C. Failure of return of cord activity within 48 hours is a very poor prognostic sign
   D. Both B and C

Ans. is 'D' Both B and C

9. **Return of Bulbocavernous reflex in spinal shock:** *(JIPMER 1999)*
   A. Sign of recovery from spinal shock
   B. Partial lesion of spinal cord
   C. Complete transection of spinal cord
   D. Incomplete transection of spinal cord A

Ans. is 'A' Sign of recovery from spinal shock

10. **Symmetrical areflexic bladder bowel and lower limb occur in:** *(MAHE 2003, NIMHANS 2002)*
    A. Cauda equina syndrome
    B. Conus medullaris syndrome
    C. Nerve root damage
    D. Brown-séquard syndrome

Ans. is 'B' Conus medullaris syndrome

11. A patient presented with Saddle anesthesia, bladder and bowel are normal and muscle power is normal. The diagnosis is: *(AMU 2000, NIMS 1998)*
    A. Cauda equina syndrome
    B. L3-L4 root involvement
    C. Conus medullaris lesion
    D. L4-L5 disc prolapsed

Ans. is 'C' Conus medullaris lesion
- **Conus medullaris** syndrome is characterized by bilateral saddle anesthesia, prominent bladder bowel dysfunction and impotence with loss of bulbocavernosus and anal reflex but with the preservation of muscle strength largely.

LEVEL OF INJURY

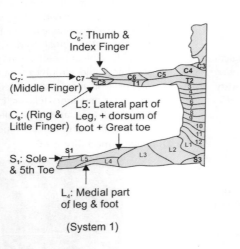
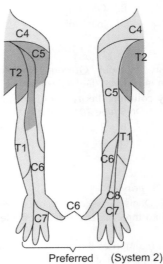

Fig. 8.2: Dermatomes (sensory supply)

Nerve root	Muscle group used for motor grading in ASIA system	Other motor	Sensory	Reflex
C5	Elbow flexion (Biceps, Brachialis)	Deltoid* (arm abduction)	Lateral shoulder Lateral arm	Biceps
C6	Wrist extension (extensor carpi radialis longus and brevis)		Thumb	Brachioradialis
C7	Elbow extensor (triceps)	Extensor digitorum* (finger extensor) Wrist flexion	Index and Middle finger	Triceps
C8	Finger flexors (flexor digitorum profundus)		Ring and little fingers	
T1	Hand intrinsics (interossei) Finger abduction		Upper anterior forearm	
L2	Hip flexors (iliopsoas)		Upper anterior thigh	
L3	Knee extensor (quadriceps)	Thigh (hip) adduction	Lower anterior thigh Anterior knee	(knee)
L4	Ankle dorsiflex or (tibialis anterior)	Quadriceps* (knee extension) Hip adduction	Medial calf, medial border of foot	(knee)
L5	**Great toe extensors (extensor hallucis longus) EHL**	Peronei (foot eversion)	**Dorsal surface foot**	
		Tibialis anterior (ankle dorsiflexion) Gluteus medius (hip abduction), Knee flexion Toe dorsiflexors	Lateral calf Great toe all aspects	
S1	Ankle plantar flexors (gastrocnemius and soleus)/FHL (Flexor Hallucis Longus)	Abductor hallucis Gluteus—maximus (hip extension)	Plantar surface foot Lateral aspect foot including 5th toe all aspects	Ankle reflex

Note: In disk prolapse usually lower nerve root is compressed.

Note: Index finger has supply from C_6 and C_7 by 2 different systems. Thus if it is asked sensory supply of thumb and Index finger C_6 and C_7 should be marked.

MULTIPLE CHOICE QUESTIONS

1. A patient is diagnosed with disc prolapse. Examination reveals paralysis of Extensor Hallucis Longus. Which nerve root is affected? *(JIPMER 2014)*
   A. L3
   B. L4
   C. L5
   D. S1

Ans. is 'C' L5

2. Root value of sensory supply of thumb and middle finger:
   A. C6, C6
   B. C7, C7 (AIIMS Nov 2013)
   C. C7, C8
   D. C6, C7

Ans. is 'D' C6, C7

3. L4–L5 disc prolapse compresses commonly:
   (NEET Pattern 2012)
   A. L3
   B. L4
   C. L5
   D. S1

Ans. is 'C' L5

4. Ankle reflex nerve root: (NEET Pattern 2016, 2012)
   A. L4
   B. L5
   C. S1
   D. S2

Ans. is 'C' S1

5. A patient involved in a road traffic accident presents with quadriparesis, sphincter disturbance, sensory level up to the upper border of sternum and respiratory rate of 35/minute. The likely level of lesion is: (AI 2010)
   A. C1 – C2
   B. C4 – C5
   C. T1 – T2
   D. T3 – T4

Ans. is 'B' C4 – C5

- C_2 dermatome – Occiput and top part of neck.
- C_3 dermatome – Lower part of neck up to the clavicle.
- C_4 dermatone – Area just below the clavicle (Area which coincide with upper border of sternum).
- Motor supply of upper-limb is $C_{5-8}\,T_1$
- Motor supply of diaphragm (Phrenic nerve) is C_{3-5}
- Thus C_4–C_5 prolapse will cause increased respiratory rate with all mentioned features.

6. A 40-year-old male after RTA, attains spinal injury. His lower limb power is greater than that of upper limb and sacral sensations are present. Type of spinal cord lesion is: (JIPMER 2005, NIMHANS 2003, AIIMS 92)
   A. Central cord syndrome
   B. Anterior cord syndrome
   C. Posterior cord syndrome
   D. Complete spinal cord injury

Ans. is 'A' Central cord syndrome

7. Complete transaction of the spinal cord at the C_7 level produces all of the following effects except: (AI 2002)
   A. Hypotension
   B. Limited respiratory effort
   C. Anesthesia below the level of the lesion
   D. Areflexia below the level of the lesion

Ans. is 'D' Areflexia below the level of the lesion

- The diaphragm is innervated by two phrenic nerves that originate as branches of the cervical plexus in neck. This motor nerve to diaphragm arise from the anterior rami of cervical nerves C_3, C_4, C_5, with major contribution coming from C_4.
- So transection of spinal cord at C_7 level is not going to stop respiration but due to involvement of thoracic intercostal muscles and abdominal muscles, there will be some weakness of respiratory effort (i.e. limited respiratory effort).
- Deep tendon reflexes above the level of complete spinal cord injury will be spared; at the level of injury will be absent and below the level of injury will be exaggerated.
- Superficial reflexes above the level of injury are spared and at the level of injury and below the level of injury are absent.

DISLOCATION OF CERVICAL SPINE

Cervical spines has highest chances of dislocation without fracture as their zygapophyseal (facet) joints slope in almost anteroposterior horizontal plane. Where as in thoracic and lumbar region facet joints are oriented vertically and inter locked.

Whiplash Injury

Hyperextension of lower cervical spine.

Jefferson's Fracture

Jefferson's fracture is burst fracture of ring of atlas (Cl) vertebrae

Burst fracture is a **vertical compression fracture.**

It is most common fracture of Atlas. There is 50% association of concomitant injury in cervical spine elsewhere.

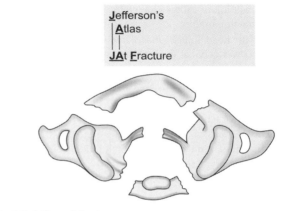

Fig. 8.3: Jefferson's fracture

Hangman's Fracture

It occurs when a fracture line passes through the neural arch of the axis (C_2) vertebrae **traumatic spondylolisthesis of axis (C_2) vertebrae on C_3–H_2** (Hangman's involves 2nd Cervical Vertebra).

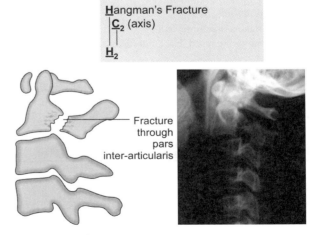

Fig. 8.4: Hangman's fracture

Note: C_1 and C_2 injuries usually do not cause neural deficit because of wide spinal canal here.

- Odontoid fracture
  Odontoid fracture. (Anderson and D'Alonzo Classification)
  Type 1 : Avulsion of tip (by alar ligaments). Unites conservatively
  Type 2 : Fracture at junction of odontoid process and axis
    Most dangerous type
    Treatment is screw fixation
  Type 3 : Fracture through the body of axis
    Conservative management
  Flexion rotation injury is the most common spinal injury followed by compression extension injury (2nd most common).
  (AIPG 2007)

  Tear drop fracture is caused by combined axial compression and flexion injury.

  In axial load injuries (compression injuries), the most common site of trauma is at the thoracolumbar junction ($D_{12} > L_1$).

  Car seat belt injury causes chance fracture- Jack-knife injury;- Flexion – Distraction injury.

  Patient with head injury, unexplained hypotension warrants evaluation of Lower cervical spine > Thoracic spine.

Fractures of spine

1. Jefferson fracture: Burst fracture of C_1
2. Hangman's fracture: Traumatic spondylolisthesis of C_2(axis) over C_3
3. Burst fracture: Vertical compression injuries
4. Whiplash injury: Sprained neck.
   Earlier were called as railroad spine/Erichsen's disease
   Hyperextension followed by flexion.
5. Flexion – Compression:
   a. Wedge compression
   b. Tear drop (may have bone fragment from antero-inferior part of vertebra).
6. Flexion – distraction: Facet dislocation
7. Clay-Shoveler's fracture: Avulsion fractures of spinous process of $C_7 > D_1$ Vertebra
8. Motor Cyclists fracture (Hinged fracture): Transverse fracture across base of skull leading to separation into anterior–posterior.
9. Undertakers fracture: Tearing of C_{6-7} disc space causing subluxation, caused by Undertaker's handling the dead body.
10. SCIWORA: Pediatric injury (<8 years of age). X-rays are normal but there is neural deficit. This is due to lax ligaments permitting traction injury to cord. Cervical spine is most commonly affected.

MULTIPLE CHOICE QUESTIONS

1. **Left-Right movement of skull occurs at:** *(NEET Pattern 2019)*
   A. Atlanto-occipital joint
   B. Atlanto-axial joint
   C. C2 – C3
   D. C6 – C7
   Ans. is 'B' Atlanto-axial joint
   Yes movement occurs at atlanto-occipital joint and **No** movement occurs at atlanto-axial joint.

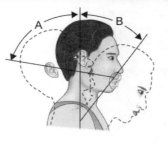 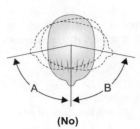
(Yes) (No)

2. **True about fractures of verterbae is/are:** *(PGI May 2017)*
   A. Wedge compression causes flexion injury
   B. Anterior longitudinal ligament runs along the posterior surface of the vertebral bodies
   C. Vertical compression force does not extend to cervical spine
   D. Chance fracture occurs due to flexion distraction injury
   E. Fracture dislocation is common in flexion rotation injury
   Ans. is 'A' Wedge compression causes flexion injury; 'D' Chance fracture occurs due to flexion distraction injury; and 'E' Fracture dislocation is common in flexion rotation injury

3. **Which of the following is not true about Jefferson's fracture?** *(NEET DEC 2016)*
   A. It is a burst fractures of the ring of atlas vertebra
   B. It is the most common type of atlas fracture
   C. Fracture definition is particularly clear on CT scan image
   D. It is associated with injury elsewhere in spine in 25% of the cases
   Ans. is 'D' It is associated with injury elsewhere in spine in 25% of the cases

4. **Most mobile segment of vertebral column is:** *(NEET DEC 2016)*
   A. Cervical   B. Thoracic
   C. Lumbar   D. Sacral
   Ans. is 'A' Cervical

5. **Most dangerous type of odontoid fracture as per Anderson and D' Alonzo classification and its respective management is:** *(NEET DEC 2016)*
   A. Type I- immobilization in rigid collar
   B. Type II- screw fixation
   C. Type III- halo vest immobilization
   D. Type IV- open reduction internal fixation
   Ans. 'B' Type II- screw fixation

6. **Mechanism underlying burst fracture is:** *(JIPMER Nov 16)*
   A. Avulsion fracture
   B. Wedge compression
   C. Vertical compression injury
   D. Whiplash injury
   Ans. is 'C' Vertical compression injury

7. **Which vertebra fracture is due to flexion Injury:** *(JIPMER Nov 16) (pg 89)*
   A. C1, C2   B. C3, C4
   C. C5, C6   D. C6, C7
   Ans. is 'C' C5, C6

Spinal Injury

8. Undertaker's fracture is: *(CET July 16)*
   A. Traumatic spondylolisthesis of C_1 over C_2
   B. Spondylolisthesis of lower cervical spine with tearing of C_6-C_7 intervertebral disc
   C. Burst fracture of C_3
   D. Spinous process fractures of lower cervical vertebrae
Ans. is 'B' Spondylolisthesis of lower cervical spine with tearing of C_6-C_7 intervertebral disc

9. Clay-Shoveler's fracture is: *(TN 2015)*
   A. Fracture of spinous process of lower cervical and upper thoracic vertebra
   B. Fracture of spinous process of mid thoracic vertebra
   C. Fracture of spinous process of lumbar vertebra
   D. Spinous process fractures of lower cervical vertebrae
Ans. is 'A' Fracture of spinous processes of lower cervical and upper thoracic vertebra

10. Chance fracture is fracture of vertebra of: *(TN 2015)*
    A. Thoracolumbar   B. Dorsolumbar
    C. Lumbosacral   D. Lumbar
Ans. is 'D' Lumbar

11. Hangman's fracture is the fracture involving which cervical vertebra? *(NEET 2015)*
    A. C1   B. C2
    C. C3   D. C4
Ans. is 'B' C2

12. Motorcyclist's fracture is: *(NEET 2015)*
    A. Stellate fracture across base of skull
    B. Transverse fracture across base of skull
    C. Lamina fracture of C_7 vertebra
    D. Spinous process fracture of C_7 vertebra
Ans. is 'B' Transverse fracture across base of skull

13. Full form of SCIWORA: *(PGI Nov 2015)*
    A. Spinal cord injury with radiological abnormality
    B. Spinal cord injury without radiological abnormality
    C. Spinal cord involvement with radiological abnormality
    D. Spinal cord involvement without radiological abnormality
    E. Spinal Cord Injury with regional ataxia
Ans. is 'B' Spinal cord injury without radiological abnormality

14. Block vertebrae are seen in: *(NEET Pattern 2013)*
    A. Paget's disease   B. Leukemia
    C. TB   D. Klippel-Feil syndrome
Ans. is 'D' Klippel-Feil syndrome

15. Most common site for trauma of spine is: *(NEET Pattern 2012)*
    A. Cervical   B. Thoracic
    C. Lumbar   D. Sacrum
Ans. is 'A' Cervical

16. Ring fracture of C_1 is called as: *(NEET Pattern 2012)*
    A. Hangman's fracture
    B. Jefferson's fracture
    C. Clay Shoveller's fracture
    D. Chance fracture
Ans. is 'B' Jefferson's fracture

17. Seat belt injury is: *(AIIMS May 2011) (PGI 93, 90, AI 90)*
    A. Tear drop fracture   B. Wedge fracture
    C. Chance fracture   D. Whiplash injury
Ans. is 'C' Chance fracture, *Car seat belt injury causes chance fracture.*

18. Burst fracture of cervical spine is due to:
    A. Whiplash injury *(NEET 2016, All India 2007, Bihar 1990)*
    B. Fall of weight on neck
    C. Vertical compression injury
    D. Car accident
Ans. is 'C' Vertical compression injury

19. Most common type of injury to spinal cord is: *(All India 2007)*
    A. Flexion   B. Extension
    C. Compression   D. Flexion-rotation
Ans. is 'D' Flexion-rotation

20. Tear drop fracture of lower cervical spine implies:
    A. Wedge compression fracture *(AIIMS 2006, SR 05, KA 2002)*
    B. Axial compression fractures
    C. Flexion-rotation injury with failure of anterior body
    D. Flexion compression failure of body
Ans. is 'D' Flexion compression failure of body
   - **Tear drop fracture** is caused by combined axial compression and flexion injury.

21. All of the following are true about fracture of the atlas vertebra, except: *(AI 2005)*
    A. Jefferson's fracture is the most common of atlas
    B. Quadriplegia is seen in 80% cases
    C. Atlanto-occipital fusion may sometimes be needed
    D. CT scans should be done for diagnosis
Ans. is 'B' Quadriplegia is seen in 80% cases.
   - There is no encroachment on the neural canal and usually no neurological damage.

22. Regarding Hangman's fracture true is: *(SGPGI 2004, AMU 2002, JIPMER 99)*
    A. High post-admission mortality
    B. Most common axis fracture
    C. Surgical treatment is necessary
    D. Union almost always occurs
Ans. is 'D' Union almost always occurs
   - Successful healing of C_2 traumatic spondylolisthesis is reported to approach 95%. This is most commonly achieved with non-operative measures, even in the presence of displacement of pars inter-articularis.

23. 'Whip-lash' injury is caused due to: *(AIIMS May 2003)*
    A. A fall from a height
    B. Acute hyperextension of the spine
    C. A blow on top to head
    D. Acute hyperflexion of the spine
Ans. is 'B' Acute hyperextension of the spine
   - Whiplash injury is caused by sudden unexpected hyperextension of cervical spine followed immediately by flexion.

24. In a Patient with head injury, unexplained hypotension warrants evaluation of: *(AI 2002)*
    A. Upper cervical spine   B. Lower cervical spine
    C. Thoracic spine   D. Lumbar spine
Ans. is 'B > C' Lower cervical spine > Thoracic spine

25. True regarding Hangman's fracture is: *(Manipal 2000)*
    A. Odontoid process fracture of C_2
    B. Spondylolisthesis of C_2 over C_3
    C. Whiplash injury   D. Fracture of hyoid bone
Ans. is 'B' Spondylolisthesis of C_2 over C_3

26. **Dislocation without fracture is seen in:** *(Delhi 1999)*
    A. Sacral spine   B. Lumbar spine
    C. Cervical spine   D. Thoracic
Ans. is 'C' Cervical spine

27. **All are true regarding whiplash injury except:** *(PGI 98, 96)*
    A. Lumbar spine is commonly involved
    B. Fractures are not common
    C. Paresthesia and chronic pain
    D. Hyperextension injury
    E. Sprains and strains without radiological findings
Ans. is 'A' Lumbar spine is commonly involved
    – Cervical spine is the commonest affected area in whiplash injury.

28. **The compression fracture is commonest in:** *(DNB 1992)*
    A. Cervical spine   B. Upper thoracic spine
    C. Lower thoracic spine   D. Lumbosacral region
Ans. is 'C' Lower thoracic spine
    – "In axial load injuries (Compression injuries), the most common site of trauma is at the thoracolumbar junction".

VERTEBROPLASTY

Vertebroplasty is percutaneous injection of bone cement (PMMA = polymethylmethacrylate) into vertebral body. It can be used for osteolytic spinal metastasis, multiple myeloma, aggressive hemangiomas, vertebral compression fractures (Osteoporotic). Its use is **contraindicated in infections, Tuberculosis.**

Vertebroplasty prevents further collapse and kyphoplasty is correction of collapse of vertebra by using high pressures (it is not preferred now).

Painful Compressed Vertebrae
- Bone Cement (PMMA) prevents further collapse — Vertebroplasty
- Bone Cement Injected after restoring the vertebral height by pressure — Kyphoplasty (Not preferred now-a-days)

MULTIPLE CHOICE QUESTIONS

1. **Normal Curvature seen in Lumbar spine:** *(AIIMS Nov 2018)*
   A. Lordosis   B. Kyphosis
   C. Scoliosis   D. Recurvatum
Ans. is 'A' Lordosis
   Lordosis: lordosis is inward curvature of spine seen at cervical and lumbar spine.

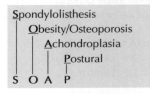

2. **Choose the correct statement about lordosis:** *(PGI Nov 2017)*
   A. Lordosis means excessive inward curvature of the spine
   B. Can be seen in Osteoporotic females
   C. Mostly seen in lumbar region and manifests as persistent back pain
   D. Poor posture is a common cause of lordosis
   E. Obesity protects against developing
Ans. is 'A' Lordosis means excessive inward curvature of the spine; 'B' Can be seen in Osteoporotic females; 'C' Mostly seen in lumbar region and manifests as persistent back pain; 'D' Poor posture is a common cause of lordosis
   Lordosis: lordosis is inward curvature of spine seen at cervical and lumbar spine. Causes of increased lordosis are SOAP.

   S — Spondylolisthesis
   O — Obesity/Osteoporosis
   A — Achondroplasia
   P — Postural

3. **Motorcyclist's fracture:** *(AIIMS Nov 2018, AI 2009)*
   A. Ring fracture
   B. Comminuted fracture
   C. Separation of suture between anterior and posterior half of skull
   D. Fracture base of skull
Ans. is 'C' Separation of suture between anterior and posterior half of skull
   – A *transverse fracture* across the floor *of the skull*, usually called a *"hinge fracture"* is sometimes referred to as *motorcyclist fracture*. At autopsy the base of the skull may be divided into two halves, each moving independent of each other like a hinge, the so-called motorcyclist fracture.

4. **What is vertebroplasty?** *(NEET Pattern 2013)*
   A. Stabilization of vertebral compression fracture
   B. Replacement of vertebral body only
   C. Replacement of vertebral body with intervertebral disc
   D. Fusion of the adjacent vertebrae
Ans. is 'A' Stabilization of vertebral compression fracture

5. **Percutaneous vertebroplasty is not done for:** *(AIIMS May 2011)*
   A. TB   B. Osteoporosis
   C. Hemangioma   D. Metastasis
Ans. is 'A' TB, vertebroplasty is contraindicated in infection or Tuberculosis

6. **Substance that is used for vertebroplasty is:** *(AIIMS May 08)*
   A. Polymethyl methacrylate
   B. Polyethyl methacrylate
   C. Polymethyl ethacrylate
   D. Polyethyl ethacrylate
Ans. is 'A' Polymethyl methacrylate
   – Vertebroplasty and kyphoplasty are interventional radiologic procedures for the treatment of the intense pain refractory to medical management or bracing caused by vertebral compression fracture associated with osteoporosis, tumors, and trauma.
   – Vertebroplasty and kyphoplasty involve intraosseous injection of acrylic cement- polymethyl methacrylate under local anesthesia and fluoroscopic guidance.

CONCEPT AND PROTOCOL OF DEFINITIVE MANAGEMENT OF SPINAL INJURIES

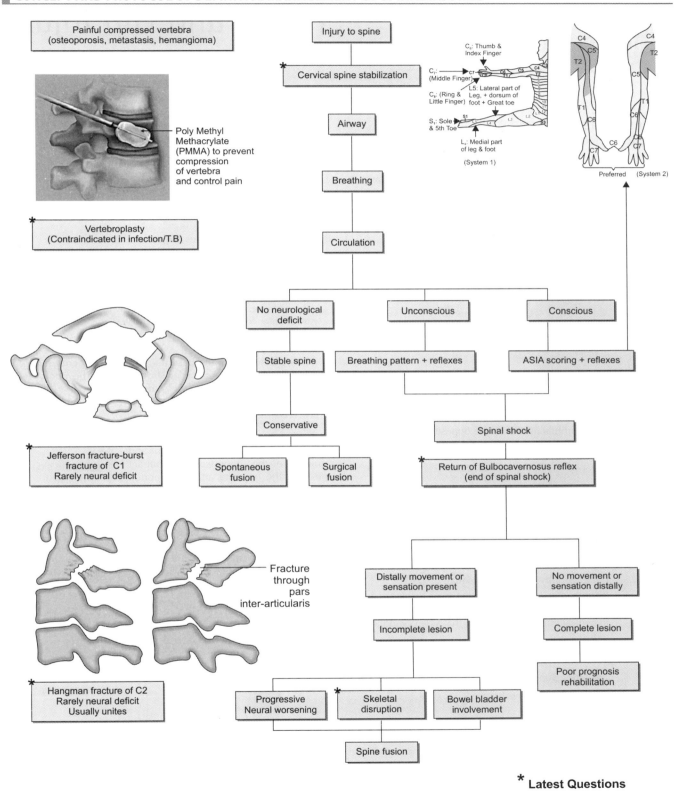

* Latest Questions

Pelvis and Hip Injury

MEASUREMENT OF SUPRATROCHANTERIC SHORTENING

Shortening of limb length produced above the level of trochanter (due to femoral head, neck and hip joint lesions) is known as supratrochanteric shortening and it is measured by following tests.

Qualitative Assessment

A. Patient lies supine and hip is extended
   1. Schoemaker's Line SchUmaker- G

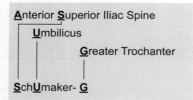

   A line joining tip of trochanter and ASIS, when prolonged on both side, should meet in the central line at or above the umbilicus. In case of proximal migration of greater trochanter the line on that side will meet its counter part below the umbilicus and on the opposite side.

   2. Morris's Bitrochanteric Test M – P – T

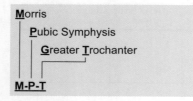

   - The distance from the tip of the trochanter to the pubic symphysis should be equal.
   - If trochanter is externally rotated or displaced back distance will increase on that side and vice versa. In central fracture dislocation that side component is reduced.

   3. Chiene's Parallelogram CAS-G

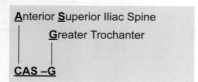

B. Nelaton's Line
   Patient lies on the normal/opposite side of the limb with preferably 90 degree flexion at hip. A line drawn from ischial tuberosity to ASIS should pass through the tip of greater trochanter. In case of supratrochanteric shortening the trochanter will be above this line.

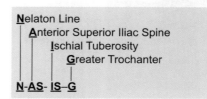

Quantitative Measurement

Bryant's Triangle: Measures Supra-trochanteric area
- The patient lies supine and tips of trochanter and ASIS are marked on both sides.
- A perpendicular is dropped from each ASIS on to the bed. From tip of greater trochanter another perpendicular is dropped on to the first one, (base of the triangle). Now join the tips of greater trochanter to ASIS on respective side. Each side of this right angled triangle is compared with its counter part on the normal side.
- **Any shortening of the base (i.e. femoral axis continuation), which may be because of shortening in the neck, head, joint or dislocation of joint can be measured.**

TRENDELENBURG SIGN

Normally when the body weight is supported on one limb, the glutei (medius and minimus) of the supported side contract and raise the opposite and unsupported side of pelvis, if the abductor mechanism is defective the unsupported side of pelvis drops and this is known as positive Trendelenburg's test.

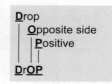

Trendelenburg's test is done to assess the integrity of abductor mechanism. It is positive in the conditions in which any of the three—fulcrum (Femoral Head), lever arm (neck length) or power (muscles/nerve) is affected.

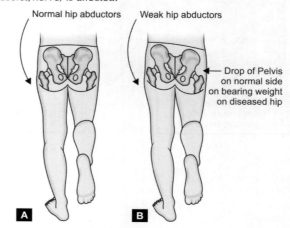

Figs. 9.1A and B: Trendelenburg test

Causes of Positive Trendelenburg Test

1. **Power-Paralysis of abductor muscles**
   - **Abductors of hip are—Gluteus medius and minimus,** Tensor fascia lata and sartorius (accessory).

   Note: Disc prolapse at L4–5 compresses L5 nerve root which supplies G.medius and minimus.

   - **Superior gluteal nerve palsy** (supply gluteus medius and minimus)
   - Polio
   - Iliotibial tract palsy
2. **Decreased lever arm**
   - Fracture neck femur
3. **Absence of stable fulcrum** about which the abductor muscles can act. Dislocation of hip, destruction of femoral head as in Perthes disease, AVN, late stages of TB hip (stage 4 and 5) and septic arthritis.

   Tuberculosis of Hip—Trendelenberg's test may be positive in TB hip only in late stages (stage 4 and 5) when the head of femur is destroyed.

   Patients walk with positive trendelenbrug sign on. **One hip-Lurching/Trendelenburg Gait and Both hip- Wadding Gait**

   Thomas test—to measure **fixed flexion deformity** of hip by neutralizing lumbar lordosis. **Up to 30 degree flexion deformity of hip can be compensated by lumbar lordosis.**

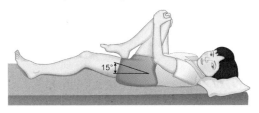

Fig. 9.2: Thomas test to assess hip flexion deformity

Shenton's line is an imaginary semicircular line joining the medial cortex of femoral neck to the lower border of superior pubic ramus. Its femoral part is of more significance. It is breeched in fracture neck femur, head femur, superior pubic rami and dislocation of hip.

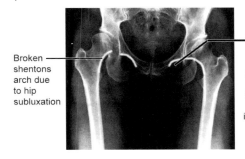

Fig. 9.3: X-ray pelvis

Telescopic Test

In supine position, hip and knee are flexed as much as 90 degrees and thigh is pulled up and pushed down. Even in normal condition a slight amount of excursion of trochanter can be felt by other hand. If excursion is more, then this indicates instability of hip joint such as: old unreduced posterior dislocation, loss of neck and or head in old fractures neck femur and paralytic hip.

MULTIPLE CHOICE QUESTIONS

SUPRATROCHANTERIC SHORTENING

1. Bryant's triangle is useful in diagnosis of except:
   (DNB Pattern 2018)
   A. Supratrochanteric shortening
   B. Infratrochanteric shortening
   C. Anterior dislocation hip
   D. Posterior dislocation hip

   Ans. is 'B' Infratrochanteric shortening

2. Line joining anterior superior iliac spine to ischial tuberosity and passes above greater trochanter:
   (AIIMS Nov 1999)
   A. Nelaton's line   B. Schoemakers line
   C. Chiene's line   D. Perkins line

   Ans. is 'A' Nelaton's line
   - *Nelaton's Line:* A line drawn from ischial tuberosity to ASIS should pass through the tip of greater trochanter. In case of supratrochanteric shortening the trochanter will be above this line.

TRENDELENBURG SIGN AND TEST

1. A 55-year-old female came with hip flexor contracture. What is the most likely test to be done in this case?
   (AIIMS May 2018)
   A. Allis test   B. Thomas test
   C. Ober test   D. Trendelenburg test

   Ans. is 'B' Thomas test

2. Trendelenburg test is positive in: *(NEET DEC 2016)*
   A. Dislocation of hip
   B. Fracture neck of femur
   C. Coxa vara   D. All the above

   Ans. is 'D' All the above

3. A patient came with complaint of difficulty in climbing upstairs. When he is made to stand on his right leg left side of pelvis fell to a lower level. When he stands on left leg then right side of pelvis can be drawn up. Which of the following nerve of him has got affected?
   (JIPMER may 2016)
   A. Right inferior gluteal   B. Right superior gluteal
   C. Left superior gluteal   D. Left inferior gluteal

   Ans. is 'B' Right superior gluteal

4. Thomas test helps to detect: *(AI Dec 15)*
   A. Adduction deformity of the hip
   B. Integrity of the abductor mechanism
   C. Fixed flexion deformity of the hip
   D. Apparent shortening at the hip Joint

   Ans. is 'C' Fixed flexion deformity of the hip

5. Trendelenburg test would be positive in the following conditions: *(AI Dec 15)*
   A. L4 L5 PIVD   B. LSSI PIVD
   C. Synovitis of the hip
   D. Femoroacetabular Impingement Syndrome

   Ans. is 'A' L4 L5 PIVD (Disc prolapse at L4–5 compresses L5 nerve root which supplies gluteus medius and minimus)

6. Identify the test being performed in the image below: *(AIIMS Nov 2015)*

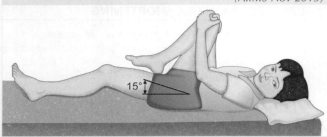

   A. Trendelenburg B. Thomas test
   C. Smith D. Narath

Ans. is 'B' Thomas test

7. Trendelenburg test is positive in palsy of: *(NEET 2015, 2012)*
   A. Gluteus maximus B. Gluteus medius
   C. Rectus femoris D. Vastus medialis

Ans. is 'B' Gluteus medius

8. Trendelenburg test is positive due to injury to: *(NEET Pattern 2013, AIIMS Nov 2008, AI 1997)*
   A. Superior gluteal nerve B. Inferior gluteal nerve
   C. Obturator nerve D. Tibial nerve

Ans. is 'A' Superior gluteal nerve

9. Trendelenburg's sign is negative in an Inter-Trochanteric fracture because of: *(AI 2000)*
   A. Gluteus medius B. Gluteus maximus
   C. Gluteus minimus D. Tensor fascia lata

Ans. is 'D' Tensor fascia lata
   – In cases of fracture intertrochanteric femur both gluteus muscles become ineffective as these are inserted in greater trochanter. Tensor fascia lata (TFL) which is inserted through the iliotibial tract on to the lateral condyle of tibia will still be in a position to affect some abduction thereby causing a negative trendelenburg test.

10. Trendelenburg's test is positive in all except:
    A. Posterior dislocation of hip *(AIIMS June 1998)*
    B. Poliomyelitis
    C. Fracture neck of femur D. Tuberculosis of hip joint

Ans. is 'D' Tuberculosis of hip joint
    – TB Hip-Trendelenburg's test may be positive in TB hip only in late stages (stage 4 and 5) when the head of femur is destroyed. Normally it is negative in TB hip.

SHENTON'S LINE

1. Shenton's line is seen in X-ray of: *(NEET DEC 2016)*
   A. Antero-posterior pelvis with both hips
   B. Antero-posterior shoulder
   C. Lateral cervical spine D. Lateral lumbosacral spine

Ans. is 'A' Antero-posterior pelvis with both hips

2. Shenton's line is: *(CET July 16)*
   A. Line joining ASIS and ischial tuberosity
   B. Line joining ASIS and tip of GT
   C. Line joining two ASIS (left & right)
   D. Curve formed by neck of femur and obturator foramen

Ans. is 'D' Curve formed by neck of femur and obturator foramen

3. All of the following names are associated with tests around the hip joint except: *(NB 1990)*
   A. Bryant B. Shenton
   C. Mc Murray E. Nelaton

Ans. is 'C' Mc Murray

TELESCOPIC TEST

1. Telescopic test is useful to diagnosis:
   A. Perthe's disease
   B. Intracapsular fracture neck of femur
   C. Malunited Trochanteric fracture
   D. Ankylosis of hip joint

Ans. is 'B' Intracapsular fracture neck of femur
   – Positive Telescopy test indicates instability of hip joint such as: old unreduced posterior dislocation, loss of neck and or head in old fractures neck femur and paralytic hip.

PELVIC FRACTURE

In pelvis fracture intrapelvic hemorrhage is by far, the most serious complication. Hemorrhage frequently results from fracture surfaces. Amount of blood loss is around 4–8 units.

Tile's Classification
A. Stable
B. Rotationally unstable but vertically stable; and
C. Rotationally and vertically unstable. This classification is widely used in the current literature.

In cases of hemodynamic instability, an external fixator should be applied immediately to decrease motion at fracture sites as well as to decrease pelvic volume and generate temponade of the pelvic venous plexus.

- Tile type A usually are treated by rest alone.
- External fixation has been widely described for the definitive treatment of Tile type B in combination with anterior fixation if pubic diastasis is >2.5 cm
- Tile type C pelvic injuries require posterior fixation to regain vertical stability. External fixation alone is not recommended as definitive treatment of vertically unstable pelvic fractures because the posterior instability cannot be controlled by this treatment method. Thus it requires posterior fixation.

Crescent Fracture, is a type II lateral compression injury that extends from posterior iliac crest, passing through iliac wing (just behind gluteal pillar), and may then exit in greater sciatic notch or more commonly may enter the sacroiliac (SI) joint. Treatment is operative. *(AIIMS May 2009)*

- *Straddle fracture:* Bilateral fracture of both pubic rami
- *Jumper's fracture:* Sacral fracture
- *Malgaigne fracture:* Fracture of pubis with a fracture of ilium near sacroiliac (SI) joint (Ipsilateral).

CRITERION OF UNSTABLE PELVIS

Radiographic factors indicating unstable pelvis are:
- Posterior sacroiliac complex displacement >1cm
- Avulsion fracture of sacral or ischial end of the sacrospinous ligament.
- Avulsion fractures of the L5 transverse process
- Disruption of pubic symphysis with pubic diastasis of 2 cm with posterior pelvic injury or injury to anterior/posterior sacroiliac ligament or sacrospinous ligaments.
- Presence of gap rather than impaction in the posterior pelvic ring.

ACETABULAR FRACTURES

The acetabulum can be described as an incomplete hemispherical socket with an inverted horseshoe-shaped articular surface surrounding the non-articular cotyloid fossa. This articular socket is composed of and supported by two columns of bone, described by **Letournel and Judet** as an inverted Y. The anterior column is composed of the bone of the iliac crest, the iliac spines, the anterior half of the acetabulum, and the pubis. The posterior column is the ischium, the ischial spine, the posterior half of the acetabulum, and the dense bone forming the sciatic notch. The shorter posterior column ends at its intersection with the anterior column at the top of the sciatic notch. The column concept is used in classification of these fractures and is central to the discussion of fracture patterns, operative approaches, and internal fixation.

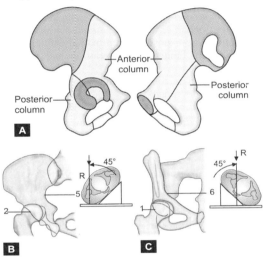

Figs. 9.4A to C: (A) Columns of acetabulum (B and C) Judet view (For Pelvis/Acetabulum-obturator and iliac views are taken)

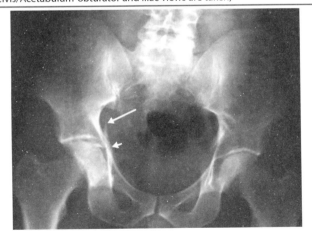

Fig. 9.5: Spur sign

The Spur sign: Triangular fragment of bone. It is seen in both anterior and posterior column acetabular fractures. (Bicolumnar fracture)

Acetabular fractures are classified by Judet and Letournel classification.

The dome, or roof, of the acetabulum is the weight bearing portion of the articular surface that supports the femoral head. Anatomical restoration of the dome with concentric reduction of the femoral head beneath this dome is the goal of both operative and non-operative treatment.

Most authors agree that displaced fractures through the weight bearing dome should be treated with operative reduction and internal fixation.

The quality of acetabular fracture reduction is the single most important factor in the long-term outcome of these patients, and such surgery should be undertaken only by surgeons with sufficient experience.

In general, operative treatment of an acetabular fracture should not be performed as an emergency except when it is part of open fracture management, vascular injury, progressive nerve injury or is performed for a fracture associated with an irreducible dislocation of the hip. Contraindications to operative treatment are Infection/suprapubic catheter/Morel Lavallee lesion/Poor bone stock.

Morel-Lavallee lesion is a **localized area of subcutaneous fat necrosis over the lateral aspect of hip** caused by same trauma that causes the acetabular fracture. The operation through it has been associated with a higher (12%) rate of post-operative infection, wound dehiscence and healing by secondary infection. The presence of a significant Morel- Lavallee lesion can be suspected by hypermobility of the skin and subcutaneous tissue in the affected area from the shear type separation of the subcutaneous tissue from the underlying fascia lata. Alternatively, some fractures can be treated through ilioinguinal approach, thus avoiding the affected area.

Complications of Fracture Acetabulum

i. *Early complications* include sciatic nerve injury and iliofemoral venous thrombosis.

   Sciatic nerve palsies as a result of the initial injury occur in approximately 10–15% of patients with acetabular fractures. Sciatic nerve injury as a result of surgery occurs in 2–6% of patients and is more often associated with posterior fracture patterns treated through the Kocher-Langenbeck and extensile exposures.

ii. Among *late complications, the common problem is development of **secondary osteoarthritis***. Other possible problems include *avascular necrosis (osteonecrosis) of femoral head*, Heterotopic ossification and joint stiffness.

Post-traumatic arthrosis (secondary aosteoarthritis) of hip is the most common late complication of acetabular fractures.

Prevention of heterotropic ossification.

Currently, for most patients treated with the Kocher-Langenbeck approach, indomethacin (25 mg three times a day for 4–6 weeks) or radiation therapy with a one-time dose of 700 cGy is used.

Kocher-Langenbeck Approach: Also used to handle Sciatic Nerve Injuries!

- This is a posterior approach used for all posterior wall, posterior column, and posterior column plus posterior wall fractures of acetabulum. It is also used for most transverse and transverse plus posterior wall fracture and many T-shaped fracture.

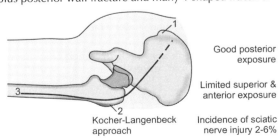

Fig. 9.6: Kocher-Langenbeck approach

- It allows complete exposure of (posterior) retroacetabular surface caudially (distally) as far as the ischial tuberosity. The greater and lesser sciatic notches are visualized. But the anterior and superior exposure is limited. Osteotomy of greater trochanter (digastric osteotomy) allows increased anterior iliac exposure but proximal (superior) access is still largely limited by superior gluteal neurovascular bundle. And if more cranial exposure of the iliac wing is thought to be necessary an anterior approach should be chosen primarily.
- Recurrent (posterior) dislocation and sciatic nerve injury indicate injury of posterior column or posterior wall; so these are approached through (posterior) Kocher-Langenbeck approach.
- The incidence of sciatic nerve injury due to this approach is 2–6%.
- Ilioinguinal and iliofemoral approach is used for anterior column fractures.
- The most common neurological injury after ilioinguinal approach is to lateral femoral cutaneous nerve.

MULTIPLE CHOICE QUESTIONS

1. Spur sign is seen in: *(PGI May 2017, Nov 2016)*
   A. Supracondylar fracture of humerus
   B. Radial head fracture   C. Fibula fracture
   D. Talus fracture   E. Acetabular fracture

   Ans. is 'E' Acetabular fracture

2. Which of the following fractures is associated with high mortality and morbidity? *(CET Nov 15)*
   A. Femur Shaft fractures   B. Pelviacetabular fractures
   C. Subtrochanteric fractures   D. Shaft tibia fractures

   Ans. is 'B' Pelviacetabular fractures

3. "Judet" view of X-ray is for: *(AIIMS May 2015)*
   A. Pelvis   B. Calcaneum
   C. Scaphoid   D. Shoulder

   Ans. is 'A' Pelvis

4. Radiological factors indicating an unstable pelvis are all except: *(NEET 2015)*
   A. Posterior sacroiliac complex displacement by > 1 cm
   B. Avulsion fracture of sacral or ischial end of the sacrospinous ligament
   C. Avulsion fractures of the L5 transverse process
   D. Isolated disruption of pubic symphysis with pubic diastasis of 2 cm

   Ans. is 'D' Isolated disruption of pubic symphysis with pubic diastasis of 2 cm

5. Pelvic fracture most serious complication is: *(AIIMS May 2013)*
   A. Hypovolemic shock   B. Neurogenic shock
   C. Bladder injury   D. Pelvic instability

   Ans. is 'A' Hypovolemic shock

6. Morel-Lavallee lesion is seen in: *(NEET Pattern 2013)*
   A. Acetabular fracture   B. Fracture femur neck
   C. Fracture lumbar spine   D. Fracture proximal tibia

   Ans. is 'A' Acetabular fracture

7. Kocher Langenbeck approach for emergency acetabular fixation is done in all except: *(AIIMS May 09)*
   A. Open fracture
   B. Progressive sciatic nerve injury
   C. Recurrent dislocation in spite of closed reduction and traction
   D. Morel-Lavallee lesion

   Ans. is 'D' Morel-Lavallee lesion

8. Which is not true about Langenbeck Kocher operation? *(AIIMS May 09)*
   A. Adequate exposure of posterior segment
   B. Anterior segment is not visualized adequately
   C. Superior exposure is limited
   D. Sciatic nerve injury in 10% in the cases

   Ans. is 'D' Sciatic nerve injury in 10% in the cases

   Kocher-Langenbeck Approach
   - This is a posterior approach used for all posterior wall, posterior column, and posterior column plus posterior wall fractures of acetabulum. It is also used for most transverse and transverse plus posterior wall fracture and many T-shaped fractures.
   - It allows complete exposure of (posterior) retroacetabular surface caudially (distally) as far as the ischeal tuberosity. The greater and lesser sciatic notches are visualized. But the anterior and superior exposure is limited. Osteotomy of greater trochanter (digastric osteotomy) allows increased anterior iliac exposure but proximal (superior) access is still largely limited by superior gluteal neurovascular bundle.
   - Incidence of sciatic nerve injury is 2–6% (older studies explain wider range).

9. Which is not true about Langenbeck Kocher operation?
   A. Adequate exposal of posterior segment *(AIIMS May 09)*
   B. Anterior segment is not visualized adequately
   C. Superior exposure is very well exposed
   D. Sciatic nerve injury in 10% in cases

   Ans. is 'C' Superior exposure is very well exposed
   - Please observe this question is not the same as previous as Kocher-Langenbeck approach is not a good approach for superior segment as its visualization is limited hence D option will be considered acceptable as nerve injuries in earlier studies were more than 6% as compared to now.

10. True about Crescent fracture is: *(AIIMS May 09)*
    A. Anteroposterior instability with rotational stability
    B. Diastasis of pubis with pubic rami fracture
    C. Antero-posterior compression is the mechanism of injury
    D. Fracture of the iliac bone with sacroiliac disruption

    Ans. is 'D' Fracture of the iliac bone with sacroiliac disruption

11. All of the following areas are commonly involved sites in pelvic fracture except: *(AI 2005)*
    A. Pubic rami   B. Alae of ileum
    C. Acetabulum   D. Ischial tuberosities

    Ans. is 'D' Ischial tuberosities

12. Open book and bucket handle injuries are seen in: *(SGPGI 2002, AMU 99)*
    A. Spine   B. Pelvis
    C. Femur   D. Humerus

    Ans. is 'B' Pelvis

13. In pelvis fracture, the amount of blood loss is around: *(Tamil Nadu 1999)*
    A. 1–2 units   B. 2–4 units
    C. 2–6 units   D. 4–8 units

    Ans. is 'D' 4–8 units

FRACTURE AROUND HIP

Deformity of Hip

- Flexion, abduction, external rotation, apparent lengthening-synovitis.
- Flexion, adduction. internal rotation, true shortening arthritis-posterior dislocation.

Pelvis and Hip Injury

- Flexion, abduction, external rotation, true lengthening-anterior dislocation.
- **External rotation, shortening-femoral neck fracture.**
- **Marked external rotation, shortening-intertrochanteric fracture femur.**

Femoral neck fractures and intertrochanteric fractures occurs with about the same frequency. They are both more common in women than in men by a margin of three to one (Campbell). Moreover fracture intertrochanteric femur occurs in elderly patients even more than fractures of femoral neck itself (Watson Jones).

Femoral Neck Fracture

MRI is more sensitive (100% sensitivity) and specific for diagnosis of occult fracture neck femur.

Garden's classification for fracture neck femur

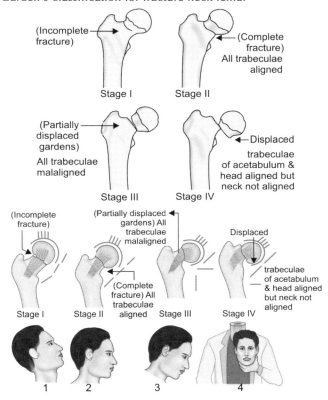

Fig. 9.7: Garden's classification for femur neck fracture

1. Stage 1: The fracture is incomplete, with head tilted in posterolateral direction, i.e. into valgus, therefore is known as valgus (abduction) impacted fracture.
2. Stage 2: Complete fracture but undisplaced.
3. Stage 3: Complete fracture with partial displacement.
4. Stage 4: Complete fracture with total displacement.

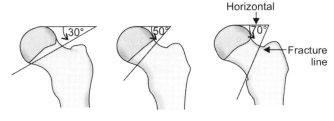

Fig. 9.8: Pauwel's angle

Pauwel's angle is the angle formed by the line of fracture with the horizontal plane

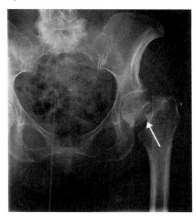

Fig. 9.9: Femur neck fracture

Delbet Classification for Pediatric Fracture Neck Femur

Type

1. Transepiphyseal
2. Transcervical
3. Cervicotrochanteric
4. Intertrochanteric

Incidence 2 > 3 > 4 > 1.

Fracture Neck of Femur—Treatment

1. < 65 years, ≤ 3 week
   - Closed reduction and internal fixation with multiple screw is the treatment of choice. In basicervical fracture, dynamic hip screw can be done.
   - If closed reduction is not possible open reduction and screw fixation is indicated.
2. < 65 years, > 3 week fracture, osteotomy/Bone grafting + fixation.
3. ≥ 65 years
   - No pre-existing arthritis—hemiarthroplasty
4. Pre-existing arthritis (any age)—total hip replacement

Complication are Osteonecrosis > Nonunion > arthritis

Chances of AVN and non-union in decreasing order is:

- Subcapital > transcervical > basal > intertrochanteric

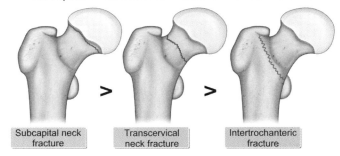

Figs. 9.10: Risk of AVN (avascular necrosis) according to location of fracture upper end femur

- Transphyseal > transcervical > cervicotrochanteric > intertrochanteric (in children)
- McMurray osteotomy (Biomechanical osteotomy) is used in case of non-union femur.

Feature	Intracapsular Neck Fracture	Intertrochanteric Fracture	
Patient profile	—	Patients are mole likely to be older, in poorer health and have comorbid conditions. (in comparison to neck femur).	
Age	Common after 50 yrs (but most common in 7th decade)	Common after 60 years (but most common in 8th decade)	
Sex	Both fractures are more common in elderly females but males are relatively more prone to develop fracture intertrochanteric femur.		
Velocity of trauma	Trivial (usually)	Significant (as compared to neck femur)	
Pain	Mild	Severe	
Swelling and Ecchymosis	Nil	Severe	
Tenderness	In scarpa's triangle	Over greater trochanter	Everything "Extra" in Extracapsular
External rotation deformity	<45 degrees	> 45 degrees (lateral border of foot touching couch)	
Shortening	<1 inch	>1 inch	
Broadening of greater trochanter	Absent	Present	
Straight leg raising and Ability to walk	May be present in impacted fractures	Absent (Not possible)	

Less lateral rotation deformity in fracture neck femur is due to attachment of capsule to the distal fracture fragment.

Intertrochanteric fracture femur

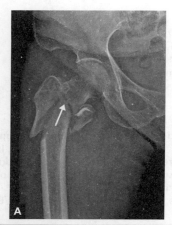

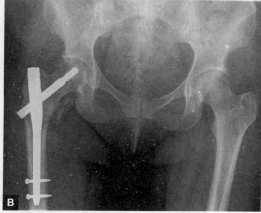

Figs. 9.11A and B: (A) Intertrochanteric fracture femur (B) Proximal femoral nail

- Treatment of choice Dynamic Hip Screw (Undisplaced fracture).
- Displaced fracture: Proximal femoral nail (Cephalo-medullary nail).
- Most common complication is malunion.

Note: Latest literature claims better results with PFN

MULTIPLE CHOICE QUESTIONS

CLASSIFICATION

1. A 75-year-old male after a fall in bathroom had hip fracture seen in the pelvic X-ray below. What will be the position of the left lower limb? *(AIIMS May 2017)*
   A. Shortened, externally rotated
   B. Shortened and adducted
   C. Extended, abducted and externally rotated
   D. Abducted and internally rotated
Ans. is 'A' Shortened, externally rotated

2. Which of the following is not true about intracapsular fracture of femur neck? *(NEET DEC 2016)*
   A. Displacement is less common than extracapsular fractures
   B. Malunion is common complication
   C. Contour of greater trochanter is normal
   D. Tenderness is mainly present over the anterior joint line
Ans. is 'B' Malunion is common complication

3. The most common type of hip fracture in childhood is:
   A. Intertrochanteric *(TN 2014)*
   B. Transcervical
   C. Transphyseal (through head)
   D. Subcapital
Ans. is 'B' Transcervical

4. Garden's classification used for which fracture? *(NEET 2015)*
   A. Surgical neck humerus   B. Shaft humerus
   C. Neck of femur   D. Shaft femur
Ans. is 'C' Neck of femur

5. McMurray's osteotomy is done for: *(NEET Pattern 2013)*
   A. Malunited intertrochanteric fracture of femur
   B. Non-union transcervical neck fracture of femur
   C. Non-union lateral condyle fracture of humerus
   D. Malunited supracondylar fracture of humerus
Ans. is 'B' Non-union transcervical neck fracture of femur

6. Fracture neck femur cause of non-union: *(NEET Pattern 2013)*
   A. Injury to blood supply with shearing stress
   B. Poor nutrition of the patient
   C. Smoking   D. Old age and osteoporosis
Ans. is 'A' Injury to blood supply with shearing stress

7. Most common fracture in elderly: *(NEET Pattern 2012)*
   A. Intertrochanteric fracture B. Neck femur fracture
   C. Colles fracture D. Supracondylar fracture
Ans. is 'C' Colles fracture

8. Garden-I fractures are also known as: *(UP 2003, Assam 97)*
   A. Complete fracture without displacement
   B. Complete fracture with minimal (partial) displacement
   C. Complete fracture with full displacement
   D. Valgus impaction fractures
Ans. is 'D' Valgus impaction fractures

9. Increase in Pauwel's angle indicate:
   A. Good prognosis *(SGPGI 2000, MAHE 2K)*
   B. Impaction
   C. More chances of displacement
   D. Trabecular alignment disrupted
Ans. is 'C' More chances of displacement

10. Pauwel's angle is: *(Rajasthan 94)*
    A. Neck shaft angle of femur
    B. The difference between neck shaft angle between two femurs of a patient
    C. Formed by joining a line extended from fracture line of femur neck to an arbitrary line depicting the horizontal plane
    D. None of the above
Ans. is 'C' Formed by joining a line extended from fracture line of femur neck to an arbitrary line depicting the horizontal plane

11. In fracture neck femur all the trabeculae of pelvis and femur are in alignment in which stage: *(AMU 94, PGI 92)*
    A. Stage I B. Stage II
    C. Stage III D. Stage IV
Ans. is 'B' Stage II

CLINICAL FEATURES

1. Occult fracture of neck femur are best diagnosed by:
   (AIIMS SR 2006, SGPGI 03)
   A. Bone Scan B. MRI
   C. X-Ray D. CT scan
Ans. is 'B' MRI
   – MRI is indicated to evaluate for occult hip fractures

2. A 60-year-old female lands up in emergency with history of fall, the attitude of limb is extension and external rotation, the most probable diagnosis is:
   (AI 2001, AIIMS Dec 1996, PGI 95) (Manipal 1998)
   (Tamil Nadu 1998)
   A. Intracapsular fracture neck of femur
   B. Posterior dislocation of hip
   C. Intertrochanteric fracture
   D. Acetabulam fracture
Ans. is 'A' Intracapsular fracture neck of femur
   – Usually if it is mentioned that 60–70 year female with fracture proximal femur the diagnosis is neck femur and if they ask about 80-year-old individual than diagnosis is intertrochanteric fracture this is subject to limited features given in question but if they mention partial external rotation of lower limb and limited shortening than it is intracapsular fracture neck femur and if it mentions complete external rotation that is lateral border of foot touches the bed than intertrochanteric fracture is a possibility.

3. The commonest hip injury in the elderly patients is:
   A. Stress fracture *(AMU 99)*
   B. Extracapsular fracture
   C. Impacted fracture neck of femur
   D. Sub capital capsular fracture neck of femur
Ans. is 'B' Extracapsular fracture
   – "The femoral neck is the common site of fracture in the elderly". "Moreover fracture intertrochanteric femur occurs in elderly patients even more than fractures of femoral neck itself".

4. A 60-year-old man fell in bathroom and was unable to stand on right buttock region echymosis with external rotation of the leg and lateral border of foot touching the bed. The most probable diagnosis is: *(UP 1998)*
   A. Extracapsular fracture neck of femur
   B. Anterior dislocation of hip
   C. Intracapsular fracture neck of femur
   D. Posterior dislocation of hip
Ans. is 'A' Extracapsular fracture neck of femur
   – Lateral border of foot touching the bed, that means there is extreme external rotation.
   – This occurs in intertrochanteric fractures.

5. 80 years old female after fall developed inability to walk with external rotation deformity on examination SLR is not possible and broadening of trochanter is present. The possible diagnosis is: *(AMU 96, PGI 93)*
   A. Fracture neck femur
   B. Fracture intertrochanteric femur
   C. Fracture subtrochanteric femur
   D. Fracture greater trochanter
Ans. is 'B' Fracture intertrochanteric femur
   – Broadening of trochanter occurs in IT fracture if the fracture causes split in GT.
   – In femoral neck fracture trochanters are normal.

COMPLICATIONS

1. Which of the following fractures of the neck of femur are associated with maximal compromise in blood supply?
   A. Intertrochanteric fractures *(AI Dec 15)*
   B. Basicervical fracture
   C. Trans cervical fracture
   D. Subcapital fractures
Ans. is 'D' Subcapital fractures

2. Most common complication of intertrochanteric fracture femur is:
   (NEET Pattern 2013, WB 99, AI 98, 88, Delhi 97)
   A. Malunion B. Non-union
   C. Osteoarthritis D. Nerve injury
Ans. is 'A' Malunion
   – Most common complications of intracapsular fracture → AVN followed by non-union.
   – Most common complication of extracapsular fracture → Malunion.

3. Nonunion is common in fracture: *(NEET Pattern 2012)*
   A. Scapula B. Talus
   C. Neck femur D. None
Ans. is 'C' Neck femur

4. The most common complication of Transcervical fracture Neck of Femur is:
   (NEET Pattern 2012) (WB 2002, TN 92)
   A. Avascular necrosis   B. Malunion
   C. Non union   D. None

Ans. is 'A' Avascular necrosis
   – AVN is the most common complication of femoral neck fracture.

5. Which of the following describes grade 2 fracture neck femur?   (NEET Pattern 2012)
   A. Incomplete fracture, medial trabeculae intact
   B. Complete fracture with undisplaced neck
   C. Complete fracture with ischemic head
   D. Moderate displacement of neck, vascularity damaged

Ans. is 'B' Complete fracture with undisplaced neck

6. Nonunion is a very common complication of intracapsular fractures of the neck of femur. Which of the following is not a very important cause for the same?
   (CMC 97, JIPMER 95)
   A. Inadequate immobilization
   B. Inadequate blood supply
   C. Inhibitory effect of synovial fluid
   D. Stress at fracture site due to muscle spasm

Ans. is 'D' Stress at fracture site due to muscle spasm
   – Causes of non-union in femoral neck fractures are posterior comminution, inadequate immobilization, inadequate vascularity, inhibition by synovial fluid, vertical fracture line and absence of cambium layer of periosteum.

MANAGEMENT IN ADULTS

1. Fracture neck of femur in 80 year old male sustained 1 week back. The treatment of choice is: (AI Dec 15)
   A. Hemiarthroplasty   B. Excision arthroplasty
   C. Closed reduction and fixation with three cancellous screws
   D. Longitudinal skin traction for 6 weeks

Ans. is 'A' Hemiarthroplasty

2. 40-year-old female history of fall complaints of pain right hip, inability to walk and on examination tenderness in scarpas triangle the X-ray is normal next investigation is:
   A. Aspiration   B. CT scan (May AIIMS 2012)
   C. MRI   D. Bone scan

Ans. is 'C' MRI

3. All the following are True except: (AIIMS 2012)
   A. Supracondylar fracture is closed reduced
   B. Lateral condyle humerus is open reduced
   C. Forearm fracture in children is closed reduced and cast applied
   D. Neck femur fracture in geriatrics is treated with open reduction and screw fixation

Ans. is 'D' Neck femur fracture in geriatrics is treated with open reduction and screw fixation. Preferred treatment in a geriatric patient that is ≥ 65 years is hemiarthroplasty.

4. A 65-year-old man presented with fracture neck femur 3 days after injury, treatment of choice is:
   (AMU 2K, AIIMS June 98, 98, UPSC 97, AI 1994)
   A. Multiple screw fixation   B. McMurray osteotomy
   C. Hemiarthroplasty   D. Total hip replacement

Ans. is 'C' Hemiarthroplasty. Preferred treatment in a geriatric patient that is ≥ 65 years is hemiarthroplasty.

5. Treatment of choice in fracture neck of femur in a 40-year-old male presenting after 2 days is:
   (UP 2K, AIIMS June 1999, AI 96)
   A. Hemiarthroplasty
   B. Closed reduction and Internal fixation by cancellous screws
   C. Closed reduction and Internal fixation by Austin Moore pins
   D. Plaster and rest

Ans. is 'B' Closed reduction and Internal fixation by cancellous screws

6. Femoral neck fracture of 4-week-old in an young adult should be best by treated one of the following:
   (Bihar 1998, Rajasthan 91, AI 1989)
   A. Total hip replacement
   B. Reduction of fracture and femoral osteotomy with fixation
   C. Prosthetic replacement of femoral head
   D. Reduction of fracture and multiple screw fixation

Ans. is 'B' Reduction of fracture and femoral osteotomy with fixation
   – >3 weeks fracture in <65 years age group–reduction and fixation along with Osteotomy/Bone grafting.

7. Best treatment for fracture neck femur in a 65-year-old lady is: (AIIMS Dec 1994)
   A. POP cast   B. Gleotomy
   C. Bone grafting and compression
   D. Hemireplacement arthroplasty

Ans. is 'D' Hemireplacement arthroplasty

8. McMurray's osteotomy is based on the following principle: (Andhra 94)
   A. Biological   B. Biomechanical
   C. Biotechnical   D. Mechanical

Ans. is 'B' Biomechanical
   – McMurray's Osteotomy is a biomechanical procedure of subtrochanteric abduction (valgus impaction) osteotomy used in young (< 65 years age) with viable femoral head (no AVN) and minimal collapse of neck. The purpose of abduction osteotomy is to turn the shaft from adducted to abducted position, which makes fracture line of neck femur more horizontal, so that the shearing stress of weight bearing and muscle retraction becomes an impaction force.

9. Trochanteric fracture of femur is best treated by:
   A. Dynamic hip screw   (PGI 1993)
   B. Inlay plates
   C. Plaster in abduction
   D. Plaster in abduction and internal rotation

Ans. is 'A' Dynamic hip screw
   – *Dynamic hip screw (DHS) plate is the implant of choice for fixation. These days proximal femoral nail (PFN)* is preferred. It is a variety of cephalomedullary fixation.

MANAGEMENT IN CHILDREN

1. In a 10-year-old male transcervical fracture neck femur is best treated by: (MAHE 2006, DNB 05)
   A. Spica   B. Austin Moore pins
   C. K-Wires
   D. Cannulated Cancellous screw

Ans. is 'D' Canulated Cancellous screw

Pelvis and Hip Injury

DISLOCATIONS OF HIP

Injuries of the hip joint may include pure hip dislocations, dislocations with fracture of the femoral head, and dislocations with fracture of the acetabulum. The position of the femoral head in relation to the acetabulum and the vector of the force at the time of impact determine the type of injury produced.

Hip joint injuries commonly are complicated by injuries to other areas also. They can damage the nerves or vessels. Late complications include osteonecrosis of the femoral head and posttraumatic arthritis of the joint.

Posterior Dislocation and Fracture-Dislocation-Dashboard injury

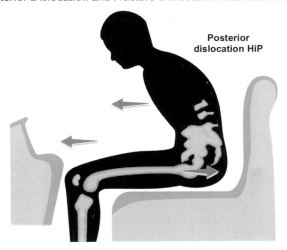

Fig. 9.12: Dashboard Injury (Posterior dislocation of hip)

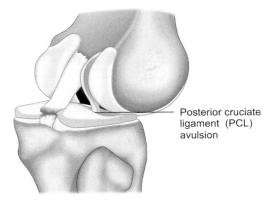

Fig. 9.13: Dashboard Injury (PCL avulsion)

> **Note:** Dashboard Injury is Post-dislocation > PCL avulsion

It is the Most common hip dislocation (90%)

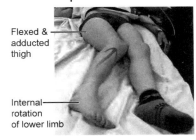

Fig. 9.14: FADIR

Patients with a posterior dislocation of the hip generally present with a **shortened, internally rotated, adducted limb in slight flexion.** This position can be altered if the femoral head is impaled on a fractured posterior acetabular wall. If the hip is adducted at the time of injury, a pure dislocation occurs, whereas a neutral position or abduction leads to fracture dislocation. It is associated with a fracture of the femoral head or acetabulum.

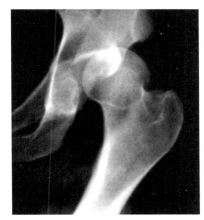

Fig. 9.15: X-ray hip showing posterior dislocation of hip

Thompson and Epstein classified posterior dislocations of the hip:

Type I: Dislocation with or without minor fracture

Type II: Dislocation with a large single fracture of the posterior acetabular rim

Type III: Dislocation with comminution of the posterior acetabular rim with or without a major fragment

Type IV: Dislocation with fracture of the acetabular floor

Type V: Dislocation with fracture of the femoral head

Type V: Thompson and Epstein is subdivided by Pipkin into four types (Pipkin classification).

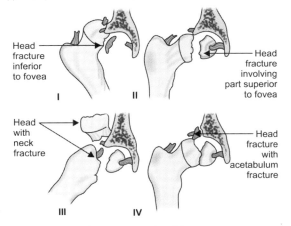

Fig. 9.16: Pipkin's classification: Femur head fractures

Type I: Femoral head fracture caudal to fovea centralis

Type II: Femoral head fracture cephalad to the fovea

Type III: Femoral head fracture associated with femoral neck fracture

Type IV: Type I, II or III with associated acetabular fracture

Associated fracture with dislocations do not have the classical deformities.

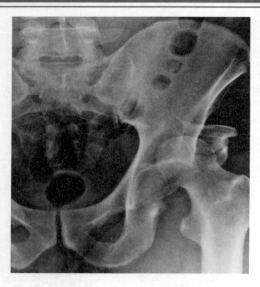

Fig. 9.17: Pipkins Type IV fracture dislocation

Position of Hip at the time of Injury	Pattern of Injury
Flexion, adduction, internal rotation	Pure posterior dislocation
Less flexion, less adduction (neutral or slight abduction), internal rotation	Posterior fracture dislocation
Hyper abduction + Flexion + External rotation	Anterior dislocation

Femoral head can be palpated posteriorly (Gluteal)

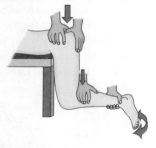

Fig. 9.18: Posterior dislocation hip-reduction

Vascular sign of Narath is positive, i.e. due to posterior dislocation of hip joint the vessels fall back unsupported so femoral arterial pulsation, which is felt against the head of the femur will be feeble or even may not be palpable.

Closed reduction Manoeuvres
1. Stimpson's gravity method
2. Allis maneuvre
3. Bigelow's maneuvre
4. East Baltimore maneuvre

The proper treatment of a dislocation or fracture-dislocation of the hip depends primarily on the type of injury, but regardless of the type of dislocation, some general guidelines apply: (1) long-term results are directly related to the severity of the initial trauma; (2) reduction, open or closed, should be performed within 12 hours; and (3) only one or two attempts at closed reduction should be made; if these fail, open reduction is indicated to prevent further damage to the femoral head.

CT scan is best investigation to judge dislocations.

Prognosis and Complications

After a dislocation of the hip, excellent function usually can be expected, provided that neither osteonecrosis of the femoral head nor traumatic arthritis of the joint develops. Early reduction has proved to be the most effective means of preventing osteonecrosis by shortening the time that the circulation of the femoral head is compromised.

Osteonecrosis painful enough to require surgery can be treated by arthrodesis or arthroplasty.

The incidence and severity of traumatic arthritis after dislocation or fracture-dislocation of the hip are related to the nature of the injury to the joint and its surrounding soft tissues.

Ectopic ossification may occur after dislocation or fracture-dislocation of the hip, especially if open reduction has been necessary, but it usually is not disabling.

Due to posterior direction of displacement sciatic nerve and superior gluteal artery injury may occur.

It is the posterior dislocation that cause maximum shortening of limb and is most commonly associated with sciatic nerve injury.

ANTERIOR DISLOCATION OF THE HIP

Anterior dislocations occur with the hip externally rotated and abducted. The degree of flexion at the time of injury determines the eventual position of the femoral head. Anterior dislocations are classified according to the position assumed by the femoral head: pubic, obturator, or perineal. **They are associated with lengthening.**

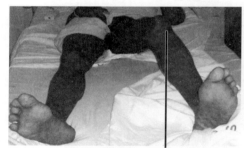

Fig. 9.19: FABER

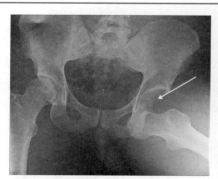

Fig. 9.20: Anterior dislocation of hip (abducted thigh)

Because of their anterior relationship to the hip, the femoral vessels and nerve may be injured, especially with pubic dislocations. An anterior dislocation usually can be reduced without surgery by pulling longitudinally on the thigh. If the dislocation cannot be reduced by these maneuvers, open reduction is performed.

CENTRAL DISLOCATION

In central fracture dislocation of hip, femoral head is forced medially through the floor of acetabulum and can be palpated on per rectal examination. There is shortening of limb. This is an extremely rare variety of dislocation. These are seen in patients with severe metabolic disorders and are usually classified under acetabular fractures.

MULTIPLE CHOICE QUESTIONS

1. Deformity seen in posterior dislocation of femur: *(PGI Nov 2018)*
   A. Flexion, abduction, external rotation
   B. Flexion, adduction, internal rotation
   C. Extension, abduction, internal rotation
   D. Extension, adduction, External rotation
   E. Shortening
   Ans. 'B' Flexion, adduction, internal rotation

2. Deformity associated with posterior dislocation of hip joint: *(PGI MAY 2018)*
   A. Flexion   B. Extension
   C. Abduction   D. Adduction
   E. Internal rotation
   Ans. 'A' Flexion; 'D' Adduction; 'E' Internal rotation

3. Most common type of hip dislocation is: *(NEET DEC 2016)*
   A. Anterior   B. Posterior
   C. Central   D. Inferior
   Ans. is 'B' Posterior

4. Patient with femur head fracture with associated fracture of acetabulum will fall into pipikin type: *(NEET DEC 2016)*
   A. I   B. II
   C. III   D. IV
   Ans. is 'D' IV

5. A patient presented after RTA with following attitude of the limb. What will be the most possible diagnosis? *(AIIMS Nov 16)*

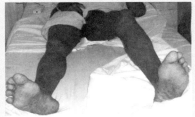

   A. Posterior dislocation of hip
   B. Anterior dislocation of hip
   C. Central dislocation of hip
   D. Lateral dislocation of hip
   Ans. is 'B' Anterior dislocation of hip

6. All of the following is true about dashboard injury except: *(CET Nov 15)*
   A. It is associated with posterior dislocation of the hip
   B. Sciatic nerve may be involved leading to foot drop
   C. Avascular necrosis of the hip could be a late complication
   D. The point of impact is on the greater trochanter
   Ans. is 'D' The point of impact is on the greater trochanter

7. Pipkin's classification system is used for: *(NEET 2015)*
   A. Fracture femur head   B. Fracture femur shaft
   C. Fracture proximal tibia D. Fracture calcaneum
   Ans. is 'A' Fracture femur head

8. Flexion, adduction and internal rotation is characteristic posture in: *(NEET Pattern 2014, AIIMS Nov 05, May 01, Nov 2K, F97, AI 2003, 02 JIPMER 95, Andhra 94, Delhi 93, 88, AMU 92, DNB 89)*
   A. Anterior dislocation of hip joint
   B. Posterior dislocation of hip joint
   C. Fracture of femoral head
   D. Fracture shaft of femur
   Ans. is 'B' Posterior dislocation of hip joint

9. Posterior hip dislocation is characterized by: *(JIPMER 2014)*
   A. Flexion, adduction, external rotation
   B. Flexion, adduction, internal rotation
   C. Extension, adduction, internal rotation
   D. Extension, adduction, external rotation
   Ans. 'B' Flexion, adduction, internal rotation

10. A patient with hip dislocation with limitation of Abduction at hip and flexion and internal rotation deformity at hip and shortening. Diagnosis is: *(AIIMS May 2013)*
    A. Central dislocation   B. Anterior dislocation
    C. Posterior dislocation D. Fracture dislocation
    Ans. is 'C' Posterior dislocation

    Explanation
    Since the question mentions limitation of abduction, hence there is adduction deformity along with flexion and internal rotation deformity. Thus this is a case of Posterior dislocation of hip.

Position of hip	Pattern of Injury
Flexion, adduction, internal rotation	Pure posterior dislocation
Less flexion, less adduction (neutral or slight abduction), internal rotation	Posterior fracture dislocation >**Central dislocation**
Hyper abduction + Flexion + External rotation	Anterior dislocation

    Some students remember an alternate format of the question 6b

11. A patient presents with lower limb in flexion, abduction and internal rotation with shortening! Diagnosis is: *(AIIMS May 2013)*
    A. Posterior dislocation
    B. Anterior dislocation
    C. Central dislocation
    D. Lateral dislocation
    Ans. is 'C' Central dislocation

Less flexion, less adduction (neutral or slight abduction), internal rotation	Posterior fracture dislocation > Central dislocation.

12. Posterior dislocation of hip can damage which nerve? *(NEET Pattern 2012)*
    A. Superior gluteal   B. Sciatic
    C. Inferior gluteal   D. Femoral
    Ans. is 'B' Sciatic

13. Posterior dislocation of hip is characterized by: *(NEET Pattern 2012)*
    A. Marked shortening of limb B. Lengthening of limb
    C. No change in limb length   D. Extension deformity
    Ans. is 'A' Marked shortening of limb

14. Pipkins classification is for Fracture of:
    (NEET Pattern 2012)
    A. Femur head   B. Femur neck
    C. Tibial plateau D. Hip dislocation
Ans. is 'A' Femur head

15. Vascular sign of Narath is positive in:
    (NEET Pattern 2016, 2012)
    A. Anterior hip dislocation
    B. Posterior hip dislocation
    C. Anterior shoulder dislocation
    D. Posterior shoulder dislocation
Ans. is 'B' Posterior hip dislocation

16. Dashboard injury results in: *(Andhra 1997)*
    A. Anterior dislocation of hip B. Posterior dislocation of hip
    C. Central dislocation of hip   D. Fracture neck femur
Ans. is 'B' Posterior dislocation of hip

17. Maximum shortening of limbs occur in:
    A. Intertrochanteric fracture femur *(AIIMS Feb 1997)*
    B. Posterior dislocation of hip
    C. Fracture neck femur
    D. Anterior dislocation of hip
Ans. is 'B' Posterior dislocation of hip

18. Which is true about dislocation of hip joint? *(KA 94)*
    A. Posterior dislocation is commoner
    B. In posterior dislocation whole lower limb is rotated medially
    C. In anterior dislocation whole lower limb is rotated laterally
    D. All of the above
Ans. is 'D' All of the above

19. Commonest dislocation of the hip is: *(TN 92, 89)*
    A. Posterior   B. Anterior
    C. Central   D. None
Ans. is 'A' Posterior

ANTERIOR DISLOCATION

1. In anterior dislocation of hip, the posture of lower limb will be: *(AIIMS N 99, Orissa 88) (Orissa 1990)*
    A. Abduction, externally rotated and extension
    B. Abduction, externally rotated and flexion
    C. Abducted externally rotated and flexion
    D. Adducted, internally rotated and flexion
Ans. is 'B' Abduction, externally rotated and flexion

CENTRAL DISLOCATION

1. In per rectal examination, femoral head is palpable in:
    A. Anterior dislocation of hip *(Andhra 1998)*
    B. Posterior dislocation of hip
    C. Central dislocation of hip
    D. Lateral dislocation of hip
Ans. is 'C' Central dislocation of hip

FRACTURE DISLOCATION

1. A 33-year-old male has history of RTA, now complaints of pain left hip. On examination there is Flexion External Rotation of left lower limb. There is 7 cm shortening of left lower limb, there is a gluteal mass felt which moves with the movement of femoral shaft, which of the following is the diagnosis? *(AI 2012)*
    A. Anterior dislocation of hip
    B. Central fracture dislocation
    C. Posterior dislocation
    D. Pipkin's type 4 fracture
Ans. is 'D' Pipkin's type 4 fracture

Anterior dislocation is ruled out because it will have Flexion Abduction External Rotation with lengthening and anterior femoral head (Mass that moves with femur shaft is femur head).

Central dislocation is ruled out because it will have shortening and femur head palpable on per rectal examination.

Posterior dislocation will have Flexion Adduction and internal rotation with shortening and gluteal femoral head.

Associated fracture with dislocations do not have the classical deformities.

Posterior dislocation with fracture of head of femur
 – Shortening
 – Classical deformities of posterior dislocation not present
 – Head posterior (Gluteal)
 – Pipkins type IV: Shortening and gluteal mass with atypical features

Type I: Femoral head fracture caudal to fovea centralis.
Type II: Femoral head fracture cephalad to the fovea.
Type III: Femoral head fracture associated with femoral neck fracture.
Type IV: Type I, II or III with associated acetabular fracture.

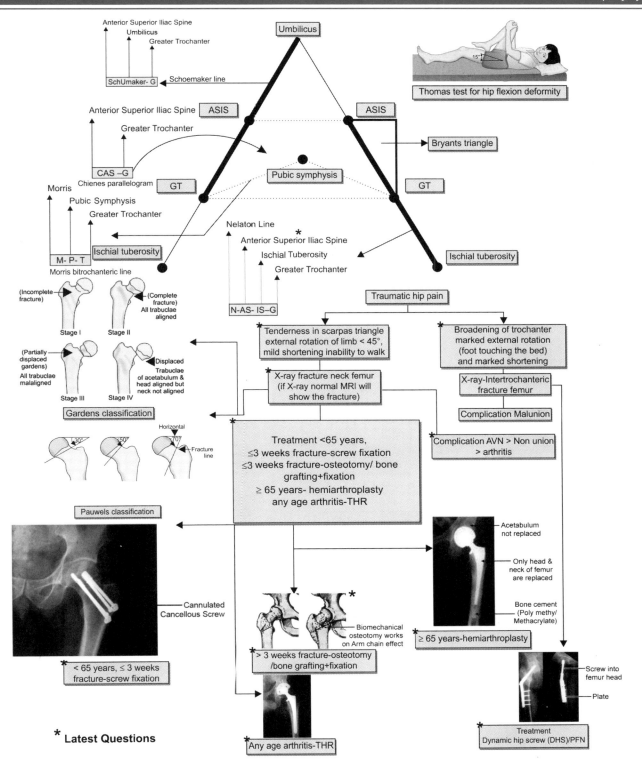

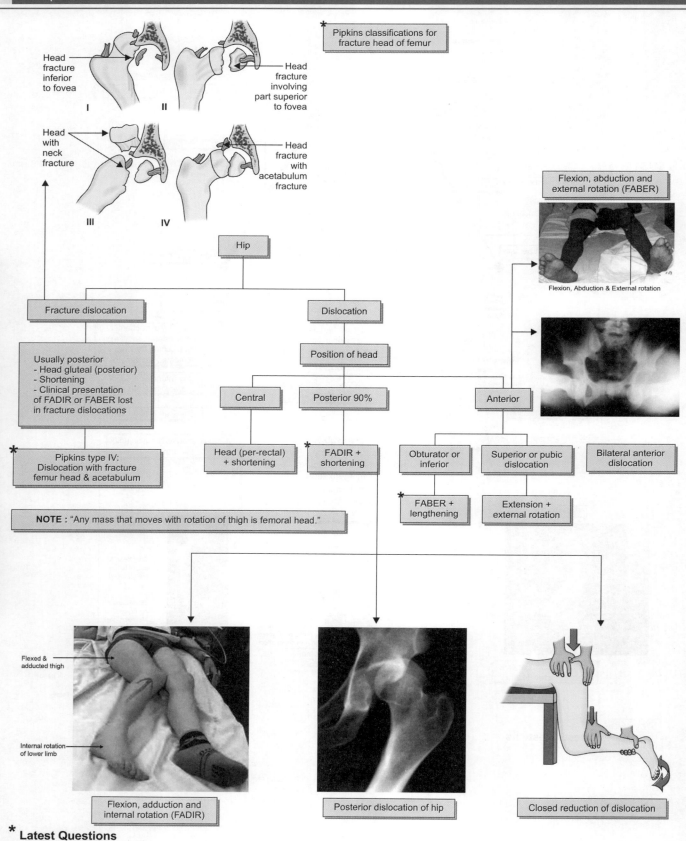

10 CHAPTER

Lower Limb Traumatology

SUBTROCHANTERIC FEMORAL FRACTURES

- Russell and Taylor classification
- There is flexion, abduction and external rotation of proximal fragment
- Treatment of choice is cephalomedullary nail
- Smith Patterson triflanged nail was used for internal fixation of fracture neck femur (not subtrochanteric femur).

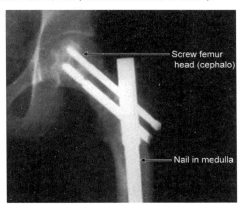

Fig. 10.1: Cephalomedullary nail or Russell Taylor reconstruction nail

MULTIPLE CHOICE QUESTIONS

1. True about proximal fragment in supratrochanteric fracture is: *(NEET Pattern 2013)*
   A. Flexion B. Abduction
   C. External rotation D. All of the above
   Ans. is 'D' All of the above

2. Subtrochanteric fractures of femur can be treated by all of the following methods except: *(AI 2005)*
   A. Skeletal traction on Thomas' splint
   B. Smith Petersen nail
   C. Condylar blade plate D. Ender's nail
   Ans. is 'B' Smith Petersen nail

FRACTURE SHAFT OF FEMUR

Fractures of the shaft of the femur are among the most common fractures encountered in orthopedic practice.

Winquist and Hansen classification is used for comminuted fractures.

Displacements in fracture shaft femur.

Proximal Third Fracture

- Proximal fragment flexes, abducts and externally rotates because of gluteus medius and iliopsoas

- Distal fragment is adducted (adductor longus, minimus, magnus and pectineus).

Middle Third Fracture

- Proximal fragments abducts relatively less because of balancing effect of gluteus medius and adductors; but flexion and external rotation by iliopsoas persists.
- Distal fragment is adducted.

Distal Third Fracture

- Proximal Fragment adducts (because adductor over power gluteus medius because of long lever arm). Distal fragment is hyperextended by gastrocnemius.
- **"Lower limb injures associated with maximum shortening are posterior dislocation of hip > fracture shaft femur > Fracture subtrochanteric femur > Intertrochanteric fracture > Fracture neck femur".**
- Possible treatment methods for fractures of the femoral shaft include the following:
   i. Closed reduction and spica cast immobilization/Skeletal traction/Femoral cast bracing.
   ii. **External fixation/Internal fixation/Intramedullary nailing with open or closed technique/Plate fixation.**

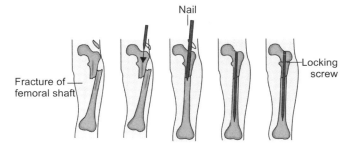

Fig. 10.2: Closed reduction and internal fixation

Management Plan of Fracture Shaft Femur in Adults

A. **Interlock intramedullary nailing** currently is considered to be the treatment of choice for most femoral shaft fractures.
B. External fixator is used in open fractures (open injuries).
C. Delayed union is treated by dynamization of nail (removal of proximal or distal screws or both) and bone grafting.
D. Non-union is treated by exchange nailing (i.e. introduction of large diameter reamed interlocking nail) and bone grafting.

Fracture shaft femur usually unites in 100 days, plus minus 20 days (3–4 months). But non-union is probably best defined by a lack of progression of healing combined with clinical symptoms of discomfort at a minimum of 9 months from the time of treatment and in last 3 months no progress in healing has taken place.

Waddell's triad: Femur fracture, intra-abdominal or intra-thoracic injury and head injury.

FRACTURE SHAFT FEMUR IN CHILDREN

Mechanism of Injury: Direct Trauma or Twisting Injury

Most common location: Upper 1/3rd of femur

Management Plan

Different available modalities of treatment are:

- Gallows traction: < 2 years of age and traction weight < 2 kg of weight can be used.
- Immediate or early spica casting is the treatment of choice in children <5 years of age for femoral fractures with < 2–3 cm of initial shortening, and stable fracture pattern.
- Femoral fractures with > 2–3 cm of shortening or marked instability, high probability of slipping of reduction and tight thigh swelling in 6 months to 5 years age group, who cannot be reduced with immediate spica casting, require 3–10 days of skin or skeletal traction before casting.
- Fixation by enders intramedullary flexible rods and plating can be used in children with multiple trauma, head injury, vascular compromise, floating knee injuries or multiple fracture, preferably in children > 6 years of age. It is important to understand that enders nail is more useful in stable fracture pattern and plating in unstable fracture pattern.

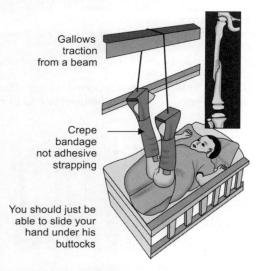

Fig. 10.3: Gallows traction for fracture shaft femur less than 2 years of age

Note: Treatment of choice for fracture shaft femur < 5-year of age is spica and not Gallows traction.

Fracture Shaft Femur – Age-wise Treatment
< 5 years: Spica
≥5 years: Nailing
5–10 years: Close reduction and internal fixation with Elastic Nails (TENS)
≥10 years: Closed interlock nailing.

FLOATING JOINT

Flail joint due to fracture of shafts of adjacent metaphysis of 2 ipsilateral bones, e.g. floating knee = femur and tibia fracture.

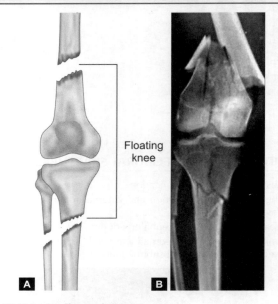

Figs. 10.4A and B: Floating knee

MULTIPLE CHOICE QUESTIONS

1. Treatment of choice for fracture shaft femur in a child less than 2 years of age: *(DNB July 2016)*
   A. Gallow's traction
   B. Hip spica
   C. Russel traction
   D. Intramedullary nail

Ans. is 'B' Hip spica

2. What is a floating knee? *(CET July 16)*
   A. Damage to both anterior and posterior cruciate ligaments
   B. Condition of knee due to tear in medial and lateral collateral ligaments
   C. Femoral shaft fracture with proximal tibia metaphyseal fracture
   D. Advanced tuberculosis of knee joint

Ans. is 'C' Femoral shaft fracture with proximal tibia metaphyseal fracture

3. True supracondylar fracture of femur: *(NEET Pattern 2013)*
   A. Type A   B. Type B
   C. Type C   D. Type D

Ans. is 'A' Type A
   – Type A – Supracondylar fracture
   – Type B – Intercondylar fracture
   – Type C – Comminuted intercondylar fracture

4. A child was given Gallow's traction. What is the diagnosis? *(AIIMS May 2013)*
   A. Fracture shaft femur   B. Fracture shaft hummers
   C. Fracture ulna   D. Spine injury

Ans. is 'A' Fracture shaft femur

5. Exsanguinating blood loss in: *(NEET Pattern 2013)*
   A. Closed humerus fracture   B. Closed tibia fracture
   C. Open femur fracture   D. Open humerus fracture

Ans. is 'C' Open femur fracture

6. Gallow's traction is most optimum for:
   (AIIMS Nov 2013; NEET Pattern 2013; 2012)
   A. Fracture shaft femur >2 years of age
   B. Fracture shaft femur <2 years of age
   C. Fracture tibia
   D. Cervical spine injuries

Ans. is 'B' Fracture shaft femur <2 years of age

7. Why fracture shaft femur is early stabilised?
   (NEET Pattern 2012)
   A. To prevent blood loss   B. ARDS
   C. Non-union   D. Compartment syndrome

Ans. is 'A' To prevent blood loss

8. Blood loss fracture shaft femur: (NEET Pattern 2012)
   A. 1 unit   B. 2 units
   C. 3 units   D. 4 units

Ans. is 'B' 2 units
   – 1 unit tibia
   – 2 units femur
   – 4–8 units pelvis

9. Thomas splint most troubling is: (NEET Pattern 2012)
   A. Ring   B. Side bars
   C. Gauze support   D. Traction attachment

Ans. is 'A' Ring, because it impinges against proximal thigh.

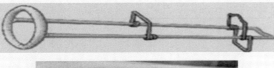
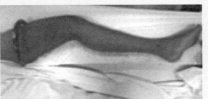

Thomas splint

10. In upper one third femoral shaft fracture, the displacement of proximal segment is: (CSE 1999, Rohtak 97)
    A. Flexion, adduction and external rotation
    B. Flexion, abduction and external rotation
    C. Flexion, abduction and internal rotation
    D. Flexion, adduction and internal rotation

Ans. is 'B' Flexion, abduction and external rotation

11. Maximum shortening of lower limb is seen in:
    A. Fracture shaft femur   (AIIMS Dec 1995)
    B. Fracture neck femur
    C. Fracture intertrochanteric femur
    D. Transcervical fracture neck femur

Ans. is 'A' Fracture shaft femur
    Lower limb injures associated with maximum shortening are posterior dislocation of hip > fracture shaft femur > Fracture subtrochanteric femur > Intertrochanteric fracture > Fracture Neck Femur

12. The femur is fractured at birth at: (Rajasthan 93)
    A. Upper third of shaft   B. Middle third of shaft
    C. Lower third of shaft   D. Neck region

Ans. is 'A' Upper third of shaft

FAT EMBOLISM SYNDROME

Fracture Femur with Breathlessness after 48 hours think of it!

Fat embolism refers to the presence of fat globules in vital organs and peripheral circulation after fracture of a long bone or other major trauma. Fat embolism syndrome reflects a serious systemic manifestation as a consequence to these emboli.

- Fat embolism is a common phenomenon. It is more commonly seen in patients with multiple fractures and in **fractures involving lower limbs especially femur.**
- Fat originates from the site of trauma, particularly from the injured marrow. **Fat globules > 10 μm are considered significant.**

Clinical Presentation

- Early warning signs are a **slight rise in temperature** and **pulse rate (tachycardia)**

  The classical triad of fat embolism syndrome is:
  1. Respiratory symptoms: Dyspnea or tachypnea.
  2. Neurological symptoms: Confusion or disorientation.
  3. Petechial rash: In axilla, neck, periumbilical area, conjunctiva of lower lid, front and back of chest, shoulder.
- Fat embolism is rare in children.

Diagnostic Criterion for Fat Embolism

Gurd's Major Criteria (4)

- Axillary or subconjunctival petechia
- PaO_2 below 60 mm Hg
- CNS depression
- Pulmonary oedema

Gurd's Minor Criteria (8)

- Tachycardia
- Fever
- Anemia
- Thrombocytopenia
- Fat globules in sputum
- Fat globules in urine (Gurd Test)
- Increasing ESR
- Retinal emboli
- **1 major + 4 minor = fat embolism**

Prevention

1. Fracture stabilization
2. Removing fat emboli from circulation by:
   a. Lipolytic agents as heparin (increase serum lipase activity)
   b. Hypertonic glucose (decrease FFA production)
3. Offset its effect by:
   a. Dextran (expand plasma volume, reduces RBC aggregation and platelet adherence)
   b. Aprotinin (protease inhibitor) decreases platelet aggregation and serotonin release.
   c. Alcohol has vasodilator and lipolytic effect.

Treatment

The aim of treatment is maintaining adequate oxygen level in the blood. If necessary by using intermittent positive pressure ventilation. **Oxygen is the only therapeutic tool of proven use.** It should be administered in sufficient amount to maintain arterial

$PO_2 > 80$ mm Hg. O_2 toxicity (pneumonitis) is avoided by using O_2 conc. below 40%.

Steroids are given to avoid pneumonitis.

Waddell's triad: Head injury; Fracture shaft femur and intra-abdominal/intra-thoracic injury.

MULTIPLE CHOICE QUESTIONS

1. Gurd's criteria for fat embolism includes:
   (PGI May 2017)
   A. Hypoxemia $PaO_2 < 60$ mm Hg, $FiO_2 = 0.4$
   B. Tachycardia < 110 bpm
   C. Central nervous system depression disproportionate to hypoxemia
   D. Axillary or subconjunctival petechiae
   E. Deep vein thrombosis

   Ans. is 'A' Hypoxemia $PaO_2 < 60$ mm Hg, $FiO_2 = 0.4$; 'C' Central nervous system depression disproportionate to hypoxemia; & 'D' Axillary or subconjunctival petechiae

2. Regarding Gurd's criteria all correct except:
   (PGI Nov 2016)
   A. Diagnostic criteria for fat embolism syndrome
   B. Pulmonary oedema is major criterion
   C. Thrombocytopenia is a major criteria
   D. 1 major + 4 minor criteria required to diagnose as Fat embolism
   E. $PaO_2 < 60$ is a major criterion

   Ans. is 'C' Thrombocytopenia is a major criteria

3. First symptom is fat embolism is:
   (TN 2015) (Jones vs Pseudojones)
   A. Tachypnea   B. Hypoxemia
   C. Rash   D. Drowsiness

   Ans. 'A' Tachypnea

4. Features of fat embolism:
   (PGI May 2015)
   A. Bradycardia   B. Hypoxia
   C. Hypotension   D. Tachypnoea
   E. Petechial rash

   Ans. is 'B' Hypoxia; 'D' Tachypnoea; and 'E' Petechial rash

5. Fat embolism syndrome is most commonly seen after:
   (NEET 2015)
   A. Femur fracture   B. Acetabular fracture
   C. Pelvis fracture   D. Calcaneal fracture

   Ans. is 'A' Femur fracture

6. Fat embolism most common fracture associated is:
   A. Humerus   B. Tibia *(NEET Pattern 2012)*
   C. Femur   D. Pelvis

   Ans. is 'C' Femur

7. Fat embolism syndrome is characterized by all except:
   (PGI June 09, Dec 07, 04, Rohtak 98)
   A. Tachycardia   B. Hypoxemia
   C. Fat globules in urine   D. Thrombocytosis

   Ans. is 'D' Thrombocytosis

   Thrombocytopenia is seen in fat embolism

8. A person with multiple injuries develops fever restlessness, tachycardia, tachypnea and subconjunctival rash after 48 hours of injury. The likely diagnosis is:
   (AIIMS Nov 2008)
   A. Air embolism   B. Fat embolism
   C. Pulmonary embolism D. Bacterial pneumonitis

   Ans. is 'B' Fat embolism

FRACTURE PATELLA: EXAMPLE OF MUSCULAR VIOLENCE

Patella

- Tube cast may be used
- Displaced transverse fracture
  – Tension band wiring by K-wires and stainless steel (SS) wire
- Comminuted fracture
  – At least proximal third of patella is intact—Partial patellectomy
  – Severe comminution—total patellectomy

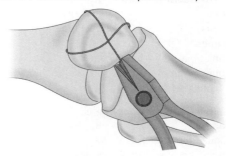

Fig. 10.5: Tension band wiring for fracture patella

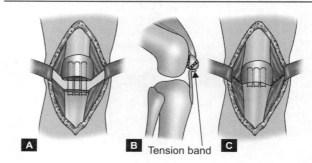

Figs. 10.6A to C: Partial patellectomy and repair

MULTIPLE CHOICE QUESTIONS

1. What is method of fixation of this fracture?
   (AIIMS May 2018, May 17, Nov 16)

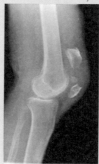

   A. Plating   B. Nailing
   C. Screws   D. Tension Band Wiring

   Ans. is 'D' Tension Band Wiring

2. **Insall-Salvati index is used for:** *(NEET Pattern 2013)*
   A. Olecranon B. Patella
   C. Talus D. Scaphoid

Ans. is 'B' Patella
   - This index is ratio of patellar tendon length to the length of patella (n) is between 0.8 to 1.2
   - <0.8 – Patella baja (low lying patella)
   - >1.2 – Patella atta (high lying patella)

3. **Bulge sign in knee joint is seen after how much fluid accumulation?** *(NEET Pattern 2013)*
   A. 100 mL B. 400 mL
   C. 200 mL D. <30 mL

Ans. is 'D' <30 mL

   Knee Effusion is tested by
   - **Patella Tap**
   - Bulge sign (10–15 mL fluid)
   - Balloon sign
   - Ballottement of patella

4. **Tube (Cylinder) cast is applied for the fracture of:**
   A. Shoulder B. Hip *(All India 2007)*
   C. Pelvis D. Knee

Ans. is 'D' Knee
   - Cylinder cast in full extension is given for undisplaced patella fractures OR knee injuries

5. **Transverse fracture of the patella with separation of fragments is best treated by:** *(PGI Dec 2006, 92, AIIMS 87, Kerala 87)*
   A. Closed reduction with cylinder cast
   B. Open reduction with screw fixation of the fragments
   C. Blind fixation of the two fragments with Kirschner-wire
   D. Open reduction with Kirschner-wire fixation of the fragment with tension band wiring

Ans. is 'D' Open reduction with Kirschner-wire fixation of the fragment with tension band wiring

6. **A comminuted fracture of the Patella should be treated by:** *(Bihar 1989)*
   A. Inserting screws and wires
   B. Physiotherapy alone
   C. Patellectomy
   D. Removal of smallest piece only

Ans. is 'C' Patellectomy

7. **Popliteal artery injury is commonly seen in which type of traumatic knee dislocation?** *(NEET DEC 2016)*
   A. Anterior B. Posterior
   C. Medial D. Lateral

Ans. is 'A' Anterior

Knee Dislocation—Popliteal Artery

Knee dislocation requires careful evaluation of Vascular Injury. Anterior knee dislocation has highest incidence of Popliteal artery damage. The incidence being 5% to 60%.

FRACTURES OF TIBIA

Most Common Bone Involved in Open Fracture

Management of Fracture Tibia

The amount of malalignment and shortening considered acceptables less than 5 degrees of varus-valgus angulation, less than 10 degrees of anteroposterior angulation, less than 10 degrees of rotation, and less than 15 mm of shortening.

Sarmiento PTB (patellar tendon bearing) plaster, is a carefully moulded patellar bearing below knee plaster which is used in fractures of shaft of tibia in the later stages of conservative treatment when the fracture is more stable (and sticky) and requires the stimulus of direct weight bearing.
- *Children*: Above knee cast
- *Adults*: Trial of conservative management is given if it fails Interlock nailing.

Locked intramedullary nailing currently is the preferred treatment for most tibial shaft fractures requiring operative fixation. Plating is used primarily for fractures at or proximal to the metaphyseal-diaphyseal junction. External fixation is useful for open fractures.

Fracture through the lower third of tibia is more liable to go onto delayed union because the lower fragment is relatively avascular.

Anterolateral approach to tibia can expose the entire tibia, provides a vascular flap to provide better healing and this approach can provide provision for secondary closure.

MULTIPLE CHOICE QUESTIONS

1. **In surgical anterolateral approach to tibia, incision is taken over the tibialis anterior muscle mass rather than over the shaft. What is/are the advantages?** *(DNB June 2017)*
   A. Medially based flap
   B. Less chances of wound dehiscence
   C. Can be converted to an extensile approach
   D. All of the above

Ans. is 'D' All of the above

2. **Mechanism of injury in lateral condylar fracture of proximal tibia:** *(NEET Pattern 2013)*
   A. Strain of valgus knee
   B. Strain of varus knee
   C. Strain of valgus knee with axial loading
   D. Rotational injury

Ans. is 'C' Strain of valgus knee with axial loading

3. **Patellar tendon bearing cast is indicated in the following fracture:** *(AI 02)*
   A. Patella B. Tibia
   C. Medial malleolus D. Femur

Ans. is 'B' Tibia

4. **A patient has 2 months POP cast for tibial fracture of left leg. Now he needs mobilisation with a single crutch. You will use this crutch on which side?** *(AIIMS Nov 2000)*
   A. Left side B. Right side
   C. Any side D. Both side

Ans. is 'B' Right side
   - Use of Single Crutch
   - In the opposite side for Fracture both bone leg and Hip Pathology

5. **In posterior compartment syndrome which passive movement causes pain?** *(AIIMS Nov 08)*
   A. Dorsiflexion of foot B. Foot inversion
   C. Toe dorsiflexion D. Toe planter flexion

Ans. is 'C' Toe dorsiflexion
   - Deeper muscles are more commonly involved and they go distal, e.g. flexor digitorum longus and flexor hallucis longus, their ischemia can be tested by toe dorsiflexion and will be more specific than foot dorsiflexion.

ANKLE AND FOOT INJURIES

Ankle Ligaments

Medial Collateral Ligament
It is also called as deltoid ligament. It is strong ligament and major stabilizer of ankle joint. It has two components superficial and deep.

Lateral Collateral Ligament
It is a weak ligament, involved in over 90% of ankle ligament injuries. It has three parts
1. Anterior talofibular—Most commonly injured
2. Middle calcaneofibular—2nd most common injured
3. Posterior talofibular—Torn in most severe injuries

Malleolar Fracture

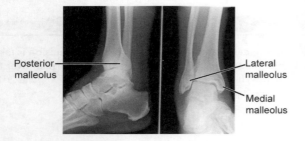

Fig. 10.7: X-ray ankle – 3 malleoli

The three malleoli are medial malleolus, lateral malleolus and posterior malleolus (the posterior part of the lower articulating surface of tibia). **Pott's fracture is bimalleolar fracture and cottons fracture is trimalleolar fracture.**

The mechanism of injury, the first word is position of foot and second word the direction of force

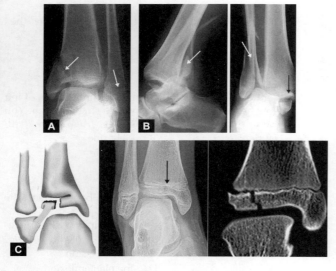

Figs. 10.8A to C: (A) Pott's fracture (B) Cotton's fracture (C) Tillaux fracture avulsion of antero-lateral part of lower tibial Epiphysis due to pull of Syndesmotic ligaments

The most common mechanism is supination-eversion (supination–external rotation), so supination is position of foot and external rotation direction of injury. Analysis of the fracture configuration, and hence the mechanism of forces producing the fracture, is especially important if closed reduction and immobilization are planned as definitive treatment. Generally, the mechanism of forces producing the fracture is reversed by the closed reduction manipulation; if the fracture is produced by a supination, eversion, or external rotation mechanism, reduction is achieved by a pronation, inversion, or internal rotation manipulation.

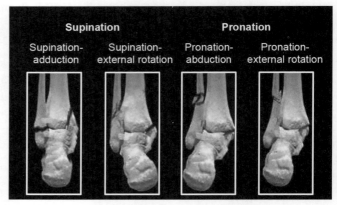

Fig. 10.9: Lauge-Hansen classification of ankle fracture

Supination adduction injury
- Avulsion of fibular tip
- **Vertical fracture of medial malleolus**

Supination external rotation (most common)
- Transverse fracture of medial malleolus/deltoid ligament injury
- Spiral fracture of fibula (Anteroinferior to Posterosuperior)

Pronation abduction
- Transverse fracture of medial malleolus/deltoid ligament injury
- Transverse fracture of fibula (above syndesmosis)

Pronation external rotation
- Transverse fracture of medial malleolus/deltoid ligament injury
- Spiral fracture of fibula (Anterosuperior to Posteroinferior)

Ottawa Ankle Rules

The Ottawa Ankle Rules were developed to decide the need for X-rays in ankle injuries. X-ray examination is called for if there is:
1. Pain around the malleolus
2. Inability to take weight on the ankle immediately after the injury
3. Inability to take four steps in Emergency Department
4. Bony tenderness at the posterior edge or tip of the medial or lateral malleolus.

If X-ray examination is considered necessary, anteroposterior, lateral and 'mortise (30 degree oblique) views of the ankle should be obtained.

Treatment Principle

1. The normal relationships of the ankle mortise must be restored,
2. The weight-bearing alignment of the ankle must be at a right angle to the longitudinal axis of the leg, and
3. The contours of the articular surface must be as smooth as possible.

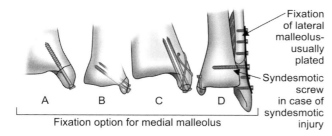

Figs. 10.10A to D: Fixation of malleolar fracture

- For most displaced bimalleolar fractures, open reduction and internal fixation of both malleoli is recommended.
- Anatomical restoration of the distal tibiofibular syndesmosis is essential.

Inversion Injury to Ankle May Lead to:

Lateral collateral ligament injury (anterior talofibular> calcaneofibular> posterior talofibular ligament)
- Peroneal tendon injury
- Avulsion fracture of tip of lateral malleolus
- Avulsion fracture of anterolateral surface of talus and calcaneum (sustentaculum tali).
- Fracture of base of 5th metatarsal.
- Medial malleolar fracture.

Tibial Pilon Fracture

The terms *tibial plafond fracture, pilon fracture,* and *distal tibial explosion fracture* all have been used to describe intra-articular fractures of the distal tibia.

Treatment is fixation.

MULTIPLE CHOICE QUESTIONS

LIGAMENTOUS INJURY

1. Ottawa ankle rules are used to: *(APPG 2015)*
   A. Diagnose rupture of Achilles tendon
   B. Decide on treatment for CTEV
   C. Decide on need of X-rays for possible fracture
   D. Decide on immediate vs. delayed treatment of ankle dislocation
Ans. is 'C' Decide on need of X-rays for possible fracture

2. Which muscle is attached to the tuberosity of navicular bone? *(PGM-CET 2015)*
   A. Adductor hallucis   B. Flexor hallucis brevis
   C. Tibialis anterior   D. Tibialis posterior
Ans. is 'D' Tibialis posterior

3. Pronation of foot the joints that become parallel are:
   A. Talonavicular and calcaneocuboid *(AIIMS Nov 2014)*
   B. Subtalar and calcaneocuboid
   C. Subtalar and navicular
   D. Subtalar and lisfrancs
Ans. is 'A' Talonavicular and calcaneocuboid

4. Pilon fracture is: *(NEET Pattern 2013)*
   A. Intra-articular fracture distal tibia
   B. Intra-articular fracture proximal tibia
   C. Fracture ulna
   D. Fracture radius
Ans. is 'A' Intra-articular fracture distal tibia

5. Which of the following is a syndesmosis? *(NEET Pattern 2012)*
   A. Superior tibiofibular joint
   B. Inferior tibiofibular joint
   C. Talocalcaneal joint
   D. Calcaneocuboid joint
Ans. is 'B' Inferior tibiofibular joint

6. Ankle sprain ligament involved is: *(NEET Pattern 2012)*
   A. Anterior talofibular ligament
   B. Posterior talofibular ligament
   C. Calcaneofibular ligament
   D. Spring ligament
Ans. is 'A' Anterior talofibular ligament

7. March fracture involves: *(NEET Pattern 2012)*
   A. 1st and 2nd metatarsal
   B. 2nd and 3rd metatarsal
   C. 3rd and 4th metatarsal
   D. 4th and 5th metatarsal
Ans. is 'B' 2nd and 3rd metatarsal

8. Runners fracture involves: *(NEET Pattern 2012)*
   A. Tibia   B. Fibula
   C. Metatarsal   D. Talus
Ans. is 'B' Fibula

MALLEOLAR FRACTURE

1. Fracture involving both the malleoli is: *(NIIMS 1992 PGI 91)*
   A. Cotton's fracture
   B. Pott's fracture
   C. Pirogoff's fracture   D. Dupuytren's fracture
Ans. is 'B' Pott's fracture
   – Pott's fracture is bimalleolar fracture and cotton's fracture is trimalleolar fracture.

FRACTURE TALUS (NECK)

Talus is the major weight bearing structure (the superior articular surface carries a greater load per unit area than any other bone in body) and it has a vulnerable blood supply and is a common site for post-traumatic ischemic necrosis.

The body of talus is supplied mainly by vessels which enter the talar neck from the tarsal canal. In fractures of the talar neck these vessels are divided; if the fracture is displaced the extraosseous plexus too may be damaged and body of talus becomes ischemic.

Hawkins Classification is used

Treatment: Undisplaced—Cast in Equinus
Displaced: Reduction and fixation

Complications

- **Secondary Osteoarthritis of Subtalar > ankle joint** occurs some years after injury in over 50% (range 47–97%) of patients. There are several causes: articular damage because of initial trauma, malunion, distortion of articular surface and AVN. This is regarded as the most common complication of fracture talus.
- Avascular necrosis of body is a common complication. The incidence varies with the severity of displacement: in type 0–15%, in type 20–50%, in type 20–100%, type IV 100% AVN. (Overall range 19–69%).

MULTIPLE CHOICE QUESTIONS

1. Fracture of talus without displacement in X-ray would lead to: *(PGI June 02)*
   A. Osteoarthritis of ankle
   B. Osteonecrosis of head of talus
   C. Avascular necrosis of body of talus
   D. Avascular necrosis of neck of talus
   E. Non-union

   Ans. is 'A' Osteoarthritis of ankle and 'C' Avascular necrosis of body of talus
   - The osseous vessels enter the talus through its neck and run postero-laterally to supply the body of talus.
   - Therefore, In displaced fracture of talus neck, the blood supply of body is cut off which results in avascular necrosis of the body of the talus.

2. Avascular necrosis is a complication of: *(AI 1999)*
   A. Fracture of talus
   B. Fracture of medial condyle of femur
   C. Olecranon fracture
   D. Radial head fracture

   Ans. is 'A' Fracture of talus

3. One of the following fracture requires plaster of Paris cast with equines position: *(PAL 96)*
   A. Distal fracture both bones leg
   B. Distal fracture fibula
   C. Bimalleolar   D. Fracture talus

   Ans. is 'D' Fracture talus

4. MC complication of fracture talus is: *(DNB July 2016, AIIMS May 1995)*
   A. Avascular necrosis   B. Non-union
   C. Osteoarthritis of ankle joint
   D. Osteoarthritis of subtalar joint

   Ans. is 'D' Osteoarthritis of subtalar joint

FRACTURE CALCANEUM OR LOVERI FRACTURE

- Calcaneum is the most commonly fractured tarsal bone
- In 5–10% of cases it is bilateral. About one fifth of these patients suffer associated injuries of the spine, pelvis or hip. With severe injuries and especially with bilateral fractures—it is essential to do X-ray of the knees, the spine and the pelvis as well.

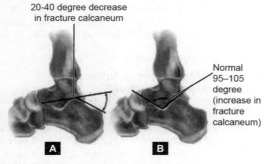

Figs. 10.11A and B: (A) Bohler angle; (B) Angle of Gissane

Calcaneal fractures can be extra-articular (not involving the subtalar joint) or intra-articular (involving the subtalar joint). Extra-articular fractures should be treated with cast or brace immobilization and non–weight bearing for the first 6 weeks.

Intra-articular fractures account for approximately 75% of calcaneal fractures.

Radiological Feature of Fracture Calcaneum (on lateral view)
- Tuber angle of Bohler (Tuber-joint angle)
- It is formed between a line drawn from highest points of anterior process and highest point of posterior facet and a line drawn tangentially to the superior edge of the tuberosity.
- It is normally between 20–40 degrees.
- Flattening /Reduction/Reversal of this angle indicates
- Weight-bearing posterior facet has collapsed (intra-articular fracture) or Degree of proximal displacement of the tuberosity (intra-articular and extra-articular fracture both).

Crucial Angle of Gissane
- Formed by two cortical struts extending laterally, one along the lateral margin of posterior facet and other extending to the beak of the calcaneus
- Normally it is an obtuse angle of 95–105 degree.
- **It increases in intra-articular fractures**

Neutral Triangle of Calcaneum
- Within the trabeculae of calcaneus lies the *neutral triangle*, an area directly below the distal edge of posterior facet. Base of the triangle is the weakest, most vulnerable portion of the calcaneum.
- Axial impaction of the talus into the calcaneum results in a vertical fracture through the neutral triangle, and it represents the primary fracture line.

Other Angles in Orthopedics
- Cobb's angle – Scoliosis
- Kite's angle – CTEV
- Meary's angle – Pes cavus deformity
- Hilgenreiner's epiphyseal angle – Congenital coxa vara
- Baumann's angle – Supra condylar fracture
- Alpha angle and beta angles in DDH

Management of Calcaneal Fractures
- Plain X-rays done for calcaneal fractures include lateral, oblique and axial views. Axial view of calcaneum is Harris view. Brodens view is also used
- CT is the investigation of choice

Treatment are:
1. Conservative treatment for non-displaced or minimally displaced fractures with early range of motion.
2. Open reduction and internal fixation for joint depression fractures.

MULTIPLE CHOICE QUESTIONS

1. Bohler's angle is decreased in the fracture. *(NEET 2016, TN 2015)*
   A. Talus   B. Calcaneum
   C. Navicular   D. Cuboid

   Ans. is 'B' Calcaneum

2. Most commonly injured tarsal bone: *(NEET Pattern 2013)*
   A. Talus   B. Navicular
   C. Cuneiform   D. Calcaneum

   Ans. is 'D' Calcaneum

3. Long compression is used for which fracture?
   (NEET Pattern 2013)
   A. Talus   B. Calcaneum
   C. Fibula   D. Femur
Ans. is 'B' Calcaneum

4. Bohler's angle is for:
   A. Talus   B. CTEV
   C. Calcaneum   D. Scaphoid
Ans. is 'C' Calcaneum

5. Fracture of calcaneus management depending upon:
   (PGI June 08)
   A. Type of fracture   B. Subtalar joint dislocation
   C. Duration of presentation D. Degree of displacement
   E. All of the above
Ans. is 'E' All of the above

6. Bohler's angle is decreased in fracture of:
   (All India 2007, AIIMS May 07; AIIMS May 2007, AIPG 2007)
   A. Calcaneum   B. Talus
   C. Navicular   D. Cuboid
Ans. is 'A' Calcaneum

Bohler's Tuber Joint Angle and Crucial Angle of Gissane are measured for Intra-articular Fractures of Calcaneum.

7. Gissane's angle in intra-articular fracture of calcaneum:
   (DNB June 2017, MAHE 04, AMU 2002)
   A. Reduced   B. Increased
   C. Not changed D. Variable
Ans. is 'B' Increased

8'. Neutral triangle is seen radiologically in: (NIMS 2003)
   A. Neck femur   B. Proximal humerus
   C. Calcaneum   D. Talus
Ans. is 'C' Calcaneum

FALL FROM HEIGHT

Calcaneum is the most commonly fractured tarsal bone and in most cases the mode of injury is fall from height over 20% of these patients suffer associated injury of Dorsolumbar spine (most common), pelvis or hip, base of skull, tibia and talus.

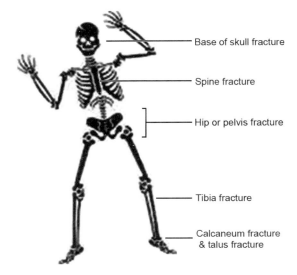

Fig. 10.12: Fall from height

MULTIPLE CHOICE QUESTIONS

1. Calcaneum is associated most commonly with which?
   (AIIMS Feb 1997, Delhi 1992)
   A. Fracture rib
   B. Fracture vertebrae
   C. Fracture skull
   D. Fracture fibula
Ans. is 'B' Fracture vertebrae

2. Least common complication of fall from height is:
   A. Fracture base of skull   (AIIMS Dec 1994)
   B. Fracture calcaneum
   C. Fracture fibula
   D. Fracture 12th thoracic vertebra
Ans. is 'C' Fracture fibula

CHRONIC ANKLE INSTABILITY

Chronic ankle instability can be satisfactorily treated by Watson-Jones procedure. In which reconstruction of ankle ligaments is carried out, using peronei tendons.

Watson Jones is also a lateral approach to the hip joint, which can be used for hip replacement (although rarely used as more commonly used approaches are Moore's posterior and Hardinge's antero-lateral approach).

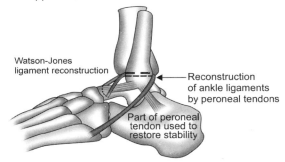

Fig. 10.13: Watson-Jone's procedure

MULTIPLE CHOICE QUESTIONS

1. Watson-Jones approach is done for? (AIIMS Nov 2008)
   A. Neglected club foot   B. Muscle paralysis
   C. Valgus deformity   D. Hip replacement
Ans. is 'D' Hip replacement

– Watson-Jones operation is anterolateral approach to the hip joint.
  There are four commonly used approaches to the hip joint:
– Anterior or Smith-Peterson- *commonly used to access the hip in cases of suspected septic arthritis*
– Anterolateral or Watson-Jones- *is used for hemi or total hip arthroplasty*
– Direct lateral or Hardinge
– Posterior or Southern approach

2. Watson-Jones procedure is done for: (AIIMS Nov 2008)
   A. Polio
   B. Muscle paralysis
   C. Neglected clubfoot
   D. Chronic ankle instability
Ans. is 'D' Chronic ankle instability

Eponym	Fractures
(I) Bumper fracture	Comminuted depressed fracture of the lateral tibial condyle
(I) Pott's fracture	Bimalleolar (medial and lateral malleolar) fracture
(I) Cotton's fracture	Trimalleolar ankle fracture (medial, lateral and posterior malleolar) fracture.
(I) Pilon fracture (Plafond)	Comminuted intra-articular fracture of distal tibial end
March fracture	Fatigue fracture of the neck of 2nd and 3rd metatarsal
Maisonneuve's fracture	An ankle fracture associated with spiral fracture of neck of the fibula
(I) Aviator's fracture	Fracture of neck of the talus
(I) Lisfranc's fracture-dislocation	A fracture dislocation through tarso-metatarsal joints.
(I) Chopart fracture-dislocation	A fracture dislocation through inter-tarsal joints
Malgaigne's fracture	(I) (1) A fracture of pelvis having a combination of ipsilateral fracture of pubic rami anteriorly and sacro-iliac joint disruption posteriorly and (2) supracondylar fracture humerus
Mallet finger	Avulsion of extensor tendon from the base of distal phalanx
(I) Dashboard fracture	Fracture of posterior lip of acetabulum with posterior dislocation of hip
Straddle fracture	Bilateral superior and inferior pubic rami fractures of the pelvis
Jefferson's fracture	Atlas vertebrae (C1)
Hangman's fracture	Axis vertebra (C2) through pars interarticularis
Clay Shoveller's fracture	Spinous process of lower cervical and upper dorsal
(I) Monteggia fracture dislocation	Fracture of proximal third of ulna with dislocation of proximal radioulnar joint
(I) Galleazzi fracture dislocation	Fracture of distal third of radius with dislocation of distal radioulnar joint
Colles fracture	Distal metaphyseal fracture of radius with dorsal displacement and angulation
Smiths fracture (Reverse Colles)	Hand and wrist displaced volarly With respect to forearm in distal metaphyseal fracture of radius.
(I) Barton's fracture	Fracture through the articular surface of distal radius with subluxation of wrist.
(I) Chauffeur's fracture	An intra-articular oblique fracture of the styloid process of the radius.
Night stick fracture	Isolated fracture of shaft ulna
(I) Bennett's fracture dislocation	Partial fracture of 1st metacarpal base with trapezium—metacarpal joint dislocation
(I) Rolando's fracture	Comminuted intra-articular (T or V) fractures of base of 1st metacarpal
Jone's fracture	Fracture of base of 5th metatarsal.
Boxer's fracture	A fracture through the neck of the 5th metacarpal.
(I) Tillaux fracture	Lower tibial epiphysis injury (anterolateral part)

I = Fractures which involves the joint surface or have concomitant joint injuries

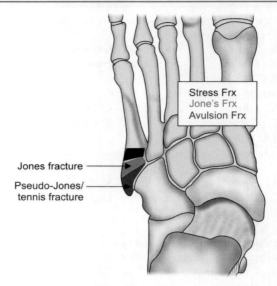

Fig. 10.14: Jone's fracture-pseudo Jones fracture

Jone's fracture occurs at the base of fifth metatarsal at metaphysio-diaphyseal junction and Pseudojones/Dancers Fractures is an avulsion fracture of the tip of 5th metatarsal

MULTIPLE CHOICE QUESTIONS

1. Lisfranc's fracture dislocation involve: (JIPMER Nov 2017)
   A. Lunate
   B. Scaphoid
   C. Trans metatarsal
   D. Capitate

Ans. is 'C' Trans Metatarsal

2. Pott's fracture is an eponym used for: (DNB June 2017)
   A. Bimalleolar ankle fracture
   B. Trimalleolar ankle fracture
   C. Fracture of distal end radius
   D. Pathological fracture in osteomalacia

Ans. is 'A' Bimalleolar ankle fracture

3. Tripod fracture is: (DNB July 2016)
   A. Displaced fracture of calcaneum
   B. Zygomaticomaxillary fracture
   C. Sphenoid Wing Fracture
   D. Coronal Shear pilon Fracture

Ans. is 'B' Zygomaticomaxillary fracture

Trauma to face causes zygomaticomaxillary fractures and its synonymous word are tripod, tetrapod or quadripod fractures

4. Which of the following is an intra-articular fracture? (PGI May 2016)
   A. Barton's fracture
   B. Bennett's fracture
   C. Colles fracture
   D. Pilon fracture
   E. Clay-shoveler's fracture

Ans. is 'A' Barton's fracture; 'B' Bennett's fracture and 'D' Pilon fracture

5. Chopart fracture involves: (AI 2016)
   A. Midtarsal
   B. Tarsometatarsal joints
   C. Base 5th metacarpal
   D. Fracture neck of talus
Ans. is 'A' Midtarsal

6. Lisfranc fracture is: (CET Nov 2015)
   A. Fracture dislocation at the tarsometatarsal region
   B. Intertarsal dislocation
   C. Avulsion of calcaneal tuberosity
   D. Fracture neck of talus
Ans. is 'A Fracture dislocation at the tarsometatarsal region

7. Jone's fracture is: (NEET 2016, TN 2015)
   A. Fracture of base of 5th metatarsal
   B. Fracture of base of 2nd metatarsal
   C. Fracture of base of 1st metacarpal
   D. Fracture of head of 5th metacarpal
Ans. is 'A' Fracture of base of 5th metatarsal

8. Chauffeur's fracture involves the: (NEET 2016, PGM-CET 2015)
   A. Radial head
   B. Radial styloid
   C. Ulnar styloid
   D. Base of I Metacarpal
Ans. is 'B' Radial styloid

9. Which of the following are intra-articular fractures? (PGI Nov 2015)
   A. Pilons fracture
   B. Bartons fracture
   C. Ronaldo fracture
   D. Hoffas fracture
   E. Bennetts
Ans. is 'A' Pilons fracture; 'B' Bartons fracture; 'C' Ronaldo fracture; 'D' Hoffas fracture and 'E' Bennetts

10. March fracture: (NEET Pattern 2013, 2012)
    A. 1st metatarsal
    B. 2nd metatarsal
    C. 3rd metatarsal
    D. 4th metatarsal
Ans. is 'B' 2nd metatarsal

11. Boxer's fracture: (NEET Pattern 2012)
    A. 1st metacarpal
    B. 3rd metacarpal
    C. 4th metacarpal
    D. 5th metacarpal
Ans. is 'D' 5th metacarpal

12. Bennett's fracture: (NEET Pattern 2012)
    A. Fracture 1st metacarpal
    B. Fracture 2nd metacarpal
    C. Fracture 3rd metacarpal
    D. Fracture 4th metacarpal
Ans. is 'A' Fracture 1st metacarpal

13. Barton's fracture occurs at: (NEET Pattern 2012)
    A. Wrist   B. Elbow
    C. Knee   D. Hip
Ans. is 'A' Wrist

14. Colle's fracture: (NEET Pattern 2012)
    A. Radius
    B. Ulna
    C. Tibia
    D. Fibula
Ans. is 'A' Radius

15. Chauffer's fracture: (NEET Pattern 2012)
    A. Distal radius fracture
    B. Distal ulna fracture
    C. Radial styloid fracture
    D. Tibial spine avulsion
Ans. is 'C' Radial styloid fracture

16. Monteggia fracture: (NEET Pattern 2012)
    A. Fracture ulna with dislocation of distal radioulnar joint
    B. Fracture ulna with dislocation of proximal radioulnar joint
    C. Fracture radius with dislocation of distal radioulnar joint
    D. Fracture radius with dislocation of proximal radioulnar joint
Ans. is 'B' Fracture ulna with dislocation of proximal radioulnar joint

17. Tillaux fracture involves: (NEET Pattern 2012)
    A. Lower end tibia
    B. Upper end tibia
    C. Lower end femur
    D. Upper end femur
Ans. is 'A' Lower end tibia

18. Aviator's fracture involves: (NEET Pattern 2012)
    A. Talus
    B. Calcaneum
    C. Tibia   D. Hip
Ans. is 'A' Talus

19. Bumper fracture involves: (NEET Pattern 2012)
    A. Medial part upper end tibia
    B. Lateral part upper end tibia
    C. Medial part lower end femur
    D. Lateral part lower end femur
Ans. is 'B' Lateral part upper end tibia

20. BosWorth fracture: (NEET Pattern 2012)
    A. Fracture distal fibula with posterior dislocation of proximal fragment
    B. Fracture distal fibula with dislocation of distal fragment
    C. Fracture distal end tibia
    D. Fracture distal end femur
Ans. is 'A' Fracture distal fibula with posterior dislocation of proximal fragment

21. Cotton's fracture: (NEET Pattern 2016, 2012)
    A. Bimalleolar fracture   B. Trimalleolar fracture
    C. Wrist subluxation   D. Knee subluxation
Ans. is 'B' Trimalleolar fracture

22. March fracture is: (NEET Pattern 2012)
    A. Stress fracture
    B. Post-osteomyelitis fracture
    C. Involves olecranon
    D. Involves tibia
Ans. is 'A' Stress fracture

23. **Malgaigne's fracture involves:** *(NEET Pattern 2012)*
    A. Pelvis
    B. Femur head
    C. Tibial spine
    D. Proximal humerus

Ans. is 'A' Pelvis

24. **Pilon fracture is:** *(NEET Pattern 2012)*
    A. Intra-articular fracture distal tibia
    B. Intra-articular fracture proximal tibia
    C. Fracture ulna
    D. Fracture radius

Ans. is 'A' Intra-articular fracture distal tibia

25. **Pellegrini-Stieda Disease is:** *(NEET Pattern 2012)*
    A. Avulsion of femoral attachment of MCL
    B. Avulsion of tibial attachment of MCL
    C. Avulsion of femoral attachment of LCL
    D. Avulsion of tibial attachment of LCL

Ans. is 'A' Avulsion of femoral attachment of MCL

26. **Toddler fracture involves:** *(NEET Pattern 2012)*
    A. Femur
    B. Tibia
    C. Fibula
    D. Talus

Ans. is 'B' Tibia

Classifications

1. Allman's: Fracture clavicle
2. Campbells/Rockwood: AC Joint
3. Neers: Proximal Humerus
4. Gartland: Supracondylar Humerus
5. Milch: Lateral Condyle Humerus
6. Masons: Head Radius
7. Bados: Monteggia
8. Frykmanns/Fernandez: Colles
9. Dennis: 3 Columns of spine
10. Young & Burges/Tiles: Pelvis
11. Judet & Lectournel: Acetabulum
12. Thompson & Epstein: Posterior dislocation
13. Pipkins: Head of femur
14. Gardens/Pauwels/Anatomical: Neck femur
15. Boyd & Griffith/Evans: Intertrochanteric fracture
16. Winquist & Hansen's: Shaft femur
17. Schatzkers: Proximal tibia
18. Ruedi and Allgower: Distal tibia
19. Hawkins: Neck talus
20. Essex Lopresti (X-ray)/Sanders (CT Scan): Calcaneum
21. Gustilo Anderson: Open fracture
22. Tscherne: Soft tissue injury in closed fracture

11 Fracture Management

MANAGEMENT OF MUSCULOSKELETAL INJURIES

Methods of Treatment of a Fracture
- Nonoperative or operative

NONOPERATIVE OPTIONS

Splints
- Any material which is used to support a fracture is called *splint*
- Splints are used for immobilizing fractures; either temporarily during transportation or for definitive treatment.
- Rule of splintage is immobilize a joint above and a joint below
- The most commonly employed splints are:
  1. Casts: Here the POP roll completely encircles the limb. **C for cast C for circumference.**
  2. Slab: It is plaster only for one surface of limb. **S for slab S for one surface.**
  3. Spica: This immobilizes limb with a trunk that is spine so **spi + ca = Cast around spine**, e.g. hip spica for fractures around hip and femur (Treatment of choice fracture shaft femur < 5 years of age).

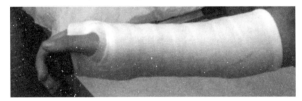

Fig. 11.1: Cast

Note: Scotach Cast (Light Weight Cast is made of epoxy resin)

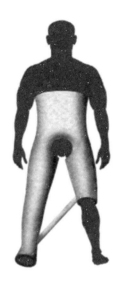

Fig. 11.2: Spica

Plaster Casts and their Uses

Name of the cast	Use
Minerva cast	Cervical and upper thoracic spine disease
Risser's cast	Scoliosis
Turn-buckle cast	Scoliosis
Shoulder spica*	Shoulder immobilization
U-slab/hanging cast	Fracture of the humerus
Hip spica	Fracture of the femur
Cylinder cast/tube cast Patellar tendon bearing	Fracture of the patella, Knee
Cast (PTB cast)	Fracture of the tibia
Colle's cast (hand shaking)	Fracture lower end radius
Glass holding cast	Fracture scaphoid

Common Splints/Braces and their Uses

Name	Use
Crammer-wire splint	Emergency immobilization
Aluminium splint	Immobilization of fingers
Upper Limb	
Cock-up splint	Radial nerve palsy
Knuckle bender splint	Ulnar nerve palsy/median nerve palsy
Volkmann's splint or Turn Buckle splint	Volkmann's ischemic contracture (VIC)
Aeroplane splint	Brachial plexus injury
Dunlop traction	Supracondylar fracture of humerus
Smith's traction	Supracondylar fracture of humerus
Figure of eight bandage	Clavicle
Velpeau sling and swathe	Acromioclavicular dislocation > shoulder dislocation
Gutter splint	Phalangeal and metacarpal fractures
Thumb spica splint	Scaphoid fracture/ Metacarpal fracture/ Game keepers thumb
Sugar tong	Humeral fracture
Distal sugar tong/Reverse sugar tong	Distal forearm fracture
Double sugar tong	Elbow fracture
Buddy strapping	Phalangeal fracture
Lower Limb	
Thomas splint	Fracture femur, knee immobilization
Böhler-Braun splint	Fracture femur, knee and tibia

Contd…

Orthopedics Quick Review

Contd...

Name	Use
Dennis Brown splint	CTEV
Toe-raising splint	Foot drop splint
Gallow's traction	Fracture shaft of femur in children below 2 years (or 12 kg body weight)
Bryant's traction	Fracture shaft of femur in children below 2 years
Russell's traction	Trochanteric fractures (described as skin traction)
Buck's traction	Conventional skin traction
Perkins traction	Fracture shaft femur in adults
90 degrees- 90 degrees traction	Fracture shaft of femur in children
Agnes-Hunt traction	Correction of flexion deformity of hip
well-leg traction	Correction of abduction deformity of hip
Pavlik harness, Von Rosen splint Ilfeld or Craig splint or Bachelor cast	Developmental dysplasia of hip
Broom stick (Petrie) cast	Legg Calve-Perthes disease
Spine	
Four- post collar	Neck immobilization
SOMI brace (Sternal occipital mandibular immobilization brace)	Cervical spine injury
ASHE (Anterior spinal hyper extension) brace	Dorsolumbar spinal injury
Taylor's brace	Dorsolumbar immobilization
Milwaukee brace	Scoliosis
Boston brace	Scoliosis
Lumbar corset	Backache
Goldthwaite brace	Lumbar spine (T.B.)
•Head-halter traction	Cervical spine injuries
Crutchfield traction	Cervical spine injuries
Halo-pelvic traction	Scoliosis
Minerva cast, Halo device	Cervical spine
Risser's cast, Milwaukee brace, Boston brace	Scoliosis (usually Idiopathic or dorsal)

Fractures for which Nonoperative Treatment is the Usual Outcome

1. Clavicle Fracture (Rarely K-wire/Plating)
2. Colle's fracture
3. Scaphoid fracture
4. Pediatric fractures except periarticular fractures or epiphyseal injuries.

SKIN AND SKELETAL TRACTION

	Skin traction	Skeletal traction
Indication	Mild to moderate force	Moderate to severe force
Weight permitted	4-5 kg	Up to 20 kg
Applied with	Buck's traction (conventional skin traction) or Gallow's/Bryant's traction for fracture femur < 2 yr	K wire, Ilizarov's wire Crutchfield's tong Steinmann pin, Denham pin are used for skeletal traction

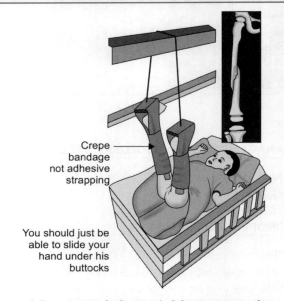

Fig. 11.3: Gallow's traction for fracture shaft femur < 2 years of age

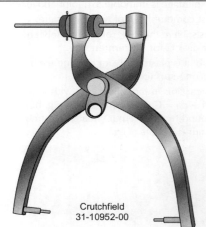

Fig. 11.4: Crutchfield traction for cervical spine traction

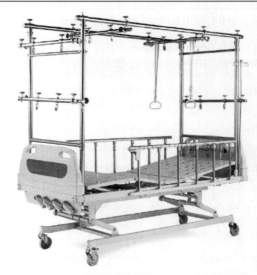

Fig. 11.5: Balkan frame for different tractions and pulley

Fracture Management

Skeletal Traction is given by:
- Steinmann's pin is nonthreaded, so used in nonosteoporotic cortical bone; Denham pin is threaded and is preferred in osteoporotic and cancellous bone, e.g. calcaneal traction.
- Crutchfield's tong is used for cervical traction. K-wires, Ilizarov wires can also be used for skeletal traction.
- Remember Rush nail is used for pediatric fracture shaft femur and not traction.

Functional Cast Bracing
- Sarmiento advocated functional cast bracing.
- Cast is moulded along the fractured limb.
- This is used for fractures of **humerus (MC)**, tibia, femur, forearm.
- Weight-bearing is permitted allowing compression at fracture site and hydrostatic pressure generated in cast keeps the fracture reduced.
- Neighbouring joints are mobilized to prevent joint stiffness
- Hence it provides enhanced rate of bone union with less chances of joint stiffness.

MULTIPLE CHOICE QUESTIONS

1. Hanging cast is used for: (PGI MAY 2018)
   A. Femur fracture   B. Radius fracture
   C. Humerus fracture   D. Tibia fracture
   E. Fibula fracture

   Ans. is 'C' Humerus fracture

2. Regarding POP cast techniques, which of the following statement is true? (PGI Nov 2017)
   A. POP should be just dipped and taken out immediately after immersion into water
   B. Leg casts moulds in 48–60 hours
   C. Using hot water takes more time to mould
   D. POP should be dipped vertically rather than horizontally
   E. Compartment syndrome is immediate complication

   Ans. is 'B' Leg casts moulds in 48–60 hours; 'D' POP should be dipper vertically rather than horizontally; & 'E' Compartment syndrome is immediate complication
   - Plaster of Paris is $CaSO_4 \cdot 1/2\ H_2O$
   - Average setting time 7–10 minutes
   - Drying time (time taken for the POP to convert from crystalline form to anhydrous from):
     - Arm cast—24–36 hours
     - Leg cast—48–60 hours
   - Dip the POP vertically
   - Cold water will maximize the moulding time

3. Agnes Hunt traction is used in: (JIPMER May 2017)
   A. Flexion deformity of hip   B. Inter-trochanteric fracture
   C. Fracture shaft femur   D. Low backache

   Ans. is 'A' Flexion deformity of hip

4. Russell's traction is used in: (JIPMER May 2017)
   A. Inter-trochanteric fracture
   B. Fracture Shaft of femur
   C. Low back ache
   D. Flexion deformity of hip

   Ans. is 'A' Inter-trochanteric fracture

5. Which splint is used in management of fracture shaft femur in age group of 2-10 years? (NEET Dec 2016)
   A. Split Russel traction   B. Gallows traction
   C. Bucks traction   D. Bryant traction

   Ans. is 'A' Split Russel traction

6. Continuous fixed traction is provided by: (NEET Dec 2016)
   A. Thomas splint   B. BB splint
   C. Hamilton Russel   D. Gallows

   Ans. is 'A' Thomas splint

7. Dunlop traction is type of traction used in management of: (NEET Dec 2016)
   A. Fracture humerus   B. Fracture radius
   C. Fracture femur   D. Fracture tibia

   Ans. is 'A' Fracture humerus

8. Tube cast is applied for injuries of: (JIPMER NOV 2017)
   A. Knee Joint   B. Spine
   C. Around Pelvis   D. Proximal Humerus

   Ans. is 'A' Knee Joint

9. Regarding cast application, Choose the correct statement: (PGI Nov 2017)
   A. In the process of applying the cast, the casting material is first dried and then applied
   B. Compartment syndrome is a major complication caused by a tight or rigid cast that constricts a limb
   C. Help in immobilizing the injured limb to keep the bone in place until it fully heals
   D. Casts are circumferential immobilization, whereas splints are noncircumferential immobilizers
   E. Plaster of Paris is $CaSO_4\ \frac{1}{2}\ H_2O$

   Ans. is 'B' Compartment syndrome is a major complication caused by a tight or rigid cast that constricts a limb; 'C' Help in immobilizing the injured limb to keep the bone in place until it fully heals; 'D' Casts are circumferential immobilization, whereas splints are noncircumferential immobilizers; 'E' Plaster of Paris is $CaSO_4\ \frac{1}{2}\ H_2O$

10. Unna boot is used for treatment of: (DNB June 2017)
    A. Diabetic foot ulcer   B. Varicose ulcers
    C. Ankle instability   D. Calcaneum fracture

    Ans. is 'B' Varicose ulcers

    Unna Boot was made by Dr Unna (dermatologist). This was designed to prevent ulcers due to varicose veins and static dermatitis.

11. All of the following are true regarding application of POP cast except: (AI Dec 2015)
    A. Putting the plaster roll in warm water hastens setting time
    B. It is anhydrous calcium phosphate
    C. It should be carefully applied in presence of swelling
    D. Gangrene is known complication of a tight plaster cast

    Ans. is 'B' It is anhydrous calcium phosphate

12. Treatment of choice for fracture shaft femur in a child less than 2 years of age: (CET July 2016)
    A. Gallows traction   B. Hip spica
    C. Russell traction   D. Intramedullary nail

    Ans. is 'B' Hip spica

13. Which of the following casts/splints is used for fracture shaft humerus? (AI Dec 2015)
    A. Hanging casts   B. Knuckle bender splint
    C. Aeroplane splint   D. Above elbow cast

    Ans. is 'A' Hanging casts

14. Brace is used in scoliosis is: *(AI Dec 2016, 2015)*
    A. Milwaukee Brace B. LS Belt
    C. Taylors Brace D. Four post collar
Ans. is 'A' Milwaukee Brace

15. Milwaukee Brace is used in: *(AI Dec 15)*
    A. Congenital kyphosis B. Scheuermann's disease
    C. Adolescent idiopathic scoliosis
    D. Spondylolisthesis
Ans. is 'C' Adolescent idiopathic scoliosis

16. Functional bracing is now the gold standard in nonoperative management of which fractures? *(CET Nov 15)*
    A. Fracture shaft humerus
    B. Fractures of both bones of the forearm
    C. Fracture shaft tibia
    D. Fracture shaft femur
Ans. is 'A' Fracture shaft humerus

17. Traction not used in lower limb: *(AIIMS May 2015)*
    A. Gallows B. Bryant
    C. Dunlop D. Perkin
Ans. is 'C' Dunlop

18. What about Denham pin is true? *(NEET 2015)*
    A. It is used to give skeletal traction
    B. It has threads in the center of pin
    C. It is used to give skeletal traction through calcaneum
    D. All of the above
Ans. is 'D' All of the above

19. Thomas splint is used for immobilizing fractures of:
    A. Femur B. Tibia *(NEET 2015)*
    C. Radius D. Ulna
Ans. is 'A' Femur

20. Functional cast bracing not used in fracture of:
    A. Humerus B. Tibia *(NEET 2015)*
    C. Ulna D. Thoracolumbar spine
Ans. is 'D' Thoracolumbar spine

21. Gallow's traction is used in management of fracture shaft:
    A. Femur B. Tibia *(NEET 2015)*
    C. Humerus D. Ulna
Ans. is 'A' Femur

22. Thomas splint was not used for: *(NEET Pattern 2013)*
    A. Injuries around knee joint
    B. Knee dislocation
    C. Infective arthritis of knee
    D. Fracture femur
Ans. is 'C' Infective arthritis of knee

23. Halopelvic traction is used for correcting which deformity? *(NEET Pattern 2013)*
    A. Spine B. Pectus carinatum
    C. Spondyloptosis D. Coxa vara
Ans. is 'A' Spine

24. Weight allowed in skeletal traction up to:
    A. 5 kg B. 10 kg *(NEET Pattern 2013)*
    C. 20 kg D. 30 kg
Ans. is 'C' 20 kg

25. Maximum weight for skin traction: *(NEET Pattern 2012)*
    A. 1–2 kg B. 4–5 kg
    C. 10–15 kg D. 15–20 kg
Ans. is 'B' 4–5 kg

26. Cast syndrome is a complication of: *(NEET Pattern 2012)*
    A. Hip spica B. Below elbow cast
    C. Above elbow case D. PTB cast
Ans. is 'A' Hip spica

Hip spica or scoliosis cast can press on superior mesenteric artery further compressing 3rd part of duodenum — cast syndrome.

27. Skeletal traction is given by: *(PGI Dec 09, 08)*
    A. K-wire B. Pavlik harness
    C. Denham pin D. Steinmann's pin
    E. Rush pin
Ans. is 'A' K-wire; 'C' Denham pin; 'D' Steinmann's pin

28. Contraindication for skin traction: *(PGI Dec 2006)*
    A. Dermatitis
    B. Compromised vascularity of limb
    C. Abrasions
    D. Hypopigmentation (vitiligo)
    E. Bony deformity
Ans. is 'A' Dermatitis; 'B' Compromised vascularity of limb; 'C' Abrasions

29. All of the following are used for giving skeletal traction, except: *(AIIMS May 2006)*
    A. Steinmann's B. Kirschner's wire
    C. Bohler's stirrup D. Rush pin
Ans. is 'D' Rush pin

Rush pin is used for fixation of fracture shaft femur in children.

PHYSIOTHERAPY

Physiotherapy means system of medicine using physical agents, mechanical and electrotherapy for diagnosis, treatment and prevention of ailments.

Heat Therapy

Superficial

Only superficial structures, i.e. skin and subcutaneous tissues are heated by:
- Hot bath/packs (kenny packs)/soaks/compresses/water bottle
- Chemical packs
- Paraffin wax bath
- Infrared lamp
- Moist air cabinet

Deep Therapy

Deeper structures, i.e. muscles are heated by:
- Shortwave diathermy
  - Heat generated by high frequency alternating current using a short-wave diathermy emitter.
- Microwave diathermy
  - This uses electromagnetic radiation energy to heat the deep tissues
- Ultrasound therapy or ultrasonic therapy
  - Uses high frequency sound energy

Electrotherapy

- Transcutaneous electrical nerve stimulation—low frequency therapy
- Interferrential therapy—high frequency therapy.

MULTIPLE CHOICE QUESTION

1. Which is not a deep heat therapy? *(AIIMS May 07)*
   A. Shortwave diathermy
   B. Ultrasound therapy
   C. Infrared therapy
   D. Microwave therapy

Ans. is 'C' Infrared therapy

OPERATIVE MANAGEMENT OF FRACTURES

Timing of Surgery

Emergency

- Emergency surgery is done for life and limb threatening problems. Examples are:
  i. *Fracture or dislocation with vascular injury (most important knee dislocation)*
  ii. *Fractures with compartment syndrome*
  iii. *Irreducible dislocation or fracture dislocation of major joint.*
  iv. *Compound (open) fractures*
  v. *Septic arthritis*
  vi. *Spinal injuries with deteriorating neurological deficit.*

Urgency

- Urgent surgery is the surgery which should be done early (within 12–36 hours).
  i. *Intra-articular fractures*
  ii. *Fracture neck femur*
  iii. *Fracture lateral condyle humerus in children*
  iv. *Displaced supracondylar fracture humerus in children.*

Elective

- Elective surgery is planned properly and can be done even after some delay (3–4 days to 3–4 weeks). Most of the surgeries in orthopedics are elective. Example are:
  i. *Closed fracture long bone*
  ii. *Joint replacement*
  iii. *Most of the arthroscopic procedures*

MULTIPLE CHOICE QUESTION

1. Which of the following condition should be given most priority in case of fracture? *(PGI Dec 2008)*
   A. Open fracture
   B. Dislocated fracture
   C. Vascular injury
   D. Malunited fracture
   E. Compartment syndrome

Ans. is 'A' Open fracture; 'B' Dislocated fracture; 'C' Vascular injury; 'E' Compartment syndrome

Operative management of fracture:

- Lambotte's principles of surgical treatment of fractures include: anatomical reduction of fracture fragments, stable internal fixation, preservation of blood supply and active pain free mobilization of adjacent muscle and joints.

Fractures are usually managed by reduction and fixation

A. *Closed reduction:* **Fracture hematoma is not exposed hence it does not interfere with fracture healing hence better prognosis.** It is used for extra-articular fractures. Closed reduction is carried out under X-ray control, Image intensifier or C-arm guidance.

Due to high remodeling potential most of the pediatric facutres are managed by close reduction as a variable amount of malalignment is acceptable. But physeal fractures and failed closed reduction with residual displacement are managed with operative treatment (open reduction and internal fixation).

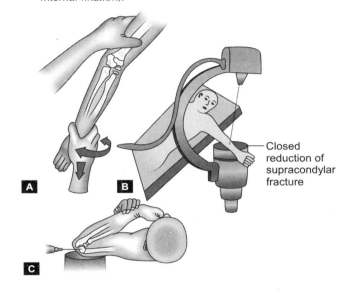

Figs. 11.6A to C: Closed reduction

B. *Open reduction:* Fracture hematoma is exposed, it is usually carried out for articular fractures as exact reduction is essential to prevent arthritis (e.g. lateral condyle fracture humerus) or open reduction is carried out, if closed reduction fails or if additional procedure like bone grafting at fracture site is required.

C. *Internal fixation the fixation device is under the coverage of soft tissues, e.g. plating or nailing.*
Tension band principle—Conversion of tensile forces to compressive forces by application of wire of plate on tensile (convex) surface (Remember plating also is on this principle).

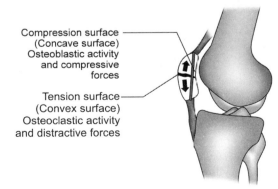

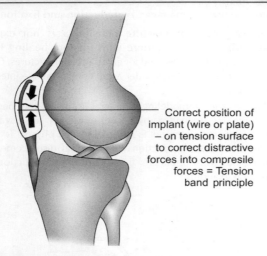

Fig. 11.7: Tension band principle

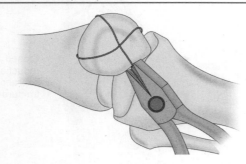

Fig. 11.8: Tension band wiring of patella

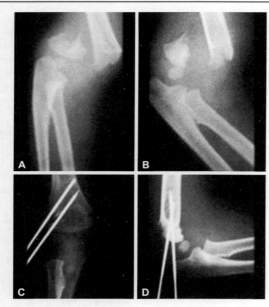

Figs. 11.9A to D: K-wire fixation

1. Tension band wiring – **Fracture Patella**, olecranon or medial malleolus may be treated by Tension Band wiring.
2. K-wire – Fractures in children, e.g. **supracondylar fracture humerus** (closed reduction) or lateral condyle fracture (open reduction).

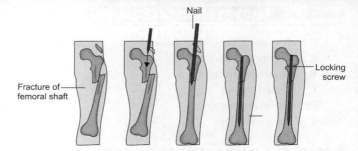

Fig. 11.10: Closed reduction and internal fixation

3. **Intramedullary nailing** (e.g. K nail, interlocking nail, Rush nail, reconstruction nail). It is done for lower limb diaphyseal fractures, e.g. femur or tibia. Nailing is preferably done by closed reduction, if closed reduction fails open reduction can be carried out.

   Kuntscher Cloverleaf Intramedullary Nail

   It is mainly useful for transverse or short oblique fractures around isthmus. It provides stability by 3 point fixation. To increase the elasticity of nail, it is hollow, has a cloverleaf cross-section and a longitudinal slot. When a straight nail passes through a curved medullary canal it is deformed (elastic deformation). (3 points are 2 ends and isthmus).

   Now-a-days interlock nail (that is having locking screws that locks nail with bone to prevent rotational malalignment) is preferred over Kuntscher nail.

4. *Plating* for upper limb fractures, e.g. humerus or radius or ulna (Plate fixation is usually done by open reduction).

TYPES OF PLATE

1. Dynamic compression plates: These are used to fix the diaphyseal region and can be used as neutralization Buttress mode or compression mode.
2. LCDCP: Limited contact–DCP It decreases the contact with bone surface hence preserving bone vascularity.
3. Locking compression plate: The screw locks in screw holes of the plates hence the name – locking plates.

The Locking Compression Plate (LCP) system is part of a stainless steel or titanium plate and screw system that merges locking screw technology with conventional plating techniques.

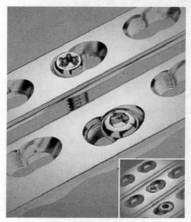

Fig. 11.11: Locking compression plate

Fracture Management

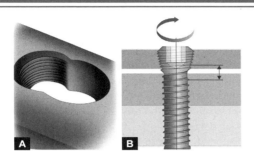

Figs. 11.12A and B: (A) Combi hole; (B) Locking screw (the threads in the head of the screw locks with the threads of the hole in plate)

Key Features and Benefits
- Combi hole allows the surgeon to choose between conventional plating techniques, locked plating techniques, or a combination of both
- Threaded hole section for locking screws provides ability to create fixed-angle constructs
- Smooth dynamic compression unit (DCU) hole section for conventional screws allows utilization of familiar AO plating techniques
- Limited-contact plate design reduces plate-to-bone contact, thus limiting vascular trauma and periosteal damage.
- Indications are for fixation of fractures, osteotomies, nonunions, malunions, replantations particularly in osteopenic bone. They are also for use in fixation of periprosthetic fractures.

Advantages of Locking Plates are:
- Osteopenic bone
- Metaphyseal areas
- Periprosthetic fractures
- Failed fixation (nonunion)

	Conventional Plate	Locking Plate
1. Adaptation to the underlying bone	Precise	Not essential
2. Blood supply to underlying bone	More disrupted	Less disrupted
3. Screw hold	Inferior	Superior
4. Fixation	Less stable	More stable (esp. Osteopenic bones)

4. Screw fixation—articular fractures where headless screws (Herbert screw) are preferred, e.g. scaphoid fracture and cannulated cancellous screw for femoral neck fracture in young.

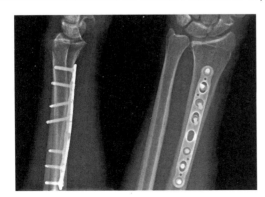

Fig. 11.13: Forearm plating

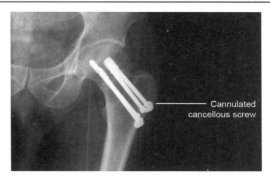

Fig. 11.14: Fracture neck femur, reduction and fixation

5. Dynamic hip screw (DHS)—For intertrochanteric fracture.

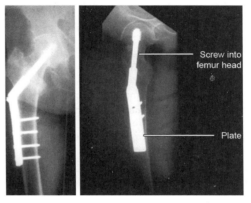

Fig. 11.15: Dynamic hip screw

D. *External fixation the fixation device is external to skin-external fixator or ilizarov fixator.*

Ilizarov fixator works on the principles of distraction osteogenesis that is an osteotomy is carried out and distracted at the rate of 1 mm per day causing distraction at the callus and subsequently lengthening can be done. It can be used for correction of deformities like malunion, shortening, shortening with discharging sinus, gap nonunion and also for CTEV.

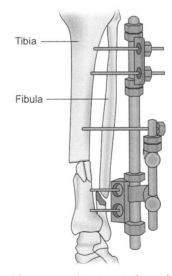

Fig. 11.16: External fixator—usual treatment of open fracture

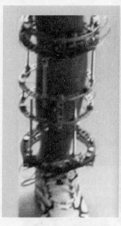
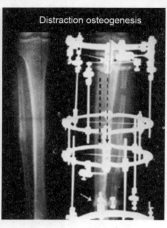

Fig. 11.17: Ilizarov external fixator

E. *Surgical excision*
   1. Done in comminuted fracture patella, olecranon and head radius (outer 1/3rd).
   2. Head and neck of femur are excised and replaced by prosthesis in fracture neck femur ≥ 65 years of age.

   Excision is contraindicated in growth plate injury, e.g. Lateral condyle fracture.

F. *Arthrodesis*—Surgical fusion rarely done for fractures sometimes grossly destroyed articular fractures
G. *Arthroplasty*—Joint replacement, e.g. fracture neck femur
H. *Bone grafting for non-union.*

BONE GRAFT

Types of bone graft are:
- **Cancellous:** If only small amount of cancellous bone is needed sites are olecranon, radial styloid, anterior aspect of greater trochanter, distal femoral condyle, proximal tibial metaphysis, Distal tibial metaphysis
- Corticocancellous – iliac crest
- Cortical – fibula
- Vascularised fibular graft
- **Ilium (Pelvis):** This is an ideal source of primary 1st order bone graft because it is relatively subcutaneous, has natural curvatures that are useful in fashioning grafts, has ample cancellous bone and has cortical bone of varying thickness. Removal of bone carries minimal risk and usually no significant residual disability.
- **Posterior superior iliac spine is the best source of cancellous bone.**
- **Anterior iliac crest is the best source of bicortical and cortico cancellous graft.**

MULTIPLE CHOICE QUESTIONS

LONG BONE FRACTURE

1. Locking compression plating is commonly indicated in the following fracture types: *(NEET DEC 2016)*
   A. Periarticular fractures
   B. Transverse of oblique fractures of long bones
   C. Intertrochanteric fractures
   D. Fracture of long bones
   Ans. is 'A' Periarticular fractures

2. K nail can be used for all of the following fractures except:
   A. Isthmic femur shaft fractures *(AI Dec 15)*
   B. Intertrochanteric fractures
   C. Low subtrochanteric fractures
   D. Distal femur shaft fractures
   Ans. is 'B' Intertrochanteric fractures

3. Bone transport can be used in the management:
   A. Gap nonunion *(AI Dec 2015)*
   B. Deformity correction
   C. Comminuted shaft femur fracture
   D. Avascular necrosis of femoral head
   Ans. is 'A' Gap nonunion

4. Which of the following requires surgical correction?
   A. Pathological fracture *(PGI Nov 2016)*
   B. Fracture humerus shaft with RN palsy
   C. Fracture humerus shaft with vascular involvement
   D. Polytrauma patient
   E. Old age
   Ans. is 'A' Pathological fracture; 'C' Fracture humerus shaft with vascular involvement; and 'D' Polytrauma patient

5. True about Locking compression plate: *(PGI May 2015)*
   A. In osteoporotic patients, it should not be used
   B. Can be used as buttress plate
   C. Usually cause periosteal injury
   D. Mechanically superior to a conventional plate
   E. Can not be used as compression plate
   Ans. is 'B' Can be used as buttress plate and 'D' Mechanically superior to a conventional plate

6. Most common bone for which nailing is done?
   A. Radius   B. Ulna *(NEET Pattern 2012)*
   C. Tibia   D. Humerus
   Ans. is 'C' Tibia

7. In the management of long bone fracture following can be done: *(PGI Dec 06,03)*
   A. Intramedullary nailing B. Plating
   C. External fixation   D. Tension band wiring
   E. Screw
   Ans. is 'A' Intramedullary nailing, 'B' Plating and 'C' External fixation

8. Action of intramedullary 'K' nail is: *(NEET 2016, AI 1996)*
   A. Two-point fixation   B. Three-point fixation
   C. Compression   D. Weight concentration
   Ans. is 'B' Three-point fixation

9. Treatment of choice for fracture lower 1/4th of tibia in non-union with multiple scarred wounds and discharging sinuses and about 4 cm shortening of leg: *(AIIMS Nov 09)*
   A. Ilizarov fixator   B. Plate
   C. External fixation   D. Intramedullary nail
   Ans. is 'A' Ilizarov fixator
   – Shortening with discharging sinus ilizarov fixator is the preferred method.

OPEN REDUCTION AND INTERNAL FIXATION

1. Tension band wiring is done in all except: *(NEET Pattern 2012)*
   A. Fracture patella   B. Fracture olecranon
   C. Fracture medial malleolus D. Colle's fracture
   Ans. is 'D' Colle's fracture

2. The contraindication to internal fixation:
 (NEET Pattern 2012)
   A. Physeal injury
   B. Active infection
   C. Intra-articular fracture
   D. Fracture dislocation

Ans. is 'B' Active infection

3. All of the following are indications for open reduction and internal fixation of fractures except: *(CSE 2000)*
   A. Compound fracture
   B. Unsatisfactory closed reduction
   C. Multiple trauma
   D. Intra-articular fracture

Ans. is 'A' Compound fracture
 – Open fractures usually external fixator is applied.

4. Open reduction and internal fixation is done for all of the following fractures except: *(AI 97, AIIMS 91)*
   A. Patella fracture
   B. Olecranon fracture
   C. Volar Barton's fracture
   D. Fracture lateral condyle of humerus

Ans. is 'C' Volar Barton's fracture
 – Volar Barton an attempt of closed reduction can be carried out if it fails open reduction and plating is done. Although recently it has been shown operative results yield better results, but for all other fractures open reduction and internal fixation is carried out.

SURGICAL EXCISION

1. 60 degree angle of Z plasty causes how much increase in length? *(NEET Pattern 2012)*
   A. 25%   B. 50%
   C. 75%   D. 100%

Ans. is 'C' 75%

Explanation

Z plasty—relationship between angle of Z plasty and elongation:
 – 30 degrees—25% elongation
 – 45 degrees—50% elongation
 – 60 degrees—75% elongation
 – 75 degrees—100% elongation
 – 90 degrees—125% elongation

2. Surgical excision is contraindicated in: *(AIIMS Dec 95)*
   A. Olecranon process   B. Patella
   C. Head of radius   D. Lateral condyle humerus

Ans. is 'D' Lateral condyle humerus
 – Lateral condyle of humerus is never excised because of if being the physeal region.

BONE GRAFTING

1. Which of the following is ideal site for harvesting bone graft? *(AI 08)*
   A. Iliac crest   B. Distal end of humerus
   C. Distal end of femur   D. Fibula

Ans. is 'A' Iliac crest
 – Iliac crest is the ideal and most common site for harvesting bone graft.

2. Cancellous bone graft taken from: *(PGI Dec 2006)*
   A. Femoral condyles   B. Pelvis
   C. Greater trochanter   D. Tibial metaphysis
   E. All of the above

Ans. is 'E' All of the above

3. Site for 1st order bone grafting: *(PGI June 03, Dec 2002)*
   A. Pelvis   B. Tibial metaphysis
   C. Medial malleolus   D. Femoral condyle
   E. Greater trochanter

Ans. is 'A' Pelvis
 – Iliac crest is the site for 1st order bone grafting

ARTICULAR FRACTURES

Principles

- Anatomical reduction and stable fixation of articular fragments is necessary to restore joint congruity.
- Immediate motion is necessary to prevent joint stiffness and to ensure articular healing and recovery.

Management

The main aim of treatment is to restore the congruity of the joint surface, to prevent further joint damage which may lead to secondary osteoarthritis. It can be done by:

Aspiration of intra-articular hematoma
- Excision of loose articular fragments
- In undisplaced fractures where only immobilization is necessary
  1. POP slab/cast
  2. Skeletal traction
- **Internal fixation:** In displaced fracture depending on age and site **(Treatment of choice)**
- **Arthrodesis:** When other measures fail or stable painless joint is required in young active labourer surgical fusion is carried out.
- Arthroplasty (joint replacement) also can be carried out for articular fractures.

MULTIPLE CHOICE QUESTIONS

1. Cobra head plate is used for: *(NEET Dec 2016)*
   A. Hip arthrodesis   B. Knee arthrodesis
   C. Elbow arthrodesis   D. Ankle arthrodesis

Ans. is 'A' Hip arthrodesis
- Schneider developed Cobra plates for hip arthrodesis
- Smith-Peterson Nail — Fracture Neck Femur
- Gamma Nail — Intertrochanteric fracture Femur

2. Commonest indication for ankle arthrodesis is:
   A. Rheumatoid arthritis *(Maharashtra PG 2016)*
   B. Post-traumatic arthritis
   C. Post infective arthritis
   D. Failed total ankle arthroplasty

Ans. is 'B' Post-traumatic arthritis

3. Which of the following is included in management of intra-articular fracture? *(PGI June 09, 04, Dec 08)*
   A. Arthrodesis   B. Excision
   C. Aspiration   D. K-wire
   E. Plaster of paris cast   F. All of the above

Ans. is 'F' All of the above

4. Identify the bone holding forceps amongst the following: *(AIIMS May 2017)*

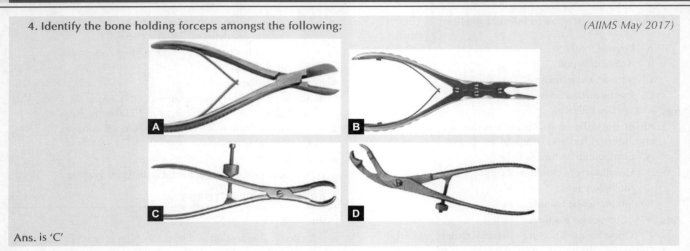

Ans. is 'C'

INSTRUMENTS AND IMPLANTS

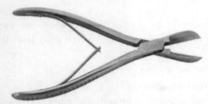
Fig. 11.18: Bone Cutter

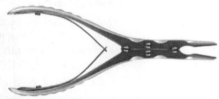
Fig. 11.19: Bone Nibbler Double Action

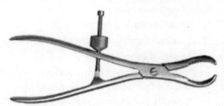
Fig. 11.20: Bone Holding Forceps

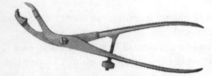
Fig. 11.21: Bone Plate Holding Forceps

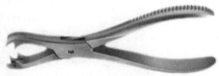
Fig. 11.22: Fergusson Bone Holding Forceps

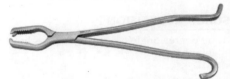
Fig. 11.23: Lane Bone Holding Forceps

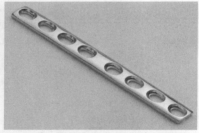
Fig. 11.24: Dynamic Compression Plate (DCP)

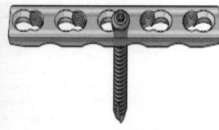
Fig. 11.25: Locking Compression Plate (LCP)

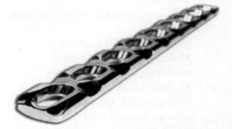
Fig. 11.26: Limited Contact Dynamic Compression Plate (LCDCP)

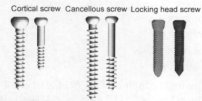
Fig. 11.27: Screws

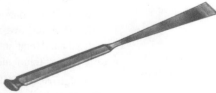
Fig. 11.28: Osteotome

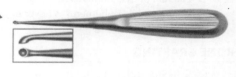
Fig. 11.29: Bone Curette

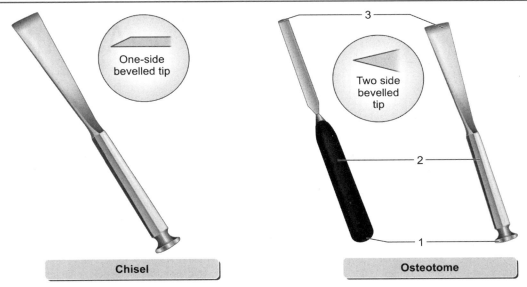

Fig. 11.30: Osteotome Versus Chisel

Amputations

AMPUTATIONS

- Amputation is a procedure where a part of the limb is removed through one or more bones.
- Disarticulation is a procedure where the limb is removed through a joint.

Indications of Amputation

Absolute
- Irreparable loss of blood supply of a diseased or injured limb
- Fulminant infection (e.g. gas gangrene)
- Microvascular ischemia (Burgers gangrene)
- Diabetic gangrene.

Relative
- Infections
- Frostbite
- Tumors
- Congenital anomalies – rare
- Chronic osteomyelitis – rare
- Burn
- Trauma
- Nerve injuries – rare

Note: Most common cause of amputation is peripheral vascular disease.

Mangled Extremity Severity Score (MESS)

Mangled extremity severity score (MESS) can be used as predictor of eventual amputation versus limb salvage in crushing injuries. Higher the score lower the chances of salvage, i.e. higher score has higher chances of amputation. However, recent studies have shown it to be inaccurate in predicting the functional outcome for mangled limb patient.

"SIVA"—the destroyer will decide survival.

Type	Points (Depending on severity)
Shock group	0–2
Ischemia group	1–4
Velocity of trauma	1–4
Age group	0–1
Total score	11

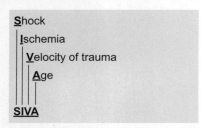

Mess Score: Total Score is 11, six or less consistent with a salvageable limb. Seven or greater amputation is generally the eventual result.

TECHNIQUES IN AMPUTATIONS

1. **Closed Amputation:**
   - Nerves are retracted and cut, so that they are not superficial on stump and cause pain.
   - Bone is kept shorter than soft tissue in flap method of amputation to facilitate closure of amputation stump.
   - Muscles usually are divided at least 5 cm distal to the intended bone resection. They may be stabilized by Myofascial flaps (muscle is attached to fascia). Myodesis (suturing muscle or tendon to bone) or by myoplasty (suturing muscle to periosteum or to fascia of opposing musculature). If possible, myodesis should be performed to provide a stronger insertion, help maximize strength, and minimize atrophy. Myodesed muscles continue to counterbalance their antagonists, preventing contractures and maximizing residual limb function. Myodesis may be contraindicated, however, in severe ischemia because of the increased risk of wound breakdown.
   - The skin and soft tissue are closed primarily.
   - Thus nerves are cut most proximal than bone and than muscles.

2. **Open or Guillotine Amputation:**
   - In guillotine amputation or open amputation, limb is transected at one level through skin, muscle and bone. The skin is not closed over the end of the stump. The operation is the first of at least two operations required to construct a satisfactory stump. It always must be followed by secondary closure, reamputation, revision, or plastic repair. The purpose of this type of amputation is to prevent or eliminate infection so that final closure of the stump may be done without breakdown of the wound. Open amputations are indicated in infections and in severe traumatic wounds with extensive destruction of tissue and gross contamination by foreign material. Appropriate antibiotics are given until the stump finally heals.

   Ideal Amputation Stump:
   1. Non-tender
   2. Well-healed
   3. Non-adherent
   4. Non-bulbous
   5. Skin at end of stump mobile sensate skin
   6. Properly constructed to allow satisfactory fitting of prosthesis.

   Cardinal rule – Preserve all possible length consistent with good coverage of stump

Type of Amputation	Traditional Length of Stump
Above knee	23 cm (9 inches)
Below knee	14 cm (5.5 inches)
Below elbow	18 cm (7 inches)
Above elbow	20 cm (8 inches)

A way to remember total of amputation stumps in upper and lower limbs is 15:

8	+	7	=	15	
↓		↓			Inches (1 Inch = 2.54 cm)
Above elbow		Below elbow			
9	+	5.5	~	15	
Above knee		Below knee		(Roughly)	

Amputations about Foot

Mid-foot Amputation

Type	Level of Amputation
Lisfranc	**Tarsometatarsal joint**
Chopart	**Intertarsal joint** (Choparts – Intertarsal = CIT)
Pirogoff	Calcaneus is rotated forward to be fused to tibia after vertical section through its middle.

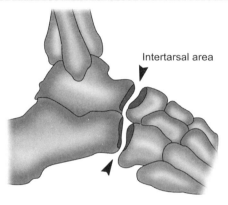

Fig. 12.1: Chopart amputation (Intertarsal area)

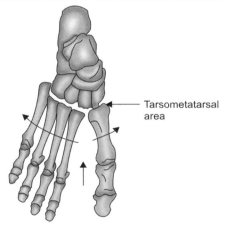

Fig. 12.2: Lisfranc's amputation (Tarsometatarsal area)

Ankle/Hindfoot Amputation

Type	Level of Amputation
Syme	Distal tibia fibula 0.6 cm proximal to the periphery of ankle joint passing through the dome of ankle
Sarmiento	Distal tibia and fibula 1.3 cm proximal to the ankle joint and excision of medial and lateral malleoli.
Boyd	Talectomy, forward shift of the calcaneus and calcaneotibial arthrodesis.

Complications of Amputation

1. Hematoma
2. Wound infection
3. **Phantom limb'** is a late complication of amputation, and is used to describe the feeling that the amputated limb is still present. Phantom limb sensations are so common after an amputation that they should be considered normal. Most patients do not find these to be bothersome. The most important part of management is simply to educate the patient regarding these sensations so that they are not surprised by their presence. **Although no one specific method is universally beneficial, some patients may benefit from such diverse measures as massage, ice, heat, increased prosthetic use, relaxation training, biofeedback, sympathetic blockade, local nerve blocks, epidural blocks, ultrasound, transcutaneous electrical nerve stimulation, and placement of a dorsal column stimulator.**
4. Amputation neuroma—The nerve ending at the stump forms a neuroma that is extremely painful A painful neuroma occurs when the nerve end is subjected to pressure or repeated irritation. A painful neuroma usually can be prevented by gentle traction on the nerve followed by sharp proximal division, allowing the nerve end to retract deep into the soft tissue. A painful neuroma usually is easily palpable and often has a positive tinel sign. Treatment initially consists of socket modification. If this fails to relieve symptoms, simple neuroma excision or a more proximal neurectomy may be required and the pain is controlled through **Transcutaneous electrical nerve stimulation (TENS) > Interferential therapy > Ultrasound.** TENS and interferential therapy works on the principle of inhibiting pain gate pathway hence are better for control of neurogenic pain. Surgical treatment is considered better than other methods.

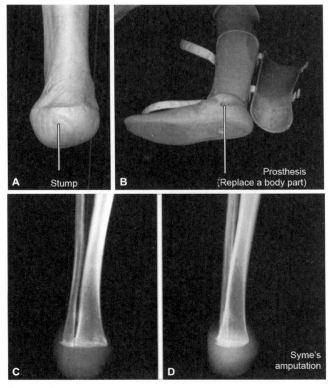

Figs. 12.3A to D: Syme's amputation

5. Sequestrum—Excessive periosteal stripping is contraindicated as it may result in formation of ring sequestrum in amputation stump.

Type of sequestrum	Found in
Ring sequestrum	Amputation stumps **Around pin tracts (external fixator)**
Tubular sequestrum	Hematogenous osteomyelitis and segmental fractures (middle segment)
Rice grain sequestrum/ Coke sequestrum/ Feathery sequestrum	**Tuberculosis**
Button sequestrum	Pheochromocytoma
Black sequestrum	Gunshot
Bombay sequestrum	Overlying skin loss
Colored sequestrum	Fungal
Linear/Flake sequestrum	Only one cortex involved

Foot Prosthesis for Amputation Stump

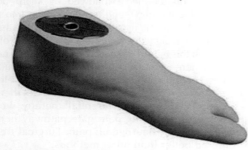

Fig. 12.4: Solid ankle cushion heel (SACH Foot)

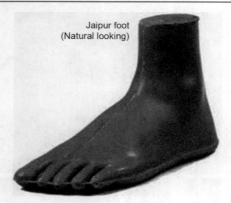

Fig. 12.5: Jaipur foot by Dr PK Sethi

SACH (Solid ankle cushion heel) foot does not allow ankle movements (required for squatting), subtalar movements (inversion and eversion movements for walking on uneven grounds). Hence more suitable for western Lifestyle and in Jaipur foot these movements are permitted. Hence more suitable for Indian scenario also Jaipur foot is appropriate for walking barefoot and in SACH foot barefoot walking is not possible.

Prosthesis	Solid ankle cushion heel (SACH)	Jaipur foot (Dr PK Sethi)
Appearance	Does not look normal, requires shoe	Looks normal, can walk barefoot
Keel	Long keel restricting movements	Small keel allowing all movements
Ankle movements	**Squatting not possible**	Possible
Inversion/ eversion	Not present so difficult to walk on uneven grounds	Present so can walk on uneven grounds
Cost	High	Low

MULTIPLE CHOICE QUESTIONS

1. Most common cause of amputation in India is: *(NEET 2015)*
   A. Diabetic gangrene
   B. Gas gangrene
   C. Road traffic accident
   D. Tumors

Ans. is 'C' Road traffic accident

2. Patient comes with crush injury to upper limb, doctor is concerned about gangrene and sepsis what can help decide between amputation and limb salvage? *(NEET 2015)*
   A. MESS
   B. GCS score
   C. Gustilo-Anderson classification
   D. ASIA guidelines

Ans. is 'A' MESS

3. Jaipur foot was invented by: *(NEET 2015)*
   A. Dr. P. K. Sethi   B. Dr. S. K. Verma
   C. Dr. B. L. Sehgal   D. Dr. H. R. Gupta

Ans. is 'A' Dr. P. K. Sethi

4. Principle of TENS for alleviating pain around joints and nerve pain: *(AIIMS Nov 2013)*
   A. Gate theory of pain control
   B. Referred pain
   C. Decreases substance P
   D. Local heat at the site

Ans. is 'A' Gate theory of pain control

5. Amputation neuroma treatment modality used is: *(AI 2012)*
   A. Ultrasound
   B. Infrared
   C. Compression bandage
   D. Interferential therapy

Ans. is 'D' Interferential therapy but if TENS is mentioned that is a better answer.

6. SACH Foot all are true except: *(AI 2012)*
   A. Solid ankle cushion heel
   B. Prosthesis
   C. Squatting is easy
   D. Does not look like a normal foot

Ans. is 'C' Squatting is easy
   – SACH foot does not allow ankle movements (required for squatting), subtalar movements (inversion and eversion movements for walking on uneven grounds). Hence more suitable for western lifestyle and in Jaipur foot these movements are permitted. Hence more suitable for Indian scenario also Jaipur foot is appropriate for walking barefoot and SACH foot barefoot is not possible.

7. A, 30-year-old male suffers from road traffic accident car run-over his right leg. His examination is vitals stable and general physical examination is okay. His right leg is crushed with exposed muscles and bones. The debate about limbs survival can be resolved to an extent by MESS score it includes all except: *(AIIMS May 2011)*
   A. BP
   B. Distal circulation
   C. Velocity of trauma
   D. Nerve injury

Ans. is 'D' Nerve injury

8. Myodesis is employed in amputations for all of the following indications except: *(AI 2009)*
   A. Trauma
   B. Tumor
   C. Children
   D. Ischemia

Ans. is 'D' Ischemia

9. Tarsometatarsal amputation is also known as: *(AIIMS SR 2006, KA 99, UP 97)*
   A. Chopart's amputation
   B. Lisfranc amputation
   C. Pirogoff amputation
   D. Syme's amputation

Ans. is 'B' Lisfranc amputation

10. In below elbow amputation the length of stump should be: *(AIIMS May 1993)*
    A. 10–15 cm
    B. 15–20 cm
    C. 20–25 cm
    D. 5–10 cm

Ans. is 'B' 15–20 cm

11. In closed method of amputation which structure is kept shorter than the level of amputation: *(DNB 1992)*
    A. Bone
    B. Muscles
    C. Nerves
    D. Skin

Ans. is 'C' Nerves "Nerves are divided proximal to the bone".

12. Ring sequestrum is seen in: *(TN 1992)*
    A. Typhoid osteomyelitis
    B. Chronic osteomyelitis
    C. Amputation stump
    D. Tuberculosis osteomyelitis

Ans. is 'C' Amputation stump

REIMPLANTATION OF AMPUTATED DIGIT (GREENS) ORDER OF REPAIR OF STRUCTURES

1. Locate and tag vessels and nerves
2. Debride
3. Shorten and fix bone
4. Repair extensor tendon
5. Repair flexor tendon
6. Repair arteries
7. Repair nerves
8. Repair veins
9. Skin coverage.

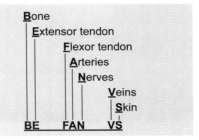

Note: Skin is preserved the first as there has to be an adequate soft tissue coverage over deeper structures and sensation of palmar skin cannot be reproduced by any skin graft.

MULTIPLE CHOICE QUESTION

1. In reconstruction of limb. What is done first? *(DNB 2017, AIIMS Nov 2010)*
   A. Bone fixation
   B. Artery anastomosis
   C. Nerve repair
   D. Vein repair

Ans. is 'A' Bone fixation
   – Remember 1st preserved is skin!

13 CHAPTER

Sports Injury

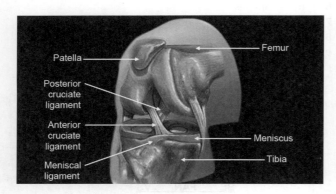

Fig. 13.1: Knee anatomy

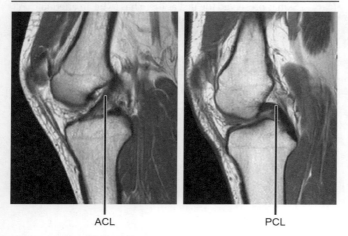

Fig. 13.2: MRI knee sagittal view

	ACL	PCL (stouter ligamentous structure)
1.	**It is intracapsular, extrasynovial**	**It is intracapsular, extrasynovial**
2.	It is major stabilizer of knee. Its mechanism is to stabilize internal rotation and extension of tibia on femur. Its function is multiple in that it limits forward gliding of tibia on femur and limits hyperextension. It makes a significant contribution to lateral stability and limits anterolateral rotation of tibia on femur. It is injured by occurrence of excessive movements which it limits.	It limits backward glide of tibia on femur (posterior translation) and checks hyperextension only after the ACL is ruptured. **PCL restricts External rotation as well.** Classically injured by high velocity trauma with posterior dislocation of tibia on a flexed knee as in a 'dash board impact' in a motor car. (Remember Dash Board Injury is posterior dislocation of hip also). Posterior cruciate ligament is active in all knee movements.
3.	**Anterior cruciate ligament (ACL) is most important for walking downhill.**	**Posterior cruciate ligament (PCL) is most important for walking downhill.**

	Anterior Cruciate Ligament:	Posterior Cruciate Ligament:

4.	• Lachman's test (most sensitive done at 20° knee flexion)
	• Anterior drawer test (done at 90° of knee flexion)
	• Pivot shift test flexion rotation drawer test (2nd best)
	• Test for ACL in decreasing order of sensitivity and specificity:
	  – Lachman's test > flexion rotation drawer test > anterior drawer test > pivot shift phenomenon tested by lateral pivot shift test of macintosh or jerk test of Hughston and loose.
	  – **Lelli test** (New test for ACL)
		• Posterior tibial sag
		• Posterior drawer test
		• Reverse pivot shift test
		• Quadriceps active test

5.	Treatment of ACL tear-Arthroscopic ACL reconstruction with hamstring graft (Remember ligaments are usually reconstructed not repaired).	Treatment is Arthroscopic reconstruction.

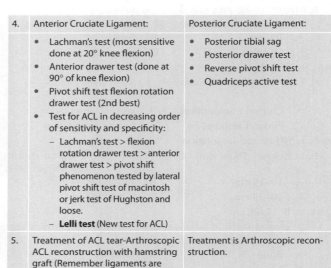

Fig. 13.3: Anterior drawer test

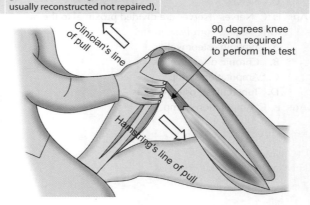

Fig. 13.4: Lachman's test

Lachman's test is the most sensitive test for anterior cruciate ligament tears. It is done with the knee, flexed at 20°. So, it can be done in acute as well as chronic injuries. (Because in acute cases with hemarthrosis more flexion is usually not possible so performing anterior drawer test is difficult as it is performed in 90° knee flexion).

Bounce Home Test: From flexed position knee is suddenly extended and than end point feel on extension is compared.

End point in Bounce Home Test normally has hard (bony) or firm (cartilage) feel. The rubbery feel indicates pathology (torn ACL or Menisci). Empty feel is not seen.

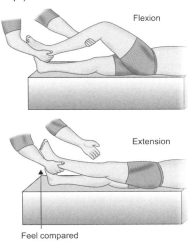

Fig. 13.5: Bounce home test of knee

Rotatory Instabilities of Knee

Anterolateral instability: ACL + LCL + Lateral half of joint capsule
1. Anterior drawer test with foot internally rotated 30°.
2. Pivot shift phenomenon.

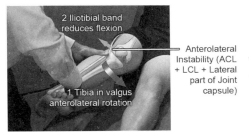

Fig. 13.6: Pivot shift test

Anteromedial rotatory instability: ACL + MCL + Medial knee capsule (posterior oblique ligament).

Test
- Anterior drawer test with foot externally rotated 15°.

Posterolateral Rotatory Instability
a. The Posterolateral Corner (PLC) is a complex that includes the lateral collateral ligament (LCL), popliteus tendon, fabellofibular ligament, arcuate ligament, popliteofibular ligament, and the short lateral ligament.

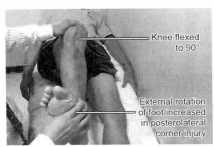

Fig. 13.7: DIAL test: Posterolateral corner injury

b. **Dial Test or Tibial External Rotation Test**
   - This is the test for **posterolateral instability**.
   - The tibia is externally rotated on femur first at 30° flexion and then at 90° flexion. Comparison is made with the normal side.
   - An increase in external rotation of greater than 10° indicates pathology.
   - Increase in external rotation at 30° of flexion but not at 90° indicates an isolated posterolateral corner injury and at both 30° and 90° of flexion indicates injury of both posterior cruciate ligament and posterolateral corner.
c. **Reverse Pivot Shift test.**

Snapping Knee Syndrome
Snapping of tendons at the posteromedial corner of the knee when knee goes into extension from flexion. Tendons of pes anserinus (Semitendinosus and Gracilis) are involved.

MULTIPLE CHOICE QUESTIONS

1. True about anterior cruciate ligament is/are: *(PGI May 2017)*
   A. Mostly occurs as a result of twisting force
   B. May occur secondary to tibial fracture
   C. Almost always associated with meniscal injury
   D. Lachman test is highly sensitive test for tear
   E. Immediate surgery needs to be done

   Ans. is 'A' Mostly occurs as a result of twisting force; 'B' May occur secondary to tibial fracture; 'C' Almost always associated with meniscal injury; & 'D' Lachman test is highly sensitive test for tear.

2. Test for anterior cruciate ligament is/are: *(PGI May 2017)*
   A. Lachman test
   B. Apley's grinding test
   C. Pivot shift test
   D. Anterior drawer
   E. KT-l000 knee arthrometer is an objective instrument for ACL reconstruction

   Ans. is 'A' Lachman test; 'C' Pivot shift test; 'D' Anterior drawer; 'E' KT-l000 knee arthrometer is an objective instrument for ACL reconstruction

   KT-1000 knee arthrometer is strapped to tibia and than with traction to tibia we can quantify the translation of tibia in millimeters.

3. Which of the following is incorrect about PCL? *(AIIMS Nov 2017)*
   A. It is the main restraint in posterior drawer test
   B. It is an extrasynovial structure
   C. It is the main restraint to internal rotation
   D. It originates from anterolateral aspect of medial femoral condyle in the area of intercondylar notch

   Ans. is 'C' It is the main restraint to internal rotation

4. A patient sustained a hyperextension injury to his knee. Which of the following ligament prevents excess movement of femur on tibia? *(JIPMER MAY 2016)*
   A. Anterior cruciate ligament
   B. Posterior cruciate ligament
   C. Medial collateral ligament
   D. Lateral collateral ligament

   Ans. is 'A' Anterior cruciate ligament

5. Not true about anterior cruciate ligament: *(NEET Dec 2016)*
   A. It begins just behind the anterior horn of lateral meniscus on tibia
   B. It is taut in extension
   C. It provides proprioceptive inputs to knee
   D. It is extra-synovial

   Ans. is 'A' It begins just behind the anterior horn of lateral meniscus on tibia

6. Which of the following is not true about ACL injury? *(NEET Dec 2016)*
   A. It is component of the O' Donoghue triad
   B. ACL is extra-synovial
   C. ACL is important for proprioceptive function
   D. Anterior drawer test is the most sensitive test

   Ans. is 'D' Anterior drawer test is the most sensitive test

7. Regarding Anterior Cruciate Ligament all are true except: *(PGI Nov 2016)*
   A. Lachman test is the most sensitive test for ACL tear
   B. Non contact pivoting injury causes ACL damage
   C. Posterolateral bundle becomes taut in flexion
   D. Almost always associated with meniscal tear
   E. Is pathognomonic of Segond's fracture

   Ans. is 'C' Posterolateral bundle becomes taut in flexion and 'D' Almost always associated with meniscal tear

8. In Complete ACL rupture the tibia moves over the femur in which direction: *(NEET 2016, CET July 16)*
   A. Forward
   B. Backward
   C. Lateral
   D. Medial

   Ans. is 'A' Forward

9. Muscle with intra-articular tendon? *(JIPMER May 2016)*
   A. Popliteus
   B. Semimembranosus
   C. Sartorius
   D. Triceps

   Ans. is 'A' Popliteus

10. All of the following are true about ACL except:
    A. Prevents anterior motion of femur over tibia *(CET Nov 15)*
    B. Prevents anterior motion of tibia over femur
    C. Also provides secondary varus-valgus stability
    D. Is taught in extension of knee

    Ans. is 'A' Prevents anterior motion of femur over tibia

11. Snapping knee syndrome is due to involvement of: *(AI Dec 15)*
    A. Pes Anserinus
    B. Quadriceps Tendon
    C. Gastrocnemius origin
    D. Lateral collateral ligament

    Ans. is 'A' Pes Anserinus

12. Posterior gliding of tibia on femur is prevented by:
    A. Anterior cruciate ligament *(NEET 2015)*
    B. Posterior cruciate ligament
    C. Medial collateral ligament
    D. Lateral collateral ligament

    Ans. is 'B' Posterior cruciate ligament

13. Lachman's test is used for: *(NEET 2015)*
    A. ACL injury
    B. PCL injury
    C. MCL injury
    D. LCL injury

    Ans. is 'A' ACL injury

14. Which of the following is the SAFEST test to be performed in a patient with acutely injured knee joint? *(NEET Pattern 2013; AI 08, 01)*
    A. Lachman's test
    B. Pivot shift test
    C. McMurray's test
    D. Apley's grinding test

    Ans. is 'A' Lachman's test

15. Lateral blow to knee with fracture in intercondylar area structured injured is: *(AIIMS Nov 2012)*
    A. MCL
    B. ACL
    C. LCL
    D. Menisci

    Ans. is 'B' ACL

    Explanation
    Mechanism of injury
    1. Valgus force MCL
    2. Varus force LCL
    3. Backward force PCL
    4. Twisting injury (medial and lateral) meniscus
    5. Anterior ACL
    6. Combination of Valgus in Flexion with twist injures the structure in following order. MCL than ACL, and last menisci.
    - Abduction or valgus force at flexed knee with rotational component is most common mechanism causing ligament injury at knee and if all forces are combined ACL is most commonly injured and if there is only rotational component than it causes menisci injury medial meniscus >lateral meniscus.
    - Thus rotation with valgus causes ACL injury
    - In this question there is a point given—fracture at intercondylar which is the site of insertion of ACL.
    - Hence ACL is the answer.

16. Injury from lateral side of knee causes damage to:
    A. MCL
    B. LCL *(NEET Pattern 2012)*
    C. ACL
    D. PCL

    Ans. is 'A' MCL

17. Anterior drawer test is for: *(NEET Pattern 2012)*
    A. ACL
    B. PCL
    C. Medial meniscus
    D. Lateral meniscus

    Ans. is 'A' ACL

18. A patient met with Road Traffic Accident and developed knee pain. DIAL test was positive. Structure injured is: *(AIIMS May 2012/Nov 2010)*
    A. Medial collateral ligament injury
    B. Medial meniscal injury
    C. Lateral meniscus tear
    D. Posterolateral corner injury

    Ans. is 'D' Posterolateral corner injury

19. In 'bounce home' test of knee 'end feels' are interference. All are 'end feels' except: *(AIIMS May 2011)*
    A. Firm
    B. Sponge block
    C. Empty
    D. Bony

    Ans. is 'C' Empty

20. Posterior cruciate ligament—true statement is:
    A. Attached to the lateral femoral condyle
    B. Intrasynovial *(All India 2007, AIIMS Nov 2006)*
    C. Prevents posterior dislocation of tibia
    D. Relaxed in full flexion

    Ans. is 'C' Prevents posterior displacement of tibia
    PCL prevents posterior gliding (subluxation) of tibia over femur.

21. Which one of the following tests will you adopt while examining a knee joint where you suspect an old tear of anterior cruciate ligament?
    (AI 2003, AIIMS May 02, PGI June 02, Rajasthan 92, Delhi 88)
    (JIPMER 2002)
    A. Posterior drawer test   B. McMurray's test
    C. Lachman's test   D. Pivot shift test
Ans. is 'C' Lachman's test is the *most sensitive test for anterior cruciate ligament tears (acute or chronic both).*

22. Which activity will be difficult to perform for a patient with an anterior cruciate deficient knee joint?
    (AIIMS May 2002)
    A. Walk downhill
    B. Walk uphill
    C. Sit cross leg
    D. Getting up from sitting
Ans. is 'A' Walk downhill

23. Positive pivot shift test in knee is because of injury to:
    A. Anterior cruciate ligament   (AIIMS June 2000)
    B. Posterior cruciate ligament
    C. Medial meniscus
    D. Lateral meniscus
Ans. is 'A' Anterior cruciate ligament

COLLATERAL LIGAMENT INJURY

- The **most common mechanism of ligament disruption of knee is abduction (valgus), flexion and internal rotation of femur** on tibia which usually occur in sports in which the foot is planted solidly on the ground and leg is twisted by rotating body.
- The medial structures medial (tibial) collateral ligament (MCL) and medial capsular ligament are first to fail, followed by ACL tear, if the force is of sufficient magnitude. The medial meniscus may be trapped between condyles and have a peripheral tear, thus producing unhappy triad of O'Donoghue.

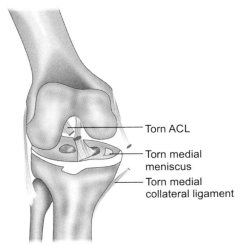

Fig. 13.8: O'Donoghue triad

- Main test for MCL (medial collateral ligament) is valgus (abduction) stress in 30° of knee flexion. (Because in full extension it is indicative of combined MCL, posterior oblique ligament injury and posterior cruciate ligament injury).

- Varus (Adduction) stress test in 30° flexion (removes the lateral stabilizing effect of iliotibial band so that the lateral collateral ligament can exclusively be examined).
- Apley's distraction test is used for **collateral** ligaments.

Mechanism of Injury

1.	Valgus force	MCL
2.	Varus force	LCL
3.	Backward force	PCL
4.	Twisting injury	(Medial and lateral) Meniscus
5.	Anterior	ACL
6.	Combination of Valgus in Flexion with twist injures the structure in following order MCL than ACL and last menisci.	

Examination

Direction of force	Position of knee	Ligament tested
Varus/Valgus	Full extension	PCL, Posterior capsule
Varus	30° flexion	LCL
Valgus	30° flexion	MCL
Posterior	90° flexion	PCL
Anterior	20° flexion (Lachman's test)	ACL
	90° flexion (anterior drawer)	ACL

Treatment of collateral ligaments is repair/reconstruction

MULTIPLE CHOICE QUESTIONS

1. A patient sustained injury to his knee with a twisting force. On examination pain is felt more on medial femoral side of knee than tibial side. Injured structure might be?
   A. Anterior cruciate ligament   (JIPMER May 2016)
   B. Posterior cruciate ligament
   C. Medial collateral ligament
   D. Lateral collateral ligament
Ans. is 'C' Medial collateral ligament

2. Which among the following is not a feature of Unhappy triad of O' Donoghue?   (NEET 2015)
   A. ACL injury
   B. Medial meniscus injury
   C. Medial collateral ligament injury
   D. Fibular collateral ligament injury
Ans. is 'D' Fibular collateral ligament injury

3. O'Donoghue triad   (PGI Nov 2015)
   A. Medical Collateral Ligament
   B. Lateral Collateral Ligament
   C. Anterior Cruciate Ligament
   D. Medial Meniscus
   E. Posterior Cruciate Ligament
Ans. is 'A' Medical Collateral Ligament; 'C' Anterior Cruciate Ligament and 'D' Medial Meniscus

4. Structural integrity of collateral ligaments are tested by:
   (MAHE 04, JIPMER 02)
   A. Varus/valgus stress test in full flexion
   B. Varus/valgus stress test in full extension
   C. Varus/valgus stress test in 30° of flexion
   D. Varus/valgus stress test in 90° of flexion
Ans. is 'C' Varus/valgus stress test in 30° of flexion

5. A twisting injury of knee in flexed position would result in injury to all except: (AIIMS May 2002)
   A. Meniscal tear
   B. Capsular tear
   C. Anterior cruciate ligament
   D. Fibular collateral ligament

Ans. is 'D' Fibular collateral ligament
   – The most common mechanism of ligament disruption of knee is *abduction (valgus) flexion and internal rotation of femur on tibia* which usually occur in sports in which the foot is planted solidly on the ground and leg is twisted by rotating body (i.e. football, soccer, basket ball, skiing).
   – The medial structures **medial (tibial) collateral ligament (MCL) and medial capsular ligament** are first to fail, followed by **ACL tears**, if the force is of sufficient magnitude. The medial meniscus may be trapped between condyles and have a peripheral tear, thus producing **unhappy triad of O' Donoghue**.

6. Torsion of knee results in injury most commonly to: (AIIMS May 2002)
   A. Anterior cruciate ligament
   B. Medial meniscus
   C. Fibular collateral ligament
   D. Tibial collateral ligament

Ans. is 'B' Medial meniscus

MENISCAL INJURY

Biochemically human meniscal tissue consists of 70% collagen. Type I collagen predominates making up about 90% of total collagen.

Predominant collage in menisci/fibrocartilage—Type I collagen

Predominant collagen in articular/hyaline cartilage—Type II collagen.

Physiological locking	Pathological locking
Physiological locking occurs in last 30° of extension when femur rotates medially (internally) over stabilized tibia. This is caused by quadriceps femoris muscle.	Pathology of knee joint can cause locking of the knee, i.e. the knee is locked in partial flexion and there is inability to extend the knee for the last few degrees. This is frequently known as locking of the knee joint.
Unlocking needed to initiate flexion is carried out by popliteus muscle, which moves femur laterally on stabilized tibia.	Causes of locking are: • Meniscal tear • Loose body in the knee • Osteochondral fracture • Osteophytes fracture in osteoarthritis • Fractures tibial spine

Note: If knee is extended from flexed position tibial tuberosity moves toward lateral border of patella. Knee extension from flexion with foot off the ground is called as open chain movement and there occurs external rotation of tibia hence tibial tuberosity moves toward lateral border of patella. This is modified Helfet test. Knee extension from flexion with foot on the ground is called as closed chain movement and there occurs internal rotation of femur causing center of patella to move medially hence tibial tuberosity moves toward lateral border of patella. This may be blocked with meniscal injury.

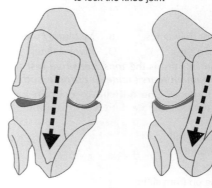

Fig. 13.9: Helfet test

Q angle provides a lateral vector to patella and is line between Quadriceps and Patellar tendon. Increase in Q angle predisposes patella to lateral overload and makes it prone to subluxate or dislocate laterally. It is best measured in 30° of knee flexion to center patella in trochlea. Its value is more in females (about 15°) than males (8–10°). Vastus medialis balances this lateral vector especially vastus medialis obliquus.

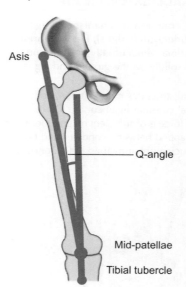

Fig. 13.10: Q-angle

Recurrent dislocation Patella predisposing factors are:
1. Hyperlaxity
2. Genu Valgum
3. External tibial torsion
4. Patella too high or too low
5. Under developed lateral femoral Condyle
6. Weak medial ligaments/structures.

The patella dislocates almost always laterally.

The twisting force (rotation) in a weight bearing flexed knee is the commonest mode of meniscal (semilunar cartilage) injury.

Medial meniscus is more frequently torn than the lateral

Medial meniscus	Lateral meniscus
Semilunar in shape (less circular).	Semicircular in shape (C shaped; more circular).
Larger in diameter but narrower in body.	Smaller in diameter but wider in body.
Anterior horn is small while posterior horn is large covers less tibial articular surface than lateral (covers about 65% of tibial articular surface).	Anterior horn and posterior horn are uniform in size (covers about 85% of tibial articular surface).
Entire periphery of the meniscus is attached to the joint capsule.	Entire periphery of meniscus is not attached to joint capsule (area where the popliteus tendon crosses the joint through the popliteus hiatus is not attached).
Is attached to the medial collateral ligament.	Is not attached to the lateral collateral ligament.
Less mobile (due to firmer attachment with joint capsule and medial collateral ligament).	More mobile (due to gaps in attachment with joint capsule and lateral collateral ligament).
More prone to injury (due to reduced mobility). The medial meniscus is three to four times more prone to injury than the lateral meniscus.	Less prone to injury (due to increased mobility).

Note: Popliteus muscle sends few fibers into the posterior margin of lateral meniscus. Thus muscle contraction withdraws and protects the lateral meniscus by drawing it posterolaterally during flexion of the knee and medial rotation of the tibia I.

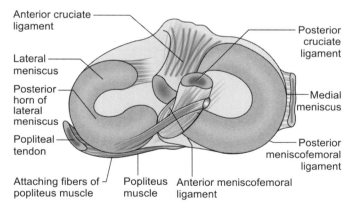

Fig. 13.11: Knee

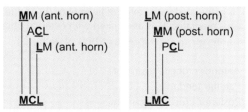

Order of Structures (anterior to posterior) on Tibia upper Surface (MCL—Medical College Lucknow; LMC—Lucknow Medical College)

MM—Medial Meniscus
LM—Lateral Meniscus
ACL—Anterior Cruciate Ligament
PCL—Posterior Cruciate Ligament

Injury to Meniscus

The commonest type of medial meniscal injury in a young adult is the bucket handle tear. **This is vertical longitudinal tear that is complete.**

Smillie Classification—Meniscus Injury

Meniscal injury	Cruciate injury/collateral ligament
1. Effusion	Hemarthrosis
2. Delayed swelling	Immediate swelling

- Symptoms include joint line pain, catching, popping and locking, usually and weakness and giving way (instability) sometimes. Deep squatting and duck walking are usually painful.
    1. McMurray's test is positive
    2. Apley's grinding test is positive
    3. Difficult to perform full squatting and Toe walk in squatting position (Payr's sign)
    4. Steinmann tenderness test
    5. Thessaly test
    6. Ege's test (weight bearing McMurray test)

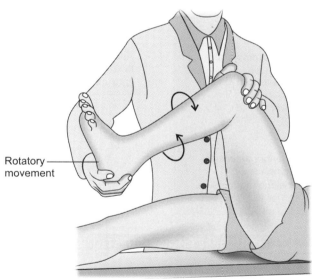

Fig. 13.12: McMurray's test—menisci

Meniscal Injury

- At birth entire meniscus is vascular, decrease in vascularity continues up to age 9 years, when the meniscus closely resembles the adult meniscus. In adults, only 10–25% of lateral meniscus and 10–30% of medial meniscus is vascular.
    – Red (Vascular) periphery of menisci
    – Red – White (border of vascular and avascular area)
    – White (avascular area) inner 2/3rd of menisci

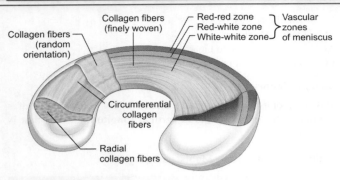

Fig. 13.13: Zones of meniscus

- Because of the avascular nature of inner two-thirds of the meniscus; cell nutrition is believed to occur mainly through diffusion or mechanical pumping. Inner avascular meniscus once torn does not heal and requires removal of torn part.
- Tears in the peripheral third of the meniscus, if small (<15 mm), may heal spontaneously because this portion in adults has good blood supply. Larger tears require repair.
- Arthroscopy is the gold standard for making diagnosis and arthroscopic repair or removal is the treatment of choice.

1. Meniscal cysts—Lateral > Medial and Pirani Sign—Cysts disappear within joint on flexion.
2. Discoid Meniscus—Lateral > Medial.

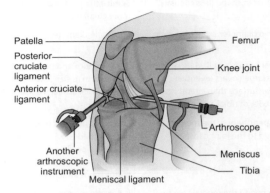

Fig. 13.14: Arthroscopy gold standard for diagnosis and management of most knee injuries

Note: Celery stalk appearance is seen in degenerated ACL and congenital Rubella.

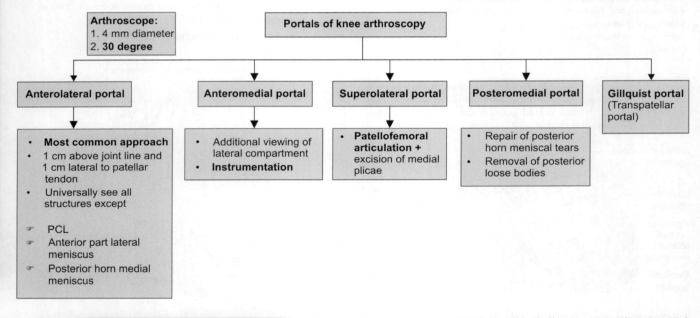

MULTIPLE CHOICE QUESTIONS

1. Patellar dislocation factors: *(PGI Nov 2017)*
   A. Genu varum
   B. Loose quadriceps femoris
   C. Ligamental laxity
   D. Femoral torsion with anteversion
   E. Lateral femoral condyle is shallow and hypoplastic

   Ans. is 'B' Loose quadriceps femoris; 'C' Ligamental laxity; 'D' Femoral torsion with anteversion; & 'E' Lateral femoral condyle is shallow and hypoplastic

2. About recurrent dislocation of patella, Choose the correct statement: *(PGI Nov 2017)*
   A. Is associated with Genu Varum
   B. Is associated with Laxity of ligaments
   C. Common in persons with Shallow/underdeveloped medial condyle
   D. Is due to defect of vastus medialis
   E. Is associated with external tibial torsion

   Ans. is 'B' Is associated with Laxity of ligaments; 'D' Is due to defect of vastus medialis; 'E' Is associated with external tibial torsion

3. Most anterior to interspinous tibial plateau is: *(PGI May 2017)*
   A. Anterior cruciate ligament
   B. Patellar tendon
   C. Posterior cruciate ligament
   D. Medial meniscus
   E. Lateral meniscus

   Ans. is 'D' Medial meniscus

4. Increased Q angle predisposes to: (NEET Dec 2016)
   A. Medial patellar subluxation
   B. Lateral patellar subluxation
   C. Superior patellar subluxation
   D. Interior patellar subluxation

Ans. is 'B' Lateral patellar subluxation

5. Jumpers knee: (NEET Dec 2016)
   A. Apophysitis of patellar tendon as it inserts in patella
   B. Apophysitis of patellar tendon as it inserts in tibia
   C. Apophysitis of quadriceps tendon as it inserts in patella
   D. Apophysitis of hamstring tendon as it inserts in tibia

Ans. is 'A' Apophysitis of patellar tendon as it inserts in patella

Jumper knee (Patellar tendonitis) is seen due to inflammation of patellar tendon as it inserts into patella.

Treatment is physiotherapy.

6. Following are the tests done for medial meniscal tear: (PGI May 2016)
   A. McMurray's test   B. Lachman test
   C. Apley's grinding test D. Ege's test
   E. Pivot shift test

Ans. is 'A' McMurray's test; 'C' Apley's grinding test; 'D' Ege's test

7. A young boy presents with swollen knee, on getting hit over lateral aspect of knee and there was a twist while playing. Joint line tenderness was present. Anterior Drawer test done was negative. X-ray shows no fracture. Which structure is most likely to be damaged in the person: (JIPMER Nov 16)
   A. ACL   B. Medial Meniscus
   C. PCL   D. Lateral Meniscus

Ans. is 'B' Medial Meniscus

Joint line tenderness goes towards medial meniscus.

Note: Some students remember a different version of the same question as Q. No 3.

8. A young boy presents with swollen knee, on getting hit over lateral aspect of knee. Anterior Drawer test done was negative. X-ray shows no fracture. Which structure is most likely to be damaged in the person: (JIPMER Nov 16)
   A. ACL   B. MM
   C. MCL   D. LM

Ans. is 'C' MCL

9. Which of the following structure are not normally visualized during the arthroscopy of the knee? (NEET 2015)
   A. Meniscus   B. Cruciate ligaments
   C. Collateral ligaments D. Patella articular surface

Ans. is 'C' Collateral ligaments

10. Anterolateral arthroscopy of knee is for:
    A. To see patellofemoral articulation (NEET Pattern 2013)
    B. To see the posterior cruciate ligament
    C. To see the anterior portion of lateral meniscus
    D. To see the periphery of the posterior horn of medial meniscus

Ans. is 'A' To see patellofemoral articulation

Explanation

Standard portals in knee arthroscopy
1. Anterolateral portal
   - Almost all the structures within the knee joint can be seen except the posterior cruciate ligament, the anterior portion of the lateral meniscus, and the periphery of the posterior horn of the medial meniscus in tight knees.
   - Located 1 cm above the joint line, 1 cm lateral to the margin of the patellar tendon.
2. Anteromedial portal
   - Used for additional viewing of lateral compartment and insertion of probe for palpation of medial and lateral compartment structures.
   - Placed 1 cm above the medial joint line, 1 cm inferior to the tip of patella, and 1 cm medial to the edge of the patella.
3. Posteromedial portal
   - Located on the soft triangular soft spot formed by the posteromedial edge of the femoral condyle and the posteromedial edge of tibia.
   - Used for viewing the posteromedial structures and for repair or removal of the displaced posterior horn of meniscal tears and for posteromedial loose body removal.
4. Superolateral portal.
   - Used for diagnostically viewing the dynamics of patella-femoral joint, excision of medial plica.
   - Located just lateral to the quadriceps tendon and about 2.5 cm superior to the superolateral corner of patella.

11. Patient presents with knee problem. He gives history of injury during playing hockey 3 months back. On testing knee was unstable anteriorly in extension but was stable in 90 degrees of flexion. Probably injury involves:
    A. ACL anteromedial fiber (AIIMS May 2013)
    B. ACL posterolateral fiber
    C. PCL
    D. Anterior portion of medial meniscus

Ans. is 'B' ACL posterolateral fiber

Explanation
- The ACL ligament is the primary restraint to anterior tibial displacement, accounting for approximately 85% of the resistance to the anterior drawer test when the knee is at 90° of flexion and neutral rotation. Selective sectioning of the ACL has shown that the anteromedial band is tight in flexion, providing the primary restraint, whereas the posterolateral bulky portion of this ligament is tight in extension. The posterolateral bundle provides the principal resistance for hyperextension.
- Thus complete tear will have instability in both flexion and extension.
- Thus anteromedial tear will have instability in flexion only and posterolateral tear will have instability only in extension.

12. All are true about menisci of knee joint except: (NEET Pattern 2013)
    A. Lateral meniscus covers more articular surface of tibia
    B. Lateral meniscus is more mobile
    C. Lateral meniscus is more prone to injury
    D. Lateral meniscus is semicircular

Ans. is 'C' Lateral meniscus is more prone to injury

13. Unlocking of knee is caused by: (NEET Pattern 2013)
    A. Rectus femoris   B. Quadriceps
    C. Hamstrings   D. Popliteus

Ans. is 'D' Popliteus

14. Menisci to tibia connection is: (AIIMS Nov 2012)
    A. Coronary ligaments   B. Wrisberg ligaments
    C. Arcuate ligaments   D. Oblique ligaments
Ans. is 'A' Coronary ligaments
    Explanation
    - The coronary ligaments of the knee (also known as meniscotibial ligaments) are portions of the joint capsule which connect the inferior edges of the fibrocartilaginous menisci to the periphery of the tibial plateaus.

15. Q angle is used for: (NEET Pattern 2012)
    A. Knee   B. Hip
    C. Elbow   D. Wrist
Ans. is 'A' Knee

16. Locking of knee can be due to: (NEET Pattern 2012)
    A. Menisci   B. Loose body
    C. Both   D. None
Ans. is 'C' Both

17. An athlete is sitting on the edge of table with knees flexed at 90 degree. When he extends his knee fully, what will happen to the tibial tuberosity in relation to patella:
    A. No change (AIIMS May 10)
    B. Movement of TT towards medial border of patella
    C. Movement of TT towards lateral border of patella
    D. Movement of TT towards center of patella
Ans. is 'C' Movement of TT towards lateral border of patella

18. Which of the following statements about 'Menisci' is not true: (AI 2010, Manipal 1994)
    A. Medial meniscus is more mobile than lateral
    B. Lateral meniscus covers more tibial articular surface than lateral
    C. Medial meniscus is more commonly injured than lateral
    D. Menisci are predominantly **made up of Type I Collagen**
Ans. is 'A' Medial meniscus is more mobile than lateral
    - Medial meniscus is less mobile, more prone to injury and covers less area of the tibia! articular surface in comparison to the lateral meniscus.

19. It is wise to keep and repair the meniscus rather than removing it when the injury is to which of the following?
    A. Medial part of meniscus (AI 08)
    B. Mid part of meniscus
    C. Peripheral part of meniscus
    D. Associated with collateral ligament injury
Ans. is 'C' Peripheral part of meniscus
    - Meniscal Repair is recommended for tears in the Red zone and the Red white zone (Periphery). Meniscal Repair is not recommended for tears in the white zone (Inner zone).
    - Tear of the inner zone are treated with arthroscopic excision.

20. Physiological locking involves: (AI 08)
    A. Internal rotation of femur over stabilized tibia
    B. Internal rotation of tibia over stabilized femur
    C. External rotation of tibia over stabilized femur
    D. External rotation of femur over stabilized tibia
Ans. is 'A' Internal rotation of femur over stabilized tibia

21. Locking of knee joint can be caused by: (PGI Dec 2005)
    A. Osgood-Schlatter   B. Loose body in knee joint
    C. Tuberculosis of knee   D. Medial meniscal partial tear
Ans. is 'B' Loose body in knee joint and 'D' Medial meniscal partial tear

22. Medial meniscus of knee joint is injured more often than the lateral meniscus because the medial meniscus is relatively: (AIIMS Nov 2002)
    A. More mobile   B. Less mobile
    C. Thinner   D. Attached lightly to femur
Ans. is 'B' Less mobile

23. McMurray's test is positive in injury of:
    A. Anterior cruciate ligament (PGI June 02, UPSC 88)
    B. Posterior cruciate ligament
    C. Medial meniscus injury
    D. Lateral meniscus injury
    E. Popliteal bursitis
Ans. is 'C'>'D' Medial meniscus injury > Lateral meniscus injury

24. An 18-year-old boy was playing football, when he suddenly twisted his knee on the ankle and he fell down. He got up after 10 minutes and again started playing, but next day his knee was swollen and he could not move it. The most probable cause is: (AIIMS May 2001)
    A. Medial meniscus tear
    B. Anterior cruciate ligament tear
    C. Medial collateral ligament injury
    D. Posterior cruciate ligament injury
Ans. is 'A' Medial meniscus tear
    - This boy has:
        i. History of twisting injury to the knee
        ii. Swelling appearing next day due to effusion
    - This is classical to the medial meniscal injury.
    In ACL injury swelling appears immediately due to hemarthrosis.

25. Athlete sustained an injury around the knee joint suspecting cartilage damage, which of the following is an investigation of choice? (Andhra 2000, AIIMS 94)
    A. Pain X-ray   B. Clinical examination
    C. Arthroscopy   D. Arthrotomy
Ans. is 'C' Arthroscopy is investigation of choice for damage to the structures of knee.

26. Which type of injury causes more damage to the semilunar cartilage in the Knee: (Andhra 1999, AI 1996)
    A. Flexion arid extension at the ankle
    B. Rotation on a flexed knee
    C. Rotation on an extended knee
    D. Squatting position
Ans. is 'B' Rotation on a flexed knee

27. Commonest dangerous complication of posterior dislocation of knee is: (AIIMS Nov 99)
    A. Popliteal artery injury
    B. Sciatic nerve injury
    C. Ischemia of lower leg compartment
    D. Femoral artery injury
Ans. is 'A' Popliteal artery injury

28. A patient gives a history of twisting strain and locking of the knee joint, the most likely diagnosis is: (PGI 97, AI 93)
    A. Avulsion of tibial tubercle
    B. Meniscal tear
    C. Tearing of lateral collateral ligament
    D. Tear of anterior cruciate ligament
Ans. is 'B' Meniscal tear
    - There is classical history of twisting injury and locking so diagnosis is meniscal injury.

29. Which is the investigation of choice for a sport injury of the knee? *(Andhra 93, TN 97)*
    A. Ultrasonography   B. Plain radiography
    C. Arthrography   D. Arthroscopy

Ans. is 'D' Arthroscopy
- The usual protocol for sports injury in a suspected case is to diagnose the injury by MRI and if diagnosis is in doubt than arthroscopy can confirm the lesion.

30. Bucket handle tear at knee joint is due to: *(Orissa 1991)*
    A. Injury to medial collateral ligament
    B. Injury to lateral collateral ligament
    C. Injury to ligamentum patellae
    D. Injury to menisci

Ans. is 'D' Injury to menisci
- The commonest type of medial meniscal injury in a young adult is the bucket handle tear. This is vertical longitudinal tear of medial menisci that is complete.

ATHLETIC PUBALGIA

Athletic pubalgia refers to chronic pain in the inguinal or pubic region in athletes that is noted primarily on exertion. It is also called as Sportman's Hernia or Gilmore's Groin.

Pathology

The primary site of pathology is the **insertion of rectus abdominis on the pubis**. Abdominal component is believed to be the initial injury in athletic pubalgia that in turn causes subtle pelvic instability/anterior pelvic tilt which predisposes to injury to proximal adductors. The conjoint tendon insertion and the adductor longus insertion on the pubis may also be involved.

Clinical Presentation

Pain in inguinal/pubic region following exercise
Tenderness at the pubic tubercle (Adductor insertion tenderness).

Management

Primary management is conservative (Rest, Ice, Anti-inflammatory medications, etc).
Surgery is indicated if conservative therapy fails. Nesovic's operation (bilateral) is reserved for resistant cases.

MULTIPLE CHOICE QUESTION

1. The primary pathology in Athletic Pubalgia is: *(AI 2009)*
   A. Abdominal muscle strain   B. Rectus femoris strain
   C. Gluteus medius strain   D. Hamstring strain

Ans. is 'A' Abdominal muscle strain

ANKLE LIGAMENT INJURY

Ankle ligamentous injuries, as classified by O'Donoghue, occur as minor ligamentous "stretch" injuries (type I sprain), incomplete ligamentous tears (type II sprain), or complete disruption of the ligament or ligaments (type III sprain).
- The most common site of ligament injury is ankle joint.
- The most common mode of ankle injury is **inversion of plantar flexed foot.**
- Over 90% of the ankle ligament injury involves lateral collateral ligament usually the **anterior talofibular ligament.**

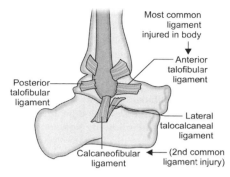

Fig. 13.15: Ligaments around ankle

Sprains are treated initially with
- **Protection**—use crutches to aid walking and minimize further tissue damage.
- **Rest**—to minimize further tissue damage and facilitate healing.
- **Ice**—to reduce swelling and provide pain relief.
- **Compression**—to reduce swelling.
- **Elevation**—to reduce swelling.

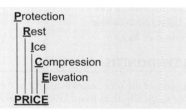

Deltoid Ligament Injury—pain around medial malleolus but normal X-rays

It has the tibial attachment and the other expansions into the following structure:
- Talus
- Navicular
- Calcaneum
- Spring ligament
- The most common mechanism of injury is **supination external rotation** or pronation external rotation

MULTIPLE CHOICE QUESTIONS

1. Sudden inversion of foot leads to rupture of which tendon? *(NEET Dec 2016)*
   A. Deltoid ligament
   B. Anterior talofibular ligament
   C. Posterior talofibular ligament
   D. Spring ligament

Ans. is 'B' Anterior talofibular ligament

2. A 23-year-old profession footballer suffered a twisting injury to his right ankle. On examination there is a lot of swelling around the medial malleolus but X-ray doesn't show any fracture. The structure injured could be:
   A. Deltoid ligament   *(CET July 16)*
   B. Anterior talofibular ligament
   C. Spring ligament
   D. Tendo Achilles

Ans. is 'A' Deltoid ligament

3. Commonest ligament injured in ankle injury:
   (NEET Pattern 2015, 2013, 2012, AI 1998)
   A. Anterior talofibular ligament
   B. Calcaneofibular ligament
   C. Posterior talofibular ligament
   D. Spring ligament

Ans. is 'A' Anterior talofibular ligament

4. When the foot is in plantar flexed position if it is suddenly inverted which of the following ligament will be injured?
   (AIIMS Nov 2012, NEET 2012)
   A. Anterior talofibular   B. Post-tibiofibular
   D. Calcaneocuboid   D. Calcaneofibular

Ans. is 'A' Anterior talofibular

5. The most common site for ligamentous injuries are those of the: (Andhra 1999)
   A. Shoulder joint   B. Elbow
   C. Knee joint   D. Ankle joint

Ans. is 'D' Ankle joint

6. Injury around the ankle joint occur due to: (Bihar 1999)
   A. Inversion of foot
   B. Eversion of foot
   C. Internal rotation of foot
   D. External rotation of foot

Ans. is 'A' Inversion of foot

ACHILLES TENDONITIS

No tendon disorders of the foot or ankle are more frustrating to treat, conservatively or surgically, than those involving the Achilles tendon.

Vascularity is supplied to the tendon through the paratenon on the deep surface of the tendon, there are arterial branches within the gastrocnemius-soleus complex proximally, and small interosseous vessels at the insertion of the tendon distally. There is a zone of **relative avascularity 2–6 cm proximal to its insertion into the calcaneus (Watershed for circulation)**. The vascular arrangement for the Achilles tendon is satisfactory for the low demand of the tendon sites in normal conditions. However, increased demand from excessive use or overuse may lead to inadequate vascular supply and subsequent degeneration and fibrosis of the involved segment of tendon.

a. **Insertional tendonitis**
   – Involves insertion site
   – May be associated with retrocalcaneal bursitis, and large exostosis on posterosuperior aspect of calcaneal tuberosity called as Haglund deformity or pump bump.
   – Overuse is the cause.

b. **Noninsertional tendenitis** with or without peritendinitis (**more common** than insertional tendonitis)
   – Involves water shed area of circulation (**2–6 cm above the insertion**)
   – **Seen in** runners and jumpers
   – It is also the **commonest site of TA rupture.**

MULTIPLE CHOICE QUESTION

1. Most common cause of noninsertional tendonitis of tendoachilles is: (AIIMS Nov 08)
   A. Overuse   B. Improper shoe wear
   C. Runners and jumpers   D. Steroid injections

Ans. is 'C' Runners and jumpers

TENDON RUPTURE

Tendon ruptures are more common in middle-aged and elderly patients. Intrinsic weakness of the tendon as a result of repetitive microtrauma and incomplete healing in watershed areas of vascularity predispose to tendon rupture in some more commonly ruptured tendons, including the **supraspinatus, biceps**, and **Achilles** tendons.

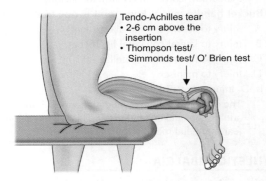

Fig. 13.16: Tendo-Achilles tear

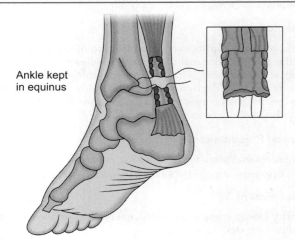

Fig. 13.17: TA repair

- Most frequent cause of partial or complete rupture of a muscle or tendon is eccentric overload of the muscle tendon unit. One factor contributing to muscle overload is fatigue in runners and jumpers.
- Strains most commonly occur in muscles that cross two joints, muscles that have higher percentage of type II fast twitch muscle fibers, and weaker muscle of an agonist antagonist muscle group, e.g. hamstring, gastrocnemius and rectus femoris.
- Achilles tendon rupture commonly occurs to otherwise healthy men between the ages of 30 and 50 years who have no previous injury or problem reported in affected leg; typically "weekend warriors" who are active intermittently.

Most TA tears occurs in left leg in the substance of TA, 2–6 cm above the calcaneal insertion (watershed zone).

The most common mechanism of injury include sudden forced plantar flexion of foot, unexpected dorsiflexion of foot and violent dorsiflexion of plantar flexed foot. Other mechanism include direct trauma and less commonly, attrition of the tendon as a result of long standing Noninsertional tendonitis with or without peritendinitis that body is unable to repair. Test for TA rupture – **Thompson test/ Simmonds test/O'Brien needle test.**

Treatment

In several comparison studies of operative and nonoperative treatment, overall results have been shown to be similar, but with a much higher rate of reruptures after nonoperative treatment.

Tendo-Achilles repair with reinforcement from tendons most commonly Plantaris and Flexor Hallucis Longus can be done.

MULTIPLE CHOICE QUESTIONS

1. High crural index is seen in: *(DNB JUNE 2017)*
   A. Jumping athletes
   B. Gymnasts
   C. Weight lifters
   D. Long distance runners

   Ans. is 'A' Jumping athletes
   Crural Index = Leg Length/Thigh Length
   High Index in Long Jumpers

2. Sudden dorsiflexion of foot may lead to which of the following injuries: *(AI Dec 15)*
   A. Anterior talofibular ligament injury
   B. Tendo-Achilles avulsion injury
   C. Rupture of deltoid ligament
   D. Tarsal tunnel syndrome

   Ans. is 'B' Tendo-Achilles avulsion injury

3. All are the common sites of tendon rupture except:
   A. Supraspinatus Tendon *(Maharashtra PG 2016)*
   B. Long head of biceps brachii
   C. Achilles tendon
   D. Extensor Hallucis longus tendon

   Ans. is 'D' Extensor Hallucis longus tendon

4. Ruptured tendon is most commonly seen in: *(AI 2000)*
   A. Stab injury
   B. Soft tissue tumor
   C. Athletes
   D. Congenital defect

   Ans. is 'C' Athletes

HAMMER TOE

It is plantar **flexion deformity of proximal interphalangeal joint** frequently associated with hyperextension of metatarsophalangeal joint.

GAME KEEPER'S/SKIER'S THUMB

Injury to the thumb metacarpophalangeal joint **ulnar collateral ligament**, commonly referred to as *gamekeeper thumb* or *skier's thumb*, is **most common injury of 1st MCP joint**. Snow skiing accidents and falls on an outstretched hand with forceful radial and palmar abduction of the thumb are the usual causes. Patients commonly report pain, swelling and ecchymosis around the metacarpophalangeal joint. Tenderness is greatest over the ulnar aspect of the joint, but is not localized. Differentiating between an incomplete and complete rupture of the ulnar collateral ligament is necessary because incomplete ruptures are treated nonoperatively, and complete ruptures require surgery. Stener described the anatomical pathology, he found the adductor aponeurosis interposed between the ruptured ulnar collateral ligament and its site of insertion on the base of the proximal phalanx. (Steners lesion) On clinical examination, a prominent lump can be palpated, which represents the ulnar collateral ligament being displaced by the adductor aponeurosis. Pathological rotation of the thumb also may be evident. If left uncorrected, this lesion prevents proper healing and leads to chronic instability and subsequent arthrosis.

MRI can distinguish complete from incomplete tears.

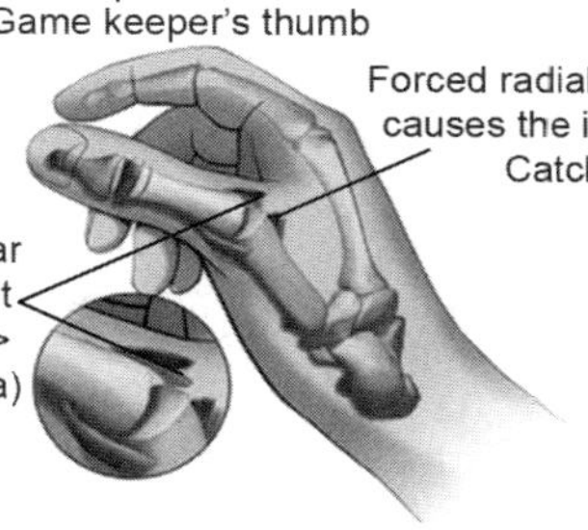

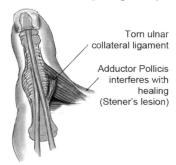

Fig. 13.18: Game Keeper's thumb (Most common injury of 1st MCP Joint)

Incomplete ruptures of the ulnar collateral ligament of the thumb are common and require only proper protection for restoration of function, although pain and swelling may persist for several months. A thumb spica cast or functional brace is recommended for 4–6 weeks. Acute complete rupture of the ulnar collateral ligament and Stener lesion should be treated with surgical repair of the ligament.

Fig. 13.19: Stener's lesion

MULTIPLE CHOICE QUESTIONS

1. Game keepers thumb is: *(NEET Pattern 2013)*
   A. Thumb metacarpophalangeal joint ulnar collateral ligament rupture
   B. Thumb metacarpophalangeal joint radial collateral ligament rupture
   C. Thumb interphalangeal joint ulnar collateral ligament rupture
   D. Thumb interphalangeal joint radial collateral ligament rupture

   Ans. is 'A' Thumb metacarpophalangeal joint ulnar collateral ligament rupture

2. Cricketer while catching a Ball gets hit on thumb. Which damage should be looked for specifically?
   (AIIMS Nov 2011)
   A. Ulnar collateral ligament
   B. Volar plate
   C. Abductor pollicis
   D. Extensor pollicis brevis

   Ans. is 'A' Ulnar collateral ligament

MALLET FINGER/BASEBALL FINGER

It is **avulsion of extensor tendon** of the distal interphalangeal joint from its insertion at the **base of distal phalanx.**

Cause

It may be due to direct trauma, but more often occurs when the finger tip is forcibly bent during active extension (i.e. sudden occurrence of passive flexion of distal interphalangeal joint).

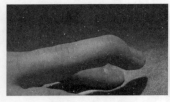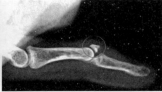

Fig. 13.20: Mallet finger

Presentation and Type

- The terminal phalanx is held flexed and patient cannot straighten it, but passive movement is normal.
- The proximal interphalangeal joint may become hyper-extended due to unbalanced extensor mechanism (Swan neck).
- Three types are a tendinous avulsion (X-ray is normal), a small flake of bone or a large dorsal bone fragment, (some times with subluxation of Joints).

Treatment

- An acute mallet finger should be **splinted** and the DIP joint is kept in **hyperextension for 6–8 weeks.**
- Surgery is not advised even with fracture dislocation, as the complication rate is very high and it is unlikely to improve outcome.
- Old lesion need treatment if deformity is marked, hand functions seriously impaired, and joint still mobile. The options include fusion, tendon reconstruction or Fowler's central slip tenotomy.

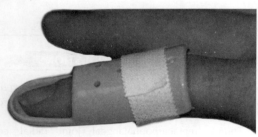

Fig. 13.21: Stack splint or mallet hypertension splint for mallet finger

Mallet finger deformities in children may be caused by traumatic separation of the epiphysis. These deformities can be readily recognized with radiographs. Early detection usually allows straightforward reduction with hyperextension of the distal interphalangeal joint. The finger is splinted for 3–4 weeks, and healing is rapid compared with injury of the extensor tendon itself. Growth disturbance is possible but rare.

JERSEY FINGER

- **It is avulsion of FDP from distal phalanx**
- There is hyperextension of a flexed finger as in finger trapped in a jersey
- **Ring finger most commonly affected**
- Treatment is surgical

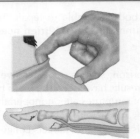

Fig. 13.22: Jersey finger

MULTIPLE CHOICE QUESTIONS

1. Identify the deformity: *(AIIMS Nov 2018)*

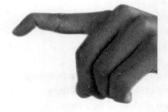

 A. Swan Neck deformity B. Boutonniere deformity
 C. Jersey Finger D. Mallet Finger
Ans. is 'D' Mallet Finger

2. Mallet finger is: *(JIPMER 2014)*
 A. Facture of proximal phalanx
 B. Avulsion of extensor tendon
 C. Rupture of flexor tendon
 D. Capsular rupture of PIP joint
Ans. is 'B' Avulsion of extensor tendon

3. Jersey finger is caused by rupture of: *(AIIMS May 2015)*
 A. Flexor digitorum profundus
 B. Extensor digiti minimi
 C. Flexor digitorum superficialis
 D. Extensor indicis
Ans. is 'A' Flexor digitorum profundus

4. Mallet finger is due to rupture of: *(PGM-CET 2015)*
 A. Central extensor slip of finger
 B. Distal end of index extensor
 C. Distal end of flexor digitorum profundus
 D. None of above
Ans. is 'B' Distal end of index extensor

Note: The central slip attaches at the base of middle phalanx, hence it is not involved in mallet finger

5. A 30-year-old man involved in a fight, injured his middle finger and noticed slight flexion of DIP joint. X-rays were normal. The most appropriate management at this stage is: *(AIIMS Nov 2004; Andhra 1999)*
 A. Ignore
 B. Splint the finger in hyperextension
 C. Surgical repair of the flexor tendon
 D. Buddy strapping
Ans. is 'B' Splint the finger in hyperextension

ZONES AND PULLEYS OF HAND

Zone	Lies between
I	Distal to insertion of flexor digitorum superficialis
II	Between flexor crease of PIP joint and distal palmar crease
III	Between end of carpal tunnel and beginning of flexor-sheath (over lumbricals)
IV	Within the carpal tunnel
V	Proximal to the carpal tunnel

Zones and Pulleys

Zone II-Situated between the opening of the flexor sheath (the distal palmar crease) and insertion of flexor superficialis (flexor crease of proximal interphalangeal joint) is known as **'no man's land'** or dangerous area of hand. **The results of flexor tendon repair is worst in this area** because both superficial and deep tendons run together in a tight sheath and passes through three pulleys.

Flexor Tendon Sheath and Pulleys

Fibrous pulleys-designated A1 to A5 holds the flexor tendons to the phalanges and prevent bowstringing during movement.

A1, 3 and 5 are attached to the palmar plate near each joint MP, PIP and DIP. A2 and A4 are opposite proximal and middle phalanx.

A1 pulley is involved in trigger thumb/finger.

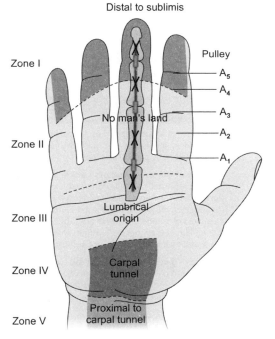

Fig. 13.23: Zones of flexor tendon of hand

It is essential, however, that at least the A2 and A4 annular pulley areas of the flexor sheath be preserved; otherwise, tendon bowstringing and flexion deformity of the finger can develop, and excursion of the tendon becomes impaired.

Cuts above the wrist (Zone V), in the palm (zone III) or distal to superficialis insertion (zone I) generally have better outcome than injuries in carpal tunnel (zone IV) or flexor sheath (zone II).

If repair is done under satisfactory conditions by an experienced surgeon, satisfactory function can be expected in 80% or more of patients even in Zone II.

Tendons – Nutrition – Synovial fluid – tenosynovium and blood supply is by Vincula longa and brevia.

"Strickland" gave characteristics for ideal tendon repair.

Timing

- < 12 hours – for repair: (Preferably up to 2 hrs)—Primary
- 24 hours to 10 days—delayed Primary
- 10–14 days—Secondary
- > 4 weeks—delayed Secondary

Donor tendons-**Palmaris longus** (Present in 85% of general population), Plantaris, Extensor Hallucis Longus (EHL) and Flexor Digitorum Superficialis (FDS) are common donor tendons.

MULTIPLE CHOICE QUESTIONS

1. No Man's land in hand surgery all are false except:
   (PGI Nov 2016)
   A. Results of flexor tendon repair & satisfactory in this area
   B. Comprises zone II
   C. Extends from distal palmar crease and flexor crease of PIP
   D. Extends from distal palmar crease and insertion of flexor superficialis
   E. It is for extensor tendons

   Ans. is 'B' Comprises zone II; 'C' Extends from distal palmar crease and flexor crease of PIP; 'D' Extends from distal palmar crease and insertion of flexor superficialis

2. In hand surgery which area is called no man's land:
   (DNB June 2017, AIIMS Nov 2000)
   A. Proximal phalanx
   B. Distal phalanx
   C. Between distal palmar crease and flexor crease of PIP
   D. Wrist

   Ans. is 'C' Between distal palmar crease and flexor crease of PIP

14 Neuromuscular Disease

DISC PROLAPSE

The commonest site of disc prolapse is lumbar spine. In more than 95% of cases lumbar disc herniation are localized at **L4–5 (50% cases)** and L5–S1 (45% cases). The next commonest site of intervertebral disc prolapse is **lower cervical spine (C5–6)**. Lumbar disc is dehydrated hence more prone.

Pathology and Types

- Small herniation of nucleus pulposus produce Schmorl's nodules
- Degenerated disc is extruded posteriorly in three patterns
  1. Central disc herniation
  2. **Paracentral (paramedian)** type annulus usually bulges to one side of posterior longitudinal ligament. **It is most common type of disc prolapse most unilateral radicular symptoms are due to this.** The nerve root may be compressed medially and backwards (when protrusion is lateral to nerve root) or laterally (when protrusion is between theca and nerve root).
  3. Far lateral disc herniation: bulge is within or just lateral to neural foramina.

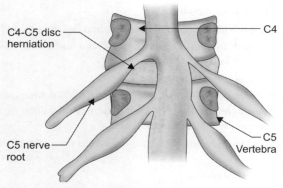

Fig. 14.1: Usually, lower nerve root is involved

Neurological Involvement: Usually Lower Nerve Root is Compressed

- Central or paracentral disc herniation at L3–4 compress L4 at L4–5 compress L5 and at L5–S1 compress S1 nerve root.
- Most unilateral radicular symptoms are due to paracentral/paramedian type disc herniation.
- Far Lateral disc herniation of L4–5 compress L4 nerve root; of L5–S1 compress L5 nerve root (less common type and compresses the above nerve root).

Please remember while answering:

"Answer according to paracentral herniation, i.e. lower nerve root compressed".

LUMBAR DISC HERNIATION

Clinical Presentation

It may occur at any age but is most commonly seen at age group 20–40 years uncommon in very young and very old. Typically patient has, **Sciatica (pain in back radiating to lower limb)** commonly preceded by back pain. Both backache and sciatica are made worse by coughing, straining, sneezing or Valsalva maneuver and prolonged sitting. Standing and supine position reduces pain.

The patient usually stands with slight tilt (list) to one side (sciatic scoliosis). If the disc protrudes medial to the nerve root the tilt is toward the painful side (to relieve pressure on the root) with the far lateral prolapse the tilt is away from painful side.

Straight leg raising is restricted (normal is up to 90°). The Lasegue sign (pain when the affected limb is elevated) is positive in 98% cases and cross Lasegue sign/crossed sciatic tension (pain radiating to affected leg when contralateral leg is elevated) is positive in 20%. Midline tenderness, paravertebral spasm and femoral stretch test is seen in upper or mid lumbar prolapse.

Neurological Features

Compression level	Symptoms and signs
L4	Weakness of quadriceps muscle, adductors. Decreased knee reflex, ankle dorsiflexion. Sensory loss on medial aspect of knee, leg, ankle and foot.
L5	**Wasting of glutei (abductors), ankle and toe (Extensor Hallucis longus) dorsiflexion and weakness of knee flexion. Knee and ankle jerks are normal. Paradoxically knee (quadriceps) reflex may appear to be increased because of weakness of antagonist (which are supplied by L5). Sensory loss on lateral aspect of lower thigh, anterolateral aspect of knee and leg and dorsum of foot and big toe on all aspects.**
S1	Wasting of glutei, hamstring and calf muscles, weakness of eversion and plantar flexion of foot and toes (Flexor Hallucis longus), ankle jerk is reduced or absent, sensory loss on sole and lateral border of foot and little toe.

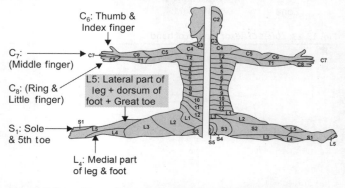

Fig. 14.2: Dermatomes (Sensory supply) (also refer to Figure 8.2)

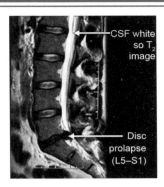

Fig. 14.3: MRI lumbosacral spine

Investigations

- Magnetic resonance imaging **(MRI) is investigation of choice.**

Treatment

1. **Rest and Anti-inflammatory Medications**
   Continuous bed rest for 2 weeks will reduce the herniation in over 90% of cases.
2. If improvement is not complete epidural injection of corticosteroid and local anesthetic may help. **Back strengthening should be started only after pain has subsided.**
3. **Operative removal of disc** options are unilateral laminectomy/laminotomy or microscopic disc removal or endoscopic disc removal.

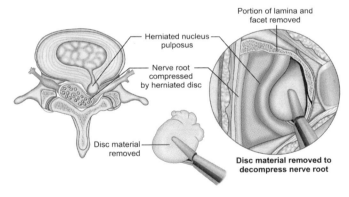

Fig. 14.4: Discectomy

4. Chemonucleolysis dissolution of nucleus pulposus by percutaneous injection of proteolytic enzyme (chymopapain) is of theoretical significance.

Indications for Surgery

Absolute indications

1. **Bladder and bowel involvement (Cauda Equina Syndrome)**
2. Increasing neurological deficit.

Relative indications

1. Failure of conservative treatment—**Up to 6 weeks of trial is usually given**
2. *Recurrent sciatica:* 1st attack 90% recover
   2nd attack 90% recover; 50% recurrent consider surgery
   3rd attack 90% recover but all recurrent propose surgery

3. Significant neurological deficit with SLR reduction
4. Disc rupture in stenotic canal
5. Recurrent neurological deficit.

Canal Stenosis Syndrome (Lumbar > Cervical)

- Affects Geriatric population
- Decrease in diameter of spinal canal
- Spinal Canal diameter < 10 mm is diagnostic
- Etiology
  - Congenital (e.g. Achondroplasia)
  - Acquired (Degenerative most common)
- Neurogenic claudication: Pain that increases on standing or walking and decreases on sitting or forward bending
- Treatment: Conservative trial is given, if it fails laminectomy or laminoplasty can be done.

LOW BACK PAIN (LBP)

Classification (based on duration)

- Acute <4 weeks
- Subacute 4–8 weeks
- Chronic > 8 weeks.

RED FLAG SIGNS OF BACKACHE—INDICATIVE OF FURTHER WORK UP AND MANAGEMENT

- Thoracic pain
- Fever and unexplained weight loss
- **Bladder or bowel dysfunction**
- **History of carcinoma**
- Ill health or presence of other medical illness
- **Progressive neurological deficit**
- Disturbed gait, saddle anesthesia
- Age of onset < 20 years or > 55 years
- **Prolonged steroid intake (> 4 weeks)**
- Radicular impingement.

YELLOW FLAG SIGNS—NO FURTHER WORK UP AND MANAGEMENT REQUIRED

- Psychosocial factors shown to be indicative of long-term chronicity and disability:
  - A negative attitude that back pain is harmful or potentially severely disabling
  - Fear avoidance behavior and reduced activity levels
  - An expectation that passive, rather than active, treatment will be beneficial
  - A tendency to depression, low morale, and social withdrawal.

Management (Most of the patients can be treated conservatively)

Proven Efficacy

Analgesic (NSAIDs) and muscle relaxants are used to manage acute and subacute exacerbation of chronic LBP. Exercise programs can reverse atrophy in paraspinal muscles and strengthen extensors of trunk.

May Benefit

Epidural injection

Unproven Benefit

- Trigger point sclerosant
- Facet joint/ligamentous injection
- Acupuncture
- Traction
- Manipulation
- TENS (Transcutaneous electrical nerve stimulation)
- Hydrotherapy.

Avoided/Harmful

Prolonged bed rest is avoided. In chronic low backache (lumbago) bed rest should not exceed 2–4 days, because bed rest for longer period may lead to debilitating muscle atrophy and increased stiffness.

MULTIPLE CHOICE QUESTIONS

1. A 55-year-old male presents with severe backache for 10 days and urinary incontinence with a H/o Intevertebral lumbar disc prolapse. There is no H/o fever or weight loss. What is the likely diagnosis? *(AIIMS May 2018)*
   A. Pott's spine
   B. Multiple myeloma
   C. Cauda equina syndrome
   D. Bone metastasis

Ans. is 'C' Cauda equina syndrome

2. In a patient with L4-L5 disc prolapse, which of the following nerve roots can get compressed? *(PGI MAY 2018)*
   A. L5
   B. S1
   C. S2
   D. S2-S4
   E. L4

Ans. is 'A' L5 'E' L4

3. Features of L5, S1 disc prolapse includes: *(PGI May 2017)*
   A. Lower back pain
   B. Pain radiation to leg
   C. Sensory loss in medial calf muscle
   D. Knee jerk is lost
   E. Bowel and bladder incontinence

Ans. is 'A' Lower back pain; 'B' Pain radiation to leg; & 'E' Bowel and bladder incontinence

4. While examining a patient in supine position the examiner keeps his hand below the heel of one foot and asks the patient to flex the other hip against resistance, while keeping the week leg straight this is known as: *(AIIMS Nov 2017)*
   A. Waddell's test
   B. O'Donoghue's test
   C. Hoover's Sign
   D. McMurray test

Ans. is 'C' Hoover's Sign

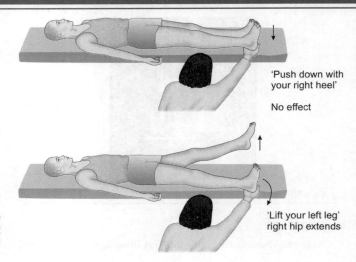

Hoover's Sign

- Hoover's sign is a maneuver to separate organic from non-organic paresis of Leg.
- **Principle:** Synergistic Contraction.
- Involuntary extension of normal leg occurs with flexion of contralateral limb against resistance.
- **Method:** Examiner places one hand under heel of normal limb and contralateral hip flexion is done by patient against resistance.

Interpretation

- **Organic Cause:** Flexion of paralyzed limb→heel of normal limb pushes the examiner's hand.
- **Functional Weakness:** Heel does not pushdown, i.e. the effort is not being transmitted.

O'DONOGHUE'S MANEUVER FOR CERVICAL SPINE

- Structures affected: Cervical spinal muscles and/or cervical spinal ligaments.
- Since resisted range of motion mainly stresses muscles and passive range of motion mainly stresses ligaments, you should be able to determine between strain and sprain or a combination thereof.

O'Donoghue's Maneuver for Knee Joint

- This maneuver can be used to diagnose meniscal pathologies in the knee.

O'Donoghue Triad

Note: The medial structures medial (tibial) collateral ligament (MCL) and medial capsular ligament are first to fail, followed by ACL tear, if the force is of sufficient magnitude. The medial meniscus may be trapped between condyles and have a peripheral tear, thus producing unhappy triad of O'Donoghue.

WADDELL'S TEST

- Tests of malingering

- Each test counts as +1 if +, 0 if –
  - Superficial skin tenderness to light pinch over wide area of lumbar spine.
  - Deep tenderness over wide area, often extending to thoracic spine, sacrum, and/or pelvis.
  - Low back pain on axial loading of spine in standing.
  - SLR test positive supine, but not when seated with knee extended to test Babinski reflex.
  - Abnormal or inconsistent neurological (motor and/or sensory) patterns.
  - Overreaction.
  - If 3+ points or more, investigate for non-organic cause.

MENISCAL INJURY

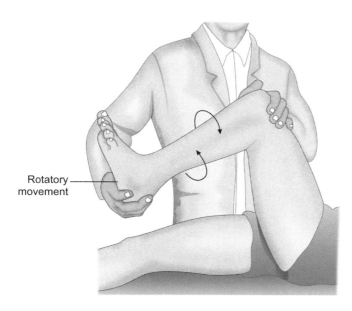

Fig. 14.6: McMurray's test—menisci

5. All of the following are red flag signs of back pain except:
   A. Previous history of malignancy *(CET July 16)*
   B. Previous history of steroid use
   C. Saddle anesthesia
   D. Age between 35–50
Ans. is 'D' Age between 35–50

6. The investigation of choice to detect a prolapsed intervertebral disc is? *(AI Dec 15)*
   A. CT Scan   B. MRI
   C. Myelography   D. Radiograph
Ans. is 'B' MRI

7. Straight leg raising test is/are positive in: *(PGI May 2015)*
   A. Spinal stenosis   B. Spinal abscess
   C. Also called as Trendelenburg test
   D. Prolapsed intervertebral disc
   E. Sciatica
Ans. is 'D' Prolapsed intervertebral disc and 'E' Sciatica

8. Removal of vertebral disc is by all these methods except: *(AIIMS May 2015)*
   A. Laminotomy   B. Laminectomy
   C. Laminoplasty   D. Hemilaminectomy
Ans. is 'C' Laminoplasty

9. When do you operate for prolapsed disc? *(NEET 2015)*
   A. Busy executive needs quick surgery
   B. Only with weakness no pain
   C. Severe pain interfering with activity and not relieved by rest and treatment of 8 weeks
   D. Patient of PID with difficulty in ambulation
Ans. is 'C' Severe pain interfering with activity and not relieved by rest and treatment of 8 weeks

10. Test used for prolapsed lumbar intervertebral disc is:
    A. Active straight leg raising test *(NEET 2015)*
    B. Lasegue test   C. Thomas test
    D. Apley's grinding test
Ans. is 'B' Lasegue test

11. Lumbar canal stenosis presents as: *(NEET 2015)*
    A. Claudication   B. Scoliotic deformity
    C. Kyphotic deformity   D. Radiculopathy
Ans. is 'A' Claudication

12. H reflex on electromyography is seen in:
    (AIIMS Nov 2014; NEET Pattern 2012)
    A. L1 Radiculopathy   B. L4 Radiculopathy
    C. L5 Radiculopathy   D. S1 Radiculopathy
Ans. is 'D' S1 Radiculopathy

   Explanation
   - The H reflex is basically an electrophysiologically recorded Achilles tendon stretch reflex.
   - It is performed by stimulating the tibial nerve in popliteal fossa.
   - It is recorded over the soleus or gastrocnemius muscles.
   - It is used most commonly to evaluate S1 radiculopathy or to distinguish it from an L5 radiculopathy.

13. Disc prolapse is common at all site except:
    A. L4–L5   B. L5–S1 *(NEET Pattern 2013)*
    C. C6–C7   D. T3–T4
Ans. is 'D' T3–T4

14. Most common nerve used for nerve conduction study in H reflex: *(NEET Pattern 2013)*
    A. Median nerve   B. Ulnar nerve
    C. Tibial nerve   D. Peroneal nerve
Ans. is 'C' Tibial nerve

15. L5–S1–Nerve involved: *(NEET Pattern 2012)*
    A. L4   B. L5
    C. S1   D. S2
Ans. is 'C' S1

16. A patient has decreased sensation on tip of middle finger and decreased triceps reflex. This presentation can be linked to disc prolapse at: *(NEET Pattern 2012)*
    A. C5–C6   B. C6–C7
    C. C8–T1   D. T1–T2
Ans. is 'B' C6–C7

17. Disc prolapsed MC Lumbar due to: *(NEET Pattern 2012)*
    A. Less hydrated   B. Posterior nucleus pulposus
    C. Weak ligamentum flavum   D. More degenerative forces
Ans. is 'A' Less hydrated

18. Most common site for lumbar disc prolapsed:
    (DNB June 2017, NEET Pattern 2012)
    A. L4–L5
    B. L5–S1
    C. L1–L2
    D. L3–L4

Ans. is 'A' L4–L5

19. A 44-year-old man presented with acute onset of low backache radiating to the right lower limb. Examination revealed SLRT < 40 degrees on the right side, weakness of extensor hallucis longus on the right side, sensory loss in the first web space of the right foot and brisk knee jerk. Which of the following is the most likely diagnosis:
    (AIIMS Nov 2011, May 2004, UPSC 90)
    A. Prolapsed intervertebral disc L4–5
    B. Spondylolysis L5–S1
    C. Lumbar canal stenosis
    D. Spondylolisthesis L4–5

Ans. is 'A' Prolapsed intervertebral disc L4–5

20. Which of the following is not recommended in the treatment of Chronic Low Back Pain: (AI 2009)
    A. NSAIDs
    B. Bed rest for 3 months
    C. Exercises
    D. Epidural steroid Injection

Ans. is 'B' Bed rest for 3 months

21. A previously healthy 45 years old laborer suddenly develops acute lower back pain with right-leg pain and weakness of dorsiflexion of the right great toe. Which of the following is true: (AI 2002)
    A. Immediate treatment should include analgesics muscle relaxants and back strengthening exercises
    B. The appearance of the foot drop indicate early surgical intervention
    C. If the neurological sign resolve within 2–3 weeks but low back pain persists, the proper treatment would include fusion of affected lumbar vertebra
    D. If the neurological signs fail to resolve within 1 week, lumbar laminectomy and excision of any herniated nucleus pulposus should be done

Ans. is 'B' The appearance of the foot drop indicate early surgical intervention
   – Bowel bladder involvement, increasing neurological deficit or failure of conservative treatment is an indication for surgery. Exercises are contraindicated acute pain and 6 weeks of trial is advised before carrying out surgical intervention.

22. Yellow flag signs are seen in: (AI 2012)
    A. Psychosocial factors of back pain
    B. Clinical factors of back pain
    C. Tuberculosis of hip
    D. Spinal metastasis

Ans. is 'A' Psychosocial factors of back pain

SPONDYLOLISTHESIS AND SPONDYLOLYSIS

Spondylolisthesis is the slippage forward of one vertebrae upon another. It nearly always occurs **between L5 and S1 (most common)** or L4 and L5. Spondylolysis is characterized by presence of bony defect at pars interarticularis, which can result in spondylolisthesis. Most common vertebra having spondylolysis is L5.

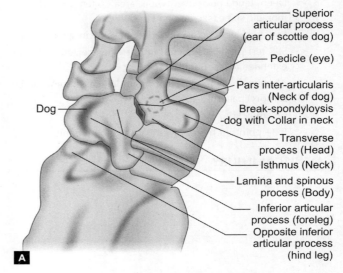

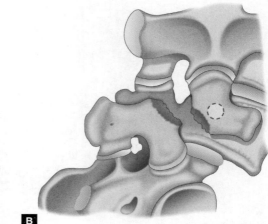

Figs. 14.7A and B: (A) Oblique view of lumbosacral spine; (B) Spondylolisthesis

Clinical Features

High incidence of spondylolysis in gymnasts and other athlete's suggest repetitive injury may be contributing mechanism.

Patient aged over 50 years are usually women. They always have backache or sciatica and claudication due to spinal stenosis. The extent of slippage may not be correlated with severity of pain. In young patient regardless of extent of slip there may be tight hamstrings and a knee bent, hips-flexed gait, the classical Phalen-Dickson sign.

On examination buttocks look flat, the sacrum appears to extend to the waist and transverse loin creases are seen.

Step off can be felt when the fingers are run down the spine, secondary to prominent spinous processes of L5. With more severe slippage the lumbosacral junction becomes more kyphotic and the trunk appears shortened with the rib cage approaching the iliac crest.

Neuromuscular Disease

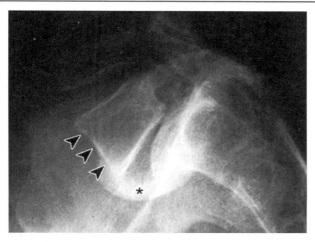

Fig. 14.8: X-ray showing spondylolisthesis

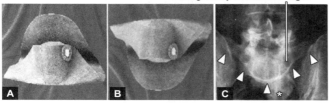

Figs. 14.9A to C: AP view in spondylolisthesis

Percentage of slippage is measured on lateral view and oblique radiograph demonstrate **collar or broken neck on the scottie dog in spondylolysis and beheaded dog in spondylolisthesis** (Beheaded Scottish terrier sign).

Spondyloptosis

A complete dislocation of one vertebra over the other is spondyloptosis (L_5 over S_1).

In last stages on (AP) view inverted Napoleon hat sign is seen when complete slip occurs. Thus AP views are for last stage otherwise oblique or lateral views are preferred.

- CT scan can diagnose early defects and slips
- MRI can diagnose cord compression.

Treatment principle is:
- Rest and Analgesics with or without brace
- Once pain subsides put patient on exercise regimen
- Epidural steroids may benefit some
- Patient may require surgery in form of fusion of spine with instrumentation and bone grafting in cases of back pain or radicular symptoms that have not improved with conservative treatment.

MULTIPLE CHOICE QUESTIONS

1. The following X-ray was taken of a 50-year-old female with chronic backache. What is the most likely diagnosis? *(AIIMS Nov 2015)*

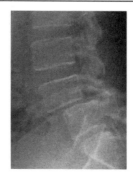

   A. Spondylolysis   B. Spondylosis
   C. Spondylolisthesis
   D. Prolapsed inter-vertebral disc
   Ans. is 'C' Spondylolisthesis

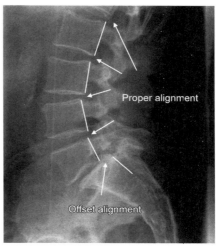

Slip of one vertebra over the other

2. In Spondylolisthesis, which of the following is NOT useful investigation? *(TN 2014)*
   A. Anteroposterior X-ray   B. Lateral view X-ray
   C. CT   D. MRI
   Ans. 'A' Anteroposterior X-ray
   - AP view will show changes only in last stages-inverted Napoleon hat sign all other are more important for diagnosis and management. CT and MRI are required in all cases.

3. Partial anterior dislocation of one segment of the spine over another is: *(NEET Pattern 2012)*
   A. Spondylosis   B. Spondylolisthesis
   C. Kyphosis   D. Scoliosis
   Ans. is 'B' Spondylolisthesis

4. Spondylolisthesis most common level: *(NEET Pattern 2012)*
   A. L4–L5   B. L5–S1
   C. C5–C6   D. C6–C7
   Ans. is 'B' L5–S1

5. In spondylolisthesis, there is fracture of vertebra in:
   A. Spinous process   *(Bihar 1998)*
   B. Neural arch pars interarticularis
   C. Transverse process   D. Body
   Ans. is 'B' Neural arch pars interarticularis

6. True about spondylolisthesis is/are: (PGI 1991)
   A. Congenital defect of posterior arch
   B. Slipping of L5 over S1
   C. Progressive slipping
   D. Abnormal congenital development

Ans. is 'A' Congenital defect of posterior arch; 'B' Slipping of L5 over S1; 'C' Progressive slipping; and 'D' Abnormal congenital development

CERVICAL SPONDYLOSIS

It is cluster of abnormalities arising from **chronic intervertebral disc degeneration.**

Like disc prolapse it usually occurs immediately above or below the 6th cervical vertebral (in lower two segments C_5–C_6 > C_6–C_7).

Pathophysiology

Degeneration of disc (loss of water and proteoglycan) cause decrease of disc height (hard disc) and converging of disc space causing

1. Segmental instability resulting in facet joint arthropathy and hypertrophic osteophyte formation by uncovertebral joint of Luschka. These spurs result in compression of existing nerve root (in intervertebral foramen) and later the spinal cord (in spinal canal).
2. Buckling of ligamentum flavum and narrowing of spinal canal.
3. Ligamentous instability.
4. Radiculopathy (more common), myelopathy or both may be seen secondarily.

Clinical Features

90% of men > 50 years and 90% of women > 60 years

Headache, neck pain and stiffness, worse in morning and improving throughout day, commonly located in occipital region and radiating to frontal area, back of shoulders, and down one or both arms.

Typically patients have proximal arm pains and distal paresthesia.

Muscles of back of neck and interscapular region may be tender and neck movements limited.

X-rays reveal spur/osteophyte formation (or lipping) at the anterior and posterior margins of disc.

Treatment is usually conservative, patient education on physiotherapy, lifestyle modifications and nonsteroidal anti-inflammatory drugs. Surgery is advocated for cervical radiculopathy in patients who have intractable pain, progressive symptoms, or weakness that fails to improve with conservative therapy.

MULTIPLE CHOICE QUESTIONS

1. Cervical spondylosis is more common at:
   A. C1–C2   B. C2–C3   (UP 99 AIIMS 90)
   C. C6–C7   D. C4–C5

Ans. is 'C' C6–C7

2. In cervical spondylosis which part of vertebral body is involved: (Delhi 1999)
   A. Inferior articular facet   B. Pars interarticularis
   C. Superior articular facet   D. All of the above

Ans. is 'D' All of the above

3. Cervical spondylosis: (Bihar 98)
   A. Most frequently results from an incidence of acute trauma
   B. Causes compression of nerve roots to produce an upper motor neuron lesion in the lower limbs
   C. Produces pain and paresthesia over the lateral aspect of the forearm and thumb when affecting the 6th cervical nerve
   D. Most frequently affects the upper cervical vertebrae

Ans. is 'C' Produces pain and paresthesia over the lateral aspect of the forearm and thumb when affecting the 6th cervical nerve

4. Osteophytes developing at the joint at Luschka characteristically compresses spinal nerves at: (NIMS 96)
   A. Intervertebral foramen   B. Anterior part of body
   C. Posterior part of body   D. Paradural areas

Ans. is 'A' Intervertebral foramen

FROZEN SHOULDER OR ADHESIVE CAPSULITIS OR PERIARTHRITIS SHOULDER

It is characterized by progressive pain and stiffness of the shoulder, which **usually resolve spontaneously after about 18 months.** There is significant restriction in both active and passive range of motion. The shoulder is stiff even when the articular surface are normal and the joint is stable.

Pathology

- Fibroblastic proliferation in rotator interval, coracohumeral ligament and anterior capsule is seen.
- Most prominently involved is rotator interval that includes coracohumeral ligament.
- Passes through three phases
  A. **Painful Inflammatory Freezing Phase**
     - Lasts 2–9 months
  B. **Phase of Progressive Stiffness**
     - Lasts 3–12 months
     - Pain decreases and stiffness increases
     - Attempt to exceed range of stiffness is accompanied by pain.
  C. **Resolution/Thawing Phase**
     - Lasts 1–3 years (can be as short as 1 month)
     - Shoulder slowly and progressively becomes more supple.

Associated Conditions

- Diabetes mellitus 10–35% of diabetics develop frozen shoulder
- Dupuytren's disease
- Hyperlipidemia
- Hyperthyroidism
- Cardiac disease
- Lung disease
- Hemiplegia
- Recovery from neurosurgery.

Clinical Presentation

The cardinal feature is stubborn lack of active and passive movement in all directions, i.e. **global restriction of movements in all planes.**

- **Often the first motion to be affected is internal rotation followed by abduction.**

Treatment

1. NSAIDs and Exercise
2. Manipulation under anesthesia
3. **Intra-articular steroids**
4. Adhesiolysis—breaking the adhesions in joint, can be done by arthroscopy.

MULTIPLE CHOICE QUESTIONS

1. All of the following are associated with frozen shoulder except: *(CET July 16)*
   A. Diabetes
   B. Hyperthyroidism
   C. Psoriasis
   D. Hemiplegia

   Ans. is 'C' Psoriasis

2. Which of the following movements are restricted in frozen shoulder? *(Andhra 2000)*
   A. Abduction and internal rotation
   B. Adduction and external rotation
   C. All range of movements
   D. Only abduction

   Ans. is 'C' All range of movements

3. Gradual painful limitation of shoulder movements in an elderly suggest that the most probable diagnosis is: *(Orissa 1990)*
   A. Arthritis
   B. Osteoarthritis
   C. Periarthritis
   D. Myositis ossificans
   E. Fracture - dislocation

   Ans. is 'C' Periarthritis

ROTATOR CUFF SYNDROME

i. **Subacute tendonitis (Painful arc syndrome-painful abduction between 60°–120°)**
ii. Chronic tendonitis (Impingement syndrome; Neer's test is used for it)
iii. Rotator cuff tears.

Treatment:
- Physiotherapy + NSAIDs
- **Local injection of steroids**
- Surgery if required for impingement syndrome or rotator cuff tears (especially in young individuals).

PAINFUL ARC SYNDROME

It is anterior shoulder pain in 60–120° of glenohumeral abduction. It can be caused by
- Chronic supraspinatus tendinitis (most common)
- Calcification of supraspinatus tendon
- Partial (not complete) tears of supraspinatus tendon
- Fracture of greater tuberosity
- Subacromial bursitis.

MULTIPLE CHOICE QUESTIONS

1. Painful arc syndrome which movement is painful. *(NEET Pattern 2019)*
   A. Initial abduction
   B. Terminal abduction
   C. Mid abduction
   D. Full range of abduction

   Ans. is 'C' Mid abduction

2. Which of the following is not true about impingement syndrome? *(NEET DEC 2016)*
   A. It is the tendinitis caused by inflammation of the rotator cuff tendons
   B. Supraspinatus tendon is most often involved
   C. Shoulder abduction in the arc of 60–120 degrees is particularly painful
   D. Surgical decompression of the subacromial space is frequently indicated

   Ans. is 'D' Surgical decompression of the subacromial space is frequently indicated

3. The following are True regarding Rotator cuff tendinitis except: *(APPG 2015)*
   A. Injection of local anesthetic helps in diagnosis
   B. Steroid injections are contraindicated
   C. Painful arc of movement causes secondary weakness
   D. Acromial beak of bone appears with age

   Ans. is 'B' Steroid injections are contraindicated

4. Causes of painful arc syndrome is/are: *(NEET 2015)*
   A. Supraspinatus tendinitis
   B. Subacromial bursitis
   C. Fracture of greater tuberosity
   D. All of the above

   Ans. is 'D' All of the above

5. Painful arc syndrome is seen in all except:
   A. Complete tear of supraspinatus *(AIIMS Nov 2011)*
   B. Fracture greater tuberosity
   C. Subacromial bursitis
   D. Supraspinatus tendinitis

   Ans. is 'A' Complete tear of supraspinatus

TENNIS ELBOW/LATERAL EPICONDYLITIS

- It is **chronic tendonitis of common extensor origin (esp. extensor carpi radialis brevis) on lateral epicondyle.**
- It may result in small tears, fibrocartilaginous metaplasia, microscopic calcification and painful vascular reaction in tendon fibers close to lateral epicondyle (degenerative changes with angiofibroblastic proliferation).

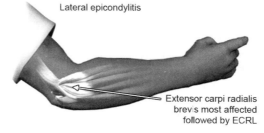

Fig. 14.10: Tennis elbow

Clinical Features

- Localized tenderness at or just below lateral epicondyle.
- Pain can be reproduced by passively stretching the extensor radialis brevis; this is done by extending the elbow, pronating the forearm and then passively flexing the wrist or active extension of wrist against resistance can produce pain (Cozen's test).

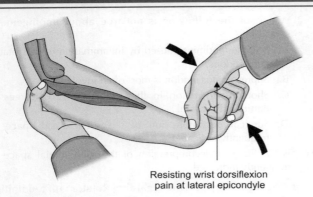

Fig. 14.11: Cozen's test

- Treatment includes trial of anti-inflammatory medications if not relieved steroid injection if not relieved detachment of common extensor origin, orbicular ligament, and synovial fringe.

Golfer's Elbow Medial epicondylitis involving common flexor pronator origin.

Baseball Pitcher's Elbow, repetitive, vigorous throwing activities can cause damage to the bones or soft tissue attachment around elbow. Hypertrophy of lower humerus and incongruity of the joint, or loose body formation and osteoarthritis.

The junior equivalent (Little leaguer's elbow) is a partial avulsion of medial epicondyle.

Javelin Throwers Elbow: It is avulsion of tip of Olecranon due to over arm action.

MULTIPLE CHOICE QUESTIONS

1. Lateral epicondylitis elbow begins in: *(AI 2016)*
   A. Flexor digitorum superficialis
   B. Flexor digitorum profundus
   C. Extensor carpi radialis brevis
   D. Extensor carpi radialis longus
Ans. is 'C' Extensor carpi radialis brevis

2. Cozen's test is used for the diagnosis of:
   A. Tennis elbow *(NEET 2016, 2015)*
   B. Golfer's elbow   C. Base bailer's pitcher elbow
   D. Carpal tunnel syndrome
Ans. is 'A' Tennis elbow

3. Tennis elbow, is characterized by:
   (AIIMS Nov 2005, AI 1997)
   A. Tenderness over the medial epicondyle
   B. Tendinitis of common extensor origin
   C. Tendinitis of common flexor origin
   D. Painful flexion and extension
Ans. is 'B' Tendonitis of common extensor origin

4. A 40-year-old man was repairing his wooden shed on Sunday morning. By afternoon, he felt that the hammer was becoming heavier and heavier. He felt pain in lateral side of elbow and also found that squeezing water out of sponge hurt his elbow. Which of the muscles are most likely involved? *(AIIMS May 2002)*
   A. Biceps brachii and supinator
   B. Flexor digitorum superficialis
   C. Extensor carpi radialis brevis
   D. Triceps brachii and anconeus
Ans. is 'C' Extensor carpi radialis brevis

de QUERVAIN'S DISEASE

The **abductor pollicis longus and extensor pollicis brevis** tendons may become inflamed beneath the retinacular pulley at the radial styloid within the first extensor compartment.

Pathognomic sign is Finkelstein's test. The examiner places patients' thumb across the palm in full flexion, and then holding the patient's hand firmly, turns the wrist sharply into adduction. In positive test this is acutely painful; repeating the movement with the thumb left free is relatively painless.

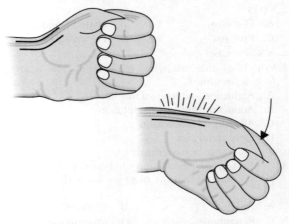

Fig. 14.12: Finkelstein's test—de Quervain's tenosynovitis

Differential diagnosis includes scaphoid non-union, arthritis at the base of thumb and intersection syndrome.

Treatment

NSAIDs with splint if it fails than steroid injection into tendon sheath and if not relieved than treatment consists of splitting the thickened tendon sheath.

MULTIPLE CHOICE QUESTIONS

1. de Quervain's tenovaginitis involves: *(NEET 2015)*
   A. Abductor pollicis-longus B. Extensor pollicis-brevis
   C. Both of the above   D. None of the above
Ans. is 'C' Both of the above

2. Finkelstein's test is used for: *(NEET Pattern 2013)*
   A. Golfer's elbow   B. de Quervain's tenovaginitis
   C. Trigger linger   D. Tennis elbow
Ans. is 'B' de Quervain's tenovaginitis

3. de Quervain's disease classically affects the:
   (NEET 2018, PGI Dec 2008, AIIMS May 2005, NIMS 2000)
   A. Flexor pollicis longus and brevis
   B. Extensor carpi radialis and extensor pollicis longus
   C. Abductor pollicis longus and brevis
   D. Extensor pollicis brevis and abductor pollicis longus
Ans. is 'D' Extensor pollicis brevis and abductor pollicis longus

DUPUYTREN'S CONTRACTURE

This is nodular hypertrophy and contracture of superficial palmar fascia (palmar aponeurosis).

Neuromuscular Disease

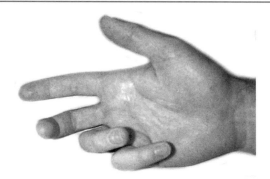

Fig. 14.13: Dupuytren's contracture ring finger and little finger involved

Epidemiology and Associations

Higher incidence in epileptics receiving phenytoin therapy, **diabetics, alcoholic cirrhosis,** AIDS, pulmonary tuberculosis.

Pathology

Proliferation of myofibroblast. Fibrous bands cause flexion deformity of MP and PIP joints and puckering of skin.

Ectopic deposits may occur in dorsum of PIP joint (Garrod's/knuckle pads), sole of feet (Ledderhose's disease) and fibrosis of corpus cavernosum (Peyronie's disease).

Clinical Features

A middle aged man usually complains of nodular thickening of palm.

Flexion contracture most commonly occurs at **MCP joint.** > PIP joint > DIP joint.

Ring finger is most commonly involved > little finger > thumb and index finger.

PIP contractures soon become irreversible.

Pain may occur but is seldom a marked feature.

Treatment

Wait and watch is the usual treatment

Primary indication of surgery is fixed contracture of >30° at MP joint or > 15° contracture at PIP joint.

Surgery does not cure the disease, it only partially corrects the deformity usually done surgery is **subtotal fasciectomy.** Closure may be done by Z plasty.

Severe or recurrent PIP joint disease may need arthrodesis.

MULTIPLE CHOICE QUESTIONS

1. Which of the following is true regarding Dupuytren's contracture? *(PGI May 2016)*
   A. It is nodular hypertrophy and contracture of Superficial palmar fascia
   B. Inherited as autosomal recessive trait
   C. Pathology is proliferation of myelofibroblasts
   D. Most commonly affected is radial nerve
   E. Pain is predominant feature throughout disease process

Ans. is 'A' It is nodular hypertrophy and contracture of Superficial palmar fascia and 'C' Pathology is proliferation of myelofibroblasts

Note: Dupuytren's contracture is autosomal dominant

2. Dupuytren's contracture is fibrosis of:*(NEET Pattern 2012)* *(Karnataka 96, AI 94, Delhi 1994, Bihar 1991, AI 88)*
   A. Palmar fascia
   B. Forearm muscles
   C. Sartorius fascia
   D. None of the above

Ans. is 'A' Palmar fascia

3. A 50-year-old diabetic/alcoholic patient, presented with 15 degree flexion deformity of the little finger. What is the most appropriate management? *(AIIMS Nov 2011)*
   A. Wait and watch
   B. Subtotal fasciectomy
   C. Total fasciectomy
   D. Percutaneous fasciotomy

Ans. is 'A' Wait and watch because indication of surgery is > 30° MCP joint contracture and > 15° contracture at PIP. Here most commonly affected joint (MCP) needs to be assumed.

4. Dupuytren's contracture occur in: *(PGI Dec 2008, PGI 1999)*
   A. Diabetes mellitus
   B. Alcohol
   C. Epilepsy
   D. Rheumatoid arthritis
   E. Chronic pulmonary disease

Ans. is 'A' Diabetes mellitus; 'B' Alcohol; 'C' Epilepsy and 'E' Chronic pulmonary disease

5. The best treatment for Dupuytren's contracture is:
   A. Fasciotomy *(Andhra 1994)*
   B. Fasciectomy
   C. Incision and release
   D. Subtotal fasciectomy + Skin transplantation

Ans. is 'D' Subtotal fasciectomy + Skin transplantation

STENOSING FLEXOR TENOSYNOVITIS (TRIGGER FINGER)

Due to stenosing tenosynovitis the flexor tendon may become trapped at the entrance to its fibrous digital sheath. The usual cause is thickening of fibrous tendon sheath or constriction of mouth of fibrous digital sheath **(mainly A1 pulley)** at the level of **metacarpophalangeal joint.**

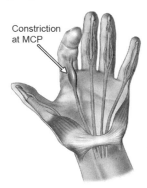

Fig. 14.14: Trigger finger

Causes

Local trauma/unaccustomed activity/rheumatoid arthritis (RA)/diabetes mellitus/gout.

Clinical Feature

Although any digit (including the thumb) may be affected, but the *ring and middle fingers* are most commonly involved.

Patient frequently notes catching/locking/triggering of affected finger after forceful flexion. In some instances, the opposite hand must be used to passively bring the finger into extension.

Patient notices that finger clicks as he or she bends it; when the hand is unclenched the affected finger remains bent at the proximal interphalangeal joint, but with further effort it suddenly straightens with a snap.

Triggering is more pronounced in morning than later in day.

A tender nodule can be felt in front of metacarpophalangeal joint.

In a child it must be distinguished from congenital clasped thumb due to insufficiency of extensor mechanism, in which both the interphalangeal joint and metacarpophalangeal joint is flexed.

Treatment

Injection of methyl prednisolone into the tendon sheath.

Surgical release of A1 pulley. A2 pulley must be spared to preserve effective digital flexion.

In patients of RA, the entire annular pulley system should be preserved to prevent further ulnar drift of fingers. These patients are treated by tenosynovectomy and excision of one slip of flexor digitorum superficialis.

In children it is worth wailing until the child is a year old, as spontaneous recovery often occurs.

MULTIPLE CHOICE QUESTIONS

1. Most common cause of trigger finger: *(NEET Pattern 2012)*
   A. Trauma
   B. Alcohol
   C. Smoking
   D. Drug abuse
Ans. is 'A' Trauma

2. In trigger finger the level of tendon sheath constriction is found at the level of: *(AIIMS May 2005, AIIMS 96)*
   A. Middle phalanx
   B. Proximal interphalangeal joint
   C. Proximal phalanx
   D. Metacarpophalangeal joint
Ans. is 'D' Metacarpophalangeal joint

3. Trigger finger is: *(NB 2000, Orissa 90)*
   A. A feature of carpal tunnel syndrome
   B. Injury to fingers while operating a gun
   C. Stenosis tenovaginitis of flexor tendon of affected finger
   D. Any of the above
Ans. is 'C' Stenosis tenovaginitis of flexor tendon of affected finger

4. Trigger finger occurs in: *(PGI 98, Delhi 94)*
   A. Rheumatoid arthritis
   B. Trauma
   C. Osteosarcoma
   D. Osteoarthritis
Ans. is 'A' Rheumatoid arthritis; 'B' Trauma

5. Cause of trigger finger is: *(AIIMS Sept 1996)*
   A. Thickening of the fibrous tendon sheath
   B. Following local trauma
   C. Unaccustomed activity
   D. All of the above
Ans. is 'D' All of the above

6. Pulley involved in trigger finger: *(AIIMS 93)*
   A. A1
   B. A2
   C. A3
   D. A4
Ans. is 'A' A1

GANGLION: MORE COMMON IN FEMALES

It is most common soft tissue tumors (swelling) of hand and wrist. It arises from leakage of synovial fluid from a joint or tendon sheath. It is a unilocular cystic structure filled with mucinous fluid but without a synovial or epithelial lining. In most cases, stalk can be identified, communicating between the cyst and adjacent joint or tendon sheath. It usually develops on **dorsal surface of scapholunate ligament.** Back of wrist is the commonest site.

The three most common location of ganglion are:
1. Dorsal wrist (from scapholunate joint > palmar wrist radioscaphoid or scaphotrapezial joint),
2. Digital flexor sheath and
3. Distal interphalangeal joint.
   Age: 20–40 years.

Treatment of ganglion

1. Usually unnecessary and it may resolve spontaneously.
2. Aspiration to reassure the patient.
3. Pressure symptoms (e.g. Nerve) – removal.

Compound palmar ganglion is chronic inflammation of common sheath of flexor tendon both above and below flexor retinaculum causing hour glass swelling. **RA and tuberculosis are the commonest cause.**

MULTIPLE CHOICE QUESTIONS

1. True about Ganglion cyst: *(PGI MAY 2017)*
   A. Most common in young male
   B. Contain synovial fluid
   C. Arise from extensor retinaculum
   D. It usually arise from the lunotriquetral joint
   E. Surgical treatment is excision of cyst
Ans. is 'B' Contain synovial fluid; 'C' Arise from extensor retinaculum; 'E' Surgical treatment is excision of cyst

2. Ganglion: *(PGI Nov 2015)*
   A. Cystic tumor of hand
   B. Solid tumor of hand
   C. Treated by enucleation
   D. Unilocular
   E. Filled with mucinous fluid
Ans. is 'A' Cystic tumor of hand; 'D' Unilocular and 'E' Filled with mucinous fluid

3. True about ganglion: *(PGI Dec 03)*
   A. Common in volar aspect
   B. Seen adjacent to tendon sheath
   C. Communicates with joints cavity and tendon sheath
   D. It is unilocular
Ans. is 'A' Common in volar aspect; 'B' Seen adjacent to tendon sheath; 'C' Communicates with joints cavity and tendon sheath and 'D' It is unilocular

4. Compound palmar ganglion is: (UP 97)
   A. Tuberculosis affection of ulnar bursa
   B. Pyogenic affection of ulnar bursa
   C. Non-specific affection of ulnar bursa
   D. Ulnar bursitis due to compound injury

Ans. is 'A' Tuberculosis affection of ulnar bursa

BURSITIS

Bursitis	Site
Student's elbow/miners elbow	Olecranon bursitis
Housemaid's knee	**Prepatellar bursitis (commonest)**
Clergyman's knee	Infrapatellar bursitis (superficial bursa)
Weaver's bottom	Ischial bursitis
Tailor's ankle	Lateral malleolus bursitis
Bunion	Medial side of great toe-1st metatarsal head bursitis
Bunionette	5th toe of foot-5th metatarsal head bursitis

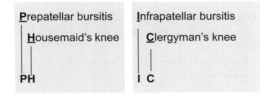

Four bursa communicate with synovial cavity of knee joint
1. Suprapatellar bursa
2. Popliteus bursa (deep to distal quadriceps)
3. Anserine bursa (deep to tendinous attachments of sartorius, gracilis and semitendinous)
4. Gastrocnemius bursa.

Tubercular bursitis is most common in trochanteric bursa (gluteal bursa) > bursa-anserine > compound palmar bursa > deltoid bursa > radial/ulnar long flexor bursa.

Swelling of Knee

In front of joint
Prepatellar bursitis/Infrapatellar bursitis

Medial Side
Bursa pes anserine is between tendons of sartorius, gracilis, semitendinosus muscles and tibial collateral ligament.

On Back of Knee
Semimembranosus bursa between semimembranosus and medial head of gastrocnemius.

Morrant Baker's cyst or popliteal cyst-centrally located in popliteal region often bilateral, in > 40 years age group
- It is pressure diverticulum of synovial membrane so it can be compressed
- Prominent on extension and reduced on flexion
- Usually secondary to osteoarthritis/RA/pigmented Villonodular synovitis/meniscal injury
- Swelling is soft and fluctuant

- No transillumination (since muscles are surrounding it)
- Excision if symptomatic.

MULTIPLE CHOICE QUESTIONS

1. Bakers cyst is a type of: (DNB June 2017)
   A. Pulsion diverticulum of knee joint
   B. Retention cyst
   C. Bursitis
   D. Benign tumor

Ans. is 'A' Pulsion diverticulum of knee joint

2. Bursa involved in Clergyman's knee: (CET July 2016)
   A. Prepatellar bursa   B. Infrapatellar bursa
   C. Olecranon bursa   D. Ischial bursa

Ans. is 'B' Infrapatellar bursa

3. Ischial bursitis is also known as: (NEET Pattern 2013)
   A. Clergyman's knee   B. Housernaid's knee
   C. Weaver's bottom   D. Student's elbow

Ans. is 'C' Weaver's bottom

4. Bunion is commonly seen at: (NEET Pattern 2016, 2013)
   A. Great toe MTP joint B. Medial malleolus
   C. Lateral malleolus   D. Shin of tibia

Ans. is 'A' Great toe MTP joint

5. Housemaid's knee is bursitis of:
   (NEET Pattern 2012)(AIIMS May 1995)
   A. Prepatellar bursa   B. Infrapatellar bursa
   C. Olecranon   D. Ischial bursa

Ans. is 'A' Prepatellar bursa

6. Prepatellar bursitis is: (NEET Pattern 2012)
   A. Housemaid's knee   B. Clergyman's knee
   C. Tailor's knee   D. Tubercular knee

Ans. is 'A' Housemaid's knee

7. Olecranon bursitis: (NEET Pattern 2012)
   A. Tennis elbow   B. Golfer's elbow
   C. Student's elbow   D. Lesser leagues elbow

Ans. is 'C' Student's elbow

8. Pes planus ligament stretched is: (NEET Pattern 2012)
   A. Calcaneonavicular   B. Talofibular
   C. Calcaneofibular   D. Deltoid

Ans. is 'A' Calcaneonavicular

9. Site of TB bursitis: (PGI Dec 07) (PGI June 03)
   A. Prepatellar   B. Subacromial
   C. Subdeltoid   D. Subpatellar
   E. Trochanteric

Ans. is 'E' Trochanteric

Tubercular bursitis is most common in trochanteric bursa (gluteal bursa) > bursa-anserine > compound palmar bursa > deltoid bursa > long flexor tendons.

10. Which of the following cysts is medially situated? (NB 1991)
   A. Housemaid's knee   B. Clergyman's knee
   C. Bursa anserine   D. Morrant Baker's cyst

Ans. is 'C' Bursa anserine

Bursa pes anserine is between tendons of sartorius, gracilis, semitendinosus muscles and tibial collateral ligament.

HALLUX VALGUS

- It is outward/lateral deviation of great toe.
- It is the **commonest of the foot deformities** (and probably of all musculoskeletal deformities).
- Splaying of forefoot, with varus angulation of 1st metatarsal, predispose lateral angulation of great toe in people who wear shoes.

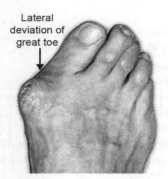

Fig. 14.15: Hallux valgus

- Overriding or under riding of 2nd toe can take place.
- Metatarsus primus varus may be congenital or result from loss of muscle tone in forefoot in elderly. It is also common in rheumatoid arthritis. Family history is obtained in 60%.

Elements of Deformity are:

- Lateral deviation and rotation of hallux, together with prominence of medial side of head of 1st metatarsal (bunion).
- Prominence of 1st metatarsal head is due to subluxation of metatarsophalangeal joint; there may be an overlying bursa and thickened soft tissue.
- In long standing cases metatarsophalangeal joint becomes osteoarthritic and osteophytes may develop.
- In adolescent and young it is wise to try conservative measures first, mainly because surgical correction in this age group carries 20–40% recurrence rate.
- Relief of pain is good after surgery in adults.
- Treatment is by change in shoewear or by brace.
- Surgery may be indicated in case of painful hallux valgus.
- The surgical options are **chevron osteotomy** or by arthrodesis.

MULTIPLE CHOICE QUESTIONS

1. Identify the abnormality shown in the following picture: *(AIIMS Nov 2015)*

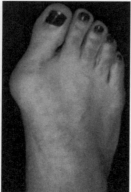

   A. Hallux valgus B. Hallux varus
   C. Rheumatoid nodule D. Subcutaneous nodule
   Ans. is 'A' Hallux valgus

2. Which of the following is true about hallux valgus? *(NEET 2015)*
   A. Great toe points laterally
   B. Great toe points medially
   C. Lateral angulation of the 1st metatarsophalangeal joint
   D. Dorsal angulation of the 1st metatarsophalangeal joint
   Ans. is 'A' Great toe points laterally

3. Hallux valgus means: *(Andhra 2000)*
   A. Outward deviation of great toe
   B. Inward deviation of great toe
   C. Outward deviation of fifth toe
   D. Inward deviation of fifth toe
   Ans. is 'A' Outward deviation of great toe

4. Hallux valgus is associated with all except: *(PGI Dec 2000)*
   A. An exostosis on the medial side of the head of the first metatarsal
   B. A bunion
   C. Osteoarthritis of the metatarsophalangeal joint
   D. Over-riding or under-riding of the second toe by the third
   Ans. is 'A' An exostosis on the medial side of the head of the first metatarsal

5. In hallux valgus surgery, the patients who are likely to be most satisfied are: *(AIIMS 95)*
   A. Those with pain
   B. Those with hammer toe
   C. Those with metatarsus primus varus
   D. Young age
   Ans. is 'A' Those with pain
   Relief of pain is good after surgery in adults of hallux valgus.

SUPRAPATELLAR PLICA OR PLICA SYNDROME

- In 5–20% knees there is a fold of plica (Synovial fold) in suprapatellar region that can undergo chronic inflammation, trauma, scarring and can cause signs and symptoms of torn meniscus (locking).
- Best diagnosis is by—Arthroscopy.
- Treatment—initially conservative—NSAIDs and quadriceps exercises if not relieved surgical excision by arthroscopy.

CHONDROMALACIA PATELLAE

- There is anterior knee pain and there is degeneration of articular cartilage of patella (basal degeneration)
- There is decrease in sulfated mucopolysaccharidosis in cartilage
- Seen in adolescent females and patient has chief complaint of difficulty in climbing stairs
   Movie sign—"Theater sign" increased pain on getting up after prolonged sitting
   Treatment—Nonoperative—NSAIDs/quadriceps/hamstrings exercises
   Operative—Release of lateral retinaculum
   Sequelae—Patellofemoral arthritis in which there is uniform pain on all knee movements.

MULTIPLE CHOICE QUESTIONS

1. Which of the following is a false statement regarding patellofemoral stress syndrome? *(JIPMER May 2016)*
   A. Difficulty in standing from prolonged sitting
   B. Difficulty in climbing stairs
   C. Pain during intense sporting activities
   D. Pain on posterior aspect of knee

Ans. is 'D' Pain on posterior aspect of knee

Patellofemoral sterss syndrome:
- Anterior knee pain
  - Increases on stairs
  - Increases after standing from prolonged sitting (Movie sign)
- Young females
- Vastus medialis obliques weakness. (Lateral structures stronger)
- Increased Q angle and genu valgus
  Rx.: Correct muscle imbalance
  Complication may develop patellofemoral arthritis.

2. A 15-year-old Female complains of anterior knee pain, increased on climbing stairs and getting up after prolonged sitting. Diagnosis is: *(AI 2011)*
   A. Chondromalacia patellae   B. Bipartite patellae
   C. Plica syndrome   D. Patellofemoral arthritis

Ans. is 'A' Chondromalacia patellae
   - Plica syndrome presents with meniscal symptoms of locking.
   - Patellofemoral arthritis will be seen at a later age and will have pain in all movements of knee.
   - Bipartite patella is congenital fragmentation of patella and is usually asymptomatic.

PLANTAR FASCIITIS

Plantar fasciitis (PF) is a **painful inflammatory process of the plantar fascia.**

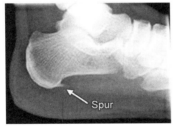

Fig. 14.16: Heel X-ray with heel spur

It is commonly associated with long periods of **weight bearing.** Among non-athletic populations, it is associated with a **high body mass index.** The pain is usually felt on the underside of the heel and is often most intense with the first steps of the day.

The diagnosis of plantar fasciitis is usually made by clinical examination.

An incidental finding associated with this condition is a **heel spur**, a small bony **calcification** on the **calcaneus** heel bone, in which case it is the underlying plantar fasciitis that produces the pain, and not the spur itself. The condition is responsible for the creation of the spur; the plantar fasciitis is not caused by the spur.

Some current studies suggest that plantar fasciitis is not actually inflamed plantar fascia, but merely an inflamed **flexor digitorum brevis muscle** (FDB) belly.

Treatment

Treatment options for plantar fasciitis include rest **physical therapy, cold therapy, heat therapy, orthotics (K.L. splint)** anti-inflammatory medications, injection of **corticosteroids** and surgery in **refractory** case.

MULTIPLE CHOICE QUESTIONS

1. K.L. splint is used for: *(NEET Pattern 2012)*
   A. Fracture tibia   B. Plantar fasciitis
   C. de Quervain's tenosynovitis   D. Tennis elbow

Ans. is 'B' Plantar fasciitis

2. Ligament stretched in flat foot: *(NEET Pattern 2012)*
   A. Calcaneonavicular ligament
   B. Anterior talofibular ligament
   C. Posterior talofibular ligament
   D. Calcaneofibular ligament

Ans. is 'A' Calcaneonavicular ligament

3. Impingement syndrome refers to: *(NEET Pattern 2012)*
   A. Nerve entrapped in closed space
   B. Soft tissues entrapment
   C. Arterial injury   D. Venous engorgement

Ans. is 'B' Soft tissues entrapment

MEARY'S ANGLE

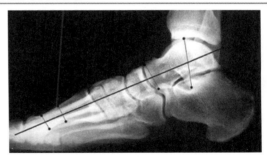

The longitudinal axis of 1st metatarsal and talus forms zero degree angle-Meary's angle

Fig. 14.17: Meary's angle

- Meary's Angle > 4 degrees (convex upward) pes cavus
- Meary's Angle > 4 degrees (convex downward) pes planus

PES PLANUS (FLAT FOOT)

- Flat foot refers to obliterated medial longitudinal arch
- Heel is often in valgus called as planovalgus
- Pes Planus is of 2 types: (Differentiated by Jack's test)
  - Flexible: Disappears on non-weight bearing. Management is conservative
  - Rigid: Due to Congenital Vertical talus or RA or Infection or tarsal coalition or tibialis posterior dysfunction. They often require surgical intervention
- Tarsal Coalition is autosomal dominant
  - Fusion of tarsal bones (Talocalcaneal, calcaneonavicular and talonavicular)

- Present at birth but becomes symptomatic later when fibrous connection becomes rigid bar
- Stiff flat foot (with spasm of peroneal muscles).

Diagnosis is by X-ray/CT scan (better)
1. Initially conservative if fails
2. Surgery: Excision of coalition bar or arthrodesis.

MULTIPLE CHOICE QUESTIONS

1. All are true regarding pes planus except: *(PGI May 2016)*
   A. There is collapse of medial longitudinal arch
   B. The heel becomes valgus and foot pronates at the subtalar-mid complex joint
   C. Jack's test differentiates between flexible and rigid deformity
   D. One of the common type of tarsal coalition is calcaneo-navicular
   E. Tarsal coalition is inherited as X-linked recessive condition

Ans. is 'E' Tarsal coalition is inherited as X-linked recessive condition

2. Pes Planus is seen in: *(PGI Nov 2015)*
   A. Perthes disease
   B. Congenital vertical talus
   C. CTEV
   D. RA
   E. Infection

Ans. is 'B' Congenital vertical talus; 'D' RA and 'E' Infection

15 Peripheral Nerve Injury

SEDDON'S CLASSIFICATION

Neuropraxia: Tinel's Sign Negative
- It is temporary physiological disruption of nerve impulse conduction. The loss of function is incomplete.
- Complete recovery takes place in 3–6 weeks and it comes back like lightening, i.e. completely recovers in one go.
- No Wallerian degeneration takes place and **Tinel's sign is negative**.
    - Crutch palsy—Pressure palsy (radial nerve or part of brachial plexus injured)
    - Saturday night palsy—Pressure palsy (radial nerve)
    - Tourniquet palsy—Pressure palsy
- Few traumatic nerve injuries are neuropraxia.

Axonotmesis: Tinel's Sign Positive and Progressive
- It is Axon breakdown, **Tinel's sign is positive**, Motor March is seen (recovery of muscles takes place in the order of their nerve supply from proximal to distal direction).
- Recovery is usually not complete.
- Seen in closed fractures and dislocations.

Neurotmesis: Tinel's Sign is Positive and Nonprogressive
- Complete anatomic section of the nerve. Tinel's sign is positive and nonprogressive.
- No recovery without surgical intervention. Even with intervention may not have complete recovery.
- Degeneration distal to injuries (Secondary or Wallerian degeneration)
- Degeneration in proximal segment (Primary or retrograde degeneration)
- At proximal end forms—Neuroma
- At distal end forms—Glioma

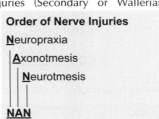

Order of Nerve Injuries
Neuropraxia
Axonotmesis
Neurotmesis
NAN

Sunderland Classification in Relation to Seddon's:

Type I	– Neuropraxia
Type II, III, IV	– Axonotmesis
Type V	– Neurotmesis

Sunderland classified nerve injuries into five types but sometimes sixth-degree (Mackinnon) or mixed injuries occur in which a nerve trunk is partially severed and the remaining part of the trunk sustains fourth, third, second, or rarely even first-degree injury.

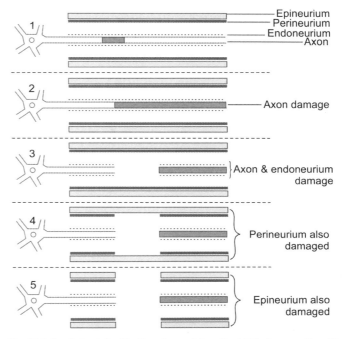

Fig. 15.1: Sunderland classification of nerve injury: **Type IV behaves as Type V**

The five grades of nerve injury

Grade		Continuity of structure				Clinical features			
Sunderland	Seddon	Epineurium	Perineurium	Endoneurium	Axon	Outcome	Treatment	Tinel's	Electrophysiology
1.	Neurapraxia	+	+	+	Block	Good	Expectant	Absent	Expectant
2.	Axonotmesis	+	+	+	Damage	Good/Fair	Expectant	Advancing	Conduction block at injury site, Denervation on EMG
3.	Axonotmesis	+	+	Damage	Damage	Fair/Poor	Expectant/repair/graft	Advancing	As2
4.	Axonotmesis	+	Damage	Damage	Damage	Poor	Repair/graft	Variable	As2
5.	Neurotmesis	Damage	Damage	Damage	Damage	Poor	Repair/graft	Static	No conduction in NCV, EMG denervation

Autonomous Zone of Nerves: Exclusively Supplied by that Particular Nerve

- Median Nerve—Tip of index finger, middle finger.
- Ulnar Nerve—Tip of little finger
- Radial Nerve—1st web space on dorsum of hand
- Deep peroneal nerve—Dorsum of 1st web space on foot

Tinel's Sign: (Records regeneration rate) by tapping on the nerve course from distal to proximal direction tingling is felt at the sprouting nerve ends till the distal course of the nerve (Law of projection) and it disappears as myelinization takes place (Rate of Recovery of Nerve is 1 mm/day) Tinel's is positive and progressive in axonotmesis and Sunderland 2 and 3.

Diagnostic Tests for Nerve Injuries:

- *EMG:* Denervation fibrillation potentials. Appears at 2–3 weeks then spontaneous fibrillation.
- **EMG is the earliest indicator of nerve recovery.**
- *Nerve conduction study:* Reduced in axonotmesis and neurotmesis but cannot differentiate between the 2. Normal nerve conduction velocity on day 10 goes toward neuropraxia. No conduction will indicate neurotmesis.
- *Sweat Test:* In autonomous area, presence of sweat rules out complete injury as sweat fibers are most resistant to compression.
- *MRI:* Value only in nerve root lesions (e.g. Brachial plexus injuries).

Management:

1. In closed injury (Neuropraxia or axonotmesis or Sunderland 1–3)
   - *Splints:*
   - Axillary N – Shoulder abduction splint
   - Radial N – Cock-up splint
   - **Median N/Ulnar N – Knuckle bender splint**
   - Common peroneal N – Foot drop splint
   - Brachial plexus injury – Aeroplane splint
2. **In open injuries**
   - *Primary repair:* Within 6–8 hrs
   - *Delayed primary repair:* 7–18 days
   - *Secondary repair:* After 18 days

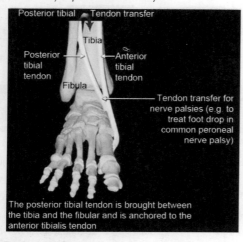

Fig. 15.2: Tendon transfer

3. Nerve that may be used as nerve donors:
   - Sural nerve: MC used
   - Saphenous nerve
4. Neurotization that is transfer of fibers of an intact nerve to a damaged nerve to augment its functions.
5. If nerve recovery does not take place tendon transfer can be carried out, e.g. modified jones transfer for radial nerve palsy and tibialis posterior transfer for foot drop. Most common tendon for transfer is Palmaris Longus.

Prognosis after Nerve Suturing

Radial nerve (best) > median nerve > *ulnar nerve* > *Peroneal nerve* > Sciatic nerve (worst prognosis).

Best prognosis after nerve repair: Radial nerve. After repair of the radial nerve the prognosis for regeneration is more favorable than for any other major nerve in the upper extremity, primarily because is **predominantly a motor nerve** and secondarily because the muscles innervated by it are not involved in the finer movements of the fingers and hand.

Worst prognosis after nerve repair in the upper extremity: Ulnar nerve: As it is mainly as sensory nerve and also is concerned with finer movements of the hands and fingers.

Worst prognosis after nerve repair: Sciatic nerve. Because of the extensive retrograde neuronal degeneration, intraneural intermixing of regenerating fibers with loss of fiber localization and degenerative changes in the distal muscles that must remain denervated for a long time.

Good Prognostic Factors

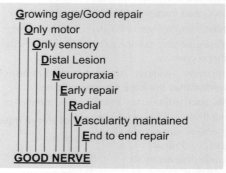

Nerve Injuries in Fractures and Dislocations

Nerve	Trauma	Effect
Axillary nerve	Dislocation of the shoulder (Anterior and Inferior)	Deltoid palsy
Radial nerve	Fracture shaft of the humerus (**lower 1/3rd**)	Wrist drop
Ulnar nerve	Fracture medial epicondyle humerus	Claw hand
Sciatic nerve	Posterior dislocation of the hip	Foot drop
Common peroneal nerve	Knee dislocation/fracture of neck of the fibula	Foot drop
Posterior interosseous nerve	Monteggia fracture	Finger drop
Anterior interosseous nerve	Supracondylar fracture humerus	Kiloh-Nevin sign
Median nerve	Supracondylar fracture of humerus	Pointing index

Iatrogenic Injuries: Usual Incidence < 3%

MULTIPLE CHOICE QUESTIONS

1. Tinel's sign used: *(NEET Dec 2016)*
   A. To assess the severity of damage of nerve
   B. To classify the type of nerve injury
   C. To locate the site of nerve injury
   D. To assess the regeneration

Ans. is 'D' To assess the regeneration

2. Tinel's sign is: *(NEET Dec 2016)*
   A. Sensation on tapping the nerve
   B. Numbness in the region of the nerve of inflating the pneumatic cuff
   C. Tingling on flexion of the joint
   D. Applying direct pressure

Ans. is 'A' Sensation on tapping the nerve

3. Following nerve injury, the injured nerve regenerates at a rate of: *(AI 2016)*
   A. 0.001 cm/day   B. 0.1 cm/day
   C. 10 mm/day   D. 0.0001 cm/day

Ans. is 'B' 0.1 cm/day

4. Seddon's Classification all are true except: *(AI 2016)*
   A. Complete anatomic division of nerve is classified as Neurotmesis
   B. Axonotmesis has Tinel's sign positive and progressive
   C. Neurotmesis has complete recovery with/without surgical intervention
   D. Saturday night palsy involves radial nerve

Ans. is 'C' Neurotmesis has complete recovery with/without surgical intervention

5. Tendon most commonly used for tendon transfer? *(JIPMER MAY 2016)*
   A. Palmaris longus   B. Flexor carpi ulnaris
   C. Patellofemoral tendon   D. Gracilis

Ans. is 'A' Palmaris longus

6. Sunderland classification is used for: *(NEET 2015)*
   A. Nerve injury   B. Muscle injury
   C. Tendon injury   D. Ligament injury

Ans. is 'A' Nerve injury

7. Nerve biopsy in leprosy is usually taken from: *(PGM-CET 2015)*
   A. Ulnar   B. Median
   C. Lateral popliteal D. Sural

Ans. is 'D' Sural

8. While performing flexor tendon graft repair, graft is taken from: *(NEET Pattern 2013)*
   A. Plantaris   B. Palmaris longus
   C. Extensor digitorum D. Extensor indicis

Ans. is 'B' Palmaris longus

9. A patient woke up in the morning with inability to extend digits rest sensory and motor examination of hand was normal. What is nerve involved in this patient?
   A. C8 T1 nerve roots *(AIIMS Nov 2013)*
   B. Posterior interosseous nerve
   C. Radial nerve
   D. Lower brachial plexus

Ans. is 'B' Posterior interosseous nerve

10. Saturday night palsy is which type of nerve injury? *(NEET Pattern 2013)*
    A. Neuropraxia   B. Axonotmesis
    C. Neurotmesis   D. Complete sect ion

Ans. is 'A' Neuropraxia

11. A politician was shot by a gun in back in political rally at T8 level, after which he developed paraplegia. The fact that the injured nerve is not able to regenerate is due to all the reasons except: *(AIIMS Nov 2012)*
    A. No endoneurial tube   B. Glial scar formation
    C. Absence of growth factors D. Lack of myelin inhibitors

Ans. is 'D' Lack of myelin inhibitors

Explanation

Potential ways to improve neuronal regeneration in the CNS:
1. Act on the secondary cell death process: so block apoptosis and help neurons survive.
2. *Neurotrophic factors:* BDNF (brain derived neurotrophic factor) is the best studied. It does help injured neurons survive. Also helps axons grow. But, should be viewed with caution since injecting a growth factor into the CNS can cause uncontrolled growth (potentially carcinogenic).
3. Remove growth inhibitors:
   - Astrocyte associated: As part of scarring process, astrocytes lay down chondroitin sulfate proteoglycears. The signal from the chondroitin sulfate proteoglycans acts as a stop signal for axon growth. Adding a chondroitinase (cleaves off chondroitin-sulfate) promotes axon regrowth in injured area.
   - Myelin-associated inhibitors (from oligodendrocytes): there are 3 diff ones that are all recognized by axons as stop signals: myelin-associated glycoprotein (MAG), oligodendrocyte myelin glycoprotein (OMgp), and Nogo. A cell surface receptor binds any one of the 3, activates a protein kinase involved in the breakdown of cytoskeletal elements that are needed for process outgrowth. A TAJ knock-out of the myelin associated inhibitors works to inhibit the inhibitor and promote axon growth.
4. *PNS nerve graft:* Provides basal lamina (called "bands of bungner"). Works to some extent. But, unclear if it is the nerve graft itself that is working, or the fact that you've caused inflammation and subsequently dumped in a bunch of activated macrophages.
5. Glial Scar inhibits nerve regeneration.

12. Which of the following is true about nerve injury? *(AIIMS Nov 2012)*
    A. In all cases of open wound with clinical signs of nerve injury, nerve exploration should always be done
    B. Nerve conduction velocity is best predictor within 48 hrs of injury
    C. Positive Tinel's sign indicates the accurate location of lesion
    D. Traction nerve injury should be repaired immediately

Ans. is 'A' In all cases of open wound with clinical signs of nerve injury, nerve exploration should always be done

Explanation
- Nerve injuries with wound should always be explored and If nerve is in continuity then it is treated like closed injury. If there is clean cut then it is primarily repaired and if ends are crushed debridement is done and then repaired later.

- Nerve conduction velocity usually predicts about nerve injury between days 10 and 14.

  Tinel's sign can predict about the rate of nerve recovery its speed of regeneration based upon the level of unmyelinated free nerve endings.

- Traction nerve injuries are managed with expectant approach of wait and watch for recovery and then if recovery does not take place then it needs exploration and repair.

13. Tinel's sign is used for: *(NEET Pattern 2012)*
    A. To assess the severity of damage of nerve
    B. To classify the type of nerve injury
    C. To locate the site of nerve injury
    D. To assess the recovery

Ans. is 'D' To assess the recover

14. Tinel's sign is positive and progressive in: *(NEET Pattern 2012)*
    A. Axonotmesis   B. Neurotmesis
    B. Neuropraxia   D. All of the above

Ans. is 'A' Axonotmesis

- *Tinel's Sign:* Records regeneration rate by tapping on the nerve course from distal to proximal direction tingling is felt at the sprouting nerve ends and it disappears as myelinization takes place (Rate of Recovery: 1 mm/day) Tinel's is positive and progressive in axonotmesis and Sunderland 2 and 3).

15. Foot drop is due to palsy of: *(NEET Pattern 2012)*
    A. Superficial peroneal nerve   B. Deep peroneal nerve
    C. Femoral nerve   D. Obturator nerve

Ans. is 'B' Deep peroneal nerve

16. Nerve with best recovery: *(NEET Pattern 2012)*
    A. Ulnar   B. Median
    C. Sciatic D. Radial

Ans. is 'D' Radial

17. Motor march is seen in: *(NEET Pattern 2012)*
    A. Axonotmesis   B. Neuropraxia
    C. Neurotmesis   D. All of the above

Ans. is 'A' Axonotmesis

18. A patient after sleeping on chair with hanging arm whole night presents with weakness in muscles supplied by ulnar nerve, causing claw hand it is managed by:
    A. Electrophysiological studies *(May AIIMS 2012)*
    B. Knuckle bender splint and wait and watch
    C. Exploration of the nerve
    D. Tendon transfer

Ans. is 'B' Knuckle bender splint and wait and watch

- Neuropraxia is physiological block in nerve conduction and this is a case of Saturday night palsy causing ulnar nerve symptoms the management is expectant, i.e. wait and watch and till the meantime splint is given that is knuckle bender splint for ulnar nerve palsy.

19. Prognosis after secondary nerve suturing is better in pure than in mixed ones. Based on this criterion, which one of the following nerves should be given the best result after suturing in identical conditions?
    (AIIMS May 2008, UP 97, Karnataka 1990, AMC 97)
    A. Common peroneal nerve   B. Radial nerve
    C. Ulnar nerve   D. Median nerve

Ans. is 'B' Radial nerve

20. A pole vaulter had a fall during pole vaulting and had paralysis of the arm. Which of the following investigations gives the best recovery prognosis. *(AIIMS Nov 2003)*
    A. Electromyography
    B. Muscle biopsy
    C. Strength duration curve
    D. Creatine phosphokinase levels

Ans. is 'A' Electromyography

- EMG (electromyography) is by far the most reliable and effective test to predict about nerve recovery.

21. Nerve suturing in a clean cut injury is done best in:
    A. 6 hours   B. 12 hours *(Delhi 1999)*
    C. After one day D. After two days

Ans. is 'A' 6 hours

22. Following indicate better prognosis in nerve injury except: *(JIPMER 1993)*
    A. Neuroproxia   B. Younger age
    C. Pure motor nerve injury D. Proximal injury

Ans. is 'D' Proximal injury

23. Rate of regeneration of severed nerve is: *(Andhra 1991)*
    A. 0.1 mm/day   B. 1 mm/day
    C. 1 cm/day   D. None

Ans. is 'B' 1 mm/day

24. Tourniquet paralysis is an unfortunate complication leads to: *(Karnataka 1990)*
    A. Neuropraxia   B. Axonotmesis
    C. Neurotmesis   D. None of the above

Ans. is 'A' Neuropraxia

25. In Seddon's classification, complete division of nerve is: *(Rohtak 1989)*
    A. Neuropraxia
    B. Axonotmesis
    C. Neurotmesis
    D. None of the above

Ans. is 'C' Neurotmesis

BRACHIAL PLEXUS INJURY

Brachial plexus is formed by confluence of **nerve roots from C5 to T1**. It is vulnerable to injury by either a stab wound or severe traction caused by a fall on the side of neck or the shoulder.

Traction injuries are generally classified as supraclavicular (65%), infraclavicular (25%) and combined (10%). Supraclavicular lesions typically occur in motorcycle accident as the cyclist collides with the ground and his neck and shoulder are wrenched apart (may be associated with subclavian artery injury). Infraclavicular lesions are usually associated with fractures or dislocations of the shoulder and axillary artery injury. Avulsion of nerve root from spinal cord is a preganglionic lesion, i.e. disruption proximal to dorsal root ganglion; this cannot recover, and it is surgically irreparable. Rupture of a nerve root distal to ganglion, or of a trunk or peripheral nerve, is a postganglionic lesion, which is surgically reparable and potentially capable of recovery.

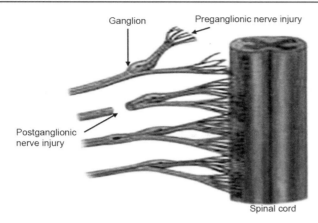

Fig. 15.3: Nerve injury

Site of Injury: Upper Trunk

Upper C_5 and C_6 roots of brachial plexus—Erb's point where 6 nerves meet.
1. Musculocutaneous N
2. Axillary N
3. Nerve to subclavius
4. Supra scapular N
5. C_5
6. C_6

Deformity and Loss of Movements 'FAbEr'S Lost in Erb's

Policeman/Waiter/Porter's tip hand

- Arm: adducted and medially rotated
- Forearm: extended and pronated
- Arm hangs limply by the side

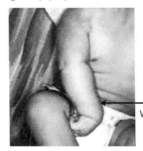

Fig. 15.4: Erb's palsy

Feature	Preganglionic lesion	Postganglionic
Site	Proximal to dorsal root ganglion, i.e. avulsion of nerve root from spinal cord	Distal to dorsal root ganglion, i.e. disruption of nerve root (distal), trunk or peripheral nerve
Surgical repair	Irreparable	Reparable
Prognosis	Poor	Better
Histamine test	Positive	Negative

Histamine test: The cutaneous axon reflexes (Histamine test) have been found useful in differentiating preganglionic Intraspinal lesions from postganglionic extra spinal lesions. These reflexes are elicited by placing a drop of histamine on the skin along the distribution of the nerve being examined. After the skin is scratched through the drop of histamine, a sequential response consisting of cutaneous vasodilatation, wheal formation, and flare response normally is seen. If the nerve is interrupted proximal to the ganglion, anesthesia exists along its cutaneous course, but the normal axon response will be seen because this **reflex is a local reflex functioning only on postganglionic region.** If the injury is distal to the ganglion, there also is anesthesia along the course of the nerve, and vasodilatation and wheal formation are seen, but the flare response is absent; this negative axonal response suggests injury at a postganglionic site where recovery might be possible. **Thus positive histamine indicates postganglionic region is intact hence the injury is preganglionic hence poor prognosis.**

- Lost movements—All movements opposite to the deformity would be lost, i.e.:
  - Loss of abduction and lateral rotation of arm
  - Loss of flexion and supination of forearm.

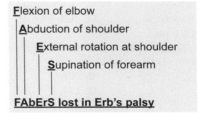

Klumpke's palsy (lower plexus injury) C8 and T1 nerve roots are involved it is much **less common, but more severe.** Wrist and finger flexors are weak and the intrinsic hand muscles are paralyzed. Sensation is lost in ulnar forearm and there may also be vasomotor impairment and unilateral Horner's syndrome. (Claw hand deformity is the usual outcome).

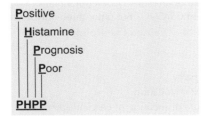

ERB'S PALSY—INJURY TO UPPER TRUNK

Erb's palsy (Best prognosis amongst brachial plexus injuries)

Erb's palsy is the commonest brachial plexus injury and commonest injury causing neurological deficit in upper limb.

Mode of Injury

Excessive downward stretching of shoulder on same side and head toward opposite side, e.g. Blow or fall on shoulder/delivery.

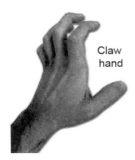

Fig. 15.5: Klumpke's palsy—claw hand

Complete plexus lesion involves all nerve roots there is flail limb and has poorest prognosis.

The best results of plexus reconstruction are obtained after early surgery. All efforts of nerve repair or nerve transfer are directed toward lesions involving C5 and C6. The objectives are to regain **shoulder abduction, elbow flexion,** wrist extension, finger flexion, and sensibility over the hand. **Aeroplane splint** is used for brachial plexus palsy.

Brachial Neuritis

Brachial neuritis consists of acute onset of severe shoulder or scapular pain followed over days to weeks by weakness of the proximal arm and shoulder girdle muscles innervated by the upper brachial plexus. The onset is often preceded by infection, recent illness, surgery, immunization, or even trauma.

Complete recovery occurs in 75% cases in 2 years.

MULTIPLE CHOICE QUESTIONS

1. What is true about Erb's Palsy? *(PGI Nov 2018)*
   A. Adduction + Internal rotation
   B. Supination seen   C. C5, C6 roots affected
   D. Lower trunk injury causes this deformity
   E. Claw hand is seen

Ans. is 'A' Adduction + Internal rotation; 'C' C5, C6 roots affected

2. Which of the following is not true about Klumpke's paralysis? *(DNB June 2017)*
   A. Involves lower trunk of brachial plexus
   B. Intrinsic muscles of hand are paralyzed
   C. Claw hand is a feature
   D. Horner's syndrome can never be associated

Ans. is 'D' Horner's syndrome can never be associated

3. Erb's palsy involves injury to: *(DNB June 2017)*
   A. C5, C6 roots   B. C6 C7 roots
   C. C7, C8 roots   D. C8, T1 roots

Ans. is 'A' C5, C6 roots

4. Brachial plexus injury with Horner's syndrome, nerve root level involved is. *(DNB June 2017)*
   A. C5   B. C6
   C. C7   D. T1

Ans. is 'D' T1

5. Which of the following deformity is evident in case of Erb's palsy? *(NEET 2015)*
   A. Policeman tip deformity   B. Winging of scapula
   C. Claw hand   D. Wrist drop

Ans. is 'A' Policeman tip deformity

6. Aeroplane splint is used in: *(NEET Pattern 2013)*
   A. Radial nerve injury   B. Ulnar nerve injury
   C. Brachial plexus injury   D. Scoliosis

Ans. is 'C' Brachial plexus injury

7. Muscles paralyzed in Erb's paralysis are all except: *(NEET Pattern 2013)*
   A. Biceps   B. Triceps
   C. Brachioradialis   D. Brachialis

Ans. is 'B' Triceps

8. Klumpke's paralysis involves: *(NEET Pattern 2012)*
   A. C1–2   B. C4–5
   C. C5–6   D. C8 T1

Ans. is 'D' C8 T1

9. Erb's palsy lesion is at: *(NEET Pattern 2012)*
   A. Upper trunk   B. Lower trunk
   C. Whole plexus   D. C5–C6

Ans. is 'A' Upper trunk

10. Erb's palsy all the movements are lost except: *(NEET Pattern 2012)*
    A. Supination
    B. External rotation at shoulder
    C. Abduction at shoulder
    D. Pronation

Ans. is 'D' Pronation

11. A 45-year-male present with abrupt onset, pain, weakness, loss of contour of shoulder and wasting of muscle of arm on 5th day of tetanus toxoid immunization in deltoid. Likely cause is: *(AIIMS May 09)*
    A. Radial nerve entrapment
    B. Thoracic outlet syndrome
    C. Brachial neuritis
    D. Hysteria

Ans. is 'C' Brachial neuritis

12. All are true regarding brachial plexus injury, except: *(AI 2006)*
    A. Preganglionic lesions have a better prognosis than postganglionic lesions
    B. Erb's palsy causes paralysis of the abductors and external rotators of the shoulder
    C. In Klumpke's palsy, Horner's syndrome may be present on the ipsilateral side
    D. Histamine test is useful to differentiate between the preganglionic and postganglionic lesions

Ans. is 'A' Preganglionic lesions have a better prognosis than postganglionic lesions
   – *Preganglionic lesions have a poor prognosis as these do not recover and are surgically irreparable. Postganglionic lesions have better prognosis than preganglionic lesions and histamine test is useful in making the distinction— Apley.*

13. All of the following muscles undergo paralysis after injury to C5 and C6 spinal nerves except: *(AIIMS Nov 04)*
    A. Biceps   B. Coracobrachialis
    C. Brachialis   D. Brachioradialis

Ans. is B' Coracobrachialis. Coracobrachialis as it receives its supply from C5/C6/C7 but other three only from C5 and C6.

14. Most common cause of neurological deficit in upper limb is: *(AIIMS Nov 1993)*
    A. Polio
    B. Erb's palsy
    C. C1–C2 dislocation
    D. Fracture dislocation of cervical spine

Ans. is 'B' Erb's palsy

MUSCULOCUTANEOUS NERVE INJURY

Musculocutaneous nerve supplies coracobrachialis, the biceps brachii and the brachialis, and is continued into the forearm as the lateral cutaneous nerve of the forearm. In its injury there is loss of flexion of elbow, supination of forearm and sensory loss on lateral aspect of forearm. It is damaged in shoulder dislocation, second common to axillary nerve.

Peripheral Nerve Injury

MULTIPLE CHOICE QUESTION

1. All of the following are features of musculocutaneous nerve injury at axilla except: *(AI 1998)*
    A. Loss of flexion of shoulder
    B. Loss of flexion at elbow
    C. Loss of supination of forearm
    D. Loss of sensation on radial side of forearm
Ans. is 'A' Loss of flexion of shoulder

AXILLARY NERVE INJURY

Axillary Nerve (C5–C6)

Injured in fracture of surgical neck humerus, shoulder dislocation (anterior and inferior) and intramuscular injections.

Motor
- Deltoid muscle palsy
- Loss of rounded contour of shoulder - giving shoulder a flattened appearance and produce hollow inferior to acromion
- Weakness of abduction (15°–90°)
- Teres minor palsy.

Sensory
- Lateral cutaneous nerve of arm
- Sensory loss over lower half of deltoid (regimental badge area).

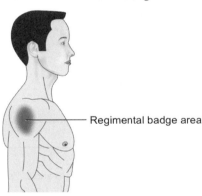
Regimental badge area

MULTIPLE CHOICE QUESTIONS

1. A patient has met with an accident and he cannot abduct his right arm. On examination there is paresthesia at the lateral aspect of right upper arm. X-ray showed fracture surgical neck of humerus. Which of the following muscle is also supplied by the involved nerve?
   (JIPMER May 2016)
    A. Subscapularis   B. Suprascapularis
    C. Infrascapularis   D. Teres minor
Ans. is 'D' Teres minor

2. Patient presented with Paresthesia and loss of sensation over lower part of deltoid. X-ray showed fracture surgical neck of humerus. Likely nerve to be involved is:
   (JIPMER Dec 2016)
    A. Musculocutaneous nerve B. Axillary nerve
    C. Radial nerve   D. Ulnar nerve
Ans. is 'B' Axillary nerve

3. Axillary nerve injury likely to be seen in: *(AI 2016)*
    A. Shoulder dislocation   B. Coracoid process fracture
    C. Hummers shaft fracture   D. Brachial plexus injury
Ans. is 'A' Shoulder dislocation

4. Child after a motor vehicle trauma is unable to abduct his arm. X-ray shows fracture around surgical neck humerus. Nerve likely to be injured: *(AI 2016)*
    A. Musculocutaneous nerve   B. Axillary nerve
    C. Radial nerve   D. Ulnar nerve
Ans. is 'B' Axillary nerve

5. A 21-year male with fracture surgical neck humerus presented with regimental badge sign and difficulty in abduction nerve most likely to be injured is:
   (JIPMER Nov 16)
    A. Axillary nerve injury   B. Suprascapular nerve injury
    C. Erb's palsy injury   D. Musculocutaneous nerve
Ans. is 'A' Axillary nerve injury

6. Axillary Nerve Injury is least likely in: *(AIIMS Nov 2015)*
    A. Shoulder dislocation
    B. Fracture proximal humerus
    C. Intramuscular injection
    D. Improper use of crutch
Ans. is 'D' Improper use of crutch

7. In axillary nerve paralysis, all the following are true except: *(NEET Pattern 2012)*
    A. Deltoid muscle is wasted
    B. Extension of shoulder with arm abducted to 90 degrees is impossible
    C. Small area of numbness is present over the shoulder region
    D. Patient cannot initiate abduction
Ans. is 'D' Patient cannot initiate abduction

8. All of the following features can be observed after the injury to axillary nerve, except: *(AI 2003)*
    A. Loss of rounded contour of shoulder
    B. Loss of sensation along lateral side of upper arm
    C. Loss of overhead abduction
    D. Atrophy of deltoid muscle
Ans. is 'C' Loss of overhead abduction

Abduction of Shoulder
Up to 15°
- Supraspinatus muscle
- Suprascapular N (C5 C6)

15° to 90°
- Deltoid muscle
- Axillary nerve **(C5 C6)**

Overhead abduction (>90°)
- Serratus anterior muscle (Nerve supply – Long thoracic nerve or N. of Bells – **C5 C6 C7**)
- Trapezius muscle (Spinal part of accessory nerve)

Axillary nerve supplies deltoid which is responsible for shoulder abduction of **15° to 90°**; so injury to axillary nerve would not affect overhead abduction.

MEDIAN/LABORER'S NERVE ($C_{5,6,7,8}T_1$)

A. **Injury at elbow level**
    1. Pronators are paralyzed so forearm is kept in supine position.

2. Long flexors are paralyzed (except FCU and FDP medial ½) so wrist flexion is weak and accompanied by adduction (paralysis of FCR and intact FCU).
3. Flexion of terminal phalanx of thumb is lost because of paralysis of FPL.
4. Flexion of interphalangeal joints of index and middle fingers is lost so there is pointing index or positive Ochsner clasp or Benediction test.

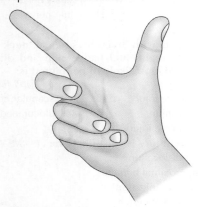

Fig. 15.6: Pointing index

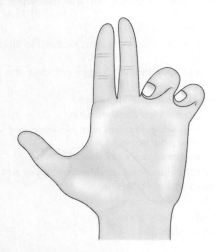

Fig. 15.7: Benediction test

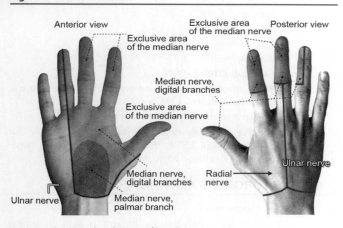

Fig. 15.8: Sensory distribution of hand

B. **Injury or compression of median nerve at wrist (e.g. Carpal tunnel syndrome) can be tested by**
1. **Pen test** for abductor pollicis brevis there is inability to touch the pen kept above the palm by thumb abduction.

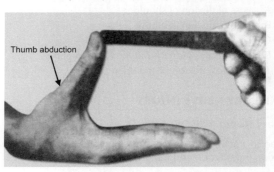

Fig. 15.9: Pen test

2. **Ape thumb deformity** (In median nerve palsy, the thumb is adducted and laterally rotated and lies in same plane as rest of finger, due to unopposed action of extensor pollicis longus (radial nerve) and adductor pollicis (ulnar nerve).

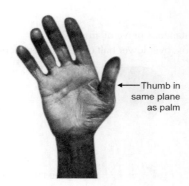

Fig. 15.10: Ape thumb deformity

3. **Loss of opposition**
4. Sensory loss lateral 3½ of digits and 2/3 palm (autonomous zone is tip of index and middle finger).
5. Anterior dislocation of lunate may cause median nerve compression, making its reduction an emergency.

Kiloh-Nevin sign (Flexor Digitorum Profundus-lateral 1/2 and Flexor Pollicis Longus) supplied by anterior interosseous nerve.

The pinch of thumb and index finger is strong if AIN is intact and this is called as Kiloh-Nevin sign.

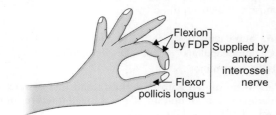

Fig. 15.11: Kiloh-Nevin sign—AIN

Note: AIN supplies: Flexor pollicis longus (FPL) + Pronator quadratus (PQ) + Flexor digitorum profundus (FDP) (Lateral 1/2)

Peripheral Nerve Injury

MULTIPLE CHOICE QUESTIONS

1. Image of dorsum of hand, which nerve gives sensory supply to this region: *(NEET Pattern 2019)*

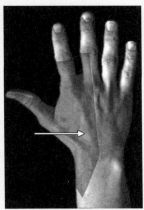

   A. PIN nerve
   B. Radial nerve
   C. Median nerve
   D. Ulnar nerve

   Ans. is 'B' Radial nerve

2. Patient presented with loss of sensations in the lateral three and a half fingers. Which of the following will be an additional finding in this patient? *(JIPMER May 2016)*
   A. Loss of sensation on thenar eminence
   B. Loss of sensation on hypothenar eminence
   C. Atrophy of adductor pollicis
   D. Opponens paralysis

   Ans. is 'D' Opponens paralysis

3. A patient can make his fist but unable to flex his index finger. Which nerve is affected in him?
   (JIPMER May 2016)
   A. Radial nerve
   A. Ulnar nerve
   C. Musculocutaneus nerve
   D. Median nerve

   Ans. is 'D' Median nerve

4. Nail bed of index finger is supplied by: *(AI 2016)*
   A. Median nerve
   B. Ulnar
   C. Palmar branch of median nerve
   D. Palmar branch of ulnar nerve

   Ans. is 'A' Median nerve

5. Damage to median nerve produces: *(NEET Pattern 2012)*
   A. Claw hand
   B. Winging of scapula
   C. Ape thumb
   D. Wrist drop

   Ans. is 'C' Ape thumb

6. Labourer's Nerve: *(NEET Pattern 2012)*
   A. Ulnar nerve
   B. Median nerve
   C. Radial nerve
   D. Musculocutaneous nerve

   Ans. is 'B' Median nerve

7. Compression of a nerve within the carpal tunnel produces inability to: *(AI 2010, 97 AIIMS May 05, 02, PGI 98)*
   A. Abduct the thumb
   B. Adduct the thumb
   C. Flex the distal phalanx of the thumb
   D. Oppose the thumb

   Ans. is 'D' Oppose the thumb

   – Abductor pollicis brevis (producing abduction of thumb) and opponens pollicis (producing opposition of thumb) are paralyzed in low median nerve palsy (in carpal tunnel). So, opposition of thumb is lost.
   – Abduction of thumb can be also carried out by abductor pollicis longus supplied by radial nerve.
   – Flexor pollicis longus will be intact to carry out flexion at thumb phalanx as it is supplied by AIN nerve branch of median nerve above carpal tunnel and adductor pollicis will cause adduction as it is supplied by ulnar nerve.

8. 'Ape thumb deformity' is observed in lesions of:
   A. Radial nerve injury *(AI 2002, Bihar 1991)*
   B. Ulnar nerve injury
   C. Median nerve injury
   D. Circumflex humeral nerve injury

   Ans. is 'C' Median nerve injury

9. Median nerve is injured during:
   A. Elbow dislocation *(PGI 2K, JIPMER 2000) (AI 1989)*
   B. Fracture lateral epicondyle of humerus
   C. Fracture medial epicondyle of humerus
   D. Supracondylar fracture of humerus

   Ans. is 'A' Elbow dislocation and 'D' Supracondylar fracture of humerus

   – Median nerve is injured in elbow dislocation, wrist dislocation, supracondylar fracture humerus and carpal tunnel syndrome.

10. Pointing index sign in seen in—nerve palsy:
    (AIIMS 97, UPSC 86, Kerala 87) (AI 97)
    A. Ulnar
    B. Radial
    C. Median
    D. Axillary

    Ans. is 'C' Median

ULNAR NERVE INJURY (MUSICIAN NERVE)

The ulnar nerve passes just behind the medial epicondyle. So, the fracture would lead to injury of ulnar nerve.

Clinical Presentation

Anesthesia is autonomous zone, i.e. tip of little finger and hypothesia in hypothenar eminence and medial 1½ fingers on volar and dorsal aspect.

Motor Supply

A. **Forearm**
   1. Flexor carpi ulnaris (weakness of ulnar deviation and flexon of wrist).
   2. Medial half of flexor digitorum profundus.

B. **Hand**
   1. Hypothenar muscles (Atrophy of hypothenar eminence)
      a. Palmaris brevis
      b. Abductor digiti minimi
      c. Flexor digiti minimi
      d. Opponens digiti minimi
   2. Thenar muscles
      a. Adductor pollicis—**Froment's sign/book test**
      b. Deep head of flexor pollicis brevis.

3. Four palmar Interossei—Tested by **card test** (loss of adduction of finger)/Wartenberg's sign
4. Four dorsal interossei—Loss of abduction of finger against resistance – **Igawa test (For middle finger)**
5. Medial two lumbricals.

Clinical Picture

1. Positive card test—weakness of palmar interosei so patient is unable to hold card firmly between fingers.

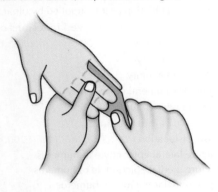

Fig. 15.12: Card test (Palmar Interossei-Adduction)

2. Wartenberg's sign is abducted position of little finger there is weakness of finger adduction.

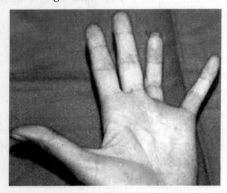

Fig. 15.13: Wartenberg's sign (Failure of adduction of little finger)

3. Book test tests the function of adductor pollicis, patient can hold the book between thumb and palm.

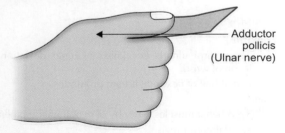

Fig. 15.14: Book test

4. **Froment Sign:** In case of ulnar nerve palsy adductor pollicis supplied by ulnar nerve is paralyzed. So, patient holds the book between thumb and palm by using flexor pollicis longus (supplied by AIN nerve). This produces flexion at interphalangeal joint, while holding book.

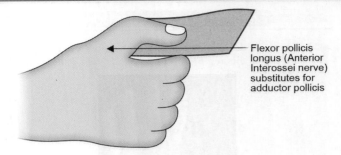

Fig. 15.15: Froment sign

5. Positive Igawa's test due to weakness of dorsal interossei, side to side movements of middle finger is weak.
6. Loss of abduction of fingers against resistance (weakness of dorsal interossei).
7. Deviation of hand toward radial side when wrist is flexed due to weakness of ulnar deviator (FCU).
8. Loss/weakness of extension of middle and terminal phalanges of medial two finger due to weakness of interossei and lumbricals (3rd and 4th).
9. Ulnar Claw Hand—clawing of little and ring fingers, i.e. hyperextension at M.P. joint and flexion at interphalangeal joint.
10. Atrophy of Hypothenar area.
11. In high ulnar nerve palsy forearm muscles are involved and the clawing is less (as compared to low ulnar nerve palsy) this phenomenon is ulnar paradox. This is due to sparing of FDP in low lesions, which causes more flexion of interphalangeal joints.
12. Disability of the hand is maximum with a lesion of ulnar nerve at wrist. Clumsiness of hand in ulnar nerve involvement is due to palsy of interosseous muscles.

*Intrinsic muscles in hands are innervated by median nerve through Martin-**Grubber** anastomosis in 7.5% of people.

Claw hand (Main en griffe)-Flexion at interphalangeal joint and hyperextension at metacarpophalangeal joint also called as intrinsic minus position.

Partial

Ulnar nerve palsy.

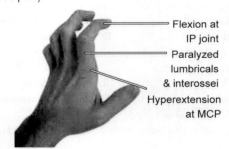

Fig. 15.16: Claw hand

Complete

Combined ulnar and median nerve palsy

Peripheral Nerve Injury

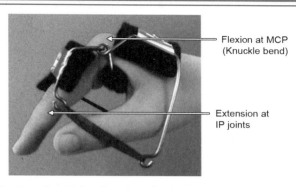

Fig. 15.17: Knuckle bender splint—for claw hand

Note: If in question it is asked Knuckle bender splint is used for choose ulnar > median.

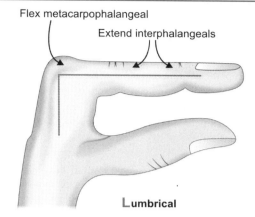

MULTIPLE CHOICE QUESTIONS

1. Identify the nerve supply of the marked muscle: *(NEET Pattern 2019)*

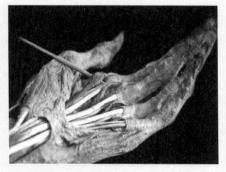

   A. Radial Nerve   B. Median Nerve
   C. Ulnar Nerve   D. Anterior Interosseous Nerve

   Ans. is 'B' Median Nerve
   The marked muscle is lumbrical (1st)
   1st and 2nd lumbrical are supplied by median nerve.
   3rd and 4th lumbrical are supplied by ulnar nerve.

2. Action of lumbricals at this joint is: *(NEET 2018)*

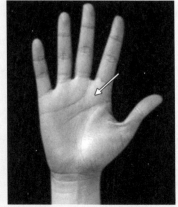

   A. Flexion   B. Extension
   C. Adduction   D. Abduction

   Ans. is 'A' Flexion

3. Adductor pollicis is supplied by: *(AI 2016)*
   A. Deep branch of ulnar nerve
   B. Median nerve
   C. Superficial branch of ulnar nerve
   D. AIN branch of median nerve

   Ans. is 'A' Deep branch of ulnar nerve

4. A patient came with complaints of difficulty in adducting his fingers and flexion of extended metacarpophalangeal joint muscles that are paralyzed are: *(JIPMER May 2016)*
   A. Interossei   B. Lumbricals
   C. Flexor digitorum profundus
   D. Flexor carpi radialis

   Ans. is 'A' Interossei

5. Ulnar paradox is seen in: *(AI Dec 15)*
   A. High ulnar nerve palsy
   B. Low ulnar nerve palsy
   C. Combined median and ulnar nerve palsy
   D. Guyon's Canal entrapment of ulnar nerve

   Ans. is 'A' High ulnar nerve palsy

6. Froment's Sign is seen in: *(AI Dec 15)*
   A. Ulnar nerve palsy
   B. Median nerve palsy
   C. Musculocutaneous nerve palsy
   D. Posterior Interosseous nerve palsy

   Ans. is 'A' Ulnar nerve palsy

7. Card test is done for testing the function of: *(AIIMS May 2015)*
   A. Lumbricals   B. Palmar interossei
   C. Dorsal interossei   D. Adductor pollicis

   Ans. is 'B' Palmar interossei

8. A patient complaints of flexion of interphalangeal joints and hyperextension of MCP of hands. He is most likely suffering from: *(AIIMS Nov 2015)*
   A. PIN palsy   B. Dupuytren's contracture
   C. Claw hand   D. Erb's palsy

   Ans. is 'C' Claw hand

9. Froment's sign is positive in cases of weakness of: *(NEET 2015)*
   A. Thumb adduction   B. Thumb abduction
   C. Thumb flexion   D. Thumb extension

   Ans. is 'A' Thumb adduction

10. A patient presents with loss of sensation of ring and littler finger with wasting of hypothenar muscles where is the lesion: *(AIIMS Nov 2012)*
    A. Deep branch of ulnar nerve
    B. Superficial branch of ulnar nerve
    C. Ulnar nerve before division into deep and superficial
    D. Median nerve

Ans. is 'C' Ulnar nerve before division into deep and superficial

Explanation
Ulnar Nerve (C8, T1)
- The Ulnar nerve is derived in most instances exclusively from the C8, T1 nerve roots although sometimes there is a minor C7 component. Nearly all ulnar fibers arise in the lower trunk of the brachial plexus and pass through the medial cord, the terminal extension of which is the ulnar nerve. It is worth remembering that a large portion of the median nerve and the medial antebrachial cutaneous nerve also arises from the medial cord. The ulnar nerve runs down the medial aspect of the arm, and there are no significant branches in the arm. At the elbow the nerve passes into the groove between the medial epicondyle and olecranon process, the ulnar groove. Just beyond the groove the nerve runs under a tendinous arch formed by the two heads of the flexor carpi ulnaris muscle. This arch is commonly referred to as the cubital tunnel but is more correctly called the humeral-ulnar aponeurosis (HUA). Muscular branches to the flexor carpi ulnaris muscle and the ulnar portion of flexor digitorum profundus are found at this site. The ulnar nerve then passes down the medial forearm with the next important branch being the dorsal cutaneous sensory branch just proximal to the wrist. This nerve supplies sensation to the dorsal medial hand and digits, whilst at the ulnar styloid there is a palmar cutaneous branch that supplies the palmar aspect of the hand. Finally the ulnar nerve passes into the hand through Guyon's canal. The ulnar nerve and artery pass superficial to the flexor retinaculum, via the ulnar canal. The course of the ulnar nerve through the wrist contrasts with that of the median nerve, which travels deep to the flexor retinaculum of the hand and therefore through the carpal tunnel.

Here it gives off the following branches:
- Superficial branch of ulnar nerve
- Deep branch of ulnar nerve

Ulnar nerve deep branch supplies
At its origin it supplies the hypothenar muscles.
- As it crosses the deep part of the hand, it supplies all the interosseous muscles and the third and fourth lumbricals. It ends by supplying the adductor pollicis and the medial (deep) head of the flexor pollicis brevis. It also sends articular filaments to the wrist-joint.
- The superficial branch of the ulnar nerve is a terminal branch of the ulnar nerve. It supplies the palmaris brevis and the skin on the ulnar side of the hand, and divides into a proper palmar digital nerve and a common palmar digital nerve.
- In the question above since sensory loss and hypothenar wasting is seen hence it involves whole ulnar nerve before division.

11. Which of the following will not take place in a patient with ulnar nerve injury in arm? *(AIIMS May 2013)*
    A. Claw hand
    B. Thumb adduction
    C. Sensory loss over medial aspect of hand
    D. Weakness of flexor carpi ulnaris

Ans. is 'B' Thumb adduction

Explanation
- In a patient with ulnar nerve palsy flexor carpi ulnaris will be paralyzed; there will be sensory loss over medial aspect of hand (area supplied by ulnar nerve) and there will be claw hand due to paralysis of intrinsic muscles of hand. Adductor pollicis is supplied by ulnar nerve hence in ulnar nerve palsy thumb adduction will not be seen.

12. Tardy ulnar nerve palsy: *(NEET Pattern 2016, 2012)*
    A. Early onset
    B. Late onset
    C. Caused by shoulder dislocation
    D. None

Ans. is 'B' Late onset

13. Knuckle-Bender splint is for: *(NEET Pattern 2012)*
    A. Median nerve injury
    B. Radial nerve injury
    C. Ulnar nerve injury
    D. None

Ans. is 'C' Ulnar nerve injury

14. Froment Sign is positive in: *(NEET Pattern 2012)*
    A. Ulnar nerve injury
    B. Radial nerve injury
    C. Median nerve injury
    D. Erb's palsy

Ans. is 'A' Ulnar nerve injury

15. Musician nerve: *(NEET Pattern 2012)*
    A. Ulnar nerve
    B. Median nerve
    C. Radial nerve
    D. Musculocutaneous nerve

Ans. is 'A' Ulnar nerve

16. Lumbricals palsy causes: *(NEET Pattern 2012)*
    A. Claw hand
    B. Erb's palsy
    C. Mallet finger
    D. Hammer toe

Ans. is 'A' Claw hand

17. Froment sign tests: *(NEET Pattern 2012)*
    A. Adductor pollicis
    B. Abductor pollicis brevis
    C. Abductor pollicis longus
    D. Extensor pollicis longus

Ans. is 'A' Adductor pollicis

18. Following an incised wound in the front of wrist, the subject is unable to oppose the tips of the little finger and the thumb. The nerve(s) involved is/are:
    (AIIMS May 08, UP 2K, PGI 2003, 98, AI 95)
    A. Ulnar nerve alone
    B. Median nerve alone
    C. Median and ulnar nerves
    D. Radial and ulnar nerves

Ans. is 'C' Median and ulnar nerves
- The patient has inability to oppose little finger (paralysis of opponens digiti minimi) and oppose thumb (paralysis of opponens pollicis).
- So, both ulnar and median nerves are paralyzed.

19. A patient with leprosy presents with clumsiness of hand. His ulnar nerve is affected. Clumsiness is due to palsy of which muscle? *(AIIMS June 2000)*
    A. Extensor carpi ulnaris
    B. Abductor pollicis brevis
    C. Opponens pollicis
    D. Interosseous muscle

Ans. is 'D' Interosseous muscle
- Clumsiness is due to paralysis of muscles which are involved in fine movement, i.e. interossei and lumbricals.

20. "Ulnar paradox" is related with the following:
(UP 1994) (PGI 1991) (PGI 1990)
   A. Lumbricals   B. Intrinsic muscle
   C. EPL   D. Ulnar half of FDP

Ans. is 'D' Ulnar half of FDP
- Disability of the hand is maximum with a lesion of ulnar nerve at wrist.

RADIAL NERVE INJURY

It is usually injured in fractures of shaft humerus, injection palsy, Saturday night palsy and Crutch palsy. Sensory loss in area supplied posterior cutaneous nerve of forearm. Wrist, thumb and finger extension is lost (i.e. wrist, thumb and finger drop). **Loss of extension of wrist is wrist drop; of thumb is thumb drop; of MCP joint of finger is finger drop.**

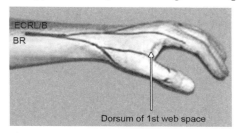

Fig. 15.18: Autonomous zone of radial nerve

*Autonomous zone for radial nerve is dorsum of 1st web space.

Type of Radial Nerve Lesion

1. Very high (i.e. above spiral groove)
   - **Total palsy, i.e.** Elbow, wrist, thumb and finger extension is lost
   - Loss of sensation over dorsum of 1st web space.
2. High (i.e. between spiral groove and lateral epicondyle)
   - Elbow extension spared
   - Brachioradialis is involved
   - Lost: Wrist, thumb, finger extension and sensation over dorsum of 1st web space.
3. Low (i.e. the elbow)
   - Elbow and wrist extension spared
   - Lost: Thumb, finger extension and sensation over dorsum of 1st web space.
4. Posterior interosseous nerve palsy (no Sensory deficit)
   - Elbow, wrist joint extension and sensations are spared
   - Loss of MP joint extension, i.e. thumb and finger drop

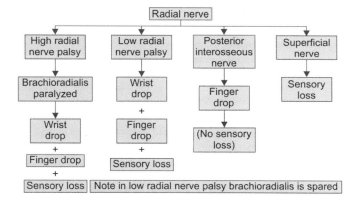

Jones Transfer—Most Important

- Pronator Teres to Extensor carpi radialis longus/Extensor carpi radialis brevis—Wrist extensors
- Flexor carpi ulnaris to Extensor digitorum communis— Finger extensors
- Flexor carpi radialis to Extensor pollicis longus (Extensor pollicis brevis and Abductor pollicis longus)— Thumb functions.

Brand Transfer

- Pronator Teres to Extensor carpi radialis brevis
- Flexor carpi radialis to Extensor digitorum longus
- Palmaris longus to rerouted Extensor pollicis longus.

Boyes Transfer

- Pronator Teres to Extensor carpi radialis longus/extensor carpi radialis brevis
- Flexor carpi radialis to Extensor pollicis brevis and Abductor pollicis longus
- Flexor digitorum superficialis Middle Finger to Extensor digitorum communis
- Flexor digitorum superficialis Ring Finger to Extensor pollicis longus and extensor indicis.

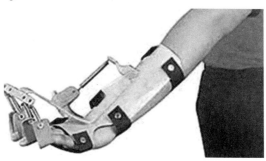

Fig. 15.19: Cock-up splint—for radial nerve

Note: MC tendon for transfer/graft: Palmaris Longus.

MULTIPLE CHOICE QUESTIONS

1. Tendon used for repair of flexor tendon injury in hand requiring reconstruction from forearm to fingertip is:
(DNB June 2017)
   A. Palmaris
   B. Plantaris
   C. Extensor digitorum communis
   D. Extensor digiti minimi

Ans. is 'B' Plantaris
   Explanation:
   Palmaris longus—Hand to fingertip } Tendon transfer.
   Plantaris—Forearm to fingertip

2. Crutch paly is injury to which nerve? (DNB JUNE 2017)
   A. Radial nerve
   B. Ulnar nerve
   C. Median nerve
   D. Musculocutaneous nerve

Ans. is 'A' Radial nerve

3. Wrist Drop is a feature of: (AI Dec 15)
   A. Superficial radial nerve
   B. Posterior interosseous nerve palsy
   C. High radial nerve palsy
   D. Avulsion of triceps tendon
Ans. is 'C' High radial nerve palsy

4. Which of the following nerve injury is most commonly associated with a humerus shaft fracture? (AI Dec 15)
   A. Radial nerve   B. Median nerve
   C. Axillary nerve   D. Ulnar nerve
Ans. is 'A' Radial nerve

5. In a patient with history of trauma of forearm and X-ray showing fracture of proximal part of medial bone with dislocation of proximal part of lateral bone. The muscles which may be paralyzed: (CET July 16)
   A. Flexor carpi ulnaris   B. Adductor pollicis
   C. Extensor pollicis longus D. Opponens pollicis
Ans. is 'C' Extensor pollicis longus

6. Dorsum of 1st web space of hand is an autonomous zone for: (DNB June 2017, AI 2016)
   A. Radial nerve   B. AIN
   C. PIN   D. Median nerve
Ans. is 'A' Radial nerve

7. A 24-year-old male presents with a humerus fracture as shown in the figure below: (AIIMS May 2016)

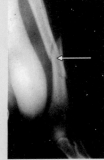

Which is the nerve likely to be involved by the fracture? (AIIMS May 2016)
   A. Ulnar   B. Radial
   C. Medial   D. Musculocutaneous
Ans. is 'B' Radial

8. A patient can't extend his wrist after he has met with an accident. He has no sensory loss. Level at which the affected nerve is injured? (JIPMER MAY 2016)
   A. Spiral groove of humerus B. Head of radius
   C. Near medial epicondyle   D. Surgical neck of humerus
Ans. is 'A' Spiral groove of humerus

9. Extensor Carpi Radialis Longus is: (AI Dec 15)
   A. Extensor and ulnar deviator of the wrist
   B. Extensor and radial deviator of the wrist
   C. Injured in posterior interosseous nerve injury
   D. Weak extensor of the wrist
Ans. is 'B' Extensor and radial deviator of the wrist

10. Saturday night palsy involves which nerve? (AI 2016)
    A. Radial   B. Median
    C. Axillary   D. Musculocutaneous
Ans. is 'A' Radial

11. Which of the following is used as a substitute for wrist extensors in radial nerve palsy? (AI Dec 15)
    A. Pronator teres   B. Palmaris longus
    C. Flexor digitorum superficialis
    D. Flexor digitorum profundus
Ans. is 'A' Pronator teres

12. A 45-year-old carpenter with a blunt trauma to his arm sustained a fracture following which he developed wrist drop, loss of extension at fingers and loss of sensations on the lateral aspect of the wrist joint. Which of the following is true? (AI Dec 15)
    A. Patient has an injury to the median nerve
    B. He should have also lost extension of the forearm
    C. Patient has injured the radial nerve in the spiral groove
    D. There is combined involvement of the radial nerve and median nerve
Ans. is 'C' Patient has injured the radial nerve in the spiral groove

13. Cock up splint is used in treatment of: (DNB June 2017, NEET 2015)
    A. Radial nerve palsy   B. Ulnar nerve palsy
    C. Median nerve palsy
    D. Posterior interosseous nerve palsy
Ans. is 'A' Radial nerve palsy

14. Extension of metacarpophalangeal joint of the hand is lost in injury to: (APPG 2015)
    A. Median nerve   B. Ulnar nerve
    C. Anterior interosseous nerve
    D. Posterior interosseous nerve
Ans. is 'D' Posterior interosseous nerve

15. Commonest cause of "Wrist Drop" is: (PGM-CET 2015)
    A. Intramuscular injection   B. Fracture humerus
    C. Dislocation of elbow   D. Dislocation of shoulder
Ans. is 'B' Fracture humerus

16. Which of the following statements about low Radial nerve palsy is not true? (TN 2014, TN 1999, 2000)
    A. Loss of nerve supply to brachioradialis
    B. Loss of nerve supply to extensor carpi radialis brevis
    C. Loss of nerve supply to extensor pollicis brevis
    D. Loss of sensation over first dorsal web space
Ans. is 'A' Loss of nerve supply to brachioradialis

17. A person is not able to extend his metacarpophalangeal joint. This is due to injury to which nerve? (NEET Pattern 2013)
    A. Ulnar nerve   B. Radial nerve injury
    C. Median nerve injury
    D. Post Interosseous nerve injury
Ans. is 'D' > 'B' Post Interosseous nerve injury > Radial nerve injury

18. A patient sustains injury in his arm following which is develops Loss of Sensation on Dorsum of Hand and Inability to Extend Wrist and Fingers? (AIIMS Nov 2012)
    A. C7 neuropathy   B. Radial nerve injury
    C. PIN injury   D. Brachial plexus injury
Ans. is 'B' Radial nerve injury

19. A 30-year-old male underwent excision of the right radial head. Following surgery, the patient developed inability to extend the fingers and thumb of the right hand. He did

not have any sensory deficit. Which one of the following is the most likely cause?

(AIIMS May 2004, Rajasthan 98, UP 94)
- A. Injury to posterior interosseous nerve
- B. Iatrogenic injury to common extensor origin
- C. Injury to anterior interosseous nerve
- D. High radial nerve palsy

Ans. is 'A' Injury to posterior interosseous nerve

20. Injury to radial nerve in lower part of spiral groove:

(AI 2003, TN 99, AI 94)
- A. Spares nerve supply to extensor carpi radialis longus
- B. Results in paralysis of anconeus muscle
- C. Leaves extensions at elbow joint intact
- D. Weakens pronation movement

Ans. is 'C' Leaves extensions at elbow joint intact
- Triceps and anconeus are supplied by radial nerve above the level of spiral groove; so these are spared in injuries of radial nerve at and below spiral groove thus leaving elbow extension intact.

21. In fracture of distal half of humerus, the nerve injured is: (UP 99, 94, ESI 1989)
- A. Axillary
- B. Median
- C. Radial
- D. Ulnar

Ans. is 'C' Radial
- Radial nerve is involved in distal part of humerus it is called as Holstein-Lewis sign.

22. Cock-up splint is used in management of:
- A. Ulnar nerve palsy (AIIMS Feb 97, Dec 95; PGI 87)
- B. Brachial plexus palsy   C. Radial nerve palsy
- D. Combined ulnar and median nerve palsy

Ans. is 'C' Radial nerve palsy
- Cock-up splint is used for radial nerve injury

23. Commonest cause of wrist drop is:

(KA 97) (AIIMS Feb 97, Dec 95)
- A. Intramuscular injection
- B. Fracture humerus
- C. Dislocation of elbow
- D. Dislocation of shoulder

Ans. is 'B>A' Fracture humerus > Intramuscular injection

24. Saturday night palsy involves nerve:

(Delhi 94, AMU 1989) (AIIMS 1989)
- A. Radial
- B. Ulnar
- C. Median
- D. Axillary

Ans. is 'A' Radial

LOWER LIMB NERVE INJURY

Sciatic nerve has two components tibial nerve centrally arranged fibers and common peroneal nerve peripherally arranged fibers. The injury to sciatic nerve sometimes can present as an injury only to common peroneal nerve because these fibers are peripheral and more prone to pressure. Sciatic nerve divides into:
1. Common peroneal nerve which further divides into superficial peroneal and deep peroneal nerve.
2. Tibial nerve which gives sural nerve supplying lateral part of foot.

COMMON PERONEAL NERVE INJURY-RELATED TO FIBULAR NECK!

Motor
- Muscles of anterior and lateral compartments of leg are paralyzed namely—tibialis anterior, extensor digitorum longus and brevis, extensor hallucis longus and peroneus tertius (supplied by deep peroneal nerve) and peroneus longus and brevis (supplied by superficial peroneal nerve)—presenting as foot drop.

Sensory
- Loss of sensation down the anterior and lateral sides of leg and dorsum of foot and toes, including medial side of big toe.

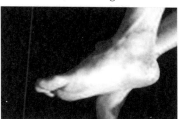

Fig. 15.20: Foot drop—CPN palsy

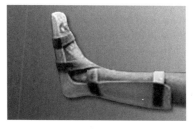

Fig. 15.21: Foot drop splint

- Lateral border of foot and lateral side of little toe are unaffected (sural nerve mainly formed from tibial nerve).
- The medial border of foot as far as the ball of big toe is completely unaffected (saphenous nerve, a branch of femoral nerve).

MULTIPLE CHOICE QUESTIONS

1. Foot drop is caused due to injury to?

(NEET Pattern 2019, Dec 2016)
- A. Common Peroneal Nerve
- B. Tibial Nerve
- C. Femoral Nerve
- D. Obturator Nerve

Ans. is 'A' Common Peroneal Nerve

2. High stepping gait is seen in: (NEET 2015)
- A. CTEV
- B. Common peroneal nerve palsy
- C. Polio
- D. Cerebral palsy

Ans. is 'B' Common peroneal nerve palsy

3. Road traffic accident, a patient lying in right lateral position with bruise on face, elbow and lateral side of knee. Which nerve injury has maximum chances in this position of the victim? (AIIMS May 2013)
- A. Trigeminal nerve
- B. Ulnar nerve
- C. Common peroneal nerve
- D. Tibial nerve

Ans. is 'C' Common peroneal nerve

Explanation
- Amongst the mentioned nerves most frequently injured nerve in lateral position will be the nerve that has maximum chances of injury due to compression against a bony prominence and that is common peroneal nerve near fibular neck.

4. Injury to the common peroneal nerve at the lateral aspect of head of fibula results in all of the following except:
   A. Weakness of ankle dorsiflexion (AIIMS Nov 06)
   B. Foot drop
   C. Loss of ankle reflex
   D. Sensory impairment on lateral aspect of leg extending to the dorsum of foot

Ans. is 'C' Loss of ankle reflex
   – Ankle reflex is mediated by tibial nerve

5. Common peroneal nerve is related to: (AIIMS Nov 06)
   A. Shaft of tibia
   B. Neck of fibula
   C. Lower tibiofibular joint
   D. Shaft of fibula

Ans. is 'B' Neck of fibula

6. A 25-year-old lady sustained a lacerated wound on the back of right thigh by a horn of a bull. The wound was sutured. Two months later she developed foot drop and an ulcer on the dorsum of the foot. The most likely diagnosis is:
   A. Chronic ischemia to limbs due to popliteal artery injury
   B. Partial injury to sciatic nerve (UPSC 1997)
   C. Complete division of sciatic nerve
   D. Injury to hamstring muscles

Ans. is 'B' Partial injury to sciatic nerve
   – The common peroneal component seems to be affected as ulcer is only on dorsum of foot supplied by common peroneal nerve.

7. Foot drop result because of injury to: (PGI 91, 90)
   A. Superficial peroneal nerve
   B. Deep peroneal nerve
   C. Posterior tibial nerve
   D. Anterior tibial nerve

Ans. is 'B' Deep peroneal nerve; 'D' Anterior tibial nerve

NERVE ENTRAPMENT SYNDROMES

This refers to nerve entrapped in closed space.

Entrapment syndrome	Nerve involved
Carpal tunnel syndrome	**Median nerve** (at wrist) **(most common)**
Pronator syndrome	**Median nerve** (proximally compressed beneath - ligament of struthers, bicipital aponeurosis or origins of pronator teres or flexor digitorum superficialis).
Cubital tunnel syndrome	**Ulnar nerve** (between two heads of flexor carpi ulnaris)
Guyon's canal syndrome	**Ulnar nerve** (at wrist)
Thoracic outlet syndrome	Lower trunk of brachial plexus, (C8 and **T1**) and subclavian vessels (between clavicle and first rib)
Piriformis syndrome	Sciatic nerve
Meralgia paresthetica	**Lateral cutaneous nerve of thigh**
Cheiralgia paresthetica	Superficial radial nerve
Tarsal tunnel syndrome	Posterior tibial nerve (behind and below medial malleolus)
Morton's metatarsalgia	Interdigital nerve compression (usually of 3rd, 4th toe)

Femoral nerve is usually not involved in Nerve Entrapment Syndrome.

Carpal Tunnel Syndrome

It is entrapment of median nerve at the wrist beneath the flexor retinaculum.

Etiology (Associated Conditions)

- **Idiopathic (most common)**
- Endocrine disorders—**Hypothyroidism**, diabetes mellitus, acromegaly
- Hyperparathyroidism, pregnancy, **rheumatoid arthritis**, gout, amyloidosis, alcoholism, sarcoidosis.
- Injury related—Synovitis of tendon sheath
- **Malunited fractures (Colles fracture)**

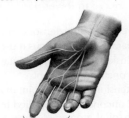

Fig. 15.22: Area of symptoms in carpal tunnel syndrome

Clinical Features

- Eight times more common in **women** than men. The usual age group is 50 years.
- Burning pain, paresthesia, tingling and numbness in the distribution of median nerve.
- Pain is increased by activities, **most troublesome in night** and relieved by hanging the arm over the side of bed, or shaking the arm. Clumsiness and weakness in tasks requiring fine manipulation.
- Sensory symptoms can often be reproduced by percussing over the median nerve (Tinel's sign) or by holding the wrist fully flexed for a minute or two (Phalen's test/Reverse Phalen's test) or tourniquet test or direct compression over median nerve. (Best clinical test).—**Durkan's test**

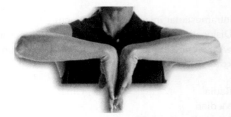

Fig. 15.23: Phalen's test for carpal tunnel syndrome

- **NCV is investigation of choice.**
- In late cases weakness of thumb abduction and wasting of thenar muscles occur.
- *Splints, NSAID's corticosteroid injection and open surgical division of transverse carpal ligament are methods of management.

MULTIPLE CHOICE QUESTIONS

1. All are true regarding carpal tunnel syndrome except: (NEET DEC 2016)
   A. Pregnancy is the most common cause
   B. More common in women
   C. Median nerve is compressed
   D. Symptoms often appear at night

Ans. is 'A' Pregnancy is the most common cause

Peripheral Nerve Injury

2. Carpal tunnel syndrome is seen in all except:
   (NEET Dec 2016)
   A. Pregnancy	B. Alcoholism
   C. Colle's fracture	D. Smith's fracture
   Ans. is 'D' Smith's fracture

3. Which of the following is not a cause for the development of carpal tunnel syndrome? (NEET Dec 2016)
   A. Alcoholism
   B. Sarcoidosis
   C. Gout
   D. Menorrhagia
   Ans. is 'D' Menorrhagia

4. Tinel's sign is seen in: (AI Dec 15)
   A. Avascular necrosis of scaphoid
   B. Kienbock's disease
   C. 1st carpometacarpal joint arthritis
   D. Carpal tunnel syndrome
   Ans. is 'D' Carpal tunnel syndrome

5. Most common cause of carpal tunnel syndrome:
   A. Pregnancy	(AI Dec 15)
   B. Idiopathic
   C. Alcoholism
   D. Occupational-excessive use of vibration instruments
   Ans. is 'B' Idiopathic

6. A person came with symptoms of tingling and burning sensation over his palm near base of his thumb. He will also have which symptoms? (JIPMER May 2016)
   A. Atrophy of hypothenar muscles
   B. Paresthesia over lateral 3 fingers
   C. Loss of adduction of thumb
   D. Loss of opposition of thumb
   Ans. is 'B' Paresthesia over lateral 3 fingers

7. Meralgia Paresthetica is due to involvement of:
   A. Lateral cutaneous nerve of thigh	(AIIMS Nov 2015)
   B. Ilioinguinal nerve
   C. Genitofemoral nerve
   D. Saphenous nerve
   Ans. is 'A' Lateral cutaneous nerve of thigh

8. Which of the following nerve is involved in 'pronator teres syndrome'? (AIIMS Nov 2015)
   A. Median nerve	B. Ulnar nerve
   C. Radius nerve	D. Anterior interosseous nerve
   Ans. is 'A' Median nerve

9. Investigation of choice for entrapment neuropathy is:
   (NEET 2015)
   A. CT scan	B. Clinical examination
   C. Ultrasonography	D. EMG NCV
   Ans. is 'D' EMG NCV

10. Causes of Carpal tunnel syndrome are all except:
    A. DM	B. RA	(NEET 2015)
    C. Leprosy	D. Gout
    Ans. is 'C' Leprosy

11. Carpal Tunnel Syndrome test used is:
    (NEET Pattern 2013, 2012)
    A. Phalen's test	B. Finkelstein test
    C. Cozen's test	D. Thompson test
    Ans. is 'A' Phalen's test

12. Cubital tunnel syndrome involves:	(NEET Pattern 2012)
    A. Median nerve	B. Ulnar nerve
    C. Tibial nerve	D. Common peroneal nerve
    Ans. is 'B' Ulnar nerve

13. Carpal tunnel syndrome nerve compressed is:
    (NEET Pattern 2012)
    A. Median nerve	B. Ulnar nerve
    C. Superficial radial nerve	D. Musculocutaneous nerve
    Ans. is 'A' Median nerve

14. Which of the following is seen in popliteal entrapment syndrome. (DNB JUNE 2017)
    A. Evidence of atherosclerosis
    B. Exercise induced calf claudications
    C. Abnormal relation between popliteal artery and lateral head of gastrocnemius
    D. Decreased ankle pulses with ankle extension
    Ans. is 'B' Exercise induced calf claudications

    Popliteal artery entrapment syndrome:
    1. Congenital abnormality between medial head of gastrocnemius and popliteal artery.
    2. Exercise induced calf claudication.
    3. Decreased ankle pulses on ankle flexion.

    Treatment:
    Release of muscular origin of medial head of gastrocnemius.

15. Compression neuropathy is:	(NEET Pattern 2012)
    A. Nerve entrapped in closed space
    B. Muscle entrapped in closed space
    C. Vein entrapped in closed space
    D. Artery entrapped in closed space
    Ans. is 'A' Nerve entrapped in closed space

16. Guyon's canal nerve is:	(NEET Pattern 2012)
    A. Median nerve	B. Ulnar nerve
    C. Radial nerve	D. Musculocutaneous nerve
    Ans. is 'B' Ulnar nerve

17. Cheralgia paresthetica involves:	(NEET Pattern 2012)
    A. Ulnar nerve	B. Median nerve
    C. Superficial radial nerve	D. Musculocutaneous nerve
    Ans. is 'C' Superficial radial nerve

18. Entrapment neuropathies commonly affect the following nerves except:	(AI 2009, 07)
    A. Tibial	B. Femoral
    C. Lateral cutaneous nerve of thigh
    D. Common digital nerve
    Ans. is 'B' Femoral

19. Sudden hyperflexion of thigh over abdomen (McRobert's procedure), which of the following nerve is commonly involved?	(AIIMS Nov 08)
    A. Common peroneal nerve
    B. Obturator nerve
    C. Lumbosacral trunk
    D. Lateral cutaneous nerve of thigh
    Ans. is 'D' Lateral cutaneous nerve of thigh
    – McRobert's maneuver to deliver babies with shoulder dystocia can cause compression of femoral nerve by overlying inguinal ligament. Occasionally lateral femoral cutaneous nerve may get damaged.

20. **Commonest cause for neuralgic pain in foot is:** *(AI 2003)*
    A. Compression of communication between medial and lateral plantar nerves
    B. Exaggeration of longitudinal arches
    C. Injury to deltoid ligament
    D. Shortening of plantar aponeurosis

Ans. is 'A' Compression of communication between medial and lateral plantar nerves

"Most common cause as pain, burning, paresthesiae or numbness in the sole of the foot, is compression of communication between medial and lateral plantar nerve".

TARSAL TUNNEL SYNDROME

The tibial nerve is compressed beneath the flexor retinaculum (laciniate ligament). It is compressive neuropathy of posterior tibial nerve as it passes behind the medial malleolus. It may arise from space occupying lesion within the tarsal tunnel (e.g. a ganglion, synovial cyst or lipoma) or distally against one of the two terminal branches: the medial or lateral plantar nerve.

Causes are **idiopathic>O.A>R.A>Ankylosing Spondylitis**

Burning pain and paresthesia over the plantar surface of foot. Pain may be precipitated by prolonged weight bearing, often worse at night, and the patient may seek relief by walking around or stamping his foot.

Percussion may elicit Tinel's sign over the posterior tibial nerves in tarsal tunnel or distally along the division of posterior tibial nerves (the medial calcaneal nerve and medial and lateral plantar nerves).

Nerve conduction velocity is reduced.

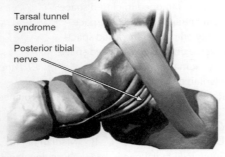

Fig. 15.24: Tarsal tunnel syndrome

Burning pain localized to plantar aspect of foot is due to tarsal tunnel syndrome with compression of posterior tibial nerve or its terminal branches medial and lateral plantar nerves.

Release of flexor retinaculum is not as effective in tarsal tunnel syndrome as release of transverse carpal ligament in carpal tunnel syndrome.

MULTIPLE CHOICE QUESTIONS

1. **Tarsal tunnel syndrome involves:** *(NEET Pattern 2013)*
    A. Lateral cutaneous nerve of thigh
    B. Posterior tibial nerve
    C. Common peroneal nerve
    D. Sciatic nerve

Ans. is 'B' Posterior tibial nerve

2. **Most common cause of tarsal tunnel syndrome:** *(AIIMS May 2009)*
    A. Osteoarthritis
    B. Ankylosing spondylitis
    C. Psoriatic arthritis
    D. Rheumatoid arthritis

Ans. is 'A' Osteoarthritis

– Amongst the given options, OA is the most common cause of tarsal tunnel syndrome. Facts about etiology of tarsal tunnel syndrome.
– Most common origin of tarsal tunnel syndrome is idiopathic (21–36%) > Osteoarthritis.

3. **In a patient with a history of burning pain localized to the plantar aspect of the foot, the differential diagnosis must include:** *(AIIMS Nov 2003)*
    A. Peripheral vascular disease
    B. Tarsal coalition
    C. Tarsal tunnel syndrome
    D. Plantar fibromatosis

Ans. is 'C' Tarsal tunnel syndrome

– Three most common caused of pain in plantar aspect of foot are plantar fasciitis, tarsal tunnel syndrome, and posterior tibial tendinopathy.
– Burning pain is characteristic of neural pain. Hence tarsal tunnel syndrome is preferred here.

THORACIC OUTLET SYNDROME

Thoracic outlet is a space between the first rib clavicle and the scalene muscle. Compression of neurovascular bundle consisting of subclavian and axillary blood vessels and brachial plexus at the thoracic outlet is included in thoracic outlet syndrome.

Causes: Narrowing of the space either due to hypertrophy of the existing muscles or due to any other cause like congenital, trauma, etc.

1. Cervical rib syndrome
2. Heavy exercises or manual Laborer's
3. Malunion/nonunion of fracture clavicle

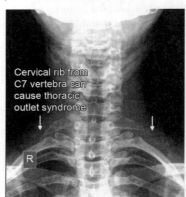

Clinical Features

- **Vascular:** Numbness of the upper limb during overhead exercises cold cyanosis, pallor and Raynaud's phenomenon that recovers on rest.
- **Neurogenic:** Commonly involves C8 and T1 nerve roots (T1 > C8).
  There is paresthesia along the medial aspect of the arm, hand and little fingers, and there is weakness of the hand.

Tests

1. *Adson's test*
2. *Wright's test*
3. *Roos test*

Note: *Allen's test:* To determine the adequacy of radial and ulnar arteries not for thoracic outlet syndrome.

Investigations

1. X-ray neck
2. Nerve conduction studies

Clinical diagnosis is very important.

Treatment

1. **Conservative:** Rest physiotherapy, exercises, etc.
2. **Surgery:** Cervical rib or 1st thoracic rib excision.

Contracture of iliotibial tract in polio results in these classical deformities

1. Lumbar scoliosis
2. Pelvic obliquity
3. Hip flexion and abduction
4. External rotation of femur
5. Triple deformity of knee
6. Flexion and valgus of knee
7. Posterior and lateral subluxation of tibia
8. External rotation of tibia
9. Foot in equinus
10. Shortening

Ober's test demonstrates iliotibial tract contracture (as in polio)

The age of patient at the time of tendon transfer is an important consideration. The child should be old enough, preferably over 4–5 years of age, to cooperate in the training of the transfer.

In musculoskeletal disorders, e.g. poliomyelitis femur is the most commonly (>50%) fractured bone, and 90% of these are supracondylar fractures and here union rate is slow because of poor muscle mass surrounding the bone hence reduced vascularity, which is required for fracture healing.

- **Post-polio syndrome (PPS, or post-poliomyelitis syndrome or post-polio sequelae)** affects 25–50% of people who have previously contracted poliomyelitis.
- Typically the symptoms appear 15–30 years after recovery from the original paralytic attack, at an age of 35–60.
- Symptoms include acute or increased muscular weakness, pain in the muscles, and fatigue. The same symptoms may also occur years after a nonparalytic polio (NPP) infection.
- The precise mechanism that causes PPS is unknown.
- It shares many features with the post-viral chronic fatigue syndrome, but unlike that disorder it tends to be progressive, and as such can cause a tangible loss of muscle strength.

Treatment is primarily limited to adequate rest, conservation of available energy, and supportive measures, such as leg braces and energy-saving devices such as powered wheelchairs, analgesia (pain relief) and sleep aids.

In normal gait, each leg goes through a stance phase and a swing phase

Stance Phase

The stance phase forms 60% of the gait and here the foot is on the ground.

- It is further subdivided into:
  - *Heel strike:* Heel striking the ground. In this *quadriceps, hamstring and ankle dorsiflexor (tibialis anterior)* are main muscles.
  - *Mid stance:* Here the foot is flat on the ground. Main muscles are *knee extensors (quadriceps), hip extensors (Hamstrings and gluteus, maximus) and ankle dorsiflexor (tibialis anterior)* to maintain posture.
  - *Push off:* Distal part of foot pushes the foot off the ground. The major muscle is *ankle plantar flexor (gastrocnemius - soleus).*

Swing Phase

This forms 40% of the gait cycle and the foot is not in contact with the ground.

It is further subdivided into *(i) Acceleration:* Leg starts to swing. The main muscle is *Quadriceps. (ii) Swing through (mid swing):* Leg continues to swing. The main muscles are *hip flexors (iliopsoas). (iii) Deceleration:* Swing slows down and the heel is ready for strike. The main muscles are *Hamstring and ankle dorsiflexors (tibialis anterior).*

> Least kinetic energy and maximum potential energy is at mid stance.

> Maximum kinetic energy and least potential energy is at double limb support.

MULTIPLE CHOICE QUESTIONS

1. Identify the given X-ray abnormality: *(AIIMS Nov 2018)*

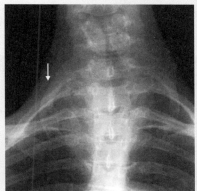

A. Costochondritis   B. Cervical Rib
C. Rib Fracture 2nd / 3rd   D. C5/C6 Spondylolisthesis

Ans. is 'B' Cervical Rib

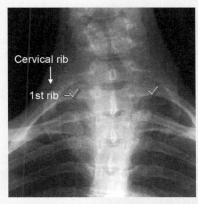

2. Nerve Roots of Long Thoracic Nerve of Bell:
A. C5   B. C6   *(PGI Nov 2018)*
C. C7   D. C8
E. T1

Ans. is 'A' C5 'B' C6 'C' C7

3. Positive Adson's test is seen in: *(DNB JUNE 2017)*
   A. Thoracic outlet syndrome B. Buerger disease
   C. Varicose veins D. Radial nerve injury
Ans. is 'A' Thoracic outlet syndrome

4. Iliotibial band contracture in patients of poliomyelitis will lead to: *(NEET DEC 2016)*
   A. Flexion at hip and knee
   B. Flexion at hip, extension at knee
   C. Extension at hip flexion at knee
   D. Extension at hip and knee
Ans. is 'A' Flexion at hip and knee

5. The root value of the long thoracic nerve is: *(AIIMS Nov 2012)*
   A. C3, 4, 5 B. C4, 5, 6
   C. C5, 6, 7 D. C6, 7, T1
Ans. is 'C' C5, 6, 7

6. Sciatic nerve palsy most common cause is: *(NEET Pattern 2012)*
   A. Fractures B. Injections
   C. Idiopathic D. Lumbar plexus injury
Ans. is 'A' Fractures

7. Winging of scapula is due to palsy of: *(NEET Pattern 2012)*
   A. Long thoracic nerve B. Nerve to latissimus dorsi
   C. Spinal accessory nerve D. Nerve to rhomboid
Ans. is 'A' Long thoracic nerve

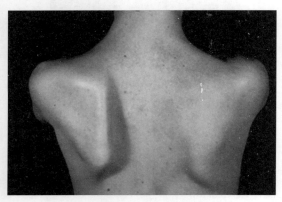

Vertebral border and inferior angle of scapula is prominent due to Serratus Anterior paralysis

8. A 45-year-old man presents with weakness, pain and fatigue in both lower limbs. He gives history of both limb paralysis 20 years back. What is the most probable diagnosis? *(AI 2012)*
   A. Poliomyositis B. Muscular dystrophy
   C. Post-polio syndrome D. Neuropathy
Ans. is 'C' Post-polio syndrome

9. A 35-year-old Female hypothyroid on treatment complaints of heaviness and tingling in left index and middle finger the pain often increases in night and she often has to get up which of the following is not a clinical test for this condition? *(AIIMS Nov 2011)*
   A. Finkelstein test B. Phalen's test
   C. Tinel's sign D. Tourniquet test
Ans. is 'A' Finkelstein test
   – Finkelstein test is for de Quervain's tenosynovitis other tests are for carpal tunnel syndrome.

10. Thoracic Outlet Syndrome is best diagnosed by:
    A. CT scan *(AI 2009)*
    B. MRI
    C. Digital subtraction angiography
    D. Clinical examination
Ans. is 'D' Clinical examination

11. You have treated the simple and undisplaced fracture of shaft of right tibia in a nine-year-girl with above knee plaster cast. Parents want to know the prognosis of union of the fractured limb which was affected by poliomyelitis four years ago. What is the best possible advice will you offer to the parents? *(AIIMS Nov 2003)*
    A. Fracture will unite slowly
    B. Fracture will not unite
    C. Fracture will unite normally
    D. Fracture will unite on attaining puberty
Ans. is 'A' Fracture will unite slowly

12. Test for tight iliotibial band is: *(AIIMS Nov 2001)*
    A. Ober's test B. Thomas test
    C. Simmond's test D. Charnley's test
Ans. is 'A' Ober's test

13. In 3-year-child with polio paralysis, tendon transfer operation is done at: *(AIIMS Dec 98)*
    A. 2 months after the disease
    B. 2 years after the disease
    C. 6–12 months after the disease
    D. After skeleton maturation
Ans. is 'B' 2 years after the disease
    – **Tendon transfers:** There are done to equalize an unbalanced paralysis or to use the motor power of working muscles for more useful functions. *It is not done before 5 years of age as the child has to be manageable enough to be taught proper exercises.*
    – As the child is 3 years old, tendon transfer should be done after 2 years (at 5 years of age).

14. What is the age of tendon transfer in post-polio residual paralysis? *(DNB June 2017)*
    A. < 6 months B. 1 years
    C. 2 years D. > 5 years
Ans. is 'D' > 5 years

	Nerve palsy	Presentation
1.	Erb's palsy	Policeman tip deformity (Porter's tip deformity)
2.	Nerve of bell (Long thoracic nerve) palsy	Winging of scapula
3.	Median nerve palsy (Labor's nerve)	Pointing index Benediction test Pen test (tests abductor pollicis brevis) Ochsner clasp test/Opposition of thumb lost/Ape thumb deformity
4.	Ulnar nerve palsy (Musician nerve)	Book test (froment sign), Card test (PAD) – Palmar Interossei, Igawa's test (DAB) – Dorsal interossei
5.	Radial nerve palsy	Wrist drop, (Finger drop and thumb drop Specifically in posterior interosseous nerve [PIN] injury)
6.	Common peroneal nerve palsy (Lateral popliteal nerve palsy) or sciatic nerve palsy	Foot drop (complete)

16 Joint Disorders

SYNOVIAL FLUID

Synovial Fluid

It is an ultra dialysate of blood plasma transudated from synovial capillaries to which hyaluronic acid protein complex (mucin) has been added by synovial B cells.

Type A synovial cells, containing numerous mitochondria in cytoplasm. They are macrophage like phagocytic cells, primarily concerned with phagocytosis of joint debris.

Type B synovial cells, which resemble fibroblasts and contain endoplasmic reticulum are **primarily responsible for the secretion of hyaluronic acid, protein and prostaglandins of synovial fluid.**

Hyaluronic acid gives synovial fluid its **thixotropic** (flow rate dependent) **non-Newtonian viscosity (i.e. viscosity changes according to rate of shear)** and lubricating property.

Fluid Kinetics

Newtonian Fluid—Newtonian fluid is a fluid whose viscosity is constant in relation to rate of shear changes. Examples are All gasses and simple fluids.

Non-Newtonian-Viscosity changes with shear. It is two types Thixotropic and Rheotropic.

Thixotropic

- Fluids whose viscosity decreases with increased rates of shear, e.g. Synovial fluid.
- Viscosity of synovial fluid is primarily because of the high levels of hyaluronate.

Rheotropic

- Fluids whose viscosity increases with increased rates of shear, e.g. printer ink
- A. **Normal Viscosity of Synovial Fluid**
  - Traumatic arthritis
  - Degenerative (osteo) arthritis
  - Pigmented villonodular synovitis
- B. **Normal/Decreased Viscosity**
  - SLE
- C. **Decreased Viscosity of Synovial Fluid**
  - Rheumatic fever
  - Rheumatoid arthritis
  - Gout
  - Pyogenic (septic) arthritis
  - Tubercular arthritis

Synovial fluid in different types of arthritis:

1. Normal synovial fluid is clear, WBC count ≤ 200/ μL
2. Non-inflammatory synovial fluid is clear, viscous, amber colored with a WBC 200-2000/μL and a predominance of mononuclear cell.
3. Inflammatory fluid is turbid, yellow, with an increased WBC count 2,000 to 50,000/μL and a polymorphonuclear leukocytic predominance.
    - 3a. **Inflammatory fluid has reduced viscosity**, diminished hyaluronate.
    - 3b. Infections (pyogenic) is purulent, WBC count > 50,000/μL, **PMN > 90%**
    - 3c. Infections **(Tuberculosis/granulomatous)** is yellow, turbid, WBC count 10,000–20,000/μL, PMN 60% and presence of lymphocytes, plasma cells and **histiocytes.**

Feature	Inflammatory arthritis	Non-inflammatory arthritis
Cardinal signs of inflammation (erythema, warmth, pain and swelling)	Present	Absent
Systemic symptoms (prolonged morning stiffness >1 hour, fatigue, fever, weight loss)	Present	Absent
Laboratory evidence of inflammation Elevated ESR Elevated C-reactive protein	Present	Absent

Causes:	• Infectious
	• Crystal induced (gout, pseudogout)
	• Immune mediated:
	  – Rheumatoid arthritis
	  – SLE
	  – Reactive, i.e. rheumatic fever, Reiter's syndrome
	• Idiopathic
		• Osteoarthritis
		• Traumatic arthritis
		• Pigmented villonodular synovitis (neoplastic)

New bone formation in form of osteophytes and osteosclerosis	Absent	Characteristically seen in osteoarthritis

Changes of articular cartilage with aging or osteoarthritis

Cartilage property	Aging	Osteoarthritis
Total water content (Hydration)	**Decreased**	**Increased** (Decreased in advanced OA)
Proteolytic enzymes:	Normal	Increased
Proteoglycan content	Decreased	Decreased

Diseases and usual joints affected

• Septic	Knee
• Syphilitic arthritis*	Knee
• Gonococcal arthritis*	Knee
• Gout*	MTP joint of Great toe

• Pseudogout*	Knee
• Rheumatoid arthritis	Metacarpophalangeal joint
• Ankylosing spondylitis*	Sacroiliac joint
• Diabetic charcot joint*	Foot joint (midtarsal)
• Senile osteoporosis*	Vertebra
• Paget's disease*	Pelvic bones > Femur > Skull > Tibia
• Osteochondritis dissecans*	Knee>elbow
• Actinomycosis*	Mandible
• Hemophilic arthritis*	Knee (children-ankle)
• Acute osteomyelitis*	Lower end of femur (Metaphysis)
• Brodie's abscess*	Upper end of Tibia

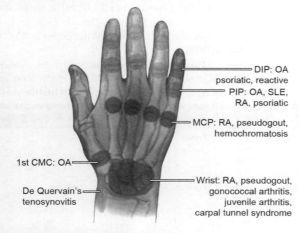

Fig. 16.1: 'The hand' (to diagnose arthritis)

PATTERN OF JOINT INVOLVEMENT

	Osteoarthritis	Rheumatoid arthritis	Psoriatic arthritis
Involved	PIP, DIP and 1'CMC (carpometacarpal) joints	PIP, MCP, wrist	DIP, PIP and any joint
Spared	MCP (metacarpophalangeal), wrist and ankle	**DIP joint usually**	Sparing of any joint

Non-Erosive arthritis—SLE
Non-deforming Arthritis-Behçet's syndrome

ZONES OF CARTILAGE

There are four zones (layers) of articular cartilage from the articular surface to subchondral bone.

Superficial zone (zone 1)
- It is the thinnest zone (10% to 20%)
- It protects deeper layers from shear
- It consists of two layer: (i) A sheet of densely packed collagen with little polysaccharide and to cells, covers the joint surface, and (ii) Flattened ellipsoid-shaped chondrocytes, with their major axis parallel to joint surface.
- It has progenitor cells (for articular cartilage)
- There is high density of chondrocytes
- There is high water content.

Transition zone (Zone 2)—40% to 60% of thickness
- Composition is intermediate between superficial zone and middle zone.
- Chondrocytes are in low density

- Proteoglycans to thicker collagen are seen
- This layer provides the 1st resistance to compressive forces.

Middle zone or radial zone or deep zone (Zone 3)—30% of thickness
- The chondrocytes are spheroidal in shape with their major axis perpendicular to joint surface.
- Chondrocytes are most active synthetically in this zone.
- This zone contains the largest diameter collagen fibrils, the highest concentration of proteoglycans and the lowest concentration of water.
- This layer provides the greatest resistance to compressive forces.

Calcified cartilage zone (Zone 4)
- It separates the middle zone from subchondral bone.
- The cells are small with small amount of endoplasmic reticulum Wand Golgi apparatus with very little metabolic activity.
- Cells are surrounded by calcified cartilage.
- Cell number is decreased.
- Chondrocytes are hypertrophic.

Note:
- Articular cartilage has no nerve supply. So there is no pain
- Capsule is the most pain sensitive structure in the joint.

MULTIPLE CHOICE QUESTIONS

1. True about articular cartilage: *(AI 2016)*
   A. Is a type of elastic cartilage
   B. Is hyaline cartilage on the articular surface of bones
   C. Is type 1 cartilage providing compressive strength
   D. Is hyaline cartilage found in growth plate of bones

Ans. is 'B' Is hyaline cartilage on the articular surface of bones

2. Choose the correct statement about articular cartilage: *(AI 2016)*
   A. Zone 2 contains articular cartilage progenitor cell
   B. Zone 4 contains calcified cartilage
   C. Zone 3 has highest proteoglycans content
   D. Zone 1 has high water content
   E. Zone 3 has chondrocytes in low density

Ans. is 'B' Zone 4 contains calcified cartilage; 'C' Zone 3 has highest proteoglycans content; and 'D' Zone 1 has high water content

3. Nutrient and oxygen reach the chondrocytes across perichondrium by: *(CET Nov 15) (TOPIC)*
   A. Capillaries   B. Diffusion
   C. Along neurons   D. Active transport

Ans. is 'B' Diffusion

4. All of the following cause erosive arthritis except:
   A. Rheumatoid arthritis   *(AI Dec 15)*
   B. Lupus Arthritis/Jaccoud arthritis
   C. Tuberculous arthritis   D. Septic arthritis

Ans. is 'B' Lupus arthritis/Jaccoud arthritis

5. In a patient with arthritis, examination of synovium aspirate, numerous lymphocytes, plasma cells and histiocytes are found. What type of arthritis it is? *(JIPMER 2014)*
   A. Acute pyogenic arthritis   B. Chronic arthritis
   C. Granulomatous arthritis   D. Rheumatoid arthritis

Ans. is 'C' Granulomatous arthritis

6. Joint erosion is not a feature in: (NEET 2015)
   A. SLE
   B. Gout
   C. Rheumatoid arthritis
   D. Psoriasis

Ans. is 'A' SLE

7. In Articular cartilage, most active chondrocytes are seen in: (NEET Pattern 2013)
   A. Zone 1
   B. Zone 2
   C. Zone 3
   D. Zone 4

Ans. is 'C' Zone 3

8. Articular cartilage, true is: (NEET Pattern 2013)
   A. Very vascular structure
   B. Surrounded by thick perichondrium
   C. Has no nerve supply
   D. Fibrocartilage

Ans. is 'C' Has no nerve supply

9. All of the following statements about synovial fluid are true, except: (AIIMS May 10, AI 2009)
   A. Secreted primarily by type A synovial cells
   B. Follows Non-Newtonian fluid kinetics
   C. Contains hyaluronic acid
   D. Viscosity is variable

Ans. is 'A' Secreted primarily by type A synovial cells
   Synovial fluid is secreted by type B synovial cells (type B synoviocytes).

10. Which of the following statements about changes in articular cartilage with aging is not true: (AI 2010)
    A. Total proteoglycan content is decreased
    B. Synthesis of proteoglycans is decreased
    C. Enzymatic degradation of proteoglycans is increased
    D. Total water content of cartilage is decrease

Ans. is 'C' Enzymatic degradation of proteoglycans is increased

11. Synovial fluid of low viscosity is seen in all except: (PGI June 05)
    A. Gout
    B. Septic arthritis
    C. Osteoarthritis
    D. Rheumatoid arthritis

Ans. is 'C' Osteoarthritis

12. Deforming polyarthritis is associated with all of the following except: (JIPMER 1999)
    A. Rheumatoid arthritis
    B. Psoriatic arthritis
    C. Behçet's syndrome
    D. Ankylosing spondylitis

Ans. is 'C' Behçet's syndrome
   – The arthritis of Behçet's syndrome is not deforming and affects knees and ankles.
   – Rheumatoid arthritis, psoriatic arthritis, ankylosing spondylitis, neuropathic arthropathy, etc. cause deforming arthritis.

13. Erosion of bone is seen with all of the following except:
    A. Gout
    B. SLE (AI 1994)
    C. Psoriasis
    D. Rheumatoid arthritis

Ans. is 'B' SLE
   – All inflammatory arthritis cause erosive arthritis, except SLE, which causes nonerosive arthritis.

INDICATIONS FOR ARTHROPLASTY

Goals of total joint replacement:
- Relieve pain
- Provide motion while maintaining stability
- Correct deformity

Absolute Contraindication: Recent or current joint sepsis

- Knee arthroplasties may be of following types:
  – *Total knee replacement (TKR):* Complete joint, i.e. both condyles of femur, both tibial plateau and patella are resected and replaced by prosthesis.
  – *Unicondylar replacement:* Only one condyle (medial or lateral) of femur and tibia is replaced.
- The primary indication is to relieve pain caused by severe arthritis with or without significant deformity.

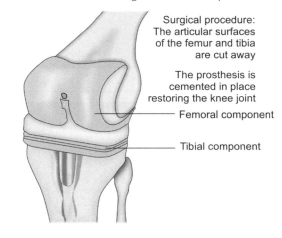

Fig. 16.2: Total knee replacement

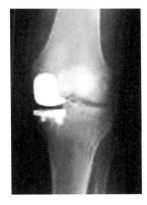

Fig. 16.3: Unicondylar knee replacement

PATELLAR CLUNK SYNDROME

It is knee popping and catching due to fibrous nodule on superior pole of patella in TKR patients that impinges on femoral component on knee extension. If symptoms are severe it requires resection of fibrous nodule (arthroscopic/open)

Types of replacement done at hip are:
- *Total hip replacement:* Both parts of joint, i.e. femoral head and acetabulum, are replaced by prosthesis.
- *Hemiarthroplasty (hemireplacement):* Only one part of the joint, i.e. femoral head, is replaced without putting acetabular component. Examples are bipolar hemiarthroplasty and unipolar hemiarthroplasty (Austin Moore hemiarthroplasty).
- *Surface replacement (resurfacing procedure):* Only diseased surface of femoral head is resected and is replaced by metal surface.

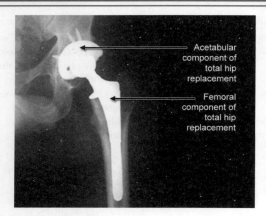

Fig. 16.4: Total hip replacement

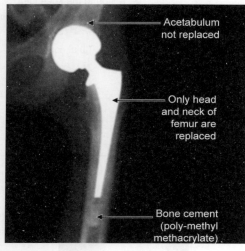

Fig. 16.5: Hemiarthroplasty

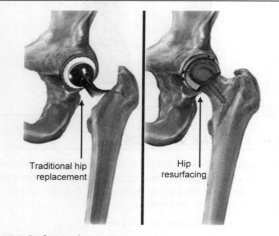

Fig. 16.6: Surface replacement

- Based on the articulating surfaces of the prosthesis, THR may be of following type:
  - *Metal on poly:* One surface is metallic (femoral side) and the other is of polyethylene (on acetabular side).
  - *Metal on metal:* Both articulating surfaces are of metal.
  - *Ceramic on ceramic:* Both articulating surfaces are of ceramic. (Aluminium compounds).

- Based on type of fixation, THR is of two types:
  - *Cemented THR:* Bone cement is used to fix the prosthesis with bone.
  - **Uncemented THR:** Prosthesis is directly inserted into the bone without using cement. After sometime osteo-integration over prosthesis takes place.

Complications of THR

- Infection < 1% incidence with current operation theater policies and laminar flow used to decrease infection rate.
- Dislocation—dislocation of a replacement is seen in < 1% cases.
- In cemented THR, there may be loosening of prosthesis. If it occurs without infection, it is called aseptic loosening (or osteolysis). Particles of metal (**titanium,** nickel, chromium, etc), cement (PMMA) and polyethylene all can produce periprosthetic osteolysis (aseptic loosening); but ***polyethylene particles are the major*** contributors.
- Mortality rates after THR ranges from 0.16% to 0.52%. Mortality is 1% for primary THA and 2.5% for revision THA. Increased mortality rates have been reported in men, patients older than 70 years, and patients with pre-existing cardiovascular disease.
- Thromboembolic disease (TED) is one of the most common serious complication. The 30-day mortality rate from pulmonary embolism in patients undergoing elective THR (at Mayo clinic) was 0.04%, behind myocardial infarction (MI) and cardiorespiratory arrest.
- Definite management of pulmonary embolism is thrombolysis.

Metal on Metal Articulations: Concerns

- Metal on metal articulation refers to the 'joint surfaces' that may be used for conventional total hip replacement or hip resurfacing procedures.

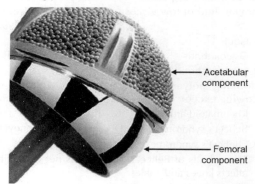

Fig. 16.7: Metal on metal surface replacement (only part of head replaced)

- The primary concern with metal on metal bearing/articulations is the release of 'metal ions', elevated levels of which, can be measured in the patient's blood and urine following implantation.

Contraindications of Metal on Metal Bearing Surfaces

- Patients with Renal Insufficiency, kidneys are chiefly responsible for eliminating metal ions from the blood.
- Young females of child-bearing age, as metal ions may cross the placenta and damage the fetus
- Patients with metal hypersensitivity
- They can also cause chromosomal changes
- Their role in carcinogenesis is under evaluation

Joint Disorders

Procedure	Metal on metal total hip replacement	Metal on metal surface replacement
Definition	Replacement of head and neck of femur and acetabulum	Replacement of the surface of femoral head and acetabulum (Neck is not replaced)
Contra-indications	Renal insufficiency, young females, hypersensitivity (metal associated)	Large femoral neck cyst or small deficient acetabulum or severe bone loss of head.
Concerns	Chromosomal abnormalities may be caused by metal articulations	• Patients with femoral head cysts > 1 cm (on preoperative radiographs) • Patients with high body mass index >35 • Care observed in rheumatoid arthritis and AVN.

Recent literature supports better results with Total hip replacements as compared to surface replacements of hip.

Note: Metal associated complications are also seen in surface replacement. The above mentioned are apart from those in Total Hip Replacement.

	Cemented arthroplasty	Uncemented arthroplasty
Interface	Implant cement bone	**Implant bone**
Weaklink	Cement bone interface	Strong construct
Good bone	No prerequisite	Normal bone stock
Longevity	Less 1/2 life	More 1/2 life
Cost	Cheaper	Costly

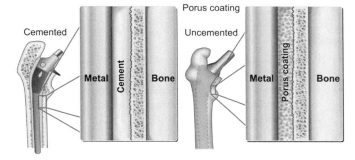

Fig. 16.8: Cemented verus uncemented arthroplasty

MULTIPLE CHOICE QUESTIONS

1. Patellar Clunk Syndrome scar is present at superior pole of patella and impinging on: *(AIIMS Nov 2018)*
   A. Femoral component during flexion
   B. Femoral component during extension
   C. Inferior pole during flexion
   D. Superior pole during extension
   Ans. is 'B' Femoral component during extension

2. In uncemented arthroplasty of the hip, the stem remains attached to the bone by: *(AI Dec 15)*
   A. Bone Ingrowth/ overgrowth over the surface of the stem
   B. Mechanical bonding between the stem and bone
   C. Press fitting of the stem in the tight canal
   D. Adhesion between the stem and bone due to adhesive properties of the stem
   Ans. is 'A' Bone ingrowth/ overgrowth over the surface of the stem

3. During performing a total hip replacement, the surgeon found destruction of the articular cartilage and multiple wedge shaped subchondral depressions. What is this called? *(AI Dec 15)*
   A. Osteolysis
   B. Osteomyelitis
   C. Osteonecrosis
   D. Osteogenesis
   Ans. is 'C' Osteonecrosis (subchondral depressions indicates avascular necrosis = Osteonecrosis)

4. Patellar clunk syndrome is a known complication of which surgery? *(CET Nov 15)*
   A. Corrective osteotomy for genu valgum
   B. Total knee Replacement
   C. Medial patellofemoral ligament reconstruction
   D. Bicondylar plating of proximal tibia fracture
   Ans. is 'B' Total knee replacement

5. Which of the following muscles seen on splitting tensor fascia lata during anterolateral approach before hip joint is exposed? *(JIPMER 2015)*
   A. Gluteus maximus
   B. Gluteus medius
   C. Gluteus minimus
   D. Superior gemellus
   Ans. is 'B' Gluteus medius

6. A patient after Total Hip Replacement develops breathlessness what is the definitive management: *(AIIMS May 2014)*
   A. Thrombolysis
   B. Bronchodilators
   C. Steroids
   D. Oxygen
   Ans. is 'A' Thrombolysis

7. After knee replacement surgery, proprioceptors of joints are altered. Effect is. *(AIIMS May 2014)*
   A. Normal movement
   B. Complete loss of sensation at joint position at resting stage
   C. Loss of sensation of joint position at dynamic stage
   D. All types of sensation lost
   Ans. is 'A' Normal movement

   Explanation
   – Joint proprioception and kinesthesia improve after total knee arthroplasty. Joint sensation is decreased in arthritic knee but improves after knee arthroplasty when compared with that of contralateral limb because, following total knee arthroplasty. The joint space and soft tissue tension are re-established. These changes may modify the response characteristics of mechanoreceptors in both capsuloligamentous and musculotendinous structures, enhancing the perception of joint motion and position.
   – The movement improves after replacement or at least is the same as preoperative range.

8. Metal on metal articulation should be avoided in: *(AI 2010)*
   A. Osteonecrosis
   B. Young female
   C. Inflammatory arthritis
   D. Revision surgery
   Ans. is 'B' Young female

9. A patient developed breathlessness and chest pain, on second postoperative after a total hip replacement. Echocardiography showed right ventricular dilatation and tricuspid regurgitation. What is the most likely diagnosis. *(AI 2010)*
   A. Acute MI
   B. Pulmonary embolism
   C. Hypotensive shock
   D. Cardiac tamponade
   Ans. is 'B' Pulmonary embolism

– *Chest pain and breathlessness,* together with echocardiographic evidence *of right ventricular dilatation and tricuspid regurgitation after a high risk procedure (for thromboembolism) like total hip replacement suggests a diagnosis of pulmonary embolism.*

10. What is the most common cause of death after total hip replacement? *(AI 09)*
    A. Infection
    B. Deep vein thrombosis
    C. Pulmonary embolism
    D. Pneumonia

    Ans. is 'C' Pulmonary embolism

    Cause of mortality after joint replacement order is myocardial Infarction > cardiorespiratory arrest > thromboembolism

11. Indications of arthroplasty: *(PGI Dec 04)*
    A. Osteoarthritis
    B. Rheumatoid arthritis
    C. Ankylosing spondylosis
    D. Gout
    E. Fracture neck femur

    Ans. is 'A' Osteoarthritis; 'B' Rheumatoid arthritis; 'C' Ankylosing spondylosis; 'D' Gout and 'E' Fracture neck femur
    – Arthroplasty can be done for any disease any joint except active infection.

12. Aseptic loosening in cemented total hip replacement, occurs as a result of hypersensitivity response to: *(AI 2004)*
    A. Titanium debris
    B. High density polyethylene debris
    C. N,N-Dimethyltryptamine
    D. Free radicals

    Ans. is 'B' High density polyethylene debris
    – Particles of metal (**titanium**, nickel, chromium, etc.), cement (PMMA) and polyethylene all can produce periprosthetic osteolysis (aseptic loosening); *polyethylene particles appear to be the major* particles causing the damage.

13. Major indication (s) for arthroplasty: *(PGI Dec 2K)*
    A. Osteoarthritis of hip
    B. Ankylosis of elbow
    C. Ununited tibial fracture
    D. Ununited femoral neck fracture
    E. TB spine

    Ans. is 'A' Osteoarthritis of hip; 'B' Ankylosis of elbow; 'D' Ununited femoral neck fracture

HIGH TIBIAL OSTEOTOMY

Biomechanics

- In normal knees, 60% of load passes through medial compartment.
- Varus and valgus deformities are common and cause an abnormal distribution of weight bearing stresses within the joint.
- Most common deformity in patients with OA of knee is a varus position, which causes stress to be concentrated medially, accelerating degenerative changes in medial part of joint. Valgus deformity causes accelerated changes on lateral compartment. (Seen in rheumatoid arthritis).

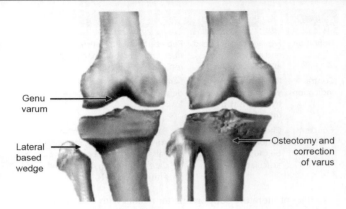

Fig. 16.9: High tibial osteotomy

Principle

- Biomechanical rationale for proximal tibial osteotomy in patients with unicompartmental osteoarthritis of knee is unloading of involved joint compartment by correcting the malalignment and redistributing the stresses on the knee joint.
- Osteotomy (corrective) is performed through cancellous bone near joint line to offer advantages of higher healing rates and to achieve better joint line inclination and limb alignment.
- In a varus knee, correction to 8–10 degrees of anatomical valgus is associated with best prognosis while knees left with residual varus have a less satisfactory result and high chances of recurrences.

Indications

- Pain and disability resulting from OA that significantly interfere with high demand employment or recreation.
- Evidence on weight bearing radiographs of degenerative arthritis that is confined to one compartment with a corresponding varus or valgus deformity.
- The ability of patient to carry out a rehabilitation program.
- Good vascular status without serious arterial insufficiency or large varicosity.

Contraindications

- **More than 20 degrees correction needed.**
- Narrowing of lateral compartment cartilage space
- Lateral tibial subluxation of > 1 cm
- Medial compartment bone loss of > 3 mm
- Flexion contracture of > 15 degrees
- Knee flexion movement of < 90 degrees
- Rheumatoid arthritis.

Complications of High Tibial Osteotomy

- Compartment syndrome
- Recurrence (5–30%) of deformity
- Infection
- Stiffness of knee
- Peroneal nerve palsy
- Nonunion of osteotomy

MULTIPLE CHOICE QUESTION

1. All of the following statements about High Tibial Osteotomy are true, except: *(AI 2009, AIIMS May 2011)*
   A. Magnitude of correction achieved is greater than 30 degree
   B. Indicated in unicompartmental osteoarthritis
   C. Performed through cancellous bone
   D. Recurrence is a long-term complication

Ans. is 'A' Magnitude of correction achieved is greater than 30 degree.

OSTEOARTHRITIS (OA): MOST COMMON JOINT DISEASE

Classification

I. Idiopathic (Primary) OA
   A. Localized (Monoarticular and Pauciarticular) OA involving:

   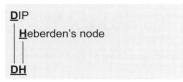

   1. **Hands:** DIP (Heberden's node), PIP (Bouchard's node), 1st carpometacarpal joint.
   2. Knee
   3. Hip **(Primary OA of Hip is Unknown in India)**
   4. Spine (apophyseal joint, inter vertebral joint).
   B. Generalized (Polyarticular) OA includes three or more of the above listed area.

II. Secondary OA
   - Trauma
   - Congenital/developmental disorders, e.g. Perthes', SCFE, DDH, varus/valgus deformity, bone dysplasias
   - Metabolic disease, e.g. ochronosis (alkaptonuria), hemochromatosis, Wilson's disease, Gaucher's disease.
   - Endocrine disorders, e.g. Acromegaly, hyperparathyroidism, **diabetes mellitus**, obesity, hypothyroidism.
   - Calcium deposition diseases, e.g. CPPD, apatite arthropathy
   - Other joint disease, e.g. fracture, AVN, gout, infection, osteopetrosis, osteochondritis, Paget's disease.

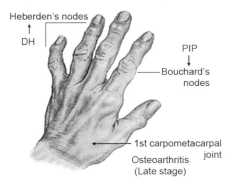

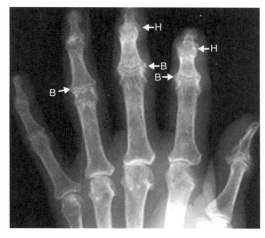

Fig. 16.10: Hand joints involved in OA (H = Heberden's node and B = Bouchard's node)

Osteoarthritis characteristically involves distal interphalangeal joint (Heberden's node), proximal interphalangeal joint (Bouchard's node), 1st carpometacarpal joint (base of thumb) of hand with sparing of metacarpophalangeal joint and wrist joint.

Pattern of Joint Involvement

- Monoarticular/Pauciarticular—Knee> Hip
- Polyarticular – DIP
- Overall DIP commonest

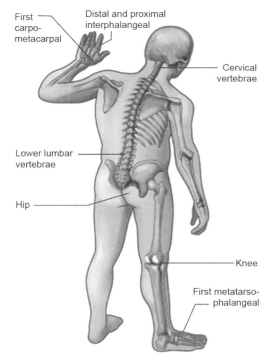

Fig. 16.11: Joints involved in osteoarthritis

Radiological Features

X-rays are so characteristic that other forms of imaging are seldom necessary. The four cardinal signs are:

1. Asymmetrical loss of Cartilage Causing Narrowing of Joint Space (earliest feature)
2. **Sclerosis of subchondral bone** under the area of cartilage loss
3. Cystic lesion close to articular surface
4. Osteophytes at the margins of joint
   Loose bodies and deformities can be there.

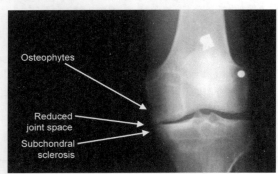

Fig. 16.12: X-ray changes in osteoarthritis knee

Quadriceps

Due to decreased loading of painful extremity quadriceps weakness is common in patients of osteoarthritis of knee. Most importantly vastus medialis is affected.

Treatment

- Maintain movement and muscle strength by physiotherapy and graded muscle exercise.
- Protects the joint from overload by giving rest and weight reduction.
- Correction of deformities if present.
- Thermal modalities, analgesic medication, wedged insoles, Orthosis and arthroscopic debridement and lavage.
- Progressive joint destruction require joint replacement in elderly and HTO in young.
- **Classification system and stage wise management for OA knee:**
  1. Initial treatment is always conservative, (exercise and glucosamines are preferred)
  2. Clinical picture is more significant than radiology or X-ray changes
  3. If activities of daily living are affected surgery is advised
  4. **Surgery for young is HTO (if not contraindicated) if contraindicated TKR is performed**
  5. **Surgery for elderly (≥ 65 years) is TKR**
  6. HTO—High Tibial Osteotomy
  7. TKR—Total Knee Replacement
  8. Usually stage 2 onwards in elderly TKR is finally carried out.

Ahlback grade	Definition	Treatment in young	Treatment in elderly
Grade 1	Joint space narrowing	Conservative if fails HTO	Conservative if fails TKR
Grade 2	Joint space obliteration	Conservative if fails HTO	Conservative if fails TKR

Contd...

Contd...

Ahlback grade	Definition	Treatment in young	Treatment in elderly
Grade 3	Minor bone attrition (0–5 mm)	Conservative if fails surgery if bone loss <3 mm HTO otherwise TKR	Conservative if fails TKR
Grade 4	Moderate bone attrition (5–10 mm)	TKR	TKR
Grade 5	Severe bone attrition (>10 mm)	TKR	TKR

* >3 mm bone loss HTO is contraindicated

Kellgren and Lawrence grade	Definition	Treatment in young	Treatment in elderly
Grade 1 "doubtful"	Minute osteophytes (doubtful joint space narrowing)	Conservative if fails HTO	Conservative if fails TKR
Grade 2 "minimal"	Definite osteophytes (possible joint space narrowing)	Conservative if fails HTO	Conservative if fails TKR
Grade 3 "moderate"	Moderate diminution of joint spaces, sclerosis and multiple osteophytes	Conservative if fails HTO	Conservative if fails TKR
Grade 4 "severe"	Joint space impaired with sclerosis of subchondral bone and bone deformities	Conservative if fails HTO	Conservative if fails TKR

MULTIPLE CHOICE QUESTIONS

1. Glucosamine supplementation is given in:
   (AIIMS Nov 2017)
   A. Arthritis   B. Diabetes
   C. Cataract   D. Asthma
   Ans. is 'A' Arthritis

2. Which of the following is not true about osteoarthritis?
   (NEET Dec 2016)
   A. Inflammation of synovial joints
   B. Most common joint disease
   C. Affects shoulder joint
   D. Narrowing of the joint space occurs
   Ans. is 'A' Inflammation of synovial joints

3. True about osteoarthritis is/are: *(PGI Nov 2017)*
   A. In knee common than hip
   B. Decreased thickness of subchondral bone
   C. Characterized by increased water content
   D. Decrease in proteoglycans
   E. It is a non-inflammatory arthritis
   Ans. is 'A' In knee common than hip; 'C' Characterized by increased water content; 'D' Decrease in proteoglycans; 'E' It is a non-inflammatory arthritis

4. About Osteoarthritis, choose the correct statement:
   (PGI Nov 2017)
   A. Thickening of synovial membrane is one of the earliest feature of the disease
   B. Weight bearing is a common etiology underlying ankle OA
   C. In India, knee OA is more common than hip OA

D. Hip arthrodesis if done, can decrease the pain associated, but will cause a decrease in joint movement
E. MCP joint is spared in OA

Ans. is 'B' Weight bearing is a common etiology underlying ankle OA; 'C' In India, knee OA is more common than hip OA; 'D' Hip arthrodesis if done, can decrease the pain associated, but will cause a decrease in joint movement; 'E' MCP joint is spared in OA.

5. Following X-ray changes are seen in: (AI 2016)

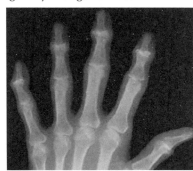

A. OA B. RA
C. Psoriasis D. Pseudogout

Ans. is 'A' OA (DIP involvement is seen—refer to Fig. 16.10 p207)

6. Pain and arthritis of distal interphalangeal joints is seen in: (CET July 16)
A. Osteoarthritis B. Rheumatoid Arthritis
C. Ankylosing spondylitis D. De Quervain's disease

Ans. is 'A' Osteoarthritis

7. Heberden's nodes are seen in: (AI Dec 15)
A. Osteoarthritis of the distal interphalangeal joints
B. Osteoarthritis of the proximal interphalangeal joints
C. Rheumatoid arthritis of the 1st carpometacarpal joint
D. Rheumatoid arthritis of the distal interphalangeal joints

Ans. is 'A' Osteoarthritis of the distal interphalangeal joints

8. Bouchard's nodes are seen in: (CET Nov 15)
A. Osteoarthritis of the distal interphalangeal joints
B. Osteoarthritis of the proximal interphalangeal joints
C. Rheumatoid arthritis of the 1st carpometacarpal joint
D. Rheumatoid arthritis of the distal interphalangeal joints

Ans. is 'B' Osteoarthritis of the proximal interphalangeal joints

9. Osteoarthritis is not seen in: (NEET 2015)
A. Ankle joints B. Knee joints
C. Hip joints D. 1st carpometacarpal joint

Ans. is 'A' Ankle joints

10. Arthritis involving DIP, PIP, 1st carpometacarpal with sparing of MCP and wrist joints is typical of: (NEET 2015)
A. Osteoarthritis B. Rheumatoid arthritis
C. Ankylosing spondylitis D. Psoriatic arthritis

Ans. is 'A' Osteoarthritis

11. Which one of the following bursae always communicates with knee joint cavity? (PGM-CET 2015)
A. Prepatellar B. Suprapatellar
C. Superficial infrapatellar D. Deep infrapatellar

Ans. is 'B' Suprapatellar

12. A 58-year-old female patient presents with one-year history of anterior knee pain on climbing stairs. On examination crepitus was present. There was severe restriction of movements beyond 110 degrees. Examination of hip and back was normal. Diagnosis is: (JIPMER 2014)
A. Osteoarthritis B. Psoriatic arthritis
C. Osteonecrosis D. Gout

Ans. is 'A' Osteoarthritis

13. Joint not involved in osteoarthritis: (NEET Pattern 2013)
A. PIP B. DIP
C. MCP D. Knee

Ans. is 'C' MCP

14. Which can cause loose body in the joint: (NEET Pattern 2013)
A. RA B. Ankylosing spondylitis
C. OA D. SLE

Ans. is 'C' OA

15. In OA one of this is beneficial: (NEET Pattern 2012)
A. Glucosamine B. Ketones
C. Glucose D. Citric acid

Ans. is 'A' Glucosamine

16. In patients with osteoarthritis of knee joint, atrophy occurs most commonly in which muscle: (AIIMS Nov 2011, May 2007, AIPG 2007)
A. Quadriceps only B. Hamstrings only
C. Both A and B D. Gastrocnemius

Ans. is 'A' Quadriceps only
Quadriceps is the most common muscle involved in OA

17. Heberden's arthropathy affects: (AI 2005, Kerala 96)
A. Lumbar spine
B. Symmetrically large joints
C. Sacroiliac joints
D. Distal interphalangeal joints

Ans. is 'D' Distal interphalangeal joints.

18. True about osteoarthritis except: (PGI Dec 03)
A. Commonly found in adult after 50 yrs.
B. Heberden's nodes are found
C. Can involve Single joint
D. Lower limb deformity is seen
E. Ankylosis is seen

Ans. is 'E' Ankylosis is seen
Ankylosis is very rare in OA it is seen in inflammatory arthritis

19. Severe disability in primary osteoarthritis of hip is best managed by: (PGI Dec 02, PGI 95)
A. Arthrodesis
B. Arthroplasty
C. McMurray's osteotomy
D. Intra-articular hydrocortisone and physiotherapy

Ans. is 'B' Arthroplasty

20. Proximal interphalangeal, distal interphalangeal and 1st carpometacarpal joint involvement and sparing of wrist is a feature of:
(AI 2001, 2K, AIIMS June 99, Dec 95, AI 1997)
A. Rheumatoid arthritis B. Pseudogout
C. Psoriatic arthropathy D. Osteoarthritis

Ans. is 'D' Osteoarthritis Involvement of PIP, DIP and 1st carpometacarpal joint (carpometacarpal joint of thumb) with sparing of wrist and metacarpophalangeal joint is characteristic of OA.

21. A 62-year-old Male complaints of pain bilateral knees R > L, he has difficulty in climbing stairs, squatting, sitting cross legged. His quadriceps muscle is wasted. On Right knee X-ray there is subchondral sclerosis, tibial spine spiking obliterated medial joint space and reduced lateral joint space. AHLBACK grade 2 stage next step is:

(AI 2011)

A. Conservative   B. Arthroscopy
C. Total knee replacement   D. High tibial osteotomy

Ans. is 'A' Conservative
- In this case next step is asked that will be a trial of conservative management, if it would have been asked best than TKR (Total Knee Replacement) would have been preferred.

RHEUMATOID ARTHRITIS (RA)

- **Women are affected 3 times more than men.** Older women (> 60 year) are 6 times more commonly involved than younger one.
- **Symmetrical** involvement of peripheral joint is more common than axial skeleton involvement.
- Felty's syndrome, osteoporosis, and increased incidence of lymphoma especially large B cell lymphoma is associated with RA.

Joint Involved in Rheumatoid Arthritis

RA can affect any diarthrodial joint and most often causes symmetrical arthritis.

Commonly Involved Joint (these 14 joints are used for diagnosis according to 1987 criterion) Right or left

1. Wrist joint
2. Metacarpophalangeal (MP) joint
3. Proximal interphalangeal (PIP) joint
4. Elbow
5. Knee
6. Ankle
7. **Metatarsophalangeal joint**

Less Common Involvement

- **Upper cervical spine** (facet joint) with Atlantoaxial subluxation: **Commonest areas affected in axial skeleton.**
- Hip joint
- Temporomandibular joint
- Subtalar and forefoot.

Usually DIP is not involved in and is not used for diagnosis **but is involved when swan neck and boutonniere deformity develops. The involvement in late stages also is not due to direct inflammatory process but due to the pull of tendons/ soft tissues in these deformities. Subsequently with altered biomechanics these joints can undergo degeneration.**

Lumbar Spine is Usually Spared in RA

Rheumatoid Arthritis Knee	Osteoarthritis Knee
Periarticular osteopenia	Subchondral sclerosis
Valgus > Varus	Varus > valgus
Marginal erosions	Marginal erosions not seen
No osteophytes are seen	Osteophytes are seen
Soft tissue swelling (pannus)	Negative
Subchondral cysts	Subchondral cysts

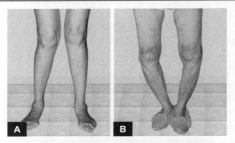

Figs. 16.13A and B: (A) RA Knee-Genu valgus; (B) OA Knee-Genu varus

Characteristic Deformities of Hand and Foot in RA

- **'Z-deformity'**, i.e. radial deviation of the wrist with ulnar deviation of the digits, often with palmar subluxation of proximal phalanges.
- **'Swan-neck deformity'**, i.e. hyperextension of PIP joints with compensatory flexion of the distal interphalangeal joints.
- **Boutonniere deformity**, i.e. flexion contracture of PIP joints and hyperextension of DIP joints. It is due to rupture of extensor tendon.
- Hyperextension of 1st interphalangeal joint and flexion of MP joint with a consequent loss of thumb mobility and pinch - Swan Neck deformity of thumb.
- Eversion at hindfoot (subtalar joint), plantar subluxation of metatarsal heads, widening of forefoot, hallux valgus, and lateral deviation and dorsal subluxation of toes; hammer toe. (Fexion of PIP).
- **Wind swept deformities of toes,** i.e. valgus deformities of toes in one foot and varus in other (as wind sweeps all the structure in one direction).

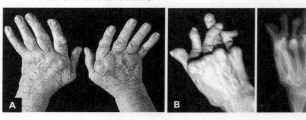

Figs. 16.14A and B: Deformities of hand in RA (A) Ulnar deviation of fingers; (B) Arthritis mutilans

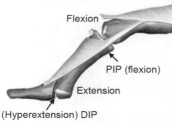

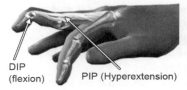

Fig. 16.15: Finger deformities in RA

Classification Criteria for Rheumatoid Arthritis–2010		Score
Joint involvement	1 large joint (shoulder, elbow, hip, knee, ankle)	0
	2–10 large joints	1
	1–3 small joints (MCP, PIP, Thumb IP, MTP, wrists)	2
	4–10 small joints	3
	>10 joints (at least 1 small joint)	5
Serology	Negative RF and negative anti-CCP antibodies	0
	Low-positive RF or low-positive anti-CCP antibodies (3 times ULN)	2
	High-positive RF or high-positive anti-CCP antibodies (>3 times ULN)	3
Acute-phase reactants	Normal CRP and normal ESR	0
	Abnormal CRP or abnormal ESR	1
Duration of symptoms	<6 weeks	0
	>6 weeks	1

Total Score 10
Score > 6 indicates – RA
RF – Rheumatoid factor

Anti-CCP antibodies—anti-Citrullinated cyclic peptide antibodies. It is positive in up to 98% of patient. 2% of general population has anti-CCP positive. It is most specific marker for RA.

The 1987 Revised Criteria for Diagnosis of RA

1. Guidelines for classification 4 of 7 criterion are required to classify a patient as having RA Patients with 2 or more criteria are not excluded.
2. Criteria (a–d must be present for at least 6 weeks and b–e must be observed by physician)
   a. **Morning stiffness**, in and around joint **lasting 1 hour** before maximal improvement.
   b. **Arthritis of 3 or more joint** areas, observed by a physician simultaneously, have soft tissue swelling or joint effusion, not just bony over growth. The 14 possible joint areas involved are right or left **proximal interphalangeal (PIP), metacarpophalangeal (MCP), wrist, elbow, knee, ankle and metatarsophalangeal joints (MTP).**
   c. Arthritis of **hand** joints, e.g. wrist, MP or PIP joints.
   d. **Symmetrical** arthritis, i.e. simultaneous involvement of same joint area on both sides of body.
   e. **Rheumatoid nodules (Pathognomonic):** Subcutaneous nodules over bony prominences, extensor surfaces or juxta-articular region.
   f. Serum rheumatoid factor.
   g. Radiological changes: bony erosion or unequivocal bony decalcification, periarticular osteoporosis and narrowing of articular (joint) space.

Note: Seronegative RA: With advent of 2010 and 1987 criterion a patient is either classified as rheumatoid arthritis or not classified as rheumatoid arthritis and seronegative RA terminology is avoided but if this comes as an option, it will be a case of RA according to criterion that has Rheumatoid factor and anti-CCP negative.

Clinical Course and Prognosis of RA

Poor Prognostic Factors Persons who present with high titers of rheumatoid factor, C-reactive protein and haptoglobin have a worse prognosis, as do individuals with subcutaneous nodules or radiographic evidence of erosions at the time of initial evaluation. Sustained disease activity of more than 1 year's duration. Also is as poor prognosis.

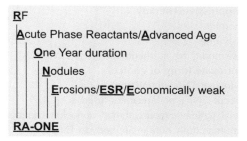

"RA one" poor prognostic factors in RA

Presence of HLA —DR b1* 0401 or DRb* 0404 has poor prognosis.

Normocytic, normochromic anemia is frequently present in active RA.

Radiological features of RA are
- Evidence of soft tissue swelling and joint effusion
- Symmetrical involvement
- **Juxta-articular osteopenia** (within weeks)
- Loss of articular cartilage and bone erosions (after months)
- Narrowing of joint space
- Articular destruction and joint deformity, e.g. subluxation of atlantoaxial and cervical joints
- Lack of hypertrophic bone changes (sclerosis or osteophyte).

Felty's Syndrome
- It consists of chronic rheumatoid arthritis, splenomegaly, neutropenia, and occasional anemia and thrombocytopenia.

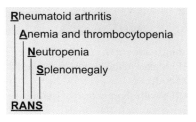

- It is most common in long standing cases. These patients frequently have high titers of rheumatoid factor, subcutaneous nodules and other manifestations of systemic rheumatoid disease. It may develop after joint inflammation has regressed.

"Pleural Effusion with Low Sugar is Seen in RA"

Management of Rheumatoid Arthritis
1. Stop synovitis
2. Keep joints moving
3. Prevent deformity
4. Reconstruction
5. Rehabilitate.

This is achieved by

Physiotherapy
- Exercise is directed at maintaining muscle strength and joint mobility.

Drug Treatment
- NSAIDs
- Glucocorticoid therapy esp. in vasculitis (mononeuritis multiplex, pericarditis and eye lesion).

Immunosuppressive Therapy
- Leflunomide
- Cyclosporine
- Disease modifying antirheumatic drugs (DMARDs)
- **Methotrexate (drug of choice)**
- Anticytokine (TNF neutralizing)
- Etanercept (TNF type II receptor fused to IgG1)
- Infliximab (chimeric mouse/human monoclonal antibody to TNF)
- Adalimumab (fully human antibody to TNF)
- Abatacept (Inhibits T-cell activation).

Surgery
- Reconstructive surgery
- Open or arthroscopic synovectomy
- Arthroplasties and total joint replacement
- Median life expectancy is shortened by 3–7 years in RA.

MULTIPLE CHOICE QUESTIONS

1. 14 years old child with pain and swelling of bilateral hand joints presents in OPD. The following is the image: *(NEET Pattern 2019)*

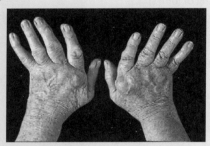

   What is the treatment?
   A. DMARDs after initial 3 months of NSAIDs
   B. Only NSAID
   C. DMARDs with short course of steroids
   D. Monotherapy with TNF drugs
   Ans. is 'C' DMARDs with short course of steroids

2. All are features of inflammatory arthritis except? *(PGI May 2018)*
   A. Morning stiffness   B. X-ray showing sclerosis
   C. Elevated ESR   D. Weight gain
   E. Swelling of joints
   Ans. is 'B' X-ray showing sclerosis & 'D' Weight gain

3. A 60 years old female previous case history of fever, fatigue, weight loss polyarthralgia. She had morning stiffness and bilateral hand pain. The radiological findings given below, what may be your diagnosis? *(DNB Pattern 2018)*

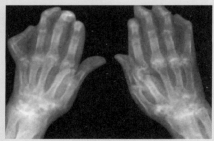

   A. Osteoarthritis   B. Rheumatoid arthritis
   C. Gout   D. Psoriatic arthritis
   Ans. is 'B' Rheumatoid arthritis

4. Which of the following is difference between Rheumatoid arthritis and osteoarthritis? *(DNB July 2016)*
   A. Osteophytes are seen in osteoarthritis
   B. Systemic symptoms are seen in osteoarthritis
   C. Rheumatoid arthritis is uncommon in hands and feet
   D. Osteoarthritis is an autoimmune disease
   Ans. is 'A' Osteophytes are seen in osteoarthritis

5. Most specific antibody seen in RA: *(DNB June 2017)*
   A. Anti CCP   B. Rheumatoid factor
   C. ANA   D. Anti dsDNA
   Ans. is 'A' Anti CCP

6. A person has injury on dorsal surface of proximal interphalangeal joint of right middle finger. Which of the following can occur? *(PGI May 2017)*
   A. Rupture of lateral ligament
   B. Buttonhole deformity   C. Mallet finger
   D. Laceration of the central slip of the extensor
   E. Swan Neck deformity
   Ans. is 'A' Rupture of lateral ligament; 'B' Buttonhole deformity; 'D' Laceration of the central slip of the extensor

7. Which of the following is not true regarding inflammatory arthritis? *(NEET Dec 2016)*
   A. Presence of morning stiffness
   B. Sclerosis on X-ray
   C. Anemia of chronic disease
   D. Presence of fever, weight loss and elevated ESR
   Ans. is 'B' Sclerosis on X-ray

8. Boutonniere deformity has: *(AI 2016)*
   A. Hyperextension of PIP joints & flexion of DIP joints
   B. Hyperextension of DIP joints & flexion PIP joints
   C. Flexion of DIP joints & Extension at metacarpophalangeal joints
   D. Flexion of DIP joints
   Ans. is 'B' Hyperextension of DIP joints & flexion PIP joints

9. True about Boutonnieres deformity is/are: *(PGI May 2016)*
   A. Rupture of extensor tendon
   B. Initially joints are mobile followed by rigidity
   C. Flexion at PIP joint and extension at DIP
   D. Seen in cases of osteoarthritis
   E. Rupture of flexor tendon
   Ans. is 'A' Rupture of extensor tendon; 'B' Initially joints are mobile followed by rigidity and 'C' Flexion at PIP joint and extension at DIP

10. In which of the following deformities is the distal interphalangeal joint flexed and proximal interphalangeal joint extended? *(DNB June 2017, CET July 16)*
    A. Boutonniere deformity B. Swan neck deformity
    C. Z deformity   D. Claw hand
    Ans. is 'B' Swan neck deformity

11. Which of the following is difference between Rheumatoid arthritis and osteoarthritis? *(CET July 16)*
    A. Osteophytes are seen in osteoarthritis
    B. Systemic symptoms are seen in osteoarthritis
    C. Rheumatoid arthritis is uncommon in hands and feet
    D. Osteoarthritis is an autoimmiune disease
    Ans. is 'A' Osteophytes are seen in osteoarthritis

12. In which of the following deformities is the distal interphalangeal joint extended? *(AI Dec 15)*
    A. Boutonniere deformity
    B. Swan neck deformity
    C. Z deformity
    D. Claw Hand

Ans. is 'A' Boutonniere deformity

13. Rheumatoid Arthritis affects which region of the spinal column? *(AI Dec 2016, 2015)*
    A. Cervical Spine
    B. Thoracic Spine
    C. Lumbosacral Spine
    D. Equally affects all regions

Ans. is 'A' Cervical spine

14. All of the following are radiological features of Rheumatoid arthritis except: *(AI Dec 15)*
    A. Decreased Joint Space
    B. Articular Erosions
    C. Periarticular osteopenia
    D. Fibrous ankylosis

Ans. is 'D' Fibrous ankylosis

15. Hammer toe deformity is seen in: *(AI Dec 15)*
    A. Rheumatoid arthritis
    B. Fracture distal phalanx of great toe
    C. Bunion
    D. Osteochondritis

Ans. is 'A' Rheumatoid arthritis

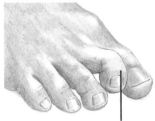

Hammer toe—flexion deformity of PIP (Compensatory hyperextension of MCP occurs)

16. Windswept deformity of the knee is seen in: *(AI Dec 15)*
    A. Osteoarthritis
    B. Rheumatoid arthritis
    C. Ankylosing Spondylitis
    D. Psoriatic arthritis

Ans. is 'B' Rheumatoid arthritis

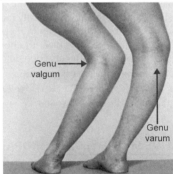

Windswept deformity = genu varum on one side and genu valgum on the other

17. Part of spine, involved in Rheumatoid arthritis is:
    A. Sacral
    B. Lumbar *(PGM-CET 2015)*
    C. Thoracic
    D. Cervical

Ans. is 'D' Cervical

18. Swan neck deformity is seen in: *(NEET 2015)*
    A. Osteoarthritis
    B. Rheumatoid arthritis
    C. Psoriatic arthritis
    D. Gout

Ans. is 'B' Rheumatoid arthritis

19. Distal interphalangeal joint involvement occur in: *(PGI Nov 2014)*
    A. Boutonniere deformity
    B. Swan neck deformity
    C. Mallet finger
    D. Trigger finger
    E. Dupuytren's contracture

Ans. is 'A' Boutonniere deformity; 'B' Swan neck deformity; 'C' Mallet finger; and 'E' Dupuytren's contracture

20. Which of the following is not a feature of rheumatoid arthritis? *(NEET 2015)*
    A. Heberden's nodes
    B. Swan neck deformity
    C. Ulnar deviation of fingers at metacarpophalangeal joint
    D. Symmetric reduction of joint space

Ans. is 'A' Heberden's nodes

21. Abatacept is used for: *(AIIMS Nov 2014)*
    A. Rheumatoid arthritis
    B. Ankylosing spondylitis
    C. Osteoarthritis
    D. SLE

Ans. is 'A' Rheumatoid arthritis

Explanation

It binds to CD80 and CD86 receptors on APC. It inhibits T cell activation by blocking CD80/86 interactions to CD28. This inhibits T cells proliferation and B cell immunological response. This normalizes inflammatory mediators in RA.

22. A middle age female of rheumatoid arthritis on treatment develops upper motor neuron signs in her limbs. The investigation required to evaluate her further is: *(AIIMS Nov 2012)*
    A. Spine lateral view flexion and extension views
    B. Open mouth view
    C. Swimmers view
    D. Broden's view

Ans. is 'A' Spine lateral view flexion and extension views

Atlantoaxial instability (AAI) is characterized by excessive movement at the junction between the atlas (C1) and axis (C2) as a result of either a bony or ligamentous abnormality. Neurologic symptoms occur when the spinal cord is involved and is upper motor neuron signs in limbs.

The causes of AAI are varied. AAI sometimes results from trauma. Other cases occur secondary to an upper respiratory infection or infection following head and neck surgery. Another cause is rheumatoid arthritis (RA), with its predilection for the upper cervical spine. In addition, congenital anomalies, syndromes, or metabolic diseases can increase the risk of AAI. The assessment involves flexion extension lateral view of cervical spine that can assess this instability. Open mouth view is for atlantoaxial area specially dens but will not demonstrate instability. Swimmers view is for cervicothoracic junction assessment. Broden's view is for subtalar joint.

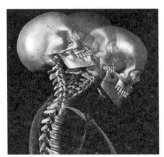

Flexion and extension of spine to show instability

23. **Earliest radiological change in RA:** *(NEET Pattern 2012)*
    A. Decreased joint space   B. Articular erosion
    C. Periarticular osteopenia D. Subchondral cyst
Ans. is 'C' Periarticular osteopenia

24. **Which arthritis causes no periosteal reaction?** *(NEET Pattern 2013)*
    A. Psoriatic arthritis   B. Reactive arthritis
    C. Neuropathic arthritis D. Rheumatoid arthritis
Ans. is 'D' Rheumatoid arthritis

25. **All are features of seronegative spondyloarthropathies except:** *(NEET Pattern 2013)*
    A. Uveitis   B. RA factor positive
    C. HLA-B27 positive D. Occur in young age
Ans. is 'B' RA factor positive

26. **All are X-ray findings of RA except:** *(NEET Pattern 2013)*
    A. Reduced joint space
    B. Soft tissue shadow
    C. Periarticular new bone formation
    D. Subchondral cyst
Ans. is 'C' Periarticular new bone formation

27. **Windswept deformity is seen in:** *(NEET Pattern 2012)*
    A. Achondroplasia B. Ankylosing spondylitis
    C. Rickets   D. Scurvy
Ans. is 'C' Rickets

28. **Joint spared in RA is:** *(NEET 2013, 2012)*
    A. Wrist B. PIP
    C. MCP   D. DIP
Ans. is 'D' DIP

29. **Pannus is seen in:** *(NEET Pattern 2012)*
    A. OA   B. RA
    C. Psoriasis D. Neurofibromatosis
Ans. is 'B' RA

30. **A burn patient develops claw hand. Joint affected will be:**
    A. Flexion at proximal interphalangeal joint
    B. Flexion at distal interphalangeal joint *(PGI Dec 2008)*
    C. Thumb abduction
    D. Flexion at metacarpophalangeal joint
    E. Extension at metacarpophalangeal joint
Ans. is 'A' Flexion at proximal interphalangeal joint; 'B' Flexion at distal interphalangeal joint and 'E' Extension at metacarpophalangeal joint.
    – **Claw hand has flexion at interphalangeal joints and hyperextension at metacarpophalangeal joints.**

31. **Boutonniere deformity occur due to:** *(PGI Dec 2008)*
    A. Flexion of proximal interphalangeal joint
    B. Flexion at distal interphalangeal joint
    C. Extension at distal interphalangeal joint
    D. Extension at metacarpophalangeal joint
    E. Flexion at metacarpophalangeal joint
Ans. is 'A' Flexion of proximal interphalangeal joint and 'C' extension at distal interphalangeal joint

32. **Joint not involved in rheumatoid arthritis according to 1987 modified ARA criterion:** *(AIIMS Nov 2008)*
    A. Knee   B. Ankle
    C. Tarsometatarsal D. Metatarsophalangeal
Ans. is 'C' Tarsometatarsal

33. **What is pathognomonic feature of rheumatoid arthritis?** *(AIIMS May 2005)*
    A. Rheumatoid factor   B. Rheumatoid nodule
    C. Morning stiffness   D. Ulnar drift of fingers
Ans. is 'B' Rheumatoid nodule

34. **Which of the following is TRUE regarding Rheumatoid arthritis?** *(AI 2002, 1994, UPSC 93, AIIMS June 97)*
    A. Typically involves small and large joints symmetrically but spares the cervical spine
    B. Causes pleural effusion with low sugar
    C. Pulmonary nodules are absent
    D. Enthesopathy prominent
Ans. is 'B' Causes pleural effusion with low sugar
    – RA causes pleural effusion with low glucose and pH.
    – Enthesopathy is not seen in RA it is a feature of Ankylosing Spondylitis.
    – Most common part of spine affected in RA is upper cervical.

35. **Distal interphalangeal joint is not involved in:** *(AI 1998)*
    A. Rheumatoid arthritis   B. Psoriatic arthritis
    C. Multicentric histiocytosis D. Neuropathic arthropathy
Ans. is 'A' Rheumatoid arthritis
    – DIP is involved in Psoriasis, Multicentric Histiocytosis and Neuropathic joints it is usually not involved in RA.

36. **"Wind-swept deformity" is seen in:** *(AIIMS Dec 1998)*
    A. Ankylosing spondylitis B. Scurvy
    C. Rheumatoid arthritis   D. Rickets
Ans. is 'D'>'C' Rickets > Rheumatoid arthritis

Wind swept deformity is classically used for knee deformity of rickets

Windswept deformity:
1. **Knee:** A valgus deformity of one knee in association of varus deformity of other knee is known as windswept deformity. It is seen in: rickets, hereditary dysplasia (epiphyseal dysplasia) of bone and rheumatoid arthritis.
2. **Foot:** Deviation of all—toes in one direction (usually laterally) is known as windswept deformity. It is seen in rheumatoid arthritis.
3. **Hand:** Deviation of all fingers (usually medially) is known as windswept deformity. It is seen in rheumatoid arthritis.

Coming to the question here we have to choose one and this terminology is classically for rickets knee deformity.

37. **Windswept deformity in foot is seen in:**
    A. Rickets   B. RA *(NEET Pattern 2013)*
    C. Hyperparathyroidism D. Scurvy
Ans. is 'B' RA

SERONEGATIVE SPONDYLOARTHROPATHIES

Feature
- Onset usually before 45 years age
- Inflammatory arthritis of spine/large peripheral joints
- Absence of autoantibodies (e.g. rheumatoid factor) in serum so known as seronegative
- HL B-27 positive/presence of uveitis

Include
1. Psoriatic arthritis.
2. Enteropathic arthritis (i.e. with IBD, e.g. Crohn's disease and UC).

3. Ankylosing spondylitis.
4. Reiter's syndrome (Conjunctivitis, Urethritis, Polyarthritis).
5. Reactive arthritis (Chlamydia, Shigella).
6. SAPHO syndrome (Synovitis, Acne, Pustulosis palmoplantar, Hyperostosis, and Osteitis).

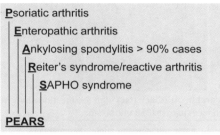

Psoriatic arthritis
 Enteropathic arthritis
  Ankylosing spondylitis > 90% cases
   Reiter's syndrome/reactive arthritis
    SAPHO syndrome
PEARS

MULTIPLE CHOICE QUESTIONS

1. True about reactive arthritis is: *(PGI Nov 2018)*
   A. Triad of arthritis, Urethritis and Conjunctivitis is seen
   B. Hyperkeratotic lesions on palms & soles are seen
   C. It is related to infections by chlamydia, shigella
   D. Anterior Uveitis is seen
   E. Does not involve spine
Ans. is 'A' Triad of arthritis, Urethritis and Conjunctivitis is seen; 'B' Hyperkeratotic lesions on palms & soles are seen; 'C' It is related to infections by chlamydia, shigella; and 'D' Anterior Uveitis is seen
   Reactive arthritis/Reiters syndrome
   – Chlamydia and shigella are associated.
   – HLA B27 positive
   – Triad: Arthritis + Conjunctivitis + Urethritis/Cervicitis (In females)
   – Mucocutaneous lesions: Circinate balanitis Keratoderma blennorrhagicum (Hyper-keratotic lesions on palms and soles)
   – Enthesitis is seen; SI joint is commonly involved
   – Anterior uveitis is seen

2. HLA B27 is not seen in: *(PGM-CET 2015)*
   A. SLE   B. Ankylosing spondylitis
   C. Reiter's syndrome   D. Psoriatic arthritis
Ans. is 'A' SLE

3. Young male having pain with daily morning stiffness of spine for 30 minutes and reduced chest movements. Most probable diagnosis is: *(AIIMS May 2014)*
   A. Ankylosing spondylitis   B. Rheumatoid arthritis
   C. Gouty arthritis   D. Osteoarthritis
Ans. is 'A' Ankylosing spondylitis

4. Oligoarthritis with ascending joint involvement seen in: *(NEET Pattern 2013)*
   A. Juvenile osteoarthritis   B. Seronegative arthritis
   C. SLE   D. Septic arthritis
Ans. is 'B' Seronegative arthritis

5. Spondyloarthropathy which is seronegative are all except: *(NEET Pattern 2012)*
   A. AS   B. Psoriasis
   C. JRA   D. Reiter syndrome
Ans. is 'C' JRA

6. Arthritis with eye involvement is seen in: *(NEET Pattern 2012)*
   A. Ankylosing spondylitis   B. Psoriasis
   C. Gout   D. Pseudogout
Ans. is 'A' Ankylosing spondylitis

7. Most common cause of reactive arthritis: *(AIIMS May 2008)*
   A. Staph aureus   B. N. gonorrhoeae
   C. S. flexneri   D. E. coli
Ans. is 'C' S. flexneri
   – Overall commonest cause of reactive arthritis is chlamydia
   – Second common is Shigella flexneri

8. Ankylosing spondylitis in associated with: *(AI 1999)*
   A. HLA-B27   B. HLA-B-8
   C. HLA-DW4/DR4   D. HLA-DR3
Ans. is 'A' HLA-B27
   – 90–95% of cases are positive for HLA-B27.

ANKYLOSING SPONDYLITIS (AS)/MARIE-STRUMPELL OR BECHTEREW'S DISEASE

It is a **seronegative spondyloarthropathy** a genetically determined generalized chronic inflammatory disease that primarily affects the axial skeleton (**sacroiliac joint** and spine) with variable involvement of root joints (shoulder and hip) and peripheral joints. The involvement is an **enthesopathy**. (Enthesis: Site of attachment of tendons and ligaments to bone thus enthesopathy is inflammation of Enthesis).

Clinical Presentation

- **Males** are affected more frequently than females (2:1 to 10:1)
- Age of onset is between **15–25 years** (late adolescence and early adulthood).
- The initial symptom is usually dull pain, insidious in onset, felt deep in lower lumbar or gluteal region, accompanied by low back **morning stiffness** of up to few hour duration that improves with activity and returns following period of inactivity.
- **Question mark (?) posture** is due to hyperkyphosis of thoracic spine and loss of lumbar lordosis. Cervical spine involvement is usually late and show forward stooping and loss of extension and rotation.
- Most serious complication of spinal disease is **spinal fracture** with even minor trauma.
- The most common extra-articular manifestation is **acute anterior uveitis** (iridocyclitis) occurring in **30%**. Cataract and secondary glaucoma are common sequela.
- Up to 60% of patients have inflammation of colon or ileum (mostly asymptomatic, only 5–10% develop IBD) 3rd degree heart block, cardiac dysfunction (Aortic incompetence), restrictive lung disease. IgA nephropathy, prostatitis and retroperitoneal fibrosis are other manifestations and may shorten life span.

Diagnostic Criteria–Modified New York Criterion

- **Essential criteria is definite radiographic sacroiliitis**
- Supporting criteria: one of these three
  Inflammatory back pain
  – Limited chest expansion (<5 cm at 4th ICS) {not a reliable criterion in elderly because of pulmonary disorders}
  – Limited lumbar spine motion in both sagittal and frontal plane (Schober test/Modified Schober test).

- Inflammatory back pain is classified if 4/5 are present
  1. Pain for > 3 months
  2. <40 years age
  3. Insidious onset
  4. Pain improves with exercise
  5. Pain at night

Etiology and Pathogenesis

- **> 90% of AS patients are HLA-B27 positive** whereas only 10% of normal population is HLA-B27 positive. 1–6% of adults inheriting B27 have been found to have AS.
- The enthesis, the site of ligamentous attachment to bone is primary site of pathology in AS particularly in pelvis and spine. It is associated with prominent edema of adjacent bone marrow and is characterized by erosive lesions that eventually undergo ossification.

Sacroiliitis is the earliest manifestation with features of both enthesitis and synovitis

Peripheral arthritis of AS (seen in 30% patients) can show synovial hyperplasia, lymphoid infiltration and pannus but lacks exuberant synovial villi, fibrin deposits, ulcers, and accumulation of plasma cells seen in rheumatoid arthritis. Central cartilaginous erosion, caused by proliferation of subchondral granulation tissue are common in AS but rare in RA.

- TNF and cytokine play central role in pathogenesis. "There is autoimmunity to cartilage proteoglycan aggrecan".
- Radiological features in chronological order.

SI Joint (more on iliac side of joint) "Never diagnose ankylosing spondylitis without sacroiliitis"

- Blurring of margins
- Juxta-articular sclerosis
- Erosions cause pseudo-widening
- Obliteration of joint (fibrous followed by bony ankylosis).

Spine

- Loss of lumbar lordosis (Straightening).
- **Enthesitis – Increased Blood flow – Cause absorption by** Erosions of anterior corners of vertebral body causing squaring of vertebral body.
- **Delicate syndesmophyte with "vertical orientation bridging vertebral bodies" "(horizontal in degenerative spine disease)".**
- **Bamboo spine, dagger sign, trolley track** syndesmophytes and paravertebral ossification.
- **Romanus sign** (shiny corner sign) it is sclerosis of margins of vertebral body.

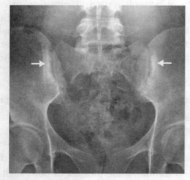

Fig. 16.16: Sacroiliitis

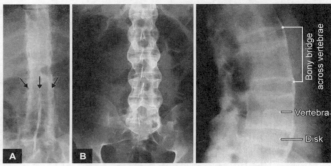

Figs. 16.17A and B: (A) Trolley track sign (ossification along supraspinous ligaments and facet joints); (B) Bamboo sign

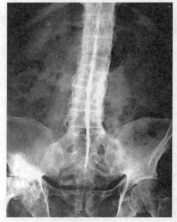

Fig. 16.18: Dagger sign (ossification along supraspinous and interspinous ligaments). Dagger is a thin knife—ossification resembles it

Clinical Examination

a: **Tests for Sacroiliitis:**
1. **Gaenslen test**
2. Patrick/Faber test
3. Figure of 4 test
4. Pump handle test
5. Side-to-side compression

b. **Lumbar spine:** Schober/Modified Schober test
c. **Cervical spine:** Fleche test.

Treatment

- Phenylbutazone is most effective drug but causes aplastic anemia so reserved for non-responsive cases.
- Indomethacin is most commonly used NSAID. Sulfasalazine and folic acid antagonist (Mtx) is used for peripheral joints.
- Anti TNF-α therapy, e.g. infliximab or etanercept are also used.

Diffuse idiopathic skeletal hyperostosis (DISH) is a *spondyloarthropathy* also known as Forestier's disease or **ankylosing hyperostosis**. It is a noninflammatory disease, with the principal manifestation being calcification and ossification of spinal ligaments and the regions where tendons and ligaments attach to bone (*entheses*). The whole spine may be involved, and bony ankylosis occurs, although the disc spaces and facet joints remain unaffected. In advanced stages, the disease may look like melted candle wax. The calcification and ossification is most common in the right side of the spine.

The distinctive radiological feature of DISH is the continuous linear calcification along the anteromedial aspect of the thoracic spine.

The disease is usually found in people in their 60's and above, and is extremely rare in people in their 40's and 30's. The disease can spread to any joint of the body, affecting the neck, shoulders, ribs, hips, knees, ankles, and hands. The disease is not fatal, however some associated complications can lead to death. Complications include paralysis, dysphagia (the inability to swallow), and pulmonary infections. Although DISH manifests in a similar manner to *ankylosing spondylitis*, these two are totally separate diseases. Ankylosing spondylitis is a genetic disease with identifiable marks, and affects organs. DISH has no indication of a genetic link, and does not affect organs other than the lungs, which is only indirect due to the fusion of the rib cage.

DISH may be discovered as a radiological abnormality, as mentioned above, without any symptoms. The usual complaint is with thoracic spinal pain. This occurs in around 80% of patients. Morning stiffness is also noticed in almost two-thirds of patients. Increased incidence of dysphagia is also reported in some cases. Similar calcification and ossification may be seen at peripheral entheseal sites, including the shoulder, iliac crest, ischial tuberosity, trochanters of the hip, tibial tuberosities, patellae, and bones of the hands and/or feet.

Treatment: NSAIDs can be helpful in relieving pain and inflammation associated with DISH.

MULTIPLE CHOICE QUESTIONS

1. True about ankylosing spondylitis: *(PGI May 2017)*
    A. Pain relives on rest
    B. Association with HLA B-27
    C. Enthesitis may occur
    D. 30% cases have acute posterior uveitis
    E. Cardiac conduction defect may present
   Ans. is 'B' Association with HLA B-27; 'C' Enthesitis may occur; 'E' Cardiac conduction defect may present

2. Which joint is rarely affected by ankylosing spondylitis? *(NEET Dec 2016)*
    A. Ankle   B. Hip
    C. Shoulder   D. Sacroiliac
   Ans. is 'A' Ankle

3. All are true about Marie-Strumpell disease *except*: *(NEET Dec 2016)*
    A. Most commonly involves the sacroiliac joints
    B. Enthesitis is common
    C. More common is males
    D. Roentgenogram is the most sensitive investigation
   Ans. is 'D' Roentgenogram is the most sensitive investigation
   • MRI is the most sensitive investigation for Sacroiliitis.

4. Correct statement regarding AS: *(PGI Nov 2016)*
    A. Young males are more commonly affected
    B. Sacroiliitis is the earliest manifestation seen
    C. Gaenslen test done
    D. Chest expansion is normal
    E. Peripheral joint involvement in 30% patients
   Ans. is 'A' Young males are more commonly affected; 'B' Sacroiliitis is the earliest manifestation seen; 'C' Gaenslen test done and 'E' Peripheral joint involvement in 30% patients

5. True regarding Ankylosing Spondylitis is: *(PGI May 2016)*
    A. Peripheral joints are involved in 70% cases
    B. Osteophytes grow in horizontal directions
    C. Earliest X-ray feature is Romanov's sign
    D. Most common extra articular manifestation is acute anterior uveitis
    E. HLA B27 is positive in more than 90% of cases
   Ans. is 'D' Most common extra-articular manifestation is acute anterior uveitis and 'E' HLA B27 is positive in more than 90% of cases

6. A young man complaints of pain lower back his X-rays are shown below. Most likely diagnosis is: *(AI 2016)*

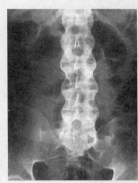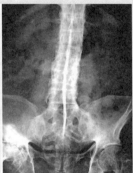

    A. AS   B. Spondylolisthesis
    C. Paget's disease D. Osteoporosis
   Ans. is 'A' AS

7. Which of the following is not the extra-articular manifestations of ankylosing spondylitis? *(NEET 2015)*
    A. Acute anterior uveitis   B. Aortic valve disease
    C. Pulmonary fibrosis   D. Dilated cardiomyopathy
   Ans. is 'D' Dilated cardiomyopathy

8. Ankylosing spondylitis all is true except: *(NEET 2015)*
    A. HLA B 27 is found 90% of sufferers
    B. Uveitis is found in 40% of sufferers
    C. Condition is commoner in females
    D. Radiological changes do not can occur in spine before symptoms
   Ans. is 'C' Condition is commoner in females

9. A 25-year-old man complaints of low backache, decreased lumbar movements, morning stiffness which clinical examination will further help: *(AIIMS Nov 2015)*
    A. Head circumference   B. Chest expansion
    C. Hyperextension of joints D. Plantar arch
   Ans. is 'B' Chest expansion

10. HLA B27 is associated with: *(AIIMS Nov 2014, NEET 2012)*
    A. Ankylosing spondylitis B. Rheumatoid arthritis
    C. Gout   D. Pseudogout
    Ans. is 'A' Ankylosing spondylitis

11. A young patient with complaints of severe low backache, with stiffness of back with reduced chest expansion is most probably suffering from: *(AIIMS May 2014)*
    A. Tuberculosis   B. Ankylosing spondylitis
    C. Rheumatoid arthritis   D. Metastasis
    Ans. is 'B' Ankylosing spondylitis

12. In a middle aged male having back pain, syndesmophytes involving 4 continuous vertebrae are seen on X-ray. The patient has: *(NEET Pattern 2013)*
    A. DISH   B. Ankylosing spondylitis
    C. Rheumatoid arthritis   D. Osteoarthritis
    Ans. is 'B' Ankylosing spondylitis

13. True about ankylosing spondylitis are all except:
    (NEET Pattern 2013)
    A. Affects males B. 30–40 years
    C. 90% HLA-B5   D. Bamboo spine
Ans. is 'C' 90% HLA-B5

14. Bamboo spine with sacroiliitis: *(NEET Pattern 2016, 2012)*
    A. Ankylosing spondylitis B. RA
    C. OA   D. Psoriatic arthritis
Ans. is 'A' Ankylosing spondylitis

15. Scleritis with autoimmune disease involving joints:
    (NEET Pattern 2012)
    A. Ankylosing spondylitis B. Rheumatoid arthritis
    C. Gout   D. Pseudogout
Ans. is 'B' Rheumatoid arthritis
    Uveitis is a feature of ankylosing spondylitis

16. Differential diagnosis of hand arthritis are all except:
    (NEET Pattern 2012)
    A. Ankylosing spondylitis B. Rheumatoid arthritis
    C. Psoriasis   D. Osteoarthritis
Ans. is 'A' Ankylosing spondylitis

17. Bechterew's Disease: *NEET Pattern 2012)*
    A. RA   B. AS
    C. Paget's D. Osteopetrosis
Ans. is 'B' AS

18. A 65-year-old man had H/o of back pain since 3 months. ESR is raised. He also has dorsolumbar tenderness on examination and mild restriction of chest movements. On X-ray, syndesmophytes are present in vertebrae. Diagnosis is: *(AIIMS May 2010)*
    A. Ankylosing spondylitis
    B. Degenerative osteoarthritis of spine
    C. Ankylosing hyperostosis D. Lumbar canal stenosis
Ans. is 'C' Ankylosing hyperostosis

	Ankylosing hyperostosis	Ankylosing spondylitis
Age	**Elderly**	Young
Sacroiliitis	**Absent**	Always present
Chest expansion	**Mild restriction**	Marked but not reliable in elderly
Tendernets	Dorsolumbar	Sacroiliac
ESR	Normal to mild rise	High
Syndesmophytes	Present	Present

19. A young male presents with joint pains and backache. X-ray of spine shows evidence of sacroiliitis. The most likely diagnosis is: *(UPSC 1998) (JIPMER 99)*
    A. Rheumatoid arthritis
    B. Ankylosing spondylitis
    C. Polyarticular juvenile arthritis
    D. Psoriatic arthropathy
Ans. is 'B' Ankylosing spondylitis

PSORIATIC ARTHRITIS–CASPAR CRITERIA

Psoriatic arthritis is characterized by seronegative polysynovitis with erosive arthritis.

CASPAR Criterion for Psoriatic Arthritis

To be classified as having PsA, a patient must have inflammatory joint disease (joint, spine, enthesitis) with ≥ 3 of the following 5

1. Evidence of psoriasis (One of these)
    a. Current psoriasis
    b. Personal history
    c. Family history
2. Psoriatic nail dystrophy
3. Negative RF
4. Dactylitis (One of a, b)
    a. Current
    b. History
5. Radiological evidence of Juxta-articular new bone formation.

Epidemiology

- Prevalence of psoriasis is 1–2% and psoriatic arthritis develops only in 5–10% of cases
- **It is associated with HLA DR7, HLA-CW6**
- A9 allele and KIR (killer immunoglobulin like receptor) alleles are associated
- **Rheumatoid factor is almost always negative**
- 60% of those with spondylitis or sacroiliitis have HLA-B27.

Clinical Features

- Sex ratio is 1:1 and usual age of onset is 30–50 years (much later than skin lesion)
- Five patterns of joint involvement are: seen
    1. **Arthritis of DIP joint**
    2. Asymmetrical oligoarthritis
    3. Symmetrical polyarthritis similar to RA
    4. Axial involvement (spine and sacroiliac joint)
    5. Arthritis mutilans
- Nail changes occurs in 90% patients of psoriatic arthritis (40% in patient without arthritis)
- Dactylitis, enthesitis and tenosynovitis are also common
- **Shortening of digitis (telescoping), because of underlying osteolysis is characteristic of psoriatic arthritis.**
- Fibrous and bony ankylosis of small joints (greater tendency than RA).
- Almost any peripheral joint can be involved.

Radiological Features

- DIP involvement, and classical **pencil cup deformity.**
- Marginal erosion with adjacent bony proliferation (whiskering).
- Osteolysis of phalangeal and metacarpal bone, with telescoping of digits.

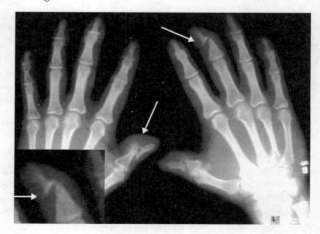

Fig. 16.19: Pencil-in-cup deformity—psoriasis

Treatment

- Anti-TNF-α agents, e.g. etanercept and infliximab are newer drugs and are effective even in longstanding cases (to previous therapy) and extensive skin lesion.
- Methotrexate is drug of choice. Other effective agents are sulfasalazine, cyclosporine, retinoic acid and psoralen and UV-A (PUVA).

Resorption of the Tuft

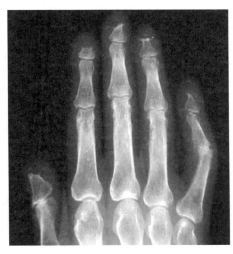

Fig. 16.20: Acro-osteolysis

1. **Scleroderma**
2. Raynaud's disease
3. Psoriatic arthropathy—can precede the skin changes
4. Neuropathic disease—diabetes mellitus leprosy myelomeningocele, syringomyelia and congenital indifference to pain
5. Thermal injuries—burns, frostbite and electrical
6. Trauma
7. Hyperparathyroidism
8. Epidermolysis bullosa
9. Porphyria—due to cutaneous photosensitivity leading to blistering and scarring
10. Phenytoin toxicity—congenitally in infants of epileptic mothers
11. Subungual exostosis
12. Snake and scorpion venom—due to tissue breakdown by proteinases.

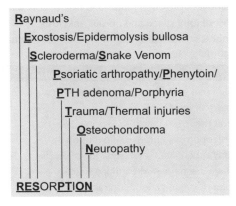

Raynaud's
Exostosis/**E**pidermolysis bullosa
Scleroderma/**S**nake Venom
Psoriatic arthropathy/**P**henytoin/
PTH adenoma/Porphyria
Trauma/Thermal injuries
Osteochondroma
Neuropathy

RESORPTION

Arthritis Mutilans

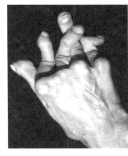 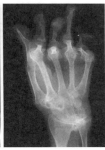

Fig. 16.21: Arthritis mutilans

A destructive arthritis of the hands and feet with resorption of bone ends and telescoping joints (main en lorgnette).
1. **Rheumatoid arthritis**
2. Juvenile chronic arthritis
3. Psoriatic arthropathy
4. Diabetes
5. Leprosy
6. Neuropathic arthropathy
7. Reiter's syndrome—in the feet.

MULTIPLE CHOICE QUESTIONS

1. CASPAR criteria is used in diagnosis of: *(NEET 2015)*
   A. Psoriatic arthritis   B. Rheumatoid arthritis
   C. Ankylosing spondylitis   D. Reactive synovitis
   Ans. is 'A' Psoriatic arthritis

2. Pencil in cup deformity is seen in: *(NEET Pattern 2013)*
   A. Rheumatoid arthritis   B. Ankylosing spondylitis
   C. AVN   D. Psoriatic arthritis
   Ans. is 'D' Psoriatic arthritis

3. Sausage digits is seen in: *(NEET Pattern 2012)*
   A. Lyme arthritis   B. Osteoarthritis
   C. Psoriatic arthritis   D. None
   Ans. is 'C' Psoriatic arthritis

4. Resorption of distal phalanx is seen in: *(NEET Pattern 2012)*
   A. Scleroderma   B. Hyperparathyroidism
   C. Reiter's syndrome   D. All
   Ans. is 'D' All

5. True about psoriatic arthritis are all expect:
   (NEET Pattern 2013; 2012)
   A. HLA-Cω6 association   B. Involvement of DIP joint
   C. More common in males   D. DOC is methotrexate
   Ans. is 'C' More common in males
   − Sex ratio is 1:1

6. Psoriatic arthritis most commonly involves:
   (NEET Pattern 2016, 2012)
   A. PIP   B. DIP
   C. MCP   D. Wrist
   Ans. is 'B' DIP

7. All are true regarding psoriatic arthritis except:
   (PGI 02, JIPMER 01)
   A. Arthritis mutilans   B. DIP involvement
   C. Ankylosis of small joints   D. Sacroiliitis
   E. Lengthening of digits called as telescoping
   Ans. is 'E' Lengthening of digit known as telescoping
   − There is shortening of digits (not lengthening).

8. A 35-year-old male develops involvements of PIP, DIP and metacarpophalangeal joints with sparing of wrist and carpo-metacarpal joints. The probable diagnosis is:
   (AIIMS June 99)
   A. Psoriatic arthropathy   B. Osteoarthritis
   C. Rheumatoid arthritis   D. Pseudogout

Ans. is 'A' Psoriatic arthropathy

9. Disease where distal Interphalangeal joint is characteristically involved: (AI 93, TN 90)
   A. Psoriatic arthritis   B. Rheumatoid
   C. SLE   D. Gout

Ans. is 'A' Psoriatic arthritis

10. In Psoriatic arthropathy, treatment of choice is:
    (AIIMS May 1993)
    A. Methotrexate   B. PUVA therapy
    C. Corticosteroids   D. Indomethacin

Ans. is 'A' Methotrexate

11. Which of the following is true about HIV related arthritis?
    (JIPMER DEC 2016)
    A. Cutaneous and mucosal lesions are rare
    B. Enthesopathy is common
    C. Associated with HLA B 27
    D. Hip is the commonest joint involved

Ans. is 'A' Cutaneous and mucosal lesions are rare

HIV related arthritis:
- Asymmetric oligoarthritis (MC) – Male and effects knee/ankle
- Symmetrical polyarthritis – Non-erosive but otherwise mimics RA.
- Enthesopathy & Mucocutaneous involvement is rare Seronegative (RA factor -ve, ANA –ve, HLAB27 -ve) NSAIDs as D.O.C
- HIV patients can develop seronegative arthropathy.

HEMOPHILIAC ARTHROPATHY

- Hemophilia is an **X-linked recessive disorder** characterized by the absence or deficiency of factor VIII (hemophilia A or classical hemophilia) or factor IX (hemophilia B or Christmas disease).
  Hemophilia A is more common accounting for ~85% cases.
- Both disorders are manifested only in males but carried by females.
  Recurrent spontaneous hemarthrosis causing chronic synovitis and progressive articular destruction occur in both.
- Plasma clotting factor 50% of the normal are compatible with normal control of hemorrhage.

Clotting Factors
- <1% – Spontaneous Hemorrhage
- 1-5% – Hemorrhage on Mild Trauma
- >5% Hemorrhage on Significant Trauma

Joints Bleeding
- Weight-bearing joints are most commonly involved, with the frequency of involvement in decreasing order, **knee**> elbow> shoulder> ankle> wrist> hip.
- Ankle is most commonly involved in children.
- Joint assumes position of minimal discomfort and minimal intra-articular pressure, which is, flexion (30–65) abduction (15) and lateral rotation (15) in hip; and slight flexion in knee.
- Pain, warmth, boggy swelling, tenderness and limited movements cause it to resemble with low grade infection.
- Joint aspiration is avoided unless distension is severe or there is a strong suspicion of infection.

Intramuscular Bleeding
- Bleeding into muscle is less common but equally harmful can cause muscle necrosis, reactive fibrosis and joint contractures.
- In **lower limbs** most common sites of bleeding is **iliopsoas**> quadriceps.
- In **upper limb** the most common site of bleeding is **deltoid**.
- Hemorrhage into iliopsoas muscle or retroperitoneum may mimic appendicitis or renal colic.

Pseudotumor
- It refers to progressive cystic swelling caused by uncontrolled hemorrhage within confined space. The hematoma increases in size and causes pressure necrosis and erosion of bone (mimicking tumor).
- It occurs in severe hemophiliacs only (clotting factor <1% of normal).
- Most **hemophilic pseudotumors** are caused by subperiosteal hemorrhage and the most common location is in **thigh (50%)**. Next in frequency are abdomen, pelvis, and tibia.
- Iliopsoas is most common muscle involved followed by Quadriceps.

Nerve Palsy
- Bleeding into peripheral nerve cause intense pain followed by sensory and muscle weakness.
- Neuropraxia is primarily due to compression of a nerve from the hematoma. The **femoral nerve** is most commonly involved as it is in closed, rigid compartment limited by iliacus fascia.

Radiological Features
- Soft tissue swelling and capsular distension.
- Juxta-articular **osteopenia** (not sclerosis).
- Overgrowth and osteoporosis of epiphysis.
- Marginal erosions and subchondral cysts.
- Narrowing of joint space (with cartilage destruction) and bony over growth.
- **Widening of intercondylar notch of femur** and squaring of distal end patella.
- Enlargement of proximal radius and trochlear notch of ulna.
- Total loss of joint space and fibrous ankylosis.

  Hemarthrosis is bleeding into a joint. Causes include trauma, bleeding disorders, etc.

Hemophiliac arthropathy (Staging)
Arnold-Hilgartner classification for knee
Stage 0 : Normal joint
Stage 1 : Soft tissue swelling
2 : Osteoporosis, epiphyseal overgrowth
3 : Early subchondral cyst, squaring of patella, widened notch
4 : Stage 3 + narrowed cartilage space
5 : Joint disorganization, contractures

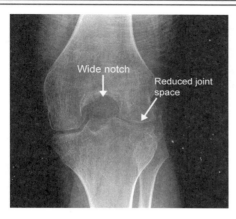

Fig. 16.22: Hemophiliac arthropathy

Treatment of acute hemarthrosis involves factor replacement (in hemophilia) joint aspiration (in severe cases), ice and analgesics (to relieve pain) rest and compressive bandage.

Arthroscopy is relatively contraindicated.

MULTIPLE CHOICE QUESTIONS

1. Hemophiliac arthropathy, which is not seen?
   A. Subchondral bone cyst formation (JIPMER 2014)
   B. Increase in intercondylar distance
   C. Juxta-articular osteosclerosis
   D. Subchondral thinning

Ans. is 'C' Juxta-articular osteosclerosis

2. Epiphyseal enlargement is seen in: (NEET Pattern 2013)
   A. Rickets   B. Hemophilia
   C. Septic arthritis D. All of the above

Ans. is 'D' All of the above

3. Fractures are more common in hemophiliac because:
   A. Joint stiffness   B. Osteopenia
   C. Both A and B   D. Vascular pulsations

Ans. is 'C' Both A and B

4. True about treatment of hemarthrosis: (PGI June 07)
   A. Aspiration   B. POP
   C. Traction   D. Compression bandage

Ans. is 'A' Aspiration; 'B' POP; 'C' Traction and 'D' Compression bandage

5. Most common muscle for pseudotumor like growth in hemophiliac arthropathy is: (AI 1998)
   A. Quadriceps femoris   B. Hamstring muscle
   C. Gastrocnemius   D. Iliopsoas

Ans. is 'D' > 'A' Iliopsoas > Quadriceps femoris

6. All are features of hemophiliac knee joint, *except*:
   A. Juxta-articular osteosclerosis (AIIMS June 1997)
   B. Subchondral cyst formation
   C. Widening of intercondylar notch
   D. Squaring of patella

Ans. is 'A' Juxta-articular osteosclerosis
   – Osteopenia is seen in hemophilia

7. Arthroscopy is contraindicated in: (NB 90)
   A. Chronic joint disease   B. Loose bodies
   C. Hemophilia   D. Meniscal tear

Ans. is 'C' Hemophilia

NEUROPATHIC JOINT DISEASE/ CHARCOT'S JOINT

- It is progressive destructive arthritis arising from **loss of pain sensation and proprioception (position sense).**
- So these joints lack normal reflex safe guards against abnormal stress or injury.

Disease	Joint involvement
Diabetes	**Midtarsal (most common)**> tarsometatarsal, metatarsophalangeal and ankle joint> knee and spine
Tabes dorsalis	Knee (most common), hip, ankle and lumbar spine
Leprosy	Hand and foot joints
Syringomyelia	**Shoulder** (glenohumeral), elbow, wrist and cervical spine
Myelomeningocele	Ankle and foot
Congenital insensitivity to pain	Ankle and foot
Chronic alcoholism	Foot
Amyloidosis	Peroneal muscle atrophy (Charcot Marie Tooth disease)

Clinical Presentation

- Joint becomes progressively enlarged from bony overgrowth and synovial effusion.
- **Loose bodies** may be palpated in the joint. Joint instability, subluxation, and crepitus occur as the disease progresses.
- Patients complain of weakness, swelling, instability, laxity and progressive deformity usually involving knee or ankle.
- **The markedly swollen joint is neither tender nor warmth.**
- The appearance suggests that movements would be agonizing and yet it is often painless.
- The paradox is diagnostic the amount of pain experienced is less than would be anticipated based on degree of joint involvement.

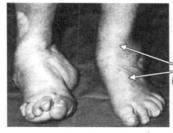

Ankle and foot joints involvement in Charcot's joints with marked deformities but they are painless

Fig. 16.23: Charcot's ankle

Radiological Features

Similar to OA, i.e. joint space narrowing, subchondral bone sclerosis, osteophytes and joint effusion marked destructive and hypertrophic changes. However, the process is usually more rapid. Joint swelling and appearance of intra-articular calcification are further clues.

- It may be difficult to differentiate it from osteomyelitis, especially in diabetic foot. **The joint margins in neuropathic joints tend to be distinct, while in osteomyelitis, they are blurred.** MRI and bone scan using indium labeled WBC/ immunoglobulin G (increased uptake in osteomyelitis but not in neuropathic joint) can differentiate. CT scan will not distinguish as increased uptake is observed in both.

- Treatment of Charcot's arthropathy is limitation of joint movements by bracing or casting, joint debridement (arthrocentesis) and fusion of joint (arthrodesis). Nowadays with advancement in replacement techniques arthroplasty–joint replacement can also be carried out for knee Charcot's joints but is not advised for ankle.

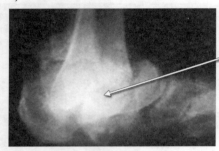

Fig. 16.24: X-ray of Charcot's ankle

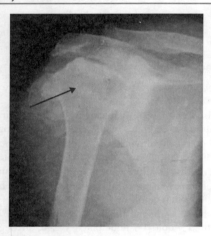

Fig. 16.25: X-ray of Charcot's shoulder

MULTIPLE CHOICE QUESTIONS

1. Examine knee X-ray carefully, Diagnosis: *(JIPMER May 2018)*

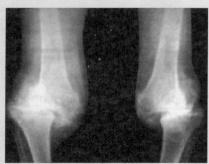

   A. TB B. Gout
   C. Charcot D. RA
Ans. is 'C' Charcot

2. Charcot's joint is another name for joint affected by:
   A. Neuropathy B. Osteoarthritis *(NEET 2015)*
   C. Rheumatoid arthritis D. Ankylosing spondylitis
Ans. is 'A' Neuropathy

3. Most common cause of neuropathic joint: *(NEET Pattern 2013)*
   A. Leprosy B. Tabes dorsalis
   C. Diabetes D. Nerve injury
Ans. is 'C' Diabetes

4. Neuropathic joint is seen in all except: *(NEET Pattern 2012)*
   A. DM B. Tabes dorsalis
   C. Syringomyelia D. Hypertension
Ans. is 'D' Hypertension

5. Neuropathic joints are seen in all except: *(NEET Pattern 2012)*
   A. Leprosy B. Syringomyelia
   C. Tuberculosis D. Diabetes Mellitus
Ans. is 'C' Tuberculosis

6. Not associated with neuropathic joint: *(NEET Pattern 2012)*
   A. DM B. Syringomyelia
   C. Friedreich's ataxia D. Tabes dorsalis
Ans. is 'C' Friedreich's ataxia

7. False about Charcot's joint in diabetes mellitus is: *(AI 08)*
   A. Limitation of movements with bracing
   B. Arthrodesis
   C. Total ankle replacement
   D. Arthrocentesis
Ans. is 'C' Total ankle replacement
   - **Treatment of** Charcot's arthropathy is *limitation of joint movements by bracing or casting, joint debridement (arthrocentesis) and fusion off joint (arthrodesis)*.
   - **Please remember that replacement is advocated now with advances in treatment but still it will be the least preferred treatment for ankle it can be carried for Knee.**

8. A 60-year-old man with diabetes mellitus presents with painless, swollen right ankle joint. Radiographs of the ankle show destroyed joint with large number of loose bodies. The most probable diagnosis is: *(AI 2003)*
   A. Charcot's joint B. Clutton's joint
   C. Osteoarthritis D. Rheumatoid arthritis
Ans. is 'A' Charcot's joint

9. Neuropathic joint may arise in: *(TN 99, 94, Manipal 94, JIPMER 93, NB 1991)*
   A. Syringomyelia B. Tabes dorsalis
   C. Leprosy D. All of the above
Ans. is 'D' All of the above

10. In a patient suffering from tabes dorsalis Charcot's joint occurs most commonly at: *(TN 99, Rajasthan 93, AI 93)*
    A. Elbow B. Tarsometatarsal
    C. Wrist D. Knee
Ans. is 'D' Knee
    - **Tabes dorsalis affects knee joints most commonly**

11. Most common Charcot's joints involved in diabetes mellitus are those of: *(AI 97)*
    A. Shoulder B. Ankle
    C. Knee D. Foot
Ans. is 'D' Foot
    - Diabetes midtarsal (most common) > tarsometatarsal

12. Clutton's joints are: *(WB 97) (AI 1995)*
    A. Syphilitic joints B. End stage tuberculous joints
    C. Associated with trauma D. Usually painful
Ans. is 'A' Syphilitic joints

Skeletal Manifestations of Syphilis

Congenital Syphilis

- Clutton's joint is painless, symmetrical, sterile effusion mostly involving knee in 8–16 years of age. Spontaneous remission is usual in several weeks.
- Parrot's joints is effusion, epiphysitis and epiphyseal separation.
- Higoumenakis' sign, i.e. periostitis with unilateral or bilateral enlargement of sternal end of clavicle.
- Saber tibia is anterior bowing of midportion of tibia because of subperiosteal apposition of bone on anterior cortical surface.
- Scaphoid scapula.
- Widened, ill-defined and irregular physis; uninvolved epiphysis and characteristic bilateral and symmetrical metaphyseal erosions and fractures.

13. Joint least affected by neuropathy: *(Delhi 1993)*
    A. Shoulder B. Hip
    C. Wrist D. Elbow

Ans. is 'D' Elbow

CRYSTAL DEPOSITION DISORDER

Gout

A disorder of purine metabolism characterized by hyperuricemia, deposition of **monosodium urate monohydrate crystals in joints and periarticular tissues** and recurrent attacks of acute synovitis. Late change include cartilage degeneration, renal dysfunction and uric acid urolithiasis.

Epidemiology

Commoner in **men** than in women (may be 20:1) Hyperuricemia term is reserved for individuals with a serum urate concentration, which is about 0.42 mmol/L (7 mg/dL) for men and 0.35 mmoL/L (5.8 mg/dL) for women.

Although the risk of developing clinical features of gout increases with increasing levels of serum uric acid, only a fraction of those with hyperuricemia develop symptoms.

Any factor that causes either an abrupt increase or decrease in the serum urate levels may provoke an acute attack, **the best correlations being factors that cause an abrupt fall.**

Serum uric acid levels can be normal or low at the time of acute attack, lowering of uric acid with hypouricemic therapy or other medications limits the value of serum uric acid determination for diagnosis of gout.

Despite these limitations, serum uric acid is almost always elevated at some time and can be used to follow the course of hypouricemic therapy.

Pathology

Tophi (= porous stone) are nodular deposits of monosodium urate monohydrate crystals, with an associated foreign body reaction. It is deposited in minute clumps in connective tissue, e.g.

- **Bursae, e.g. olecranon bursa/periarticular tissue**
- Tendons
- Synovium and joints
- Pinnae (cartilage) of ear
- Ligaments
- Articular ends of bone
- Subcutaneous tissue
- Kidney
- Tophi may ulcerate through skin or destroy cartilage and periarticular bone

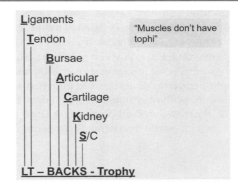

Arthritis with Soft-tissue Nodules

1. Gout
2. Rheumatoid arthritis
3. Pigmented villonodular synovitis
4. Multicentric reticulohistiocytosis
5. Amyloidosis
6. Sarcoidosis

Clinical Features

- Usually patient is obese, hypertensive, **alcoholic** and high protein eater **(nonvegetarian)**.
- The commonest sites are **metatarsophalangeal joint of big toe** > ankle and finger joints and olecranon bursae.
- The skin is red, shiny, swollen, hot and extremely tender suggesting a cellulitis or septic arthritis.

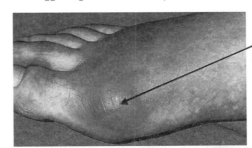

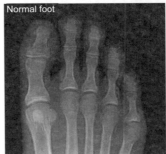 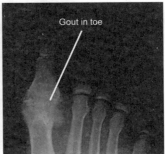

Fig. 16.26: Clinical picture—gout

- Sometimes only feature is acute pain and tenderness. Hyperuricemia is present at some stage, though not necessarily during acute attack. However, whilst a low serum uric acid level makes gout unlikely; hyperuricemia is not diagnostic and is often seen in normal middle aged men.
- **Characteristic negatively birefringent urate crystals in the synovial fluid examined by polarizing microscopy**

is diagnostic. During acute gouty attack strongly negatively birefringent needle shaped mono sodium urate (MSU) crystals are seen (diagnostic).

- During acute attack X-rays show only soft tissue swelling. Chronic gout may result in joint space narrowing and secondary OA. **Tophi appear as characteristic punched out cysts or deep erosions with over hanging bony edges (Martel's or G' sign).** These well-defined erosions are larger and slightly further from joint margin than typical RA erosions.

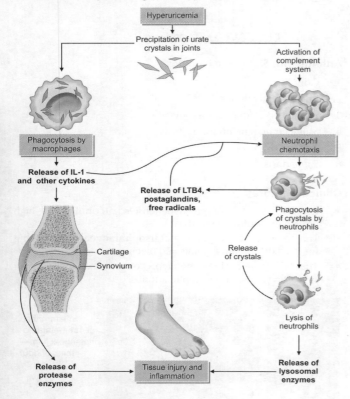

Fig. 16.27: Pathophysiology of gout

Treatment

- Mainstay of treatment during acute attack is administration of anti-inflammatory drug such as colchicine, NSAIDs (except aspirin) or glucocorticoids. NSAIDs and colchicine may be toxic in elderly particularly in renal insufficiency and GI disorders. So glucocorticoids may be preferred.
- Resting joint, icepacks, losing weight, decreasing alcohol, eliminating diuretics, low purine diet and increase in liquid ingestion may be preventive.

Chronic Cases

- **Uricosuric drugs (probenecid or sulfinpyrazone) can be used if renal function is normal. Allopurinol,** a xanthine oxidase inhibitor is usually **preferred if renal functions are compromised.** These drugs should never be started in acute attack, and they should always be **covered by an anti-inflammatory preparations or colchicine;** otherwise they may precipitate an acute attack by causing sudden fall in uric acid levels. In chronic tophaceous gout and in all patients with renal complications, allopurinol is drug of choice.

MULTIPLE CHOICE QUESTIONS

1. Martel's sign is seen in which of the following condition? *(DNB June 2017)*
   A. Rheumatoid arthritis   B. Osteoarthritis
   C. Gouty arthritis   D. Ochronosis
   Ans. is 'C' Gouty arthritis

2. 42 yrs male with frequent attacks of joint pain, underwent an X-ray showing soft tissue swelling. The likely diagnosis is: *(NEET 2016)*

   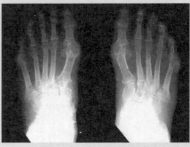

   A. Gout   B. Parathyroid adenoma
   C. Psoriasis   D. RA
   Ans. is 'A' Gout

3. 50 yr alcoholic male with complaints of recurrent pain & swelling in foot joints. On examination red, shiny swollen joints seen which is the most appropriate investigation to be first done considering the X-ray showing: *(AI 2016)*

   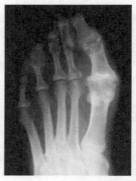

   A. HLA-B27   B. PTH levels
   C. Uric acid levels   D. Calcium levels
   Ans. is 'C' Uric acid levels

4. Most common joint involved in gout is: *(NEET 2015)*
   A. Knee   B. Hip
   C. MP joint of great toe   D. MP joint of thumb
   Ans. is 'C' MP joint of great toe

5. Drug of choice for the treatment of acute gout in patients in whom NSAIDs are contraindicated is: *(NEET 2015)*
   A. Colchicine   B. Allopurinol
   C. Xyloric acid   D. Paracetamol
   Ans. is 'A' Colchicine

6. Needle shaped crystals negatively birefringent on polarized microscopy is characteristic of which crystal associated arthropathy? *(NEET 2015)*
   A. Gout   B. CPPD
   C. Neuropathic arthropathy   D. Hemophilic arthropathy
   Ans. is 'A' Gout

7. This elderly male came with a history of recurrent attack of pain and swelling in the great toe in the past. This is the present X-ray of the hand. The diagnosis can be confirmed by: *(APPG 2015)*

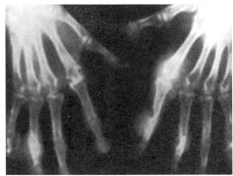

   A. X-ray of lumbosacral spine
   B. Polarized microscopy of tissue fluid aspirate
   C. Anti-CCP antibodies
   D. HLA B27

Ans. is 'B' Polarized microscopy of tissue fluid aspirate

8. A 40-year-old man presents with acute onset pain left great toe. On investigating punched out lesion is seen on phalanx and adjacent soft tissue. Most likely diagnosis is: *(AIIMS Nov 2014; 2013)*
   A. Reiter's arthritis   B. Psoriasis
   C. Rheumatoid   D. Gout

Ans. is 'D' Gout

9. A middle-aged male, known case of chronic renal failure develops MTP swelling the test to be performed is: *(AIIMS Nov 2012)*
   A. Uric acid   B. HLAB 27
   C. RA Factor   D. Calcium

Ans. is 'A' Uric acid

10. Acute Gouty arthritis drug used is:
    A. Probenecid   B. Allopurinol
    C. Colchicine   D. Sulfinpyrazone

Ans. is 'C' Colchicine

11. A 35-year-old businessmen presents suddenly with severe pain, swelling and redness in left big toe in early morning. Most likely diagnosis is:
    (PGI June 09, AIIMS 95, PGI 94, Andhra 92, AI 92)
    A. Rheumatoid arthritis   B. Gouty arthritis
    C. Pseudogout   D. Septic arthritis

Ans. is 'B' Gouty arthritis

Middle aged male with 1st MTP pain = gout

12. In a gouty arthritis, the characteristic X-ray findings includes: *(NIMS 2000)*
    A. Osteoporosis   B. Erosion of joint
    C. Soft tissue calcification D. Narrowing of joint space

Ans. is 'C' Soft tissue calcification

Soft tissue calcification is seen early followed by joint erosions.

13. Which of the following is not affected in gout?
    (PGI Dec 2K) (PGI June 03)
    A. Muscle   B. Skin
    C. Cartilage   D. Tendon
    E. Bursa

Ans. is 'A' Muscle

14. In a patient of gouty arthritis best investigation is:
    A. Serum uric acid   *(AI 98, AIIMS Sept 1996)*
    B. Uric acid in urine
    C. Urate crystal in synovial fluid
    D. Serum calcium level

Ans. is 'C' Urate crystal in synovial fluid

Monosodium urate crystals in synovial fluid are diagnostic of gout

15. What is not true about gout? *(AIIMS May 95)*
    A. Abrupt increase in serum urate levels is more common a cause for acute gout than an abrupt fall in urate levels
    B. Patient may be asymptomatic with high serum uric acid for years
    C. Development of arthritis correlates with level of serum uric acid
    D. Uric acid crystals are best seen by polarizing light microscope

Ans. is 'A' Abrupt increase in serum urate levels is more common a cause for acute gout than an abrupt fall in urate levels.

Fall of uric acid levels is more commonly associated with acute attack of gout.

PSEUDOGOUT

Feature	Gout (Protein alcohol intake)	Pseudogout (Hypothyroidism associated)
Synovial fluid analysis	Uric acid crystal Needle or rod shaped crystal, **negatively birefringent crystals**	**Calcium pyrophosphate crystal**, rhomboid shaped crystal, **Positive birefringent crystals**
Involved joint	Smaller joints (most commonly **metatarsophalangeal joint of big toe**)	Larger joints most commonly, **knee**
Clinical presentation	Intense pain	Moderate pain
Associated with	ACTH, glucocorticoid withdrawal, hypouricemic therapy, Hyperuricemia. **"Alcohol and Protein intake"**	Four 'H's i.e. hyperparathyroidism, hemochromatosis, hypophosphatasia, hypomagnesemia are associated. **Most common association is hypothyroidism; chondrocalcinosis**, i.e. appearance of calcific material in articular cartilage and menisci is seen.

ALKAPTONURIA

Heritable metabolic disorder characterized by the appearance of **homogentisic acid in urine**, dark pigmentation of the connective tissues **(ochronosis)** and calcification of hyaline and fibrocartilage. Inborn error is an absence of homogentisic acid oxidase in the liver and kidney. Those affected usually remain asymptomatic until the 3rd and 4th decade when they present with pain and stiffness of the **spine** and (later) larger joints.

Dark pigmentation of ear cartilage and sclera and staining of clothes by homogentisic acid in sweat. **Urine turns dark brown** when it is alkalinized or if it is left to stand for some hours. X-ray reveal narrowing and calcification of inter vertebral discs. Peripheral joints show chondrocalcinosis and severe osteoarthritis.

Treatment is Vitamin C.

CHONDROCALCINOSIS

It is deposition of calcium containing salts in articular cartilage. It is found in:

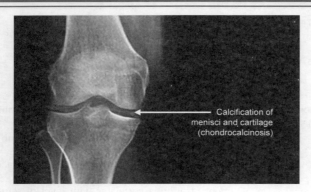

Fig. 16.28: X-ray knee

- Pseudogout (CPPD) – most important.
- Alkaptonuria (ochronosis)
- Hemochromatosis
- Hyperparathyroidism
- Hypothyroidism
- Acromegaly
- Diabetes mellitus
- Wilson's disease
- Gout.

INTERVERTEBRAL DISC CALCIFICATION

1. Degenerative spondylosis
2. **Alkaptonuria**
3. Calcium pyrophosphate dehydrate deposition disease (Pseudogout)
4. **Ankylosing spondylitis (AS)**
5. Juvenile chronic arthritis
6. Hemochromatosis
7. Diffuse idiopathic skeletal hyperostosis (DISH) or Ankylosing Hyperostosis (AH)
8. **Gout**
9. Idiopathic
10. Following spinal fusion.

CRANIOVERTEBRAL (CV) JUNCTION ANOMALIES: (BASE OF SKULL + C1 + C2)

Malformation of Occipit Bone:
- Basilar invagination
- Condylar hypoplasia

Malformation of Atlas (C1)

Malformation of Axis (C2)
OS odontoideum (dysgenesis of odontoid in which upper portion of odontoid is separated from base by a gap resembling ununited fracture).

Other causes are:
- Spondyloepiphyseal dysplasia
- **Achondroplasia**
- Mucopolysaccharidosis storage disease
- **Down's syndrome**
- **Klippel-Feil syndrome**
- **Neurofibromatosis**
- **Osteogenesis imperfecta**

- Rheumatoid arthritis
- Ankylosing spondylitis (rarest cause)
- CV Junction anomalies/instability is best judged by flexion and extension views of spine.

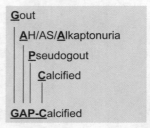

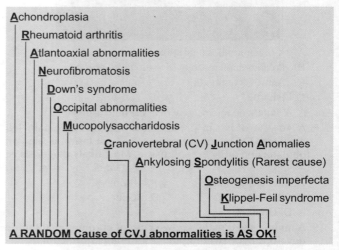

A RANDOM Cause of CVJ abnormalities is AS OK!

MULTIPLE CHOICE QUESTIONS

1. A 40-year-old female presents with urine darkening on standing, joint and stiffness, and pigment deposition in joints. What is the most probable diagnosis?
   (DNB June 2017)
   A. Phenylketonuria   B. Tyrosinemia
   C. Alkaptonuria   D. Tyrosinemia
   Ans. is 'C' Alkaptonuria

2. Which joint is most commonly affected in pseudogout?
   A. Knee   B. Hip   *(NEET 2015)*
   C. MP joint great toe D. MP joint thumb
   Ans. is 'A' Knee

3. Craniovertebral joint contains all except? *(AIIMS Nov 2015)*
   A. Wings of sphenoid B. Basiocciput
   C. Atlas   D. Axis
   Ans. is 'A' Wings of sphenoid

4. The pathognomonic finding in pseudogout is:
   A. CPPD crystals under microscope *(NEET Pattern 2013)*
   B. Polyarthritis with urinary sediment
   C. Juxta-articular osteopenia
   D. Bone spurs
   Ans. is 'A' CPPD crystals under microscope

5. Periarticular calcification is seen in: *(NEET Pattern 2013)*
   A. RA   B. Pseudogout
   C. OA   D. None of the above
   Ans. is 'B' Pseudogout

6. What change will be seen in vertebral column in ochronosis? *(NEET Pattern 2012)*
   A. Calcification of disc B. Bamboo spine
   C. Increased disc space D. None

Ans. is 'A' Calcification of disc

7. Heterotopic ossification occurs around:
   A. Bone B. Joint *(NEET Pattern 2012)*
   C. Soft tissue D. None

Ans. is 'B' Joint

8. Calcification of menisci is seen in: *(NEET Pattern 2012)*
   A. Hyperparathyroidism B. Pseudogout
   C. Renal osteodystrophy D. Acromegaly

Ans. is 'B' Pseudogout

9. A lady presents with right knee swelling, aspiration was done in which CPPD crystals were obtained. Next best investigation is: *(AIIMS May 2010)*
   A. ANA B. RF
   C. CPK D. TSH

Ans. is 'D' TSH
   - Finding CPPD crystal in aspirated synovial fluid is diagnostic of CPPD arthropathy.
   - CPPD arthropathy in some patients may be associated with: **Hypothyroidism (most common)** Primary hyperparathyroidism, Hemochromatosis, Hypomagnesemia, Hypophosphatasia.

10. X-ray of a young man shows heterotopic calcification around bilateral knee joints. Next investigation would be:
    A. Serum phosphate *(AIIMS May 07)*
    B. Serum calcium C. Serum PTH
    D. Serum Alkaline phosphatase

Ans. is 'A' Serum phosphate

Tumoral Calcinosis
   - Tumoral calcinosis is a rare condition which primarily, but not exclusively affects black people in otherwise good health.
   - This disease usually presents in the second decade of life and is characterized by deposition of painless calcific masses bilaterally around knee, hip, elbow or shoulder.
   - The primary defect responsible for this metastatic calcification appears to be hyperphosphatemia resulting from the increased capacity of renal tubule and intestines to absorb phosphate.
   - The most common laboratory findings are hyperphosphatemia and elevated serum 1,25-dihydroxy vitamin-D levels. Serum calcium, parathyroid hormone and alkaline phosphatase levels are usually normal.
   - Surgical excision is the most successful form of treatment if indicated although recurrences are common. Medical treatment to control the hyperphosphatemia (e.g. a low phosphate diet and oral estimation of phosphate binders) is an important adjuvant to surgical excision.

Parameter	Myositis ossificans	Tumor calcinosis
Etiology	Traumatic	Idiopathic/Familial
Side/Site	Unilateral-Elbow	Bilateral-Knee
Symptom	Painful	Painless
Marker	ALP increased	Increased PO_4

11. Heterotrophic ossification-most important investigation you would do for management: *(AIIMS Nov 2011)*
    A. Alkaline phosphatase B. Serum potassium
    C. Acid phosphatase D. Calcium

Ans. is 'A' Alkaline phosphatase
    - Most common marker for heterotrophic ossification and an indicator of osteoblastic activity is alkaline phosphatase

12. All of the following are associated with CV junction anomalies except: *(AI 07)*
    A. Rheumatoid arthritis B. Ankylosing spondylosis
    C. Odontoid dysgenesis D. Basal degeneration

Ans. is 'B' Ankylosing spondylosis

13. Chondrocalcinosis is seen in: *(AIIMS May 2002)*
    A. Ochronosis B. Hypoparathyroidism
    C. Rickets D. Hypervitaminosis

Ans. is 'A' Ochronosis
    - Alkaptonuria (ochronosis) can cause chondrocalcinosis.

14. The earliest manifestation of Alkaptonuria is: *(UP 02)*
    A. Ankylosis of lumbodorsal spine
    B. Ochronotic arthritis C. Prostatic calculi
    D. Pigmentation of tympanic membrane
    E. All of the above

Ans. is 'B' Ochronotic arthritis

15. How to differentiate gout with pseudogout: *(PGI June 2K)*
    A. Large joint involvement
    B. Birefringent (Particles) crystals
    C. Serum uric acid normal
    D. Associated with hyperparathyroidism
    E. Pain is very intense in pseudogout

Ans. is 'A' Large joint involvement; 'B' Birefringent (Particles) crystals; 'D' Associated with hyperparathyroidism

16. Characteristic crystals in pseudogout are: *(AI 1997)*
    A. Calcium pyrophosphate B. Sodium monourate
    C. Potassium urate D. Sodium pyrophosphate

Ans. is 'A' Calcium pyrophosphate

17. The most commonly involved joint in pseudogout:
    A. Knee B. Great toe *(Rajasthan 1993)*
    C. Hip D. Elbow

Ans. is 'A' Knee
    Knee is the commonest affected joint in pseudogout.

18. Subluxation of atlanto-occipital joint is seen in all except: *(Delhi 1991)*
    A. Gout B. Odontoid dysgenesis
    C. Rheumatoid arthritis D. Ankylosing spondylitis

Ans. is 'A' Gout very rarely causes craniovertebral anomalies.

19. Soft tissue calcification around the knee is seen in:
    A. Scurvy B. Scleroderma *(PGI 90)*
    C. Hyperparathyroidism D. Pseudogout

Ans. is 'D' Pseudogout

20. Calcification of menisci is seen in: *(AI 89)*
    A. Hyperparathyroidism B. Pseudogout
    C. Renal osteodystrophy D. Acromegaly

Ans. is 'B' Pseudogout
    - It can be seen in hyperparathyroidism and acromegaly also but pseudogout is commonest cause.

CLASSIFICATION AND CAUSES OF LOOSE BODIES IN JOINTS

Osteocartilaginous

These are composed of bone and cartilages hence are detected radiologically. It may originate from:
- Osteochondritis dissecans (most common cause in young)
- Osteochondral fracture
- Osteophyte (osteoarthritis) (most common cause/elderly)
- Synovial osteochondromatosis.

Cartilaginous

Radiolucent loose bodies usually are traumatic cartilaginous and originate from articular surface of tibia, femur or patella.

Fibrous

Radiolucent loose bodies occur less frequently and result from hyalinized reaction originating usually from synovium secondary to trauma, or more commonly from chronic inflammatory condition, such as tuberculosis (rice bodies).

Others

- Intra-articular tumors such as lipoma and localized nodular synovitis.
- Bullets, needles, and broken arthroscopic instruments.

SYNOVIAL CHONDROMATOSIS/SYNOVIAL OSTEOCHONDROMATOSIS

Synovial chondromatosis is characterized by the formation of metaplastic and **multiple foci of hyaline cartilage in the intimal layers of synovial membrane of joint (most common)**, bursae or tendon sheath. The term synovial osteochondromatosis is used when the cartilage is ossified.

Etiopathology

- **Etiology is unknown;** cytogenetic studies suggest it as clonal proliferation. Trauma is a possible stimulus of metaplasia of synovial cells into chondrocytes.
- Hyaline cartilage forms in stratum synoviale of synovial membrane, particularly at the points of reflection. The nodule initially confined within the synovial lining gradually is extruded into joint cavity, where it is attached at first by a synovial pedicle and later on may be torn free to become a loose body.
- The cartilage body may remain unchanged or may become calcified or ossified particularly at center by metaplasia or by endochondral ossification. Bony center undergoes aseptic necrosis.
- Nutrition (so growth) carried through pedicle and synovial fluid.
- Malignant change to chondrosarcoma is exceedingly rare.

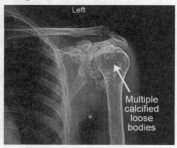

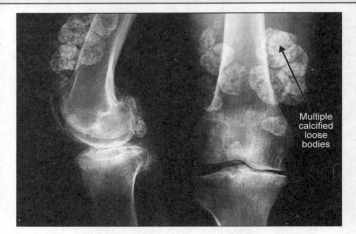

Fig. 16.29: Synovial chondromatosis

Radiology

Only calcified or ossified bodies are visible; so the number is always much greater than seen in X-rays.

Clinical Features

- This benign neoplasm is very rare. It usually occurs in persons >40 years old but occasionally occurs in adolescents with female preponderance.
- It has no hereditary predisposition and patients are usually between 30–50 years. Large diarthrodial joints especially **Knee is most commonly affected.** The condition is usually monoarticular but in 10% case there may be bilateral involvement.
- In order of decreasing frequency: Knee> Elbow >Ankle> Hip > shoulder are involved.
- Dull ache, swelling, stiffness, transient locking episode and grating sensations are usual complains. Generalized joint tenderness, thickening of soft tissues through which nodules (loose bodies) and crepitus may be palpable.
- Characteristic appearance of joint full of cartilaginous loose bodies produces **snow storm appearance.**

Treatment

Removal of loose bodies and partial synovectomy, can be done (arthroscopically).

MULTIPLE CHOICE QUESTIONS

1. True statement regarding Mseleni joint disease is:
   (JIPMER May 2018)
   A. Should, elbow wrist involvement is characteristic
   B. Elderly males are commonly involved
   C. Height is unaffected
   D. Endemic to northern Kwazulu Natal area in South Africa

   Ans. is 'D' Endemic to northern Kwazulu Natal area in South Africa

   Mseleni joint disease: Epigenetic chondrodysplasia
   - This disease affects indigenous Bantu Population in Mseleni, Kwazulu Natal area, South Africa.
   - More common in females.
   - Hip is the commonest joint affected causing its arthritis.
   - The disease is often bilateral.
   - Severe short stature has been reported

2. Loose body in joint most common site is: *(NEET 2015)*
   A. Knee
   B. Hip
   C. Elbow
   D. Ankle

Ans. is 'A' Knee

3. Multiple loose bodies are seen maximum in:
   (PGI June 2001) (PGI June 08)
   A. Osteochondritis dissecans
   B. Synovial chondromatosis
   C. Osteoarthritis
   D. Rheumatoid arthritis
   E. Osteochondral fracture

Ans. is 'B' Synovial chondromatosis

Causes of loose bodies include:
   i. *Osteoarthritis*
   ii. Osteochondral fracture (injury)
   iii. **Synovial chondromatosis**
   iv. **Osteochondritis dissecans**
   v. Charcot's disease

Among these, osteochondral fracture causes single loose bodies, while all other can cause multiple loose bodies, maximum by synovial chondromatosis (up to hundreds).

4. One of the following is to be considered as differential diagnosis for foreign body in plain X-ray of knee joint:
   (NIMS 2000)
   A. Fabella
   B. Calcified bursa
   C. Patella
   D. Chondromatosis

Ans. is 'D' Chondromatosis

5. The following is the commonest cause of loose body in knee joint: *(Bihar 1990)*
   A. Osteoarthritis
   B. Osteochondral fracture
   C. Synovial chondromatosis
   D. Osteochondritis dissecans

Ans. is 'A' Osteoarthritis
   – Commonest cause of loose bodies in knee joint is osteochondritis dissecans in young
   – **Osteoarthritis is commonest cause in elderly and overall.**

17 Metabolic Disorders of Bone

CONSTITUTION OF BONE

Inorganic Constituents of Bone
- Calcium and phosphate, which in an adult is primarily crystalline (hydroxyapatite crystals).
- Only about 65% of calcium is in an exchangeable form.
- Magnesium, sodium, potassium.

Organic Constituents of Bone
- 95% is collagen;
- Polysaccharides (mucoproteins or glycoproteins)
- Lipids (including phospholipids)

A. **Calcium homeostasis:**
   Bone serves as a store house for 99% of the body's calcium.
   When the serum level of calcium falls below its normal value, the body can react in three specific ways:
   i. It may increase intestinal absorption
   ii. It may decrease urinary excretion
   iii. It may increase the release of calcium from bone (by osteoclast).

   The factors responsible for monitoring these activities are parathyroid hormone (PTH), vitamin D and calcitonin. Calcitonin and PTH related peptide (PTHrp) are important primarily in the fetus.

B. **Vitamin D physiology:**

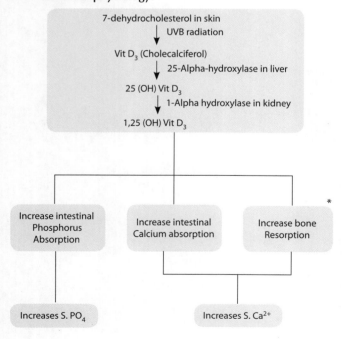

C. **PTH physiology:**

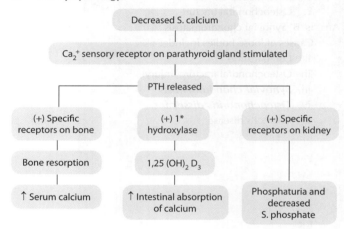

D. There are four types of metabolic bone diseases:
   - *Osteopenic diseases:* These diseases are characterized by a generalized decrease in bone mass (i.e. loss of bone matrix), though whatever bone is there, is normally mineralized (e.g. osteoporosis).
   - *Osteosclerotic diseases:* There are diseases characterized by an increase in bone mass (e.g. fluorosis).
   - *Osteomalacia diseases:* These are diseases characterized by an increase in the ratio of the organic fraction to the mineralized fraction, i.e. the available organic matter is demineralized.
   - *Mixed diseases:* These are diseases that are a combination of osteopenia and osteomalacia (e.g. hyperparathyroidism).

> Note:
> - *Rickets:* Lack of adequate mineralization of growing bones.
> - *Osteomalacia:* Lack of adequate mineralization of trabecular bone.
> - *Osteoporosis:* Proportionate loss of bone volume and mineral.
> - *Scurvy:* Defect in osteoid formation.

RICKETS AND OSTEOMALACIA

Increase in Osteoid Maturation Time

Osteoid matrix is secreted at normal rate but the mineralization is decreased (i.e. decrease in mineral apposition rate). This leads to increased osteoid maturation time. **(Maturation of osteoid means mineralization of osteoid).** Osteoid is increased in thickness, volume and total surface area. Bone tissue throughout skeleton is incompletely calcified and therefore softened. **Rickets** refers to condition where it occurs **before closure of growth plates** so that abnormalities of skeletal growth are superimposed.

Metabolic Disorders of Bone

Pathology of Rickets

Osteoid is laid down irregularly with widened osteoid seams and osteoid islets may even persist down into the diaphysis. The new trabeculae are thin and weak (as bundle of collagen fibers instead of running parallel to Haversian canal, coarse perpendicularly) and with joint loading the juxta-epiphyseal metaphysis becomes broad and cup shaped'.

- **A** – **A**bdomen protuberant
- **B** – **B**owing of bones (on weight bearing)
- **C** – **C**ostochondral junction prominent - (Rosary), **C**raniotabes (open fontanelles)
- **D** – **D**iaphragm pull - Harrison's groove (lateral indentation of chest due to pull of diaphragm on ribs)/**D**ouble malleolus
- **E** – **E**namel defect of teeth and delayed dentition
- **F** – **F**orward sternum - Pigeon chest (Pectus carinatum)
- **G** – **G**rowth plate - widening
- **H** – **H**ypocalcemia causing **H**yper PtH
- **I** – **I**rritability
- **J** – **J**oint deformities - Genu valgum/genu varum/coxa vara
- **K** – **K**yphosis
- **L** – **L**oosers zones
- **M** – **M**ilestone delayed **M**uscle weakness
- **R** – **R**ickets

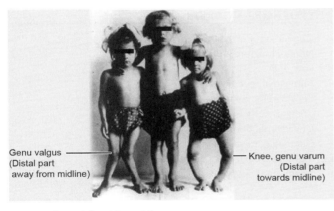

Fig. 17.1: Knee deformities—rickets

Serum alkaline phosphatase is an index of osteoblastic activity.

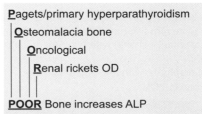

Pagets/primary hyperparathyroidism
Osteomalacia bone
Oncological
Renal rickets OD
POOR Bone increases ALP

Normal in osteoporosis, multiple myeloma and hypoparathyroidism (normal or decreased).

Causes of Rickets

1. Vit D disorders
    a. Nutritional
    b. Secondary, malabsorption, decrease in liver (25) hydroxylase activity, CRF
    c. **VDDR Type I**
       Deficiency of 1 alpha hydroxylase
    d. **VDDR Type II**
       End organ resistance to 1.25 $(OH)_2$ Vit D_3 (High prevalence of alopecia, ectodermal defects)
2. Calcium deficiency
3. Phosphorus deficiency
4. Renal losses
    i. Fanconi syndrome
    ii. Distal RTA
    iii. X-linked dominant (commonest), it is due to PHEX gene mutation, autosomal dominant and autosomal recessive are 3 varieties of hypophosphatemic Rickets (vitamin D resistant rickets)—increase incidence of skeletal deformities, no hypocalcemia, hypophosphatemia, phosphaturia, PTH is normal, vitamin D is normal and ALP is high.
5. Tumor associated with rickets:
    – Soft tissues – Hemangiopericytoma
    – Bone tumors – Non-ossifying fibroma, giant cell tumors, osteoblastoma, fibrous dysplasia, and neurofibromatosis.

Hypophosphatemic rickets has normal PTH and calcium

	Calcium	Phosphate	ALP	PTH
Osteoporosis	Normal	Normal	Normal	Normal
Rickets/osteomalacia	N or low	Low	High	High
Primary hyperparathyroidism	High	Low	High	High
Paget's disease	Normal	Normal	High	Normal

Lab Findings in Rickets	Calcium (Usually N↓)	Phosphorus (Usually ↓)	PTH (Usually ↑)	ALP (Usually ↑)	25 (OH) D	1,25 $(OH)_2$ D
Vit D deficiency	N↓	↓	↑	↑	↓	↓N↑
VDDR Type I	N↓	↓	↑	↑	N	↓
VDDR Type II	N↓	N↓	↑	↑	N	↑↑
CRF	N↓	↑	↑	↑	N	↓
Dietary P deficiency	N	↓	N	↑	N	↑
XLH-Hypophosphatemic Rickets	N	↓	N	↑	N	↓
ADHR-Hypophosphatemic Rickets	N	↓	N	↑	N	↓
Fanconi syndrome (Proximal RTA)	N	↓	N	↑	N	↓
Dietary Ca deficiency	N↓	↓	↑	↑	N	↑

RADIOGRAPHIC FINDINGS

- The characteristic feature of rickets are thickening and widening of growth plate (physis). Indistinct and hazy metaphysis that is abnormally wide (splaying) with cupping or flaring (Brush like appearance).
- Bowing of diaphysis, with thinning of cortices.
- Looser's zone in 20%.

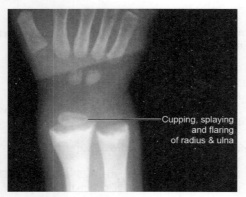

Fig. 17.2: X-ray wrist—rickets

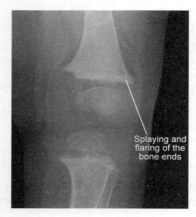

Fig. 17.3: Rickets knee

- Persistent hypocalcemia may cause secondary hyperparathyroidism.

Therapy

1. Nutritional rickets:
   - Two strategies for administration of vitamin D. Stoss therapy, 300,000–600,000 I.U. of vitamin D are administered orally or intramuscularly. The alternative is daily high dose vitamin D, 2000–5000 I.U./day over 4–6 week. Followed by 400 I.U. Vit D/Day and supplements of calcium for 2–4 months
2. Hypophosphatemic Rickets:
   - Oral phosphate and Vit D supplements
   - Joule's solution—Dibasic sodium phosphate, phosphoric acid is given in hypophosphatemic Rickets.
3. VDDR I:
   - Calcitriol, calcium, phosphate supplements
4. VDDR II:
   - Treatment not satisfactory large doses of calcitriol and calcium, phosphate supplements.
5. Renal tubular acidosis:
   - Bicarbonate supplements (**Shohl's solution**—Citric acid, sodium citrate) and phosphate supplementation.
6. CRF:
   - Calcitriol, calcium supplements and phosphate restriction.

HEALING RICKETS

Healing rickets: On treatment at metaphysis white line of Frankel is seen.

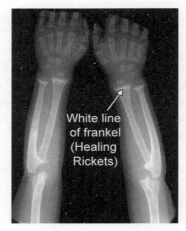

HYPOPHOSPHATASIA—DIFFERENT FROM HYPOPHOSPHATEMIA!

- Genetic error in synthesis of ALP
- Normal calcium and phosphate levels
- Low ALP
- Autosomal recessive
- Phosphoethanolamine in urine/serum
- Changes early in life
- Delayed dentition
- Genu valgum/varum
- Mortality 50–70%
- Treatment is supportive

OSTEOMALACIA: MORE COMMON IN FEMALES

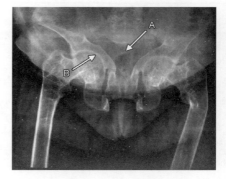

Fig. 17.4: Osteomalacia— (A) Triradiate pelvis and (B) protrusio acetabuli

Adult onset bone softening and muscle weakness. Low back and thigh pain, proximal muscle weakness. **Triradiate pelvis, protrusio acetabular** (acetabulum protrudes into pelvis due to bone softening when bilateral called as **Otto Pelvis**), **pseudofracture**. There is **waddling gait** due to muscular weakness.

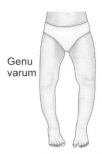
Genu varum
"Bowed legs"

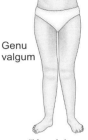
Genu valgum
"Knock knees"

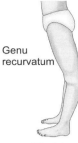
Genu recurvatum
"Back knee"

MULTIPLE CHOICE QUESTIONS

1. X-ray changes seen in rickets are: *(PGI Nov 2018)*
   A. Metaphyseal cupping & fraying
   B. Calcification of Epiphysis
   C. Metaphyseal Widening
   D. White Sclerotic ring around Epiphysis
   E. Osteopenia

Ans. is 'A' Metaphyseal cupping & fraying 'C' Metaphyseal Widening 'E' Osteopenia

2. True about Pectus excavatum: *(PGI May 2017)*
   A. More common in female
   B. In severe cases, mitral valve prolapse may occur
   C. May be present at birth
   D. Seen in Marfan syndrome
   E. Impairment of respiratory function

Ans. is 'B' In severe cases, mitral valve prolapse may occur; 'C' May be present at birth; 'D' Seen in Marfan syndrome; 'E' Impairment of respiratory function

Pectus Excavatum:
- Body of sternum is curved inwards
- Decreased chest expansion
- Decreased total lung capacity

Associations:
- Prematurity
- Congenital heart disease
- Fetal Alcohol Disease
- Homocystinuria
- Marfan syndrome
- Poland syndrome
- Noonan syndrome

3. True about Osteomalacia: *(PGI May 2017)*
   A. More common in male
   B. Low PTH
   C. ↑alkaline phosphatase
   D. ↓ed Calcium level
   E. Looser's zone on X-ray

Ans. is 'C' ↑alkaline phosphatase; 'D' ↓ed Calcium level; 'E' Looser's zone on X-ray

4. Genu recurvatum is seen in: *(NEET Dec 2016)*
   A. Rheumatoid arthritis   B. Poliomyelitis
   C. Rickets   D. All of the above

Ans. is 'D' All of the above

Genu Recurvatum or hyperextension of knee is seen in:
- Trauma
- R.A
- Rickets
- Poliomyelitis
- Charcots
- Congenital (Due to Intrauterine positioning) – self resolving

5. Child diagnosed with hypophosphatemic rickets; choose the correct statement: *(PGI Nov 2016)*
   A. Serum calcium levels are mostly normal
   B. Raised levels of alkaline phosphate seen
   C. Has XLD inheritance   D. PTH is markedly raised
   E. Pigeon chest is one of the characteristic skeletal deformity

Ans. is 'A' Serum calcium levels are mostly normal; 'B' Raised levels of alkaline phosphate seen; 'C' Has XLD inheritance; 'E' Pigeon chest is one of the characteristic skeletal deformity

6. Biochemical abnormality in rickets: *(PGI May 2016)*
   A. High calcium   B. High PO_4
   C. Low ALP   D. ALP is high
   E. Low calcium

Ans. is 'D' ALP is high and 'E' Low calcium

7. Wrist X-ray: *(AIIMS Nov 16)*

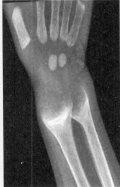

   A. Rickets   B. Colles fracture
   C. Scaphoid fracture   D. Osteoporosis

Ans. is 'A' Rickets *(Refer to Fig. 17.2)*

8. X-Ray hand, most probable diagnosis: *(AI 2016)*

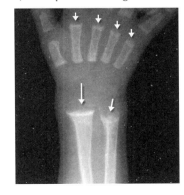

A. Scurvy B. Rickets
C. Hyper PTH D. Achondroplasia

Ans. is 'B' Rickets *(Refer to Fig. 17.2)*

9. Which of the following features are seen in pediatric Vit D deficiency? *(PGI Nov 2015)*
   A. Rachitic rosary B. Harrison's sulcus
   C. Wimberger sign D. Pigeon chest
   E. Widening near the joints

Ans. is 'A' Rachitic rosary; 'B' Harrison's sulcus; 'D' Pigeon chest and 'E' Widening near the joints

10. A 2-year-old child with rickets is on calcium supplements and has a foot deformity. The child will be referred to a surgeon for the correction of the deformity when: *(AIIMS May 2013, Nov 2012)*
    A. Serum calcium levels are normal
    B. Serum vitamin D levels are normal
    C. Growth plate healing becomes normal
    D. Serum ALP becomes normal

Ans. is 'C' Growth plate healing becomes normal

Explanation
- Corrective osteotomy in rickets should only be done once radiological healing has taken place otherwise the osteotomy will not unite due to defective mineralization.

11. Osteomalacia is due to: *(NEET Pattern 2012)*
    A. Vitamin C deficiency B. Vitamin D deficiency
    C. Vitamin E deficiency D. None

Ans. is 'B' Vitamin D deficiency

12. In Rickets all are seen except: *(NEET Pattern 2012)*
    A. Bowing of legs B. Rachitic rosary
    C. Bleeding D. Craniotabes

Ans. is 'C' Bleeding

13. A 30 years female has low serum calcium and phosphate with elevated parathormone. Diagnosis is:
    A. Vitamin D deficiency *(NEET Pattern 2012)*
    B. Primary hyperparathyroidism
    C. Osteoporosis D. Paget's diseases

Ans. is 'A' Vitamin D deficiency

14. Pectus carinatum is seen in: *(NEET Pattern 2012)*
    A. Scurvy B. Rickets
    C. Hemophilia D. Osteogenesis imperfect

Ans. is 'B' Rickets

15. Test for vitamin D deficiency: *(NEET Pattern 2012)*
    A. Vitamin D levels B. ALP levels
    C. Calcium levels D. Phosphate level

Ans. is 'A' Vitamin D levels

16. Hypophosphatemic Rickets mode of inheritance is: *(NEET Pattern 2012)*
    A. Autosomal dominant B. Autosomal recessive
    C. X-linked dominant D. X-linked recessive

Ans. is 'C' X-linked dominant

17. Which of the drugs cause osteomalacia? *(NEET Pattern 2012)*
    A. Phenytoin B. Valproate
    C. Carbamazepine D. Aspirin

Ans. is 'A' Phenytoin

18. Looser zone is a feature of: *(NEET Pattern 2012)*
    A. Osteoporosis B. Osteomalacia
    C. Metastasis D. Scurvy

Ans. is 'B' Osteomalacia

19. Osteomalacia is associated with: *(PGI Nov 2009; AI 2003)*
    A. Decreases in osteoid volume
    B. Decrease in osteoid surface
    C. Increase in osteoid maturation time
    D. Increase in mineral apposition rate

Ans. is 'C' Increase in osteoid maturation time

20. Rickets in infancy is characterised by the following except: *(AIIMS May 07)*
    A. Craniotabes B. Rachitic rosary
    C. Wide open fontanelles D. Bow legs

Ans. is 'D' Bow legs
- Long bones of legs get deformed when the child starts bearing weight. Therefore deformities of legs are unusual before the age of one year.

21. Decreased mineralisation of epiphyseal plate in a growing child is seen in: *(AI 2000)*
    A. Rickets B. Osteomalacia
    C. Scurvy D. Osteoporosis

Ans. is 'A' Rickets

22. Osteomalacia/Rickets maybe seen in A/E: *(JIPMER 99)*
    A. Neurofibroma B. Osteoblastoma
    C. Hemangiopericytoma D. Ewing's sarcoma

Ans. is 'D' Ewing's sarcoma

23. Basic pathological defect in rickets is: *(AI 99, RA 98, UP 98, 97, AIIMS 91)*
    A. Decreased osteoblastic activity
    B. Nonfunctional osteoclast
    C. Defective osteoclastic resorption of uncalcified osteoid and cartilage
    D. Defective proliferation of physis.

Ans. is 'C' Defective osteoclastic resorption of uncalcified osteoid and cartilage
- Osteoid formation is normal in rickets. With defective mineralization, however, osteoclastic resorption of the uncalcified osteoid does not take place. Therefore, osteoid is laid down irregularly with widened osteoid seams and osteoid islets.

24. A patient with raised serum alkaline phosphatase and raised parathormone level along with low calcium and low phosphate level is likely to have: *(AIIMS June 99)*
    A. Primary hyperparathyroidism
    B. Paget's disease C. Osteoporosis
    D. Vitamin D deficiency

Ans. is 'D' Vitamin D deficiency
- In osteoporosis all these parameters are normal.

25. Action of vitamin D is that it: *(UPSC 99, AMC 1991)*
    A. Stimulates bone marrow
    B. Increases calcium loss
    C. Stimulates absorption of calcium
    D. Stimulates osteoclasts

Ans. is 'C' Stimulates absorption of calcium; 'D' Stimulates osteoclasts

HYPERPARATHYROIDISM

- Hyperparathyroidism maybe primary (due to adenoma or hyperplasia), secondary (due to persistent hypocalcemia) or tertiary (when secondary hyperplasia leads to autonomous overactivity).

Metabolic Disorders of Bone

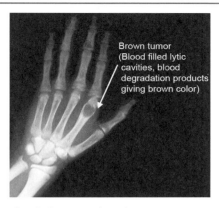

Fig. 17.5: X-ray hand—hyperparathyroidism

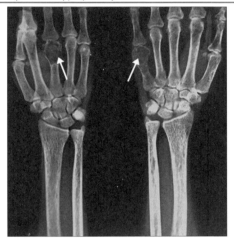

Fig. 17.6: Brown tumor

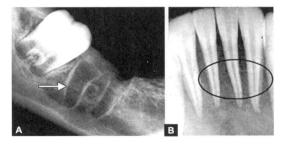

Figs. 17.7A and B: (A) Lamina dura and (B) Resorption of lamina dura

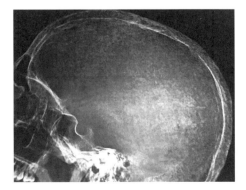

Fig. 17.8: Salt pepper skull

- Parathyroid adenoma is most common cause of primary hyperparathyroidism. It presents with subperiosteal resorption, and replacement of endosteal cavitation marrow by vascular granulation and fibrous tissue (osteitis fibrosa cystica). Classical and pathognomic feature of hyperparathyroidism is subperiosteal cortical resorption of middle phalanges on radial aspect.
- Clinical features—Abdominal **groans** (dyspepsia), psychic **moans**, renal **stones** and weak **bones** (Groans, moans, stones and Bones).
- Parathyroid hormone and S. alkaline phosphate are raised. Calcium is high, serum phosphate is low. These parameters (calcium and phosphate) are variable in secondary hyperparathyroidism.

	Primary (adenoma)	Secondary (usually due to osteomalacia)
Clinical features	More	Less
Ca	High	Low or normal
PTH	Very high	High

Hyperparathyroidism causes diffuse rarefaction of bone (osteopenia) and osteitis fibrosa cystica.

> Note: von Recklinghausen's disease of bone is also called as osteitis fibrosa cystica (it should not be confused with von Recklinghausen's disease – Neurofibromatosis type 1): In Osteitis fibrosa cystica there is fibrosa that is bony trabeculae are replaced by fibrous tissue and there is cystica that is cystic cavity in bone filled with blood and blood degradation products gives it brown color.

Radiological Features of Hyperparathyroidism

- Subperiosteal resorption of terminal tufts of phalanges, lateral end of clavicle and symphysis pubis.
- Loss of lamina dura (i.e. thin cortical bone of tooth socket surrounding teeth is seen as thin white line, is resorbed).
- Irregular, diffuse rarefaction of bones, i.e. generalized osteopenia, thinning of cortices, and indistinct bony trabeculae.
- Brown tumor.
- Salt pepper appearance of skull
- SCFE maybe seen avascular necrosis
- **Rarely AVN**

Treatment is usually conservative and includes adequate hydration and decreased calcium intake. The indications of parathyroidectomy are marked hypercalcemia, recurrent renal calculi, progressive nephrocalcinosis and severe osteoporosis.

MULTIPLE CHOICE QUESTIONS

1. A 70-year-old male, known case of chronic renal failure suffers from a pathological fracture of Right femur, the diagnosis is: *(DNB JULY 2016)*
    A. Primary Hyperparathyroidism
    B. Secondary Hyperparathyroidism
    C. Scurvy
    D. Vitamin D Resistant rickets

Ans. is 'B' Secondary Hyperparathyroidism

2. A 28-year-old lady presented with Nausea, vomiting and abdominal pain. X-Ray done showed, centrally located lytic lesions in metacarpals. Next line of management will be:
   A. Bone curettage with bone grafting
   B. Extended curettage with phenol
   C. Extended curettage with bone grafting
   D. Parathyroid hormone and serum calcium levels measurement
Ans. is 'D' Parathyroid hormone and serum calcium levels measurement

3. Primary Hyperparathyroidism is associated with:
   A. Increased serum PTH and hypercalcemia (CET Nov 15)
   B. Decreased serum PTH and hypercalcemia
   C. Increased serum PTH and hypocalcemia
   D. Decreased serum PTH and hypocalcemia
Ans. is 'A' Increased serum PTH and hypercalcemia

4. A middle aged female has resorption of 2nd and 3rd metacarpal and multiple lytic lesions in pelvis femur ribs clavicle: (AIIMS Nov 2014)
   A. Hyperthyroidism   B. Hyperparathyroidism
   C. Osteomalacia   D. Renal osteodystrophy
Ans. is 'B' Hyperparathyroidism

5. Osteitis fibrosa cystica is seen in: (NEET 2013 2012)
   A. Hyperparathyroidism   B. Hypoparathyroidism
   C. Hypothyroidism   D. Hyperthyroidism
Ans. is 'A' Hyperparathyroidism

6. Salt pepper skull is a feature of: (NEET Pattern 2013)
   A. Paget's syndrome   B. Eosinophilic granuloma
   C. Primary hyperparathyroidism
   D. Multiple myeloma
Ans. is 'C' Primary hyperparathyroidism

7. Hyperparathyroidism causes: (NEET Pattern 2012)
   A. Multiple bone cysts
   B. Subperiosteal bone resorption
   C. Brown's tumor
   D. All of the above
Ans. is 'D' All of the above

8. Subperiosteal bone resorption is seen in: (NEET Pattern 2012)
   A. Hypothyroidism   B. Hyperthyroidism
   C. Hypoparathyroidism   D. Hyperparathyroidism
Ans. is 'D' Hyperparathyroidism

9. Hyperparathyroidism is characterized by: (NEET Pattern 2012)
   A. Hypocalcemia   B. Osteoprotegerin
   C. Hyperphosphatemia   D. Multiple bone cyst
Ans. is 'D' Multiple bone cyst

10. Brown tumor is seen in: (AIPG 2010) (AIIMS Nov 09)
    A. Hyperparathyroidism   B. Hypoparathyroidism
    C. Hypothyroidism   D. Hyperparathyroidism
Ans. is 'A' Hyperparathyroidism

11. A 50-year-old man presented with multiple pathological fractures. His serum calcium was 11.5 mg/dl and phosphate was 2.5 mg/dl. Alkaline phosphatase was 940 I.U./dl. The most probable diagnosis is: (AIIMS Nov 2005)
    A. Osteoporosis   B. Osteomalacia
    C. Multiple myeloma   D. Hyperparathyroidism
Ans. is 'D' Hyperparathyroidism

12. Soft tissue calcification with hypercalcemia is observed in:
    A. Hyperparathyroidism   B. Alkaptonuria (Bihar 1998)
    C. Gout   D. Cushing's disease
Ans. is 'A' Hyperparathyroidism

13. Absence of lamina dura in the alveolus occurs in: (TN 91)
    A. Rickets   B. Osteomalacia
    C. Deficiency of vitamin   D. Hyperparathyroidism
Ans. is 'D' Hyperparathyroidism

14. Hyperphosphatemia is seen in: (PGI May 2017)
    A. Vitamin D intoxication   B. Renal failure
    C. Fanconi's anemia   D. Tumor lysis syndrome
    E. Hyperparathyroidism
Ans. is 'A' Vitamin D intoxication; 'B' Renal failure; & 'D' Tumor lysis syndrome

Hyperphosphatemia: $\uparrow PO_4^{3-}$ Levels are associated with:
a. Increased oral intake
b. Vitamin D intoxication
c. Renal failure
d. Hypoparathyroidism
e. Pseudohypoparathyroidism
f. Tumor calcinosis
g. Tumor Lysis Syndrome
h. Rhabdomyolysis
i. Acute hemolysis

PSEUDOFRACTURE

Milkman's/Increment fractures also known as looser's zones or osteoid zones are pseudofracture, seen at the sites of mechanical stress or nutrient vessel entry (pulsation). These represent incomplete (insufficiency) stress fractures that have healed by callus consisting of osteoid tissue lacking calcium (i.e. unmineralized woven bone).

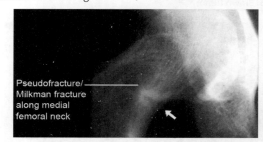

Fig. 17.9: X-ray hip—pseudofracture

It is Characteristically Seen in:
- Osteomalacia (most characteristic)
- Renal osteodystrophy
- Hyperparathyroidism
- Neurofibromatosis
- Paget's disease
- Polyostotic fibrous dysplasia
- Osteogenesis imperfecta
- Hereditary Hypophosphatasia

Common Locations
- Femoral neck (most common)
- Pubic rami
- Axillary edge of scapula immediately below the glenoid
- Scapula lateral and superior border
- Ribs and clavicle

Typical Features
- Thin (narrow) translucent band about 2–3 mm in width running perpendicular (at the right angle) to cortex is seen. It is often multiple and bilaterally symmetrical.

Treatment
Rest and treat the primary cause.

MULTIPLE CHOICE QUESTIONS

1. Pseudofracture can be seen in the following conditions: *(DNB June 2017)*
   A. Hereditary hypophosphatasia
   B. Paget's disease
   C. Fibrous dysplasia
   D. All of the above

Ans. is 'D' All of the above

2. Loosers zone are seen in which of the following conditions? *(CET Nov 15)*
   A. Osteoporosis
   B. Osteomalacia
   C. Rickets
   D. Scurvy

Ans. is 'B' Osteomalacia

3. Loosers zone/Pseudofractures are commonly seen in the following areas except: *(CET Nov 15)*
   A. Scapula
   B. Ribs
   C. Pelvis
   D. Radius

Ans. is 'D' Radius

4. Looser's zones are seen in: *(NEET Pattern 2013)*
   A. Osteomalacia
   B. Paget's disease
   C. Renal osteodystrophy
   D. All of the above

Ans. is 'D' All of the above

5. Short 4th metacarpal is a feature of: *(NEET Pattern 2013)*
   A. Hyperparathyroidism
   B. Hypoparathyroidism
   C. Pseudohypoparathyroidism
   D. Scleroderma

Ans. is 'C' Pseudohypoparathyroidism

6. Milkman's fracture is: *(AI 09)*
   A. Pseudofracture in adults
   B. Fracture of clavicle in children
   C. Fracture humerus
   D. Fracture first metacarpal

Ans. is 'A' Pseudofracture in adults

RENAL OSTEODYSTROPHY

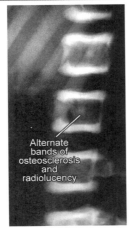

Fig. 17.10: Rugger-Jersey spine

Renal Osteodystrophy: Bony changes are combination of **Rickets + Hyperparathyroidism + Osteoporosis + Osteosclerosis**.
- Renal osteodystrophy is more common in **CRF. It is driven by presence of secondary hyperparathyroidism**.
- Pathophysiology begins with damaged glomerulus's inability to excrete phosphorus.
- Hyperphosphatemia shuts down the production of vit D thus causing decreased calcium absorption from small intestine. Hypocalcemia triggers release of PTH which enables the demineralization of bone to increase serum calcium level.
- Osteosclerosis when present, is most common at the base of the skull and in vertebra causing horizontal stripped Rugger Jersey appearance.
- 'Rugger Jersey vertebrae' appears like sandwiches, with osteosclerosis adjacent to the end plates but relative radiolucency in the middle of vertebrae. It is seen in renal osteodystrophy and osteopetrosis. In patients of renal osteodystrophy, Rugger Jersey appearance is due to hyperparathyroidism and osteosclerosis.
- Renal abnormalities precede the bony changes by several years. Children are stunted and myopathy is common. Epiphysiolysis (displacement of epiphysis) may be seen. **Low calcium and high phosphate is seen** treatment is high dose of vit D (5,00,000 IU daily), in resistant cases small doses of 1,25 DHCC may be effective.

MULTIPLE CHOICE QUESTIONS

1. "Rugger Jersey spine" is seen in: *(AI 2006)*
   A. Fluorosis
   B. Achondroplasia
   C. Renal osteodystrophy
   D. Marfan's syndrome

Ans. is 'C' Renal osteodystrophy

2. Rugger Jersey spine in CRF is due to: *(PGI Dec 04)*
   A. Osteomalacia
   B. Trauma
   C. Hyperparathyroidism
   D. Aluminium osteodystrophy

Ans. is 'C' Hyperparathyroidism

SCURVY

Scurvy: Deficiency of vitamin C, causing **defect in osteoid formation**.

Pathology
- Vit C is necessary for **hydroxylation of lysine and proline** to hydroxylysine and hydroxyproline, two amino acids crucial for proper cross-linking of triple helix of collagen. So deficiency causes **failure of collagen synthesis or primitive collagen formation**, throughout the body, including in blood vessels, predisposing to hemorrhage.
- **In bones zone of proliferation is affected primarily.**
- Hemorrhage, is capillary in origin and occurs from gums, alimentary tract, subcutaneous tissue, and bone especially at the most actively growing metaphysis and beneath periosteum.
- Hemorrhage and fractures are common, but attempts of repair is disordered. The provisional zone of calcification is weak leading to epiphyseal separations.
- Dysfunctional osteoblast (flat resembling fibroblast) causes failure of osteoid formation resulting in generalized osteoporosis.
- Chondroblast and mineralization is unaffected leading to **persistence of calcified cartilage approaching metaphysis seen radiologically as opaque white line at junction of physis and metaphysis (Frankel's line).**
- Osteoclasts are normal, thin and fragile trabeculae and cortices of bone are seen.

- **Dentin formation in teeth is abnormal** due to defective collagen.

Clinical Feature

- It develops after 6–12 months of dietary deprivation thus not seen in neonates.
- Earliest features are restlessness, fretfulness, irritability, loss of appetite and failure to thrive
- **Gums maybe spongy and bleeding.**
- Subperiosteal hemorrhage is a distinct sign occurring most commonly in distal femur and tibia and proximal humerus, causing excruciating tenderness pain near the large joints. The child lies still to minimize pain or minimally move the affected limb (pseudoparalysis) - **(Frogs like posture is attained by child).**
- **Hemorrhage** in soft tissue, joint, kidney, gut and petechiae maybe seen.
- Anemia and impaired wound healing is seen.
- Beading of ribs at costochondral junction (Scorbutic rosary).
- Systemic reaction (fever) is absent initially.

Note: In **R**ickets—Rosary is **R**ound and non-tender, and in **S**curvy it is **S**harp and tender.

Radiological Feature

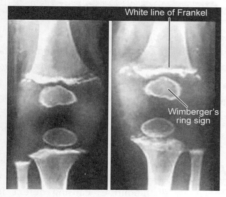

Fig. 17.11: Scurvy (sclerosed margins of epiphysis)

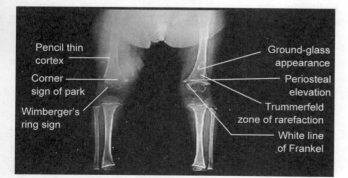

Fig. 17.12: Scurvy

- **Osteopenia (ground glass appearance) (1st sign)** with thinning of cortex (pencil thin cortex).
- Metaphysis maybe deformed or fractured.
- **Frankel's line** (zone of provisional calcification increases in width and opacity) due to failure of resorption of calcified cartilage and stands out compared to the severely osteopenic metaphysis.
- Scurvy line or scorbutic zone (Trummerfeld zone) is radiolucent transverse band adjacent to the dense provisional zone.
- **Margins of the epiphysis appears relatively sclerotic, termed ringing of epiphyses or Wimberger's sign (Ring sign) - most Important.**
- Lateral metaphyseal spur (Pelkan spur) at ends of metaphysis is produced by outward projection of zone of provisional calcification and periosteal reaction.
- Corner or angle sign is peripheral metaphyseal cleft.
- Subperiosteal hemorrhage.

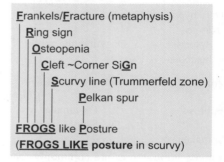

Frankels/**F**racture (metaphysis)
Ring sign
Osteopenia
Cleft ~Corner Si**G**n
Scurvy line (Trummerfeld zone)
Pelkan spur
FROGS like **P**osture
(**FROGS LIKE** posture in scurvy)

Treatment: Vitamin C

MULTIPLE CHOICE QUESTIONS

1. A female eating only junk food, pinpoint ecchymoses around hair follicle. Bleeding into joints and subperiosteal hemorrhages, swollen tongue and gingivitis. What is the defect? *(AIIMS Nov 2013)*
   A. Hydroxylation of lysine and proline
   B. Carboxylation of clotting factors
   C. Deficiency factor VIII   D. Deficiency factor IX

Ans. is 'A' Hydroxylation of lysine and proline

2. Wimberger ring sign is seen in: *(NEET Pattern 2013)*
   A. Scurvy   B. Syphilis
   C. Paget's   D. Hemophilia

Ans. is 'A' Scurvy

*Wimberger corner sign: Congenital syphilis

3. Barton's disease is:
   A. Scurvy and rickets   B. Scurvy and fracture
   C. Rickets and fracture   D. Scurvy and syphilis

Ans. is 'A' Scurvy and rickets

4. Vitamin C deficiency leads to: *(AIIMS May 2010, NIMS 98)*
   A. Defective mineralisation
   B. Defective osteoid formation
   C. Normal collagen and bone matrix
   D. X-ray shows normal evidence

Ans. is 'B' Defective osteoid formation

5. A young patient presents with enlargement of costochondral junction and with the white line of Frankel at the metaphysis. The diagnosis is: *(KA 2000)*
   A. Scurvy   B. Rickets
   C. Hyperparathyroidism   D. Osteomalacia

Ans. is 'A' Scurvy

Enlargement of costochondral junction (rosary) and white line of Frankel is seen in scurvy.

6. Vitamin required for collagen is: (PGI 97), NB 1990)
   A. Vitamin A B. Vitamin C
   C. Vitamin D D. Vitamin E

Ans. is 'B' Vitamin C

7. Metaphyseal fracture is commonly seen in: (Delhi 92)
   A. Osteogenesis imperfecta B. Scurvy
   C. Rickets D. None

Ans. is 'B' Scurvy

OSTEOPOROSIS

Osteoporosis is reduction in bone mass (density) i.e. there is quantitative decrease of units of bone formation but each unit has qualitatively normal configuration. So, osteoporosis characteristically has normal calcium, phosphate and alkaline phoshatase levels.

Bone Mineral Density is measured by DEXA (Dual Emission X-ray Absorptiometry) Scan and it is matched to Dexa scan of 30 year old individual and T score is calculated. WHO classification.

- **T score 0 to –1 is normal**
- T score –1 to –2.5 is osteopenia
- T score less than –2.5 is osteoporosis
- **Osteoporosis with a fracture is severe osteoporosis**

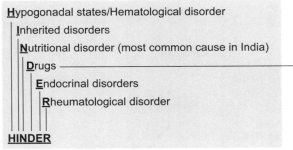

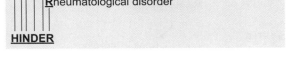

2. Inherited, e.g. osteogenesis imperfecta, Marfan syndrome.
3. Nutritional, e.g. malnutrition, malabsorption
4. Drugs, e.g. <u>A</u>nticonvulsants, <u>A</u>lcohol, <u>H</u>eparin, <u>L</u>ithium, aluminium, cytotoxic drugs, excessive thyroxine.
5. Endocrinal disorders, e.g. hyperparathyroidism, thyrotoxicosis IDDM, Cushing syndrome
6. Rheumatological disorders:
   Rheumatoid arthritis,
   Ankylosing spondylitis

Etiologies of Osteoporosis

- Radiological features are loss of vertical height of vertebrae (collapse), codfish appearance and pencillin G of vertebrae.
- Singh's Index is used for osteoporosis grading.

Treatment

1. Drug used in osteoporosis
   Inhibit resorption: Bisphosphonates, **Denosumab**, calcitonin, estrogen, SERMS, gallium nitrate.
2. *Stimulate formation:* **Teriparatide (PTH analogue)**, calcium, calcitriol, **fluorides**.
3. *Both actions:* Strontium ranelate.

Z Score

- Z score compares the patients BMD with that of adult of the same race, age and sex.
- Z Score indicates possible secondary osteoporosis.
- A Z Score of – 2 or below should trigger investigation for underlying disease.

The fractures that are most common (in decreasing order) are vertebral fracture, hip (neck femur) and lower end radius.

Most of the vertebral fractures are asymptomatic and are identified incidentally during radiograph for other purpose. Few of these present as backache of varying degree. **Up to 70 years order of fracture incidence is vertebral > Colle's. Overall and > 70 years age it is vertebral > Hip > Colle's.**

- **Bone mineral density in Hemiplegic patient is reduced maximum in Humerus**

Factors that Hinder Bone Cause—Osteoporosis

1a. **Hypogonadal states,** e.g. Turner syndrome, Klinefelter's syndrome.
1b. **Hematological:** Leukemia, lymphoma

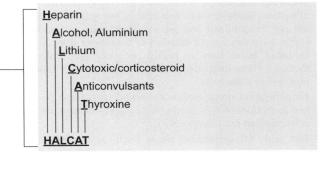

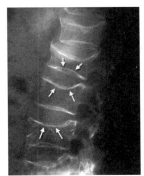

Fig. 17.13: X-ray of osteoporotic spine: **Codfish vertebra (Biconcave vertebra)**

A. Drugs decreasing bone resorption initially increase bone mineral density (BMI), but it reaches a plateau in 2–3 yrs because bone formation also decreases. On the other hand, drugs promoting bone formation can increase BMD throughout the period of treatment.
B. Calcium (1500 mg/day)
C. Vitamin D (400–800 IU per day) Initially Vit. D deficient patients are treated with active metabolite 1,25, dihydroxy Vit D3 (short half-life 4 hours and expensive)

then changing over to longer lasting and less expensive Vit D2 or D3 (t ½ up to 2½ months).

D. The principle goal of treatment is prevention. In treatment of children, adolescents, and young adults, an emphasis on attaining maximum peak bone mass during age of 20–30 years must be stressed. By adequate nutrition, weight bearing exercises, adequate vit D and Calcium intake, and maintenance of normal menstrual cycle. Young men have a much greater peak bone mass on average than do young women, which may account in part for the lower rate of osteoporosis in men.

E. Hormone replacement therapy—The mainstay of bone loss prevention in postmenopausal osteoporosis is estrogen treatment. Daily dose of 0.625 mg of conjugated estrogen in combination with progestins are recommended. Progestin is essential (even though it has no independent effect on bone) to reduce the risk of developing endometrial cancer (due to estrogen).

F. Selective estrogen receptor modulator (SERM)—These act as estrogen antagonist in breast tissue and as an agonist in bone. Raloxifene selectively stimulates estrogen receptor in bone and is used in treatment of osteoporosis. It reduces risk of breast cancer also. Tamoxifen is not used in osteoporosis.

- **Bisphosphonases** (pyrophosphate analogs) bind to the surface of hydroxyapatite crystals and inhibits resorption. These drugs are not metabolized and are excreted intact in urine. Their t 1/2 is 1–10 years and **cessation of treatment does not lead to rapid bone loss** (as occurs with estrogen replacement therapy). These drugs decrease the incidence of vertebral and non vertebral fractures.
- 1st generation drugs etidronate inhibit both bone resorption and formation, so it is approved for Paget's disease and hyper calcemia (but not osteoporosis).
- 2nd and 3rd generation drugs such as alendronate and risedronate inhibit bone resorption at rates 1000 times greater than their effect on bone formation. So, these are used in postmenopausal osteoporosis and treatment of steroid induced osteoporosis.

Note: Risedronate is used for prevention of steroid induced osteoporosis.

- Risedronate, and alendronate are approved for treatment of osteoporosis in men.
- Zoledronate (yearly) and Ibandronate (monthly) are also used
  Prolonged used of Bisphosphonates has been reported with increased incidence of fractures of proximal femur. Hence a patient on Bisphosphonates with hip pain requires X-rays to evaluate and diagnose these fractures.
- Calcitonin is approved for Paget's disease, hypercalcemia, and osteoporosis in women > 5 years past menopause. **Calcitonin is not indicated for prevention of osteoporosis** and is not sufficiently potent to prevent bone loss in early post-menopausal women. Calcitonin 200 IU daily as nasal spray has an analgesic effect also.

Recent Drugs for Osteoporosis

A. Daily low dosing of PTH (Parathyroid hormone) and PTHrP in low doses stimulate osteoblast. PTH (mild elevation) are associated with, maintenance of trabecular bone mass. So, PTH is approved for treatment of patients with osteoporosis (both men and women) at high-risk of fracture (usually in combination with estrogen as single daily injection to maximum 2 years).

B. Sodium fluoride is mitogenic for osteoblasts. Low dose with calcium produced gain in bone density. Higher doses cause production of abnormal unmineralized bone with decreased bending strength (fluorosis.)

C. RANKL-Inhibitor: RANKL (receptor activator of nuclear factor - KB ligand) a protein expressed by osteoblastic stromal cells, binds to RANK (receptor activator of nuclear factor KB) and is primary mediator of osteoclast differentiation, activation and survival. So RANKL is responsible for osteoclast mediated bone resorption. Osteoprotegerin, a soluble RANKL receptor, is a key regulator of RANKL-RANK pathway of osteoclastic resorption.

D. Denosumab is a fully human monoclonal antibody (Ig C2) that binds RANKL (mimicking osteoprotegerin) and blocks interaction of RANKL with RANK and it inhibits osteoclast function.

E. Estrogen suppress pathway through which RANKL and M—CSF (macrophage colony stimulating factor) induce monocyte precursors to develop into osteoclasts.

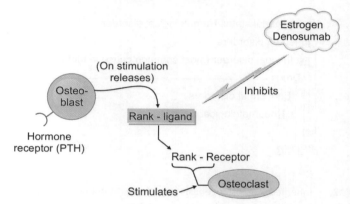

Fig. 17.14: RANK-RANK-Ligand

Note: Bisphosphonates are drug of choice for osteoporosis.

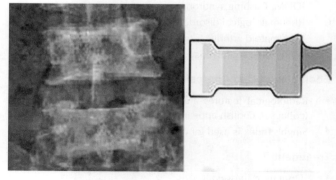

Fig. 17.15: H-shaped vertebra

H-shaped vertebra (also known as Lincoln long vertebra = sharply delimited central end plate depression which is classically seen in patients of sickle-cell anaemia (~10% cases) and results from microvascular end plate infraction)

MULTIPLE CHOICE QUESTIONS

1. A 75-year-female has chronic backache. X-ray spine is shown. What is the most likely diagnosis:
   (NEET Pattern 2019)

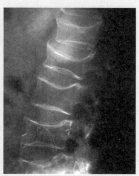

   A. Pott's spine B. Osteoporosis
   C. Spondylolisthesis D. Spondylodiscitis
   Ans. is 'B' Osteoporosis

2. A 70-year-old lady got compression fracture of L1 vertebra. There is no neurological deficit to this patient. What advise will you give for this patient?
   A. Vitamin D supplementation (PGI MAY 2016)
   B. Do MRI scan
   C. Go for screw fixation of L1 vertebra
   D. To take Dexamethasone E. To take Alendronate
   Ans. is 'A' Vitamin D supplementation; 'E' To take Alendronate
   • MRI is indicated in osteoporotic collapse in case of neural deficit. Decompression and fixation is done for unstable spine and compromised spinal canal. Steroids are given in spinal 2injuries to reduce edema associated with the trauma.

3. Osteoporosis is seen in all the following except:
   (NEET DEC 2016)
   A. Hyperprolactinemia B. Thalassemia
   C. Homocystinuria D. Systemic sclerosis
   Ans. is 'D' Systemic sclerosis

4. Drugs decreasing bone resorption in osteoporosis are all except:
   A. Raloxifene B. Teriparatide
   C. Strontium D. Risedronate
   Ans. is 'B' Teriparatide

5. Which bisphosphonate is approved for the treatment of osteoporosis and is given on yearly basis? (AI 2016)
   A. Alendronate B. Zoledronate
   C. Risedronate D. Ibandronate
   Ans. is 'B' Zoledronate

6. All the following are used in osteoporosis except:
   A. Denosumab B. Strontium (AIIMS Nov 16)
   C. PTH D. Milnacipran
   Ans. is 'D' Milnacipran
   This drug is used for fibromyalgia

7. A 70-year-old female present to OPD after a trivial trauma, MRI shows L1 collapse. Next best management is:
   A. Vitamin D therapy B. CT (PGI May 2016)
   C. Bisphosphonates D. Screw fixation
   E. Aggressive physiotherapy
   Ans. is 'A' Vitamin D therapy and 'C' Bisphosphonates

8. A 60-years-female with long term steroid intake, presents with backache X-ray spine done as shown below, next investigation to be done is: (AI 2016)

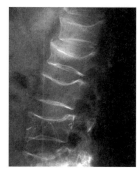

   A. DEXA B. PTH
   C. Calcium D. Calcitrol
   Ans. is 'A' DEXA

9. In Osteoporosis which of these is seen? (AIIMS May 2015)
   A. Normal calcium, decreased ALP
   B. Decreased calcium, increased ALP
   C. Normal calcium, normal ALP
   D. Decreased calcium, decreased ALP
   Ans. is 'C' Normal calcium, normal ALP

10. Most common site for the osteoporotic vertebral fracture is: (NEET 2016, 2015)
    A. Dorsolumbar spine B. Cervical spine
    C. Lumbosacral spine D. Dorsal spine
    Ans. is 'A' Dorsolumbar spine

11. Z score measures the bone mineral density compared to:
    A. Age, race and sex matched individuals (NEET 2015)
    B. Race and sex matched individuals
    C. Sex matched individuals
    D. None of the above
    Ans. is 'A' Age, race and sex matched individuals

12. Osteoporosis is characterized by all the following except:
    A. Decreased bone mineral density (NEET 2015)
    B. Decreased serum calcium, phosphorus and alkaline phosphatase is seen
    C. Glucocorticoids can cause osteoporosis
    D. Dorsolumbar spine is the most common site of osteoporotic fracture
    Ans. is 'B' Decreased serum calcium, phosphorus and alkaline phosphatase is seen

13. The bodies of spine are biconcave and are called "codfish spine" most commonly seen in: (Maharashtra PG 2016)
    A. Scurvy B. Osteomalacia
    C. Fluorosis D. Hyperparathyroidism
    Ans. is 'B' Osteomalacia

    Explanations
    Codfish Vertebra is seen in
    1. Osteoporosis > Osteomalacia
    2. Sickle cell disease
    3. Hereditary spherocytosis
    4. Homocystinuria
    5. Renal osteodystrophy
    6. Osteogenesis imperfecta
    7. Gaucher's disease

14. Hemiplegic patient maximum loss of bone mineral density is seen in: *(AIIMS Nov 2014)*
    A. Vertebra
    B. Femur neck
    C. Radius
    D. Humerus
    Ans. is 'D' Humerus

15. Osteoporosis which of the following is false? *(AIIMS Nov 2013)*
    A. Osteoporosis is defined, if T score is less than –1.5
    B. Severe osteoporosis PTH is used for treatment
    C. Calcitonin decreases the bone pain
    D. Bisphosphonates are cornerstone of treatment
    Ans. is 'A' Osteoporosis is defined, if T score is less than –1.5

16. Osteoporotic female on prolonged bisphosphonates has hip pain next investigation is: *(AIIMS May 2013; 2012, NEET 2012)*
    A. X-rays
    B. Vitamin D
    C. ALP
    D. Dexa
    Ans. is 'A' X-rays

17. Osteoporosis is caused by all except: *(NEET Pattern 2013)*
    A. Fluorosis
    B. Hypogonadism
    C. Hyperthyroidism
    D. Hyperparathyroidism
    Ans. is 'A' Fluorosis

18. Gold standard for diagnosis of osteoporosis: *(NEET Pattern 2013)*
    A. DEXA
    B. Single beam densitometry
    C. Quantitative computed tomography
    D. Bone histomorphometry
    Ans. is 'A' DEXA

19. Most common cause of kyphotic deformity: *(NEET Pattern 2013)*
    A. Trauma
    B. Osteoporosis
    C. Ankylosing spondylitis
    D. Rickets
    Ans. is 'B' Osteoporosis

20. Most common site of osteoporosis: *(NEET Pattern 2012)*
    A. Humerus
    B. Vertebrae
    C. Scapula
    D. Flat bones
    Ans. is 'B' Vertebrae

21. Decreased osteoid content is a feature of: *(NEET Pattern 2012)*
    A. Osteoporosis
    B. Osteopetrosis
    C. Osteomalacia
    D. Paget's disease
    Ans. is 'A' Osteoporosis

22. MC fracture in post-menopausal women: *(NEET Pattern 2012)*
    A. Spine
    B. Hip
    C. Radius
    D. Tibia
    Ans. is 'A' Spine

23. Osteoporosis treatment in 60 years female is: *(NEET Pattern 2012)*
    A. Estrogen
    B. Tamoxifen
    C. Alendronate
    D. Calcitonin
    Ans. is 'C' Alendronate

24. Steroids have the following effect on bone: *(NEET Pattern 2012)*
    A. Osteomalacia
    B. Osteoporosis
    C. Calcific deposits
    D. Myositis ossificans
    Ans. is 'B' Osteoporosis

25. Which of the following is used in osteoporosis for decreasing bone resorption and increasing bone formation? *(AIPG 2009)*
    A. Teriparatide
    B. Calcitonin
    C. Strontium ranelate
    D. Bisphosphonate
    Ans. is 'C' Strontium ranelate

26. Osteoporosis is seen in: *(PGI Dec 07, AI 1994)*
    A. Thyrotoxicosis
    B. Cushing's disease
    C. Menopause
    D. All of the above
    Ans. is 'D' All of the above

27. Treatment of postmenopausal osteoporosis: *(PGI June 2006)*
    A. Tamoxifen
    B. Progesterone
    C. Estrogen
    D. Alendronate
    E. Calcitonin
    Ans. is 'C' Estrogen; 'D' Alendronate; 'E' Calcitonin

28. Denosumab—a monoclonal antibody against RANKL receptor is used in treatment of: *(AIIMS Nov 06)*
    A. Rheumatoid arthritis
    B. Osteoporosis
    C. Osteoarthritis
    D. SLE
    Ans. is 'B' Osteoporosis

29. Osteoporosis is characterized by: *(PGI June 05)*
    A. Increased serum alkaline phosphatase
    B. Decreased bone density
    C. Wasting of muscles
    D. Looser's zone seen
    E. Decreased serum calcium
    Ans. is 'B' Decreased bone density

30. Treatment of postmenopausal osteoporosis: *(PGI Dec 04, KA 92)*
    A. Calcitonin
    B. Alendronate
    C. Progesterone
    D. Tamoxifen
    E. Androgen
    Ans. is 'A' Calcitonin; 'B' Alendronate
    – Calcitonin and alendronate are used in osteoporosis.

31. Which of the following is seen in osteoporosis? *(AIIMS June 2K)*
    A. Low Ca, high PO_4, high alkaline phosphatase
    B. Low Ca, low PO_4, low alkaline phosphatase
    C. Normal Ca, normal PO_4, normal alkaline phosphatase
    D. Low Ca, low PO_4, normal alkaline phosphatase
    Ans. is 'C' Normal Ca, normal PO_4, normal alkaline phosphatase
    – Serum calcium, phosphate and alkaline phosphatase are normal in osteoporosis.

32. The most common manifestation of osteoporosis is: *(AI 1999, 94)*
    A. Compression fracture of the spine
    B. Asymptomatic, detected incidentally by low serum calcium
    C. Bowing of legs
    D. Loss of weight
    Ans. is 'A' Compression fracture of the spine
    Remember most common presentation is asymptomatic (Calcium is normal).

FLUOROSIS

- Fluorine in very low concentration **1 part per million (ppm) or less is used to reduce the incidence of dental caries.**
- At slightly higher levels (2–4 ppm) it may produce mottling of teeth.

- In some parts of India and Africa, where fluorine concentration in the drinking water maybe **above 10 ppm—chronic fluorine intoxication (fluorosis)** is endemic and results in skeletal anomalies.
- **Fluorine stimulates osteoblastic activity;** fluorapatite crystals are laid down in bone and these are usually resistant to osteoclastic resorption. This leads to calcium retention and secondary hyperparathyroidism.
- Characteristic pathological feature is **subperiosteal new bone accretion** and osteosclerosis (increased bone density) most marked in vertebrae, ribs, pelvis, forearm and leg bones, together with **hyperostosis at the bony attachments of ligaments, tendons and fascia.**
- Despite the apparent thickening and density of skeleton, tensile strength is reduced and the bones fracture more easily. First clinical manifestation is usually a stress fracture, back pain, bone pain, joint stiffness and neurological defects (due to hyperostosis encroaching on vertebral canal).
- Characteristic X-ray features are osteosclerosis, osteophytosis and ossification of ligamentous and fascial attachments.
- Radiologically can be mistaken for other osteosclerotic conditions as Paget's disease, osteopetrosis, renal osteodystrophy, idiopathic skeletal hyperostosis, etc.

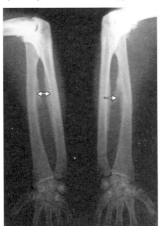

Fig. 17.16: Ossification of interosseous membrane in fluorosis

MULTIPLE CHOICE QUESTIONS

1. Increase bone density with hyperostosis seen in skeletal fluorosis is likely to occur when fluorine concentration in drinking H₂O is above: *(AI 2016)*
   A. 6 ppm
   B. 10 ppm
   C. 15 ppm
   D. 20 ppm
   Ans. is 'B' 10 ppm

2. Increased bone density occurs in:
   A. Cushing syndrome
   B. Hypoparathyroidism
   C. Fluorosis
   D. Hyperthyroidism
   Ans. is 'C' Fluorosis

3. What is the diagnostic radiological finding in skeletal fluorosis? *(JIPMER 2000, 98)*
   A. Sclerosis of sacroiliac joint
   B. Interosseous membrane ossification
   C. Osteosclerosis of vertebral body
   D. Ossification of ligaments of knee joint
   Ans. is 'B' Interosseous membrane ossification

   – Osteosclerosis, osteophytosis and ossification of ligamentous and fascial attachments is characteristic of fluorosis and amongst them most important is Interosseous membrane ossification.

4. Increased density in skull vault is seen in: *(PGI 90) (UP 88)*
   A. Hyperparathyroidism
   B. Multiple myeloma
   C. Fluorosis
   D. Renal osteodystrophy
   Ans. is 'C' Fluorosis

5. Manifestations of fluorosis include: *(PGI 90)*
   A. Stiffness of back ligaments
   B. Caries teeth
   C. Genu valgum
   D. Dental changes
   E. Stiffness of bones and tendons
   Ans. is 'A' Stiffness of back ligaments; 'D' Dental changes
   – Fluorosis causes mottling of teeth.

CAFFEY'S DISEASE

Infantile cortical hyperostosis (Caffey's disease) is a self-limiting disorder characterized by soft tissue swelling, rapid subperiosteal new bone formation, **cortical thickening of underlying bones,** fever and irritability. Classically, the onset of disease occurs before 6th month of life with resolution by 3 years of age.

- In sporadic cases, mandible is the most common site of involvement presenting as jaw tumor or swelling, i.e. is firm, tender without heat or redness. Presence of raised ESR and alkaline phosphatase and anemia mimic infection.
- In familial form Tibia > ulna are most frequently involved.
- **Hands and feet are spared. In the long bones the epiphyses and metaphyses are spared.**
- **Increased density of bones is due to massive periosteal new bone.**

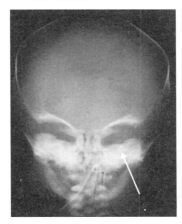 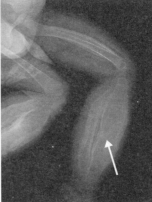

Fig. 17.17: Hyperostosis

- Treatment is Penicillin G.

MULTIPLE CHOICE QUESTIONS

1. Caffey's disease is: *(UP 2003)*
   A. Renal osteodystrophy
   B. Infantile cortical hyperostosis
   C. Osteomyelitis of jaw in children
   D. Chronic osteomyelitis in children
   Ans. is 'B' Infantile cortical hyperostosis
   – Caffey's disease is also called as infantile cortical hyperostosis.

2. **Caffey's disease occurs in:** *(NIMS 96)*
   A. Infants below 6 months   B. Above 5 years
   C. Above 10–20 years   D. 20–40 years

Ans. is 'A' Infants below 6 months
   – Age group affected is usually < 6 months and resolves by 3 years

3. **Jaw swelling is seen in:** *(AIIMS 1992)*
   A. Osteoporosis   B. Osteomalacia
   C. Osteopetrosis   D. Caffey's disease

Ans. is 'D' Caffey's disease

HYPERVITAMINOSIS—BONY ABNORMALITIES

1,25 (OH) Vit D has an antiproliferative effect on several cell types, including keratinocytes, breast cancer cells, and prostate cancer cells. Alopecia is seen in Vit D hypervitaminosis and VDRR (Vit D receptor mutation). It exerts a PTH like effect and so, as in underlying rickets, calcium is withdrawn from bones but metastatic calcification occurs.

Chronic hypervitaminosis A - >1 year of age, clinical features are failure to thrive, hepatosplenomegaly, jaundice, **alopecia** and hemoptysis. **Cortical thickening of long and tubular bones, especially in the feet.**

MULTIPLE CHOICE QUESTIONS

1. **A bald child with swollen abdomen, hyperosseous bones has:** *(NEET Pattern 2012, KA 98)*
   A. Hypervitaminosis C   B. Hypervitaminosis D
   C. Down's syndrome   D. Tuberous sclerosis

Ans. is 'B' Hypervitaminosis D

2. **Hypervitaminosis of which of the following will cause bony abnormalities?** *(PGI June 09, 01, Dec 2006)*
   A. Vit. A   B. Vit. D
   C. Vit. C   D. Vit. E
   E. Vit. K

Ans. is 'A' Vit. A; and 'B' Vit. D

PAGET'S DISEASE/OSTEITIS DEFORMANS

It is characterized by **excessive disorganized bone turnover,** that encompasses excessive osteoclastic activity initially followed by disorganized excessive new bone formation. It is the **osteoclast that appears larger and irregular** whereas **osteoblast are relatively normal.**

- The new bone formed is abnormal, very vascular and larger (deforms and fractures) than preexisting bone which leads to cortical widening and contributes to the deformity.

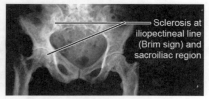

Fig. 17.18: X-ray pelvis: Paget's disease

- The diagnostic histological feature of Paget's disease is irregular area of lamellar bone fitting together like a jigsaw with randomly distributed cement lines.
- It either occurs in one bone (monostotic Paget's disease) or multiple bones (polyostotic Paget's disease).

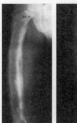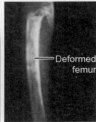

Fig. 17.19: X-ray femur Paget's disease

Etiology

- Genetic infection by paramyxovirus (measles and respiratory syncytial virus) has been linked.
- *Pathophysiology:* Increased bone resorption accompanied by accelerated bone formation is characteristic feature.
- Initial osteolytic phase involves prominent bone resorption and marked hypervascularization (Radiologically seen as advancing lytic wedge or **blade of grass lesion)** 2nd phase of active bone formation and resorption replaces normal lamellar bone with structurally weak woven bone that bend, bow and fracture easily.
- In 3rd sclerotic (burnt out) phase, bone resorption declines progressively and leads to hard, dense, less vascular pagetic or **mosaic bone.**

Clinical Features

- **Most people are asymptomatic**
- The sites most commonly involved are—**pelvis**, tibia, followed by skull, spine, clavicle and femur
- **Affects men more commonly**
- Affects **> 50 years** incidence increases with age.
- **Pain is most common presenting symptom**
- Limb looks bent and feels thick, and skin is unduly warm due to high vascularity hence the name **osteitis deformans**. Skull show frontal bossing and platybasia.

Complications

1. Pagetoid bone lacks the strength of normal bone. As a result it deforms and **fractures** more easily.
2. Cranial nerve ~ 2nd, 5th, **7th**, 8th palsy is seen.
3. Nerve compression and spinal stenosis is seen.
4. *Deafness due to nerve compression > otosclerosis*
5. High output cardiac failure, **hypercalcemia** (if immobilized).
6. **Osteosarcoma** (< 1% cases and has poorest prognosis), other malignancies arising but with lesser frequency are benign GCT or chondrosarcoma.
7. **Steal syndrome**, i.e. blood is diverted from internal organs to skeleton system, may lead to cerebral ischemia and spinal claudication.
8. Osteoarthritis of hip and knee is common.

Diagnosis

A. Serum calcium and phosphate levels are usually normal.
B. Increased marker of bone formation (e.g. S. alkaline phosphatase and S. osteocalcin) **(ALP levels are used for monitoring Paget's).**
C. Increased markers of bone resorption

Serum and urinary deoxypyridinoline, N-telopeptide and C-telopeptide:
- Urinary hydroxyproline
- Urinary deoxypyridinoline (24 hours assessment) is most valuable.

Radiological Features

- Long bone X-ray shows deformity, enlargement or expansion of bone with cortical thickening coarsening of trabecular markings and lytic and sclerotic changes.
- Blade of grass lesion is seen

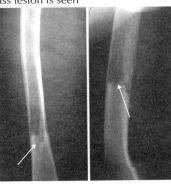

Fig. 17.20: Blade of grass

- Skull X-ray reveal "cotton wool" or osteoporosis circumscripta, thickening of diploic area. **Increasing Hat Size!**

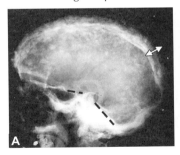 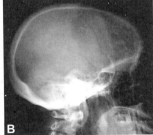

Figs. 17.21A and B: (A) Paget's disease cotton wool skull; (B) Osteoporosis circumscripta

- Vertebral cortical thickening at superior and inferior end plates creates a picture frame vertebrae and diffuse sclerosis causing ivory vertebrae.

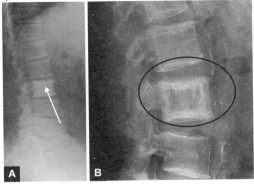

Figs. 17.22A and B: (A) Ivory vertebra and (B) Picture frame vertebra

- Pelvic radiograph shows sclerotic iliopectineal line (Brim sign), fusion or disruption of sacroiliac joints, etc.

Treatment

Indications are:
A. To control symptoms of active disease as bone pain, fracture, neurological complications or pain from radiculopathy or arthropathy.
B. To decrease local blood flow and minimize operative blood loss in patients undergoing surgery.
C. To decrease hypercalciuria.
D. To decrease complications—When site of involvement involves weight bearing bones, skull, vertebral bodies and major joints.
E. **Bisphosphonates are drug of choice** and **calcitonin is used to relieve pain.**
F. Surgery is done for pathological fracture, osteoarthritis, nerve entrapment and spine decompression.

MULTIPLE CHOICE QUESTIONS

1. Ivory Vertebra is seen in: *(PGI Nov 2018)*
   A. Pagets
   B. Osteporosis
   C. Osteopetrosis
   D. Osteomalaia
   E. Hyper PTH
Ans. is 'A' Pagets

Ivory vertebra causes are:

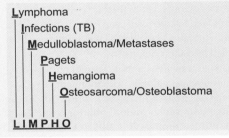

2. Osteosclerosis is a feature of which of the following? *(AI Dec 15)*
   A. Rickets
   B. Hyperparathyroidism
   C. Paget's disease
   D. Osteogenesis imperfecta
Ans. is 'C' Paget's disease

3. All of the following are true regarding Paget's disease except: *(AI Dec 15)*
   A. Pelvis is the most common site
   B. Cranial nerve involvement may be seen
   C. High output cardiac failure is one of the complications
   D. It may progress to a secondary chondrosarcoma
Ans. is 'D' It may progress to a secondary chondrosarcoma

4. Paget's disease commonly develops in which age group?
   A. 1st decade
   B. 3rd decade *(NEET 2015)*
   C. 5th decade
   D. 7th decade
Ans. is 'D' 7th decade

5. Blades of grass lesion is found in: *(APPG 2015)*
   A. Paget's disease
   B. Thalassemia
   C. Osteoporosis
   D. Carcinoma prostate
Ans. is 'A' Paget's disease

6. Picture frame vertebra is seen in: *(NEET Pattern 2013)*
   A. Paget's disease
   B. Osteopetrosis
   C. Osteoporosis
   D. Ankylosing spondylitis
Ans. is 'A' Paget's disease

7. Increased alkaline phosphatase is seen in:
   (NEET Pattern 2013)
   A. Osteoporosis
   B. Multiple myeloma
   C. Paget's disease
   D. Osteolytic metastasis
   Ans. is 'C' Paget's disease

8. All are features of Paget's disease except:
   (NEET Pattern 2013)
   A. Defect in osteoclasts
   B. Common in female
   C. Can cause deafness
   D. Can cause osteosarcoma
   Ans. is 'B' Common in female

9. Paget's disease after 10 years develops into:
   (NEET Pattern 2012)
   A. Osteosarcoma
   B. Fibrous cortical defect
   C. Osteoid osteoma
   D. Ankylosing spondylitis
   Ans. is 'A' Osteosarcoma

10. Pain in Paget's disease is relieved best by:
    (NEET Pattern 2012)
    A. Simple analgesics
    B. Narcotic analgesics
    C. Radiation
    D. Calcitonin
    Ans. is 'D' Calcitonin

11. All of the following statements regarding Paget's disease are correct except: (PGI Nov 2009, Manipal 97, Bihar 90)
    A. Females are affected more than males
    B. It can lead to osteogenic sarcoma
    C. Serum alkaline phosphates level is increased
    D. Called as osteitis deformans
    Ans. is 'A' Females are affected more than males
    – Males are affected more commonly in Paget's.

12. A 60-year-old male with bony abnormality at upper tibia associated with sensorineural hearing loss. On laboratory examination serum alkaline phosphatase levels are (440 mU/l) elevated and serum Ca^{++} and PO_4 are normal. Skeletal survey shows ivory vertebrae and cotton wool spots in X-ray skull. Diagnosis is: (AIIMS May 07)
    A. Fibrous dysplasia
    B. Paget's disease
    C. Osteosclerotic metastasis
    D. Osteoporosis
    Ans. is 'B' Paget's disease

13. Paget's disease of bone commonly affects:
    (PGI Dec 06, Dec 2K, June 01)
    A. Skull
    B. Vertebra
    C. Pelvis
    D. Femur
    E. Humerus
    Ans. is 'A' Skull; 'B' Vertebra; 'C' Pelvis; 'D' Femur
    – The pelvis and tibia being the commonest sites, and femur, skull, spine (vertebrae) and clavicle the next commonest.

14. Treatment of choice for Paget's disease of the bone is:
    (KA 2001, Manipal 97, AI 1995, AIIMS 91, 86)
    A. Vitamin D
    B. Immobilization of the limb
    C. Surgical treatment
    D. Calcitonin
    Ans. is 'D' Calcitonin
    – Bisphosphonates are drug of choice 2nd best is calcitonin

15. Which of the following is a primary defect in Paget's disease? (NB 2K)
    A. Osteoblast
    B. Osteoclast
    C. Osteocyte
    D. Fibroblast
    Ans. is 'B' Osteoclast

16. A 67-year-old man on biochemical analysis found to have three fold rise of level of serum alkaline phosphatase that of upper limit of normal value during a routine checkup but serum calcium and phosphorous concentration and liver function test results are normal. He is asymptomatic. The probable cause is:
    (AIIMS 1999, Andhra 91, KA 96, Kerala 90)
    A. Multiple myeloma
    B. Paget's disease of bone
    C. Primary hyperparathyroidism
    D. Osteomalacia
    Ans. is 'B' Paget's disease of bone
    – Paget's disease can have asymptomatic presentation with high ALP, normal calcium and phosphate.
    – Multiple myeloma will have normal ALP.
    – Osteomalacia and hyperparathyroidism will have abnormality in calcium and phosphorus levels

17. Deafness in cases of Paget's disease is due to:
    A. Thickened cranium (DNB 89, PGI 81)
    B. Narrowing of foramina of skull
    C. Brain compression
    D. Otosclerosis
    Ans. is 'B' Narrowing of foramina of skull
    – Sensorineural hearing loss > otosclerosis

18. The histopathologic feature of Paget's disease includes:
    A. Simultaneous osteoblastic activity at places (Bihar 89)
    B. Osteoclastic resorption
    C. Replacement of bone marrow by fibrovascular tissue
    D. All of the above
    Ans. is 'D' All of the above

ACHONDROPLASIA

A primary **defect of endochondral bone formation**. Autosomal dominant (but 80% are spontaneous mutations). The effect of excessive growth hormone on the mature skeleton.

Genetics and Pathophysiology

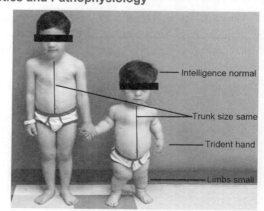

Fig. 17.23: Achondroplasia

- Inherited as autosomal dominant trait; however because few achondroplastic people have children, **80–90% of cases are sporadic** as a result of spontaneous point mutation in the gene coding for fibroblast growth factor receptor 3 **(FGFR-3)**, which apparently play role in endochondral cartilage growth to regulate linear growth. Glycine to arginine substitution (point

mutation) in FGFR-3 gene on chromosome 4p is most mutable single nucleotide in human genome.
- **Paternal age >36 year is linked with new mutation.**
- Endochondral ossification responsible for longitudinal growth is abnormal resulting in short bones.
- Intramembranous ossification are undisturbed causing normal clavicles and skull vault.

Clinical Features

- **It is most common form of disproportionate dwarfism.**
- Disproportionate rhizomelic micromelia, i.e. short stature which is most severe in proximal limbs. Trunk height tends to be normal, but arm span and standing height are diminished. This is apparent at birth and can be documented on fetal ultrasound by measuring femoral length.
- Ultimate height is about 4 feet 4 inches (131 cm) for males and 4 feet 1 inch (124 cm) for females; with midpoint of stature shifted up to inferior end of sternum (normally at umbilicus)
- Skull is large with prominent forehead (frontal bossing), saddle shaped nose (flat and depressed nasal bridge), small maxilla, prominent mandibles and normal dentition.

Usually have normal intelligence

- Hands are short and broad. The middle finger is shorter than usual resulting in all of the digits being of equal length **(Starfish hand).**
- There is separation between middle and ring fingers, described as **trident hand or main en trident.**

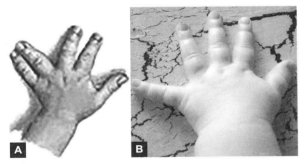

Figs. 17.24A and B: (A) Trident hand; (B) Star fish hand

Radiological Features

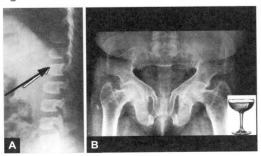

Figs. 17.25A and B: (A) Bullet shaped vertebra; (B) Champagne glass pelvis (width > depth)

- Tubular long bones are short with an **apparent increase in bony diameter and density.**
- Because the width of pelvis is greater than its depth it takes on an appearance of **champagne glass.**
- Posterior vertebral bodies in lumbar spine may be scalloped. **The pedicles are short and broad, vertebra are flat and have beak.**

MULTIPLE CHOICE QUESTIONS

1. True regarding achondroplasia is? (PGI MAY 2018)
   A. Autosomal recessive
   B. Disproportionate dwarfism
   C. Subnormal intelligence
   D. Bullet shaped vertebral bodies on radiology
   E. Abnormal sexual development
   Ans. is 'B' Disproportionate dwarfism & 'D' Bullet shaped vertebral bodies on radiology

2. Hooked vertebrae seen in: (NEET Dec 2016)
   A. Achondroplasia
   B. Osteogenesis imperfecta
   C. Congenital hypothyroid
   D. All of the above
   Ans. is 'D' All of the above

3. The characteristic mutation seen in Achondroplasia (AI 2016)
   A. Fibrillin -1
   B. FGFR-3
   C. NOTCH 1 gene
   D. COL5A1 gene
   Ans. is 'B' FGFR-3

4. The following is false about Achondroplasia: (UP 02, JIPMER 91)
   A. Autosomal dominant
   B. Mental retardation
   C. Due to gene mutation
   D. Shortening of limbs present
   Ans. is 'B' Mental retardation

5. A short statured patient brought to Orthopedics OPD with a X-ray showing flattened vertebra with beak. The probable diagnosis is: (NIMS 2K)
   A. Achondroplasia
   B. Ochronosis
   C. Eosinophilic granuloma
   D. Calve's disease
   Ans. is 'A' Achondroplasia

6. "Trident hand" seen in: (AIIMS Dec 1998)
   A. Achondroplasia
   B. Mucopolysac charidosis
   C. Diaphyseal achalasia
   D. Cleidocranial dysostosis
   Ans. is 'A' Achondroplasia

CLEIDOCRANIAL DYSOSTOSIS

It is an **autosomal dominant** (AD) disorder caused by CBFA1 gene on chromosome 6p21 responsible for osteoblast specific transcription factor and regulation of osteoblastic differentiation. In this disorder bones formed by intramembranous ossification are abnormal **(primarily clavicles, cranium and pelvis).**

Clinical and Radiological Features are:

- Skull Involvement Elfin faces, i.e. skull is wider than normal but the face appears small and flat looking (hypoplastic bones). Wider Foramen magnum is seen.
- The eyes are slightly wide set. Deciduous teeth erupt normally, but permanent teeth are delayed and maldeveloped.
- Clavicles maybe underdeveloped or absent. The most common defect is loss of lateral 1/3rd > loss of middle third of clavicle. Due to absence of clavicle shoulders look droopy and chest appears narrow. **When it is bilateral clavicle hypoplasia, child can touch the shoulders together in front of the chest.**

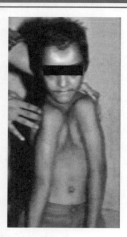

Fig. 17.26: Cleidocranial dysostosis

- Pelvis symphysis pubis remains quite wide.
- Pubic rami and iliac wings are small and thin. Rami are also incompletely fused.

Limbs

- Coxa vara is seen
- **2nd metacarpal is usually long**
- Mild dwarfism (short stature).

MULTIPLE CHOICE QUESTIONS

1. Absent lateral 1/3rd of clavicle is seen in:
   (PGI Dec 2002, AIIMS 1990)
   A. Hyperparathyroidism B. Turner's syndrome
   C. Fibrous dysplasia   D. Cleidocranial dysostosis
   Ans. is 'D' Cleidocranial dysostosis

2. A 9-year-old child with high arched palate has shoulders meeting in front of his chest. He has: (ESI 1989)
   A. Erb's palsy   B. Cleidocranial dysostosis
   C. Chondro-osteodystrophy D. Cortical hyperostosis
   Ans. is 'B' Cleidocranial dysostosis

3. Cleidocranial dysostosis may show: (AMU 87, PGI 81)
   A. Wide foramen magnum B. Absence of clavicles
   C. Coxa vara   D. All of the above
   Ans. is 'D' All of the above

OSTEOGENESIS IMPERFECTA

- Osteogenesis Imperfecta/Lobstein Vrolik's/Brittle Bone Disease.
- It is a genetic disorder of connective tissue determined by **quantitative qualitative defect in type I collagen formation.** So there is alteration in the structural integrity, or a reduction in the total amount of type I collagen, one of the major components of fibrillar connective tissue in skin, ligaments, bones, sclera, and teeth.
- It is inherited from a parent in **autosomal dominant (AD)** fashion, may occur as spontaneous mutation, or, rarely as autosomal recessive (AR) trait.
- The defining clinical features are osteopenia causing repeated propensity to fracture, generally after minor trauma and often without much pain or swelling.
- **Any fracture pattern maybe seen, and no particular fracture pattern is specifically diagnostic. Fractures heal at a normal rate.**

- According to the severity of disease fractures may occur in uterus, at birth, or after birth prior to or after walking age.
- **Lower limb fractures are more common than upper limb. Femur is commonest bone fractured followed by tibia.**
- Frequency of fractures decline sharply after adolescence or puberty, although it may rise again in postmenopausal (climacteric) women.
- Hyperlaxity of ligaments, with resultant hypermobility of joint is common.
- **Rarely recurrent dislocation of patella, radial head and hip joint dislocation and DDH can occur.**

Radiological Feature

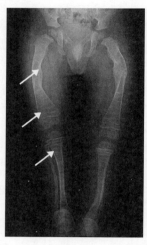

Fig. 17.27: Osteogenesis imperfecta deformed bones with fractures in different areas in different stages of healing

- Wormian bones, are detached portions of primary ossification centers of adjacent membrane bones. These are seen in skull X-ray. To be significant, it should be more than 10 in number, measure at least 6 mm 4 mm, and be arranged in general mosaic pattern.
- Wormian bones are present in osteogenesis imperfecta, other bone dysplasias such as cleidocranial dysplasia, congenital hypothyroidism, and some trisomies.
- Ring shaped epiphysis is seen

Causes of wormian bones
Pyknodysostosis
Osteogenesis imperfecta
Rickets
Kinky Hair Menke's syndrome
Cleidocranial disorder
Hypothyroidism/hypophosphatasia
Otopalatodigital syndrome
Primary Acroosteolysis
Syndrome of Down's
PORKCHOPS

Ocular Involvement

- "Blue or gray sclerae", is because of **uveal pigment showing through thin collagen layer.**

- **Saturn's ring is white sclera** immediately surrounding the cornea.
- Arcus juvenilis or embryotoxon, is opacity in periphery of cornea.
- Hyperopia and retinal detachment may occur.

Auditory Involvement
Deafness, usually onsetting in adolescence or adulthood maybe either of the conductive type due to otosclerosis or of nerve type, caused by pressure on the auditory nerve as it emerges from the skull.

Dentinogenes Imperfecta/Crumbling of Teeth: Dentine affected
- The enamel is essentially normal, as it is of ectodermal origin, not mesenchymal.
- Both deciduous and permanent teeth are involved. They break easily and are prone to carries. Yellowish brown or bluish gray discoloration of teeth is common.
- The lower incisors, which erupt first are more severely affected.

Skin and Muscle Involvement
- Skin is thin and translucent. Subcutaneous hemorrhages may occur.
- Muscles are hypotonic mostly due to multiple fractures and deformities. Hernias may occur.

Metabolic Features
- Excessive sweating, heat intolerance are due to hypermetabolic state.
- Susceptible to malignant hyperthermia during general anesthesia.

Diagnosis of Osteogenesis Imperfecta
- A molecular defect in type I procollagen can be detected in 2/3 of patients by incubating skin fibroblasts with radioactive amino acids and then analyzing the pro-al(I) chains by polyacrylamide gel electrophoresis.
- Sillence classification: Type I to IV.

Treatment
- Bisphosphonates (Decrease osteoclastic bone resorption): One of the few indications of bisphosphonates growing age.
- Ideal treatment replace COLIAI or COLIA2 gene.

MULTIPLE CHOICE QUESTIONS

1. Osteogenesis imperfecta, true is: *(AI 2016)*
   A. Marble bone disease is another name of it
   B. Hyperlaxity of ligaments with hypermobile joints
   C. Cranial nerve compression may occur
   D. Treatment involves bone marrow transplantation
   Ans. is 'B' Hyperlaxity of ligaments with hypermobile joints

2. Which of the below is a feature of osteogenesis imperfecta? *(CET July 16)*
   A. Blue sclera   B. Cataract
   C. Anterior uveitis D. Retinal detachment
   Ans. is 'A' Blue sclera

3. Osteogenesis imperfecta has abnormality in which type of collagen? *(CET July 16)*
   A. Collagen 3   B. Collagen 2
   C. Collagen 4   D. Collagen 1
   Ans. is 'D' Collagen 1

4. A child presented with hip pain: *(AIIMS Nov 16)*

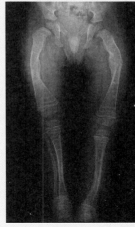

   A. Osteogenesis imperfecta   B. Osteoporosis
   C. Osteopetrosis   D. Osteopoikilocytosis
   Ans. is 'A' Osteogenesis imperfecta *(Refer to Fig. 17.27)*

5. Ring shaped epiphyses is seen in: *(NEET 2015)*
   A. Osteogenesis imperfecta   B. Morquio's syndrome
   C. Zellweger syndrome   D. Multiple epiphyseal dysplasia
   Ans. is 'A' Osteogenesis imperfecta

6. Brittle bone disease is: *(NEET Pattern 2013)*
   A. Osteogenesis imperfecta   B. Osteopetrosis
   C. Paget's disease   D. Osteoporosis
   Ans. is 'A' Osteogenesis imperfecta

7. Prenatal determination of osteogenesis imperfecta is done by: *(PGI June 07)*
   A. Acid phosphatase   B. Alkaline phosphatase
   C. Abnormal Pro-a chain D. FGF3 mutation
   Ans. is 'C' Abnormal Pro-a chain

8. All are features of osteogenesis imperfecta except:
   (PGI Dec 2003, UP 2K, TN 98, MP 98, AIIMS June 1997)
   A. Blue sclera   B. Multiple fractures
   C. Cataract   D. Hearing loss
   Ans. is 'C' Cataract
   – Multiple fractures, deafness (hearing loss) due to otosclerosis and blue sclera is seen. Cataract is not a feature.

9. Not true about osteogenesis imperfecta: *(UP 2000)*
   A. Impaired healing of fracture
   B. Deafness
   C. Laxity of joints   D. Fragile fracture
   Ans. is 'A' Impaired healing of fracture
   – Fracture union is normal in osteogenesis imperfecta

10. In which of the following condition bilateral symmetrical fractures occur? *(NIMS 2000, Delhi 98)*
    A. Rickets   B. Osteopetrosis
    C. Osteogenesis imperfecta   D. Fluorosis
    Ans. is 'C' Osteogenesis imperfecta

11. All are commonly seen in osteogenesis imperfecta except: *(AI 1998)*
    A. Blue sclera   B. Bilateral hip dislocation
    C. Lax ligament   D. Osteoporosis
    Ans. is 'B' Bilateral hip dislocation
    – Although dislocations are also seen but their frequency is less than other mentioned choices.

12. Osteogenesis imperfecta is due to the following:
    A. Excessive osteoblastic activity   (Tamil Nadu 1994)
    B. Defective osteoid formation
    C. Defective osteoclast function
    D. Defective mineralisation of bone

Ans. is 'B' Defective osteoid formation
- Collagen synthesis is defective in osteogenesis imperfecta hence osteoid formation is defective.

13. Wormian bones are seen in: (Delhi 94, Andhra 93)
    A. Osteogenesis imperfecta   B. Scheuermann's disease
    C. Paget's disease   D. Osteoclastoma

Ans. is 'A' Osteogenesis imperfecta

14. Osteogenesis imperfecta: (PGI 1990)
    A. Autosomal dominant (AD)   B. Autosomal recessive (AR)
    C. Both AD and AR   D. Sex-linked dominant
    E. None of the above

Ans. is 'C' Both AD and AR

OSTEOPETROSIS (MARBLE BONE DISEASE OR ALBERS SCHONBERG DISEASE)

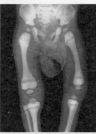
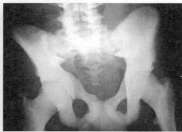
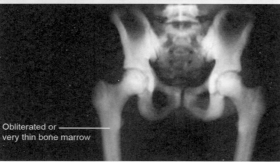

Fig. 17.28: X-ray of osteopetrotic bone—marble bone

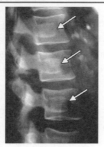

Fig. 17.29: X-ray of osteopetrotic bone—bone with in a bone appearance

Etiopathology

- It is a **diaphyseal dysplasia** characterized by failure of bone resorption due to **functional deficiency of osteoclast**. The bone contains increased number of osteoclasts but these do not resorb bone as evidenced by absence of ruffled borders and clear zones and are unable to respond to PTH. Due to functional deficiency of osteoclasts, calcified chondroid (cartilage) and primitive woven bone persists down into metaphysis and diaphysis leading to osteosclerosis and increased brittleness of bones (marble bone disease).
- Inheritance depends on form of disease: Malignant osteopetrosis (congenital form) is autosomal recessive (AR, 11q13) and late onset osteopetrosis tarda (adolescence/adult form) is AD (1P 21).
- Intermediate form is AR.

Clinical Presentation

- Autosomal dominant, benign or tarda osteopetrosis is often diagnosed in adult asymptomatic patients. It may present with mild anemia, pathological fractures premature osteoarthritis, and rarely osteomyelitis of mandible.
- Autosomal recessive malignant (congenital) osteopetrosis clinically presents at birth or in early infancy because of obliteration of marrow cavity by bony overgrowth resulting in inability of bone marrow to participate in hematopoiesis. Pancytopenia develops resulting in abnormal bleeding, easy bruising, progressive anemia, and failure to thrive
- Severe infections esp. Mandible
- Extramedullary hematopoiesis causing hepatosplenomegaly.
- Cranial nerve palsies (bony overgrowth of cranial foramen) 2nd, 7th and 8th—blindness and deafness
- Fragile brittle bones
- Pathological fractures.
- **Laboratory parameters are serum calcium low, serum PTH high, serum phosphate low and serum ALP high**
- Radiological hallmark is increased radiopacity of bones. There is no distinction between cortical and cancellous bone, because intramedullary canal is filled with bone.
- Endobones (os in os or bone within bone appearance) and rugger jersey spine.
- Treatment is bone marrow transplant.

MULTIPLE CHOICE QUESTIONS

1. Osteopetrosis, false is: (AI 2016)
   A. Low levels of serum calcium
   B. Raised levels of alkaline phosphatase
   C. Low levels of PTH
   D. Low levels of serum phosphate

Ans. is 'C' Low levels of PTH

2. Marble bone disease is: (NEET Pattern 2013, 2012)
   A. Pagets   B. Ankylosing spondylitis
   C. Osteopetrosis   D. Melorheostosis

Ans. is 'C' Osteopetrosis

3. Albers Schonberg disease is also known as:
       (NEET Pattern 2012)
   A. Osteoporosis   B. Osteopetrosis
   C. OI   D. Paget's disease

Ans. is 'B' Osteopetrosis

4. Regarding osteopetrosis all the following statements are true except: (AIIMS May 2008)
   A. Pancytopenia   B. Delayed fracture healing
   C. Cranial nerve compression D. Osteomyelitis of mandible

Ans. is 'B' Delayed fracture healing
- Cranial nerve compression due to bone encroachment on foramina may occur.

- Osteomyelitis of the mandible is common due to pancytopenia.
- Bone encroachment on marrow results in bone marrow failure with resultant pancytopenia.
- Fractures usually heal at slower rates in osteopetrosis but few studies have shown fracture healing is normal.
- Thus all 4 options are correct in case we have to choose one it will be delayed healing of fracture as there is no debate about other features.

5. Raju, a 10-year-old child, presents with predisposition to fractures, anemia, hepatosplenomegaly and a diffusely increased radiographic density of bones. The most likely diagnosis is: *(AI 2002)*
   A. Osteogenesis imperfecta B. Pycnodysostosis
   C. Myelofibrosis D. Osteopetrosis

Ans. is 'D' Osteopetrosis
- Increased density with hepatosplenomegaly, fractures, anemia is diagnostic of osteopetrosis.

6. Albers Schonberg disease is: *(PGI June 2K, 98, JIPMER 97)*
   A. Osteopetrosis B. Osteoporosis
   C. Osteochondritis D. Osteomalacia

Ans. is 'A' Osteopetrosis

7. A 3-year-old male presented with progressive anemia hepatosplenomegaly and osteomyelitis of jaw with pathological fracture, X-ray shows chalky white deposits on bone, probable diagnosis is: *(AIIMS 93)*
   A. Osteopetrosis
   B. Osteopoikilocytosis
   C. Alkaptonuria
   D. Myositis ossificans progressiva

Ans. is 'A' Osteopetrosis

CONGENITAL ABSENCE OF PECTORALIS MUSCLES

Congenital variations occur more frequently in the pectoralis than in any other of the skeletal muscles. **Pectoralis major** and minor are the most common congenitally absent muscles.

Agenesis is often partial and maybe part of a syndrome associated with other anomalies—**Poland syndrome.** Patients typically present with a flattened chest wall, with hypoplastic ribs, an elevated nipple and may present with unilateral hyper radiolucency of the lung on a roentgenogram. Diagnosis is often established on ultrasound and is mainly based on the absence of a muscle belly or tendon.

MULTIPLE CHOICE QUESTION

1. Muscle most commonly affected by congenital absence is: *(AI 2009)*
   A. Pectoralis major B. Semimembranosus
   C. Teres minor D. Gluteus maximus

Ans. is 'A' Pectoralis major
Pectoralis major and minor muscles are the most common congenitally absent muscles in human.

INCREASED BONE DENSITY (RADIOLOGICAL)

Pathogenetic Mechanism
- Periosteal reaction (seen in tumors and infections)
- Thickening and expansion of cortex
- Thickening of cancellous bone seen in traumatic collapse
- Increased (and coarse) trabeculae
- Sclerosis and dead bone (e.g. sequestrum seen in osteomyelitis)

Causes

Children:
- Caffey's disease craniotubular dysplasia and hyperostosis
- Osteopetrosis
- Poisoning-lead (Pb)
- Hypervitaminosis A and D
- Renal osteodystrophy
- Diaphyseal dysplasia (Engelmann's/Camurati disease)
- Pycnodysostosis candle bone disease or melorheostosis (Leris disease)
- Osteopoikilosis—Spotted bone disease

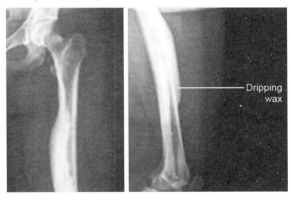

Fig. 17.30: Candle bone disease (Melorheostosis)

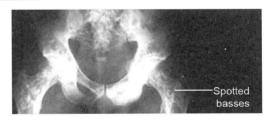

Fig. 17.31: Osteopoikilosis—the bony spots are periarticular, symmetrical and uniform in size

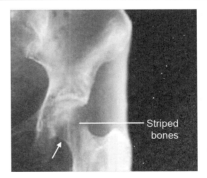

Fig. 17.32: Osteopathia striata

Adult
- Avascular necrosis/Paget's disease/myelosclerosis/fluorosis/mastocytosis/lymphoma

- Osteoblastic metastasis/renal osteodystrophy
- Idiopathic skeletal hyperostosis

MULTIPLE CHOICE QUESTIONS

1. Generalized osteosclerosis is seen in: (PGI Nov 2015)
   A. Osteoporosis   B. Osteochondritis
   C. Osteogenesis imperfecta   D. Osteopetrosis
   E. Osteomalacia

Ans. is 'D' Osteopetrosis

2. Dripping candle wax lesion on spine:
   (DNB July 2016, NEET Pattern 2013)
   A. Metastasis   B. TB spine
   C. Osteopetrosis   D. Melorheostosis

Ans. is 'D' Melorheostosis

3. Increased bone density in X-ray seen in: (PGI June 08)
   A. Collapse cancellous bone   B. Periosteal reaction
   C. Paget's disease   D. AVN
   E. Osteomyelitis

Ans. is 'All' 'A' Collapse cancellous bone; 'B' Periosteal reaction; 'C' Paget's disease; 'D' AVN and 'E' Osteomyelitis

4. Increased bone density in X-ray seen in: (PGI Dec 08)
   A. Increased thickening of trabeculae
   B. Fracture and Collapse of cancellous bone
   C. Defective mineralization
   D. Myositis ossificans
   E. Relative disuse atrophy and surrounding bone response

Ans. is 'A and B' Increased thickening of trabeculae and Fracture and Collapse of cancellous bone

METABOLIC BONE DISEASES

Coarse Trabecular Pattern—HOP-G

Haemoglobinopathies/Haemangioma
   Osteoporosis/Osteomalacia
      Paget's disease
         Gaucher's disease
HOP-G

Bone within a Bone Appearance NaNha GOPAL

Normal
   Neonate
      Growth arrest/recovery lines
         Osteopetrosis
            Paget's disease/**P**rostaglandin E, therapy
               Acromegaly
                  Lead poisoning
                     Sickle cell anemia
NaNha GOPALS

Erlenmeyer Flask Deformity GOL POT—It is flask like deformity of lower end of femur

Gaucher's disease
   Osteopetrosis
      Lead poisoning
         Pyle's disease (metaphyseal dysplasia)
            Osteodysplastic (Melnick-Needles syndrome)
               Thalassemia
GOL-POT

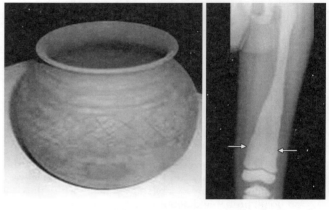

Fig. 17.33: GOL POT = Erlenmeyer flask

Short Metacarpal(s) or Metatarsal(s)—TIP

Turner's syndrome
   Idiopathic
      Pseudohypoparathyroidism/**P**ost-traumatic/**P**ostinfarction
TIP

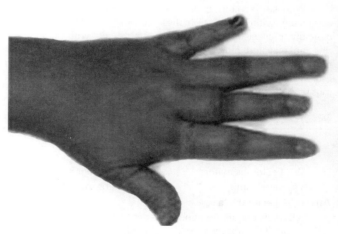

Fig. 17.34: Short metacarpal = TIP

- Pyle's disease: Metaphyseal dysplasia.
- Engelmann's disease: Diaphyseal dysplasia.
- Trevor's disease: Dysplasia epiphyseal hemimelica
- Most common skeletal dysplasia: Osteogenesis imperfecta

Metabolic Disorders of Bone

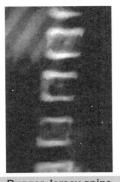

Rugger Jersey spine
Chronic renal failure
osteopetrosis

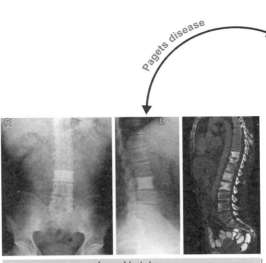

Ivory Vertebra

Pagets disease

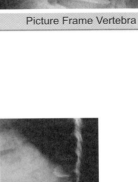

Picture Frame Vertebra

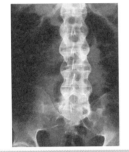

Bamboo spine
Ankylosing spondylitis

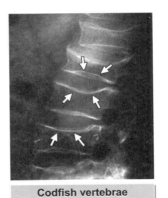

Codfish vertebrae
Osteoporosis > Osteomalacia

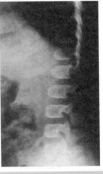

Bullet nose vertebra
Achondroplasia

18 CHAPTER

Pediatric Orthopedics

PEDIATRIC HIP PROBLEM

Differential Diagnosis of Limping Child
Painless Limp
1–3 years age group:
   (i) DDH (Developmental dysplasia of hip)
   (ii) Cerebral palsy
   (iii) Muscular dystrophy
   (iv) Infantile coxa vara
- 4–10 years age: Limb length discrepancy, Poliomyelitis

Painful Limp
1. Legg Calve Perthes disease (NOTE: Classically perthes is described as painless limp)
2. Slipped capital femoral epiphysis
3. Osteochondritis dissecans (knee) (Lateral surface of medial femoral condyle)
4. Arthritis/Synovitis/Osteomyelitis
   Order of investigation in Limping child X-ray followed by ultrasound followed by MRI.

MULTIPLE CHOICE QUESTIONS

1. All the following are causes of a painful limp except:
   A. Slipped femoral epiphysis   (AI 1995)
   B. TB of the hip
   C. Perthes disease   D. Infantile Coxa Vara
   Ans. is 'D' Infantile Coxa Vara
   Infantile (congenital) coxa vara causes painless limp.

2. Causes of a painless limp in infancy includes:
   A. Congenital dislocation of hip   (Tamil Nadu 1992)
   B. Infantile coxa vara
   C. Poliomyelitis   D. All of the above
   Ans. is 'D' All of the above

COXA VARA

It is reduced angle between neck and shaft of femur due to some growth anomaly at upper femoral epiphysis (infantile type) or secondary to various other pathologies (acquired).

The normal femoral neck shaft angle is 160° at birth, decreasing to 135 degrees in adult life. An angle of <120 degrees is called coxa vara.

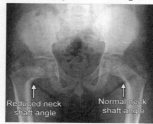

Fig. 18.1: Coxa Vara

Classification (Causes) of Coxa Vara
Congenital Coxa Vara
- Congenital femoral deficiency with coxa vara
- Developmental coxa vara

Acquired Coxa Vara
- SCFE (slipped capital femoral epiphysis)
- Sequelae of avascular necrosis of femoral epiphysis
- Legg-Calve Perthes disease
- Femoral neck fracture, Intertrochanteric fracture
- Rickets

CONGENITAL COXA VARA

Clinical Presentation
- Painless limp in a child who has just started walking
- Shortening-Limitation of abduction and internal rotation

Radiological
- Reduced neck shaft angle (coxa vara)
- Vertical epiphysis plate
- Separate triangle of bone in infero-medial part of metaphysis called as Fairbank's triangle

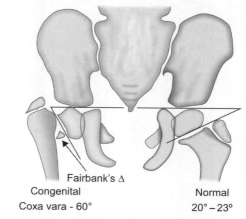

Fig. 18.2: Hilgenreiner's epiphyseal angle

- Hilgenreiner's epiphyseal angle; angle between horizontal line joining center (triradiate cartilage) of each hip (Hilgenreiner's line) and line parallel to physis; the normal angle is about 30 degrees.

Treatment (based on HE Angle)—Hilgenreiner's epiphyseal angle
>40° but <60° Observation
>60° or if shortening is progressive. Subtrochanteric valgus osteotomy

Triangles
- Babcocks Δ: T.B hip origin in femur metaphysis

Pediatric Orthopedics

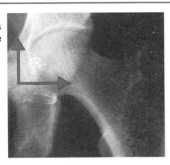

Fig. 18.3: Babcock's triangle

- Wards Δ: To assess bone density in osteoporosis

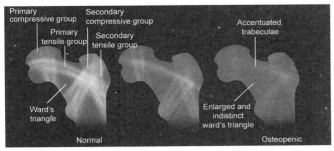

- Fairbank's Δ: Congenital Coxa Vara

MULTIPLE CHOICE QUESTIONS

1. What is the likely diagnosis of the image shown below?
 (AIIMS Nov 2018)

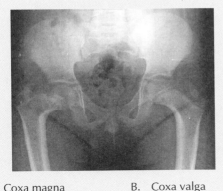

   A. Coxa magna B. Coxa valga
   C. Coxa vara D. Coxa sultans

   Ans. is 'C' Coxa vara

2. Cause of Coxa vara: *(NEET Pattern 2013)*
   A. Congenital B. Perthe's disease
   C. SCFE D. All of the above

   Ans. is 'D' All of the above

3. Fairbanks Δ is seen in: *(NEET Pattern 2016, 2012)*
   A. CTEV B. DDH
   C. SCFE D. Coxa Vara

   Ans. is 'D' Coxa Vara

4. Congenital Coxa vara is treated by: *(PGI June 04)*
   A. Fixation by SP Nail B. Osteotomy
   C. Bone grafting D. Traction

   Ans. is 'B' Osteotomy
   - Treatment is by a subtrochanteric corrective osteotomy.

5. Coxa vara is found in: *(PGI 86)*
   A. Perthe's disease
   B. Tuberculosis
   C. Rickets
   D. Rheumatoid arthritis

   Ans. is 'A' Perthe's disease; 'C' Rickets

LEGG-CALVE-PERTHES DISEASE/OSTEOCHON-DRITIS DEFORMANS JUVENILIS/COXA PLANA

It can be defined as osteonecrosis of the proximal femoral epiphysis in a growing child caused by poorly understood (non-genetic) factors.

Etiology

- The precipitating cause is unknown but the cardinal step in the pathogenesis is ischemia of femoral head. Between 4 and 8 years of age femoral head depends for its blood supply and venous drainage almost entirely on the lateral epiphyseal vessels whose situation in retinacula makes them susceptible to stretching and to pressure from an effusion.

Clinical Presentation

- 4–8 years of age
- Male > Female
- Bilateral in 10% cases
- Most frequent symptom is limp that is exacerbated by activity and alleviated with rest
- 2nd most frequent complaint is pain
- During the very early phase, joint is irritable so extremes of all movements are diminished and painful
- Later on most movements are full, but abduction (especially in flexion) is nearly always limited and usually internal rotation also. When the hip is flexed it may go into obligatory external rotation (Catterall's sign) and knee points towards axilla. (Normally goes towards midclavicular region)

Course of Disease

Most consistent factor affecting course is patient's age at onset of disease. Younger age better prognosis. Outcome is also affected by duration from onset to complete resolution; the shorter the duration the better the final results.

Head at Risk sign in perthes are: (These indicate poor development of femur head from femur epiphysis)

- Lateral subluxation of the femoral head
- Speckled calcification lateral to the capital epiphysis
- Gage sign-a radiolucent 'V' shaped defect in the lateral epiphysis and adjacent metaphysis
- Sagging Rope Sign—metaphyseal sclerotic band

INVESTIGATION

MRI is the Investigation of Choice

At first X-ray may seem normal, though subtle changes such as widening of joint space and slight asymmetry of ossification centers are usually present (isotope scan may show void in anterolateral part of femoral head). The classical feature of increased density (sclerosis) of the ossification nucleus occurs later and may be accompanied by fragmentation or crescentic subarticular fracture (best seen in lateral view). The head tends to flatten and enlarge. (coxa plana).

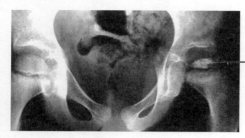

Fig. 18.4: Perthes disease

Perthes classification
- Catterall classification
- Salter-Thompson classification
- Herring's lateral pillar classification
- Stulberg classification

Management

The main aim of treatment is containment of femoral head in acetabulum. Nonsurgical containment is achieved by orthotic braces. All braces abduct the affected hip, most allow for hip flexion, and some control rotation of the limb. Broomstick or petrie cast issued.

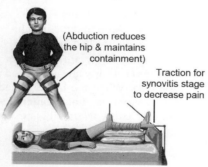

Fig. 18.5: Treatment of Perthes

Surgical containment is through (1) Femoral varus derotation osteotomy, (2) Chiari osteotomy and chielectomy (Surgically removing protruding fragments of femoral head usually anterolateral).

MULTIPLE CHOICE QUESTIONS

1. Risk factor(s) for Leg-calve-Perthe's diasease is/are: *(PGI MAY 2018)*
   A. Accelerated skeletal growth
   B. Growth hormone abnormalities
   C. Positive family history
   D. Female sex
   E. Passive smoking

Ans. is 'C' Positive family history; & 'E' Passive smoking

2. Which of the following is X-ray feature of perthes disease? *(DNB JUNE 2017)*
   A. Increased medial joint space
   B. Metaphyseal cysts and rarefaction
   C. Lateral extrusion of femur head
   D. All of the above

Ans. is 'D' All of the above

3. Which of the following is not true about perthes disease? *(NEET DEC 2016)*
   A. It is also called coxa plana
   B. Occurs more commonly in females
   C. It is caused by interruption in the blood supply of the capital femoral epiphyses
   D. Abduction, internal rotation and flexion of hip are restricted

Ans. is 'B' Occurs more commonly in females

4. Regarding Legg-Calve-Perthes disease all are correct except: *(PGI May 2016)*
   A. Osteonecrosis Osteochondritis
   B. Male predominance
   C. Restricted abduction
   D. Narrow joint space
   E. Age of onset is not related to disease severity

Ans. is 'D' Narrow joint space and 'E' Age of onset is not related to disease severity

5. All of the following are true regarding Perthes disease except: *(AI Dec 15)*
   A. It is avascular necrosis of the femoral head
   B. Commonly affects children in the first decade
   C. Limp and restricted rotations of the hip are common clinical features
   D. MRI is not a good confirmatory investigation

Ans. is 'D' MRI is not a good confirmatory investigation

6. Which of the following are true about Perthes Disease?
   A. Self-limiting condition *(PGI Nov 2015)*
   B. Bilateral in 20% cases
   C. Painful condition
   D. Femoral head is displaced laterally
   E. More common in females

Ans. is 'A' Self-limiting condition; 'B' Bilateral in 20% cases and 'D' Femoral head is displaced laterally

7. Radiological sign in case of Perthes disease:
   A. Epiphyseal calcification *(NEET Pattern 2013)*
   B. Organized calcification
   C. Lateral subluxation femur head
   D. Restriction of abduction

Ans. is 'C' Lateral subluxation femur head

8. Which of the following movements is restricted in Perthes disease? *(NEET Pattern 2013)*
   A. Adduction and external rotation
   B. Abduction and external rotation
   C. Adduction and internal rotation
   D. Abduction and internal rotation

Ans. is 'D' Abduction and internal rotation

Pediatric Orthopedics

9. True about perthes disease is: *(PGI Nov 2009, PGI 95)*
   A. Avascular necrosis of femoral head
   B. Onset before 10 years of age
   C. Osteotomy is used for treatment
   D. Limb shortening
   E. Joint space obliterated

Ans. is 'A' Avascular necrosis of femoral head; 'B' Onset before 10 years of age; 'C' Osteotomy is used for treatment; and 'D' Limb shortening

Joint space is not obliterated in Perthes till arthritis sets in.

10. Which one of the following is the investigation of choice for evaluation of suspected Perthes' disease? *(AI 2005)*
    A. Plain X-ray
    B. Ultrasonography (US)
    C. Computed Tomography (CT)
    D. Magnetic Resonance Imaging (MRI)

Ans. is 'D' Magnetic Resonance Imaging (MRI)

MRI is the *investigation of choice* as it can diagnose Perthe's disease in early stages when X-ray is normal.

11. The commonest cause of limp in a child of seven years is:
    A. T.B. hip *(UP 02)*
    B. C.D.H
    C. Perthe's disease
    D. Slipped upper femoral epiphysis

Ans. is 'C' Perthe's disease

Perthes is the most common cause of limp in age group 4–8 years.

12. An 8-year-old male with painless limp on examination and restricted abduction and internal rotation left hip, probable diagnosis is: *(AIIMS Nov 99)*
    A. Septic arthritis of hip   B. Tuberculosis arthritis of hip
    C. Cong dislocation of hip   D. Perthe's disease

Ans. is 'D' Perthe's disease

Restriction of *abduction and internal rotation in age group 4–8 years* is seen in Perthes disease.

13. Perthes disease is treated by: *(AIIMS Nov 93)*
    A. High dose of calcium with steroids
    B. Total hip replacement
    C. Supervised containment of femoral head in acetabulum
    D. Relieving weight bearing

Ans. is 'C' Supervised containment of femoral head in acetabulum. The head is required to be kept inside the acetabulum while the revascularization takes place *(head containment)*.

SLIPPED CAPITAL FEMORAL EPIPHYSIS

During a period of rapid growth, due to weakening of upper femoral physis and shearing stress from excessive body weight, there is upward and anterior movement of femoral neck on the capital epiphysis. So the epiphysis is located primarily posteriorly and medially relative to the femoral neck, although neck moves epiphysis does not.

Etiology
- The cause is unknown in vast majority of patients.

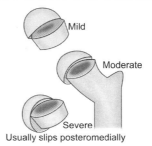

Fig. 18.6: Slipped capital femoral epiphysis

- Many of the patients are either fat and sexually immature or excessively thin and tall.
- Endocrinopathies such as Hypothyroidism (most common)
- Growth hormone excess caused by growth hormone deficiency conditions treated by growth hormone administration.
- Chronic renal failure (Hyperparathyroidism)
- Primary hyperparathyroidism
- Pan hypopituitarism associated with intracranial tumors
- Craniopharyngioma
- MEN 2 B
- Turner's syndrome
- Klinefelter's syndrome
- Rubinstein-Taybi syndrome
- Prior pelvic irradiation
- Many a times it presents in growth spurt.

Pathogenesis and Pathology

Slip occurs through hypertrophic zone of growth plate.

Clinical Picture

- Males are more commonly affected
- An adolescent child (boys 13–15 and girls 11–13) typically overweight or very thin and tall presents with pain some times and Antalgic limp, with the affected side held in a position of increased external rotation, (turning out of leg). Restriction of internal rotation, abduction and flexion.
- A classical sign is tendency of thigh to rotate in to progressively more external rotation, as the affected hip is flexed called as Axis deviation. (Similar to Perthes)
- Slipping usually occurs as a series of minor events rather than a sudden, acute episode. Patient with unstable acute or acute on chronic SCFE characteristically present with sudden onset of severe, fracture like pain usually as a result of a relatively minor fall or twisting injury.
- Chondrolysis complicating SCFE presents with more continuous pain, hip held in an external rotated position at rest, with flexion contracture and global restriction of hip motion. The patient usually complain of pain through out the arc of motion rather than just at its extremities.
- 20% cases will have evidence of contralateral slip. 60% of patients will have bilateral involvement when associated with endocrinopathies.
- Chondrolysis (Destruction of Cartilage) and avascular necrosis are possible complications.

Investigation

A line drawn tangential to superior femoral neck (**Klein's line**) on AP view will intersect a portion the lateral capital epiphysis normally. With typical posterior displacement of capital epiphysis this line will intersect a smaller portion of the epiphysis or not at all **Trethowan's sign**.

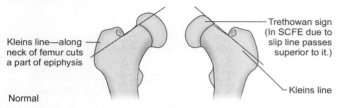

Fig. 18.7: Radiological diagnosis of slipped capital femoral epiphysis

Steel's metaphyseal sign is a crescent shaped area of increased density overlying metaphysis adjacent to physis (on AP view). It is due to overlapping of femoral neck and posteriorly displaced capital epiphysis.

A frog leg's lateral view is best for detecting mild slip.

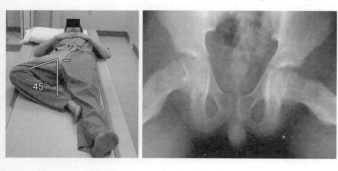

Fig. 18.8: Frog leg lateral view

Tc 99 scan show increased uptake in capital femoral physis in SCFE, decreased uptake within epiphysis is highly specific for AVN. When chondrolysis is present, there is increased uptake of isotope on both sides of the joint.

MRI is useful investigation for diagnosis.

Treatment

SCFE is usually a progressive disease that requires prompt surgical treatment. Because the changes in the chronic form occurs so slowly it is impossible to manipulate the femoral head into a better position. So treatment consists of fixing the slip in its current position and preventing progression. This is done by inserting one or more screws or pins across the growth plate (pinning in Situ). Acute slips, if unstable may be gently reduced before fixation but it increases the chances of AVN.

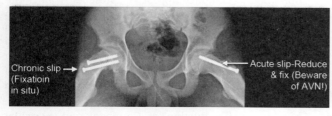

Fig. 18.9: Treatment of slipped capital femoral epiphysis

MULTIPLE CHOICE QUESTIONS

1. Which of the following is not true about SCFE?
   (NEET DEC 2016)
   A. Males are affected more frequently
   B. Extension is restricted
   C. Commonly occurs during adolescence
   D. Varus, adduction and external rotation deformities are present

Ans. is 'B' Extension is restricted

2. All are true about Slipped capital femoral epiphysis except: (PGI Nov 2014)
   A. Avascular necrosis may occur
   B. Usually occur after 10-year of age
   C. Obesity is a risk factor
   D. Frog-leg lateral view is helpful
   E. More common in girls

Ans. is 'E' More common in girls

3. Slipped capital femoral epiphysis is seen most commonly in which age group? (NEET Pattern 2012)
   A. Infants   B. Adolescents
   C. Old age   D. Childhood

Ans. is 'B' Adolescents

4. Slipped capital femoral epiphyses slips in which direction? (NEET Pattern 2012)
   A. No slip   B. Posteromedial
   C. Anterolateral   D. Medial

Ans. is 'A' No slip

5. An 11-year-old 70 kg child presents with limitation of abduction and internal rotation. There is tenderness in Scarpa's triangle. On flexing the hip the limb is externally rotated. The diagnosis is:
   (AIIMS May 2012, AIPG 2012, AIIMS Nov 2001)
   A. Perthes disease
   B. Slipped capital femoral epiphyses
   C. Observation hip
   D. Tuberculosis hip

Ans. is 'B' Slipped capital femoral epiphyses
   – Limitation **of abduction and Internal rotation**
   – 4–8 years Perthes Disease
   – 11–20 years Slipped Capital Femoral Epiphysis

6. 14-year-old boy with 78 kg weight and hypothyroidism developed sudden onset of severe pain and tenderness on left hip as a result of minor fall. Most likely diagnosis is: (JIMPMER 2002, PGI 95)
   A. Fracture neck femur   B. SCFE
   C. Perthes   D. Hip Dislocation

Ans. is 'B' SCFE
   Adolescent (14 years) male, Obese (78 kg)
   Hypothyroidism are indicators for SCFE

7. Trethowan's sign is seen in: (AMU 99)
   A. Perthe's disease   B. CDH
   C. SCFE   D. Fracture neck femur

Ans. is 'C' SCFE

DEVELOPMENTAL DYSPLASIA OF HIP (DDH) SHALLOW ACETABULUM

DDH is failure of maintenance of femoral head due to malformations of acetabulum or femur **80% of cases of DDH occur in girls**. DDH is more common in **first born child**, oligohydramnios The crowding phenomenon is the cause of its association with **torticollis** and **metatarsus adductus**. Breech presentation is another strong association factor. Familial association is seen. **But the twin pregnancy does not increase the risk.**

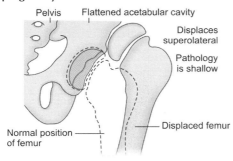

Fig. 18.10: Displaces superolateral

Clinical Diagnosis

1. Abduction is limited (especially in flexion)
2. Asymmetric thigh folds
3. **Barlow's Test**

1st part—In position of 90 degree flexion of hips and knees, the hip is adducted and pushed.

And this will lead to dislocation of hip (but not if already dislocated).

"*BAAHARLO! "DAd", i.e. Barlow's test—Dislocation By Adduction (DAd)"

Thus in Barlows we dislocate hip joint. (Provocative test)

IInd part—Now the hip is abducted and pulled. This will cause 'clunk' indicating reduction of hip.

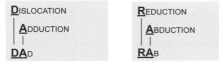

Some consider only 1st part as Barlow's test

4. Ortolani's Test—the first two alphabets **O** and **R** (Ortolani for Reduction) and for Reduction we do abduction of hip.
   It is similar to 2nd part of Barlow's test

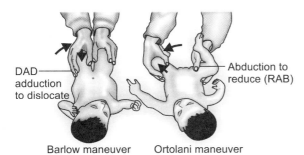

Fig. 18.11: Test for DDH

5. Short limb as shown by—Higher buttock folds, Galeazzi or Allis sign is lowering of knee on affected side in a lying child with hip and knees flexed.

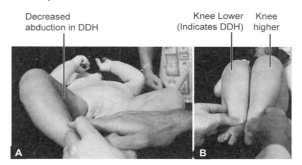

Figs. 18.12A and B: (A) Decreased abduction in DDH; (B) Galeazzi or Allis test

6. Trendelenberg's test, telescopy and vascular sign of Narath is positive.

Radiological Features

- In Von Rosen's view following parameters should be noted
- Perkin's line; Vertical line drawn at the outer border of acetabulum.
- Hilgenreiner's line; Horizontal line drawn at the level of tri-radiate cartilage.
    Shenton's line: Smooth curve formed by inferior border of neck of femur with superior margin of obturator foramen.
    Acetabular Index: Angle between Hilgenreiners line and line from triradiate epiphysis to lateral edge of acetabulum. Normal value is 20–40 degrees. (Centre edge) angle of Wiberg normal values upto 20–30 degree is angle between Perkin's line and a line joining centre of epiphysis to edge of acetabulum.

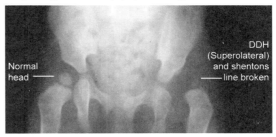

Fig. 18.13: DDH X-ray

- Normally the head lies in the lower and inner quadrant formed by two lines (Perkin's and Hilgenreiner's). In DDH the head lies in outer and upper quadrant.

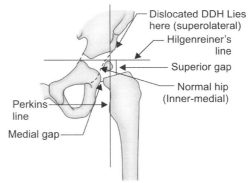

Fig. 18.14: DDH-related anatomy

- Shenton's line is broken
- Delayed appearance and retarded development of ossification of head of femur
- Sloping shallow acetabulum
- Superior and lateral displacement of femoral head.
- **Acetabular index increases and CE angle reduces in DDH.**

Alpha and Beta angles are measured for DDH and alpha angle decreases with severity whereas beta angle increases with severity of DDH. (Measured on USG).

Screening Criteria for DDH

- All neonates Should have a clinical examination for hip instability.
- Babies with risk factors associated with DDH should receive more careful screening, risk factors include family history, breech, birth position, torticollis, metatarsus adductus, oligohydramnios, talipes equino varus and genu recurvatum Because the incidence is higher in females, these factors assumes greater importance in female infants and first born caucasiAns. Twin pregnancy is not a risk factor.
- Because the ultrasound findings improve with age, diagnosis and treatment is based on USG at 6 weeks.
- Plain X-ray will usually demonstrate a frankly dislocated hip in any age. However in newborn and child <6 months with typical DDH, the hip may appear radiologically normal Hence USG is preferred in <6 months child with hip problem.

  MRI nowadays is considered a very specific and sensitive investigation for location of ossific nucleus and diagnosing DDH.

Clinical Presentation of Bilateral DDH

- In a bilateral dislocation the gait is described as **'duck like waddle' or 'sailor's gait'** and consists of an inclination to the side on which the weight is born (lurching gait on both side). In unilateral cases the child lurches towards affected side. This is known as abductor lurch or Trendelenburg gait (pelvis drops on opposite side).
- Lordosis is Particularly noticeable in bilateral cases and is often presenting complaint.
- In bilateral cases legs appear too short for the body, the perineal space is broadened, the trochanter are unduly prominent, and the buttocks are broad and flat. In unilateral cases one leg is short which can be demonstrated by Galeazzi/Allis test.
- In bilateral cases, there is no asymmetry on abduction; and flexed knees are at the same level. Combined abduction is limited but this is difficult to detect because the limitation is symmetrical.
- **Klisic test can recognize bilateral DDH.**
- In bilateral cases trendelenburg's sign is Positive on both sides and shenton's line is broken bilaterally.
- **Compensatory genu Valgum is seen.**

Treatment Plan of DDH

A. **Neonate and Young Child (1–6 month)—Closed reduction. Wide abduction and forced internal rotation must always be avoided due to fear of Avascular Necrosis of Femur head.**

   Pavlik harness after hip reduces, is treatment of choice

   Ilfeld - craig splint, Von-Rosen splint and Freika pillow can also be used.

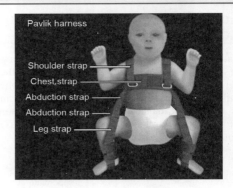

Fig. 18.15: Pavlik harness

B. **6–18 months**
   Beyond 6 months closed reduction is difficult as an inferior capsule of hip assumes hourglass shape and may prevent a successful closed reduction, Hypertrophy of ligamentum teres, Pulvinar (Fibrofatty tissues), Iliopsoas, capsular Interposition are other obstructions to closed reduction.

   All can hinder the closed reduction so usually in this age open reduction is carried out.

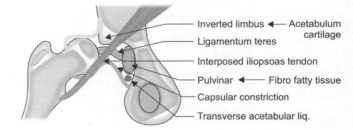

Fig. 18.16: Structures interfering with closed reduction

C. **18–36 months**
   Open reduction + femoral rotation osteotomy ± pelvic osteotomy (Femur is osteotomized and rotated after 18 months).

Walking Child (3 years–6 years)

- Beyond 3 years acetabulum needs augmentation to provide stable hip.
- Open reduction (anterolateral approach), femoral shortening with rotation and **Acetabular reconstruction procedure** are carried out. Salter's, osteotomy Chiari's pelvic displacement and Pemberton osteotomy are acetabular procedures.
- **6–10 years:** Treatment should be avoided (fear of AVN), in bilateral DDH, in unilateral same as above.
- **>11 years:** In cases of painful hips due to Osteoarthritis, THR may be done (but should be delayed till skeletal maturity).

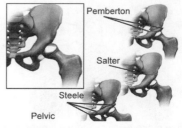

Fig. 18.17: Pelvic osteotomy to provide acetabulam coverage to femur head in DDH

Pediatric Orthopedics

MULTIPLE CHOICE QUESTIONS

1. Which of the following is true about DDH? *(DNB June 2017)*
   A. Male gender is risk factor
   B. Limbs are in adduction, internal rotation and flexion in old children
   C. Femur neck is retroverted
   D. Ligamentum teres is atrophied
   Ans. is 'B' Limbs are in adduction, internal rotation and flexion in old children

2. Following is not a part of Ortolani test: *(NEET Dec 2016)*
   A. Examiners thumb rests on the medial thigh
   B. Examiners finger li on the greater trochanter
   C. Hips are flexed to 90 degrees and gently abducted
   D. Jerk is given to the knee to dislocate the femur head jerk of exit
   Ans. is 'D' Jerk is given to the knee to dislocate the femur head jerk of exit

3. A female with H/o Oligohydramnios during her pregnancy, brings her newborn baby to OPD, on noticing asymmetric thigh folds in her child. The examiner performs flexion, IR and abduction, which produces a click sound. Which is the test done by the examiner?
   A. Ortolani test
   B. Von Rosen test
   C. Mc Murray's test
   D. Barlow's test
   Ans. is 'A' Ortolani test

4. All of the following are true regarding congenital dislocation of hip except: *(CET Nov 15)*
   A. Asymetric Thigh folds may be seen
   B. Galleazi sign and Ortolani test may be positive
   C. It may be bilateral
   D. Polyhydramnios is a known risk factor
   Ans. is 'D' Polyhydramnios is known risk factor

5. The following pelvic X-ray was seen in a patient. All the following signs will be present except: *(AIIMS May 2016)*

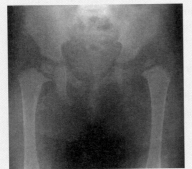

   A. Ortolani
   B. Barlow
   C. Narath
   D. Gaenslen's
   Ans. is 'D' Gaenslen's Test *(Refer to Fig. 18.10)*

6. A 4-month-child diagnosed with DDH, cast used after closed reduction is: *(AI 2016)*
   A. Hip spica
   B. Pavlik harness
   C. Minnerva cast
   D. Riser's cast
   Ans. is 'A' Hip spica

7. Pavlik harness is used to treat: *(CET July 16)*
   A. Developmental dysplasia of hip
   B. Perthe's disease
   C. Slipped Capital femoral epiphysis
   D. Congenital coxa vara
   Ans. is 'A' Developmental dysplasia of hip

8. Irregular thigh folds are seen in: *(CET July 16)*
   A. Developmental dysplasia of hip
   B. Perthe's disease
   C. Slipped Capital femoral epiphysis
   D. Congenital coxa vara
   Ans. is 'A' Developmental dysplasia of hip

9. Which of the following is not seen in a child with DDH?
   A. Waddling gait *(JIPMER May 2016)*
   B. Feeling of femoral artery pulsation is difficult
   C. Decreased growth hormone
   D. Ortolani test is positive
   Ans. is 'C' Decreased growth hormone

10. Ortolani's test is used to diagnose: *(CET Nov 15)*
    A. Congenital coxa vara
    B. Slipped Capital femoral epiphysis
    C. Developmental dysplasia of the hip
    D. Perthe's disease
    Ans. is 'C' Developmental dysplasia of the hip

11. Positive Galeazzi Sign is seen in: *(TN 2015)*
    A. Unilateral DDH
    B. Bilateral DDH
    C. Distal radioulnar dislocation
    D. Distal radius fracture
    Ans. is 'A' Unilateral DDH

12. Perkin's line on X-ray is used for diagnosis of:
    A. Perthe's disease
    B. CDH *(NEET 2015)*
    C. CTEV
    D. AVN Hip
    Ans. is 'B' CDH

13. Ortolani test is positive when the examiner hears the: *(NEET 2015)*
    A. Clunk of entry on abduction and flexion of hip
    B. Clunk of entry on extension and adduction of hip
    C. Click of exit on abduction and flexion of hip
    D. Click of exit on extension and adduction of hip
    Ans. is 'A' Clunk of entry on abduction and flexion of hip

14. Which of the following is NOT a feature of DDH?
    A. Smaller epiphysis of femoral head *(TN 2014)*
    B. Inclination of acetabular roof is increased
    C. Shenton's line disrupted
    D. Femoral head is anteverted
    Ans. is 'D' Femoral head is anteverted

15. Salter's pelvic osteotomy is done for treatment of:
    A. CTEV
    B. SCFE *(NEET Pattern 2013)*
    C. DDH
    D. None
    Ans. is 'C' DDH

16. Von-Rosen's sign is positive in: *(NEET Pattern 2013)*
    A. Perthe's disease
    B. SCFE
    C. DDH
    D. CTEV
    Ans. is 'C' DDH

17. Bachelors' cast is used in: (NEET Pattern 2013)
    A. Fracture radius   B. Club foot
    C. DDH   D. Fracture calcaneum
Ans. is 'C' DDH

18. Provocative Test for detecting CDH: (NEET Pattern 2012)
    A. Peterson test   B. Barlow test
    C. Perkin's test   D. Von Rosen tests
Ans. is 'B' Barlow test

19. Dysplastic hip in a child, investigation of choice:
    A. X-ray   B. MRI (NEET Pattern 2012)
    C. USG   D. CT Scan
Ans. is 'B' MRI

20. Primary pathology in CDH: (NEET Pattern 2012)
    A. Large head of femur   B. Shallow acetabulum
    C. Excessive retroversion   D. Everted limbus
Ans. is 'B' Shallow acetabulum

21. Alpha angle in DDH: (NEET Pattern 2012)
    A. Decreases   B. Increases
    C. Constant   D. Variable
Ans. is 'A' Decreases

22. True about Bilateral DDH:
    (PGI Dec 09, 07, 06, June 01, 90, AMC 89, Andhra 89)
    A. Exaggerated lordosis   B. B/L genu valgum
    C. Wadding gait   D. Shenton's line broken
    E. Short stature   F. All of the above
Ans. is 'F' All of the above

23. All of the following statements are true about development dysplasia (DDH) of the hip, except: (AI 2006)
    A. It is more common in females
    B. Oligohydramnios is associated with a higher risk of DDH
    C. The hourglass appearance of the capsule may prevent a successful closed reduction
    D. Twin pregnancy is a known risk factor
Ans. is 'D' Twin pregnancy is a known risk factor

24. Barlow's test is done for testing: (PGI 99, UP 99, Bihar 98)
    A. CDH in child   B. DDH in infancy
    C. Femoral neck fracture   D. Slipped femoral epiphysis
Ans. is 'B' DDH in infancy

25. In a newborn child, abduction and internal rotation produces a click sound. It is:
    (UP 99, AI 1994, Andhra 93, Delhi 1993)
    A. Ortolani's sign   B. Telescoping sign
    C. Lachman's sign   D. Mc Murray's sign
Ans. is 'A' Ortolani's sign

Barlow's test
– Part 1—Click sound (clunck) of dislocation on adduction.
– Part 2—Click sound (clunck) of reduction on abduction.

Ortolani's test
– Click sound (clunk) of reduction on abduction.

26. Commonest deformity in congenital dislocation of hip:
    A. Small head of femur   (PGI 97)
    B. Angle of torsion
    C. Decreased neck shaft angle
    D. Shallow acetabulum
Ans. is 'D' Shallow acetabulum
Primary pathology in DDH is dysplasia of the acetabulum—shallow acetabulum.

FRACTURE SEPARATION OF DISTAL FEMORAL EPIPHYSIS

- In childhood or adolescent equivalent of a supracondylar femur fracture, the lower femur epiphysis may be displaced.
- **Valgus force caused by blow to the lateral side of distal femur is causative.**
- Salter Harris type II or III injury with distal femoral epiphysis displaced laterally with a lateral fragment of the metaphysis
- Hyper-extension type injury. Distal femoral epiphysis displaced anteriorly. The triangular metaphyseal fragment and intact periosteal hinge are anterior in location.
- Nearly 70% of femur's length is derived from the distal physis, so early arrest can present a major problem.

MULTIPLE CHOICE QUESTION

1. Traumatic dislocation of epiphyseal plate of femur occurs:
   A. Medially   B. Laterally (PGI Dec 2002)
   C. Posteriorly   D. Rotationally
   E. Anteriorly
Ans. is 'B' Laterally; 'E' Anteriorly

CONGENITAL DISLOCATION OF KNEE

Etiology and Pathology

- Abnormal fetal position, i.e. feet become locked beneath the mandible or the axilla causing hyperextension of knees.
- Proximal end of tibia is displaced anteriorly and laterally on femur.
- Congenital absence of cruciate ligament and fibrosis of quadriceps and fascia lata is seen.
- Patella is small or absent and has fibrous adhesion to the femur.

Clinical Features

Congenital hyper extension (genu recurvatum) is the most common presentation.

Clinical appearance is alarming and has been described as **"knees on back wards".**

In most cases reduction of deformity is possible but the knees cannot be brought into flexion.

Associated Disorders

- Larsen's syndrome/Ehler's Danlos syndrome/Streeter's syndrome
- Myelodysplasia
- Arthrogryposis Multiplex Congenita
- DDH (ipsilateral)
- CTEV (Congenital Talipes Equino Varus)

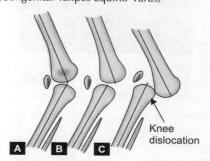

Figs. 18.18A to C: Congenital dislocation of knee–genu recurvatum

Treatment: Conservative if can be reduced and can achieve knee flexion up to 90 degrees. Surgery if persistent dislocation.

MULTIPLE CHOICE QUESTION

1. Commonest presentation of congenital dislocation of knee is: *(AIIMS Sept 1996)*
   - A. Varus
   - B. Valgus
   - C. Flexion
   - D. Hyperextension

Ans. is 'D' Hyperextension
   - The patient presents with hyperextension deformity of the knee.

GENU VALGUM (KNOCK KNEE)

It is abnormal approximation of knees with abnormally divergent ankles. It can be estimated by measuring the distance between the medial malleolus, when the knees are touching with the patella facing forwards; it is usually < 8 cm. Valgus alignment of lower extremities is normal in child between 2 and 8 years of age (Known as physiological valgus and is maximum between 2 and 4 years).

Causes

1. **Idiopathic (Physiological is most common).**
2. Post-traumatic (Lateral Side) Fractures of the lateral condyles of tibia or femur (arrest of growth on lateral side).
3. Post-infection
4. *Neoplastic:*
5. Metabolic bone disease Rickets (mostly renal osteodystrophy type is most likely to produce valgus as it is acquired in physiological valgus age group).
6. Rheumatoid arthritis, osteoarthritis of lateral compartment of knee, charcot's disease and paralytic disease are other causes seen in adults.
7. **Usually OA Causes Genu Varum and RA causes Genu Valgum**

Treatment

After 8 years age, correction of excessive physiological genu valgum may be indicated when there is gait disturbance, difficulty in running, knee discomfort, patellar malalignment, evidence of ligamentous instability or excessive cosmetic concern.

In children who have significant growth remaining (boys <12 years girls <10 years), reversible or transient hemiepiphysiodesis by staples is done. Corrective osteotomy for excessive genu valgus is appropriate when the patient present near or after skeletal maturity. It is mostly close wedge osteotomy in the distal femur.

MULTIPLE CHOICE QUESTIONS

1. A 7-year-old young boy, had fracture of lateral condyle of femur. He developed malunion as the fracture was not reduced anatomically. Malunion will produce: *(AI 2002)*
   - A. Genu valgum
   - B. Genu varum
   - C. Genu recurvatum
   - D. Dislocation of knee

Ans. is 'A' Genu valgum
   - Injury to lateral femoral condyle causes genu valgum and injury to medial femoral condyle causes genu varum.

2. Most common cause of genu valgum in children is:
   - A. Osteoarthritis
   - B. Rickets *(AIIMS Nov 1993)*
   - C. Paget's disease
   - D. Rheumatoid arthritis

Ans. is 'B' Rickets
   - Commonest type of genu valgum is idiopathic.
   - Amongst the given options, most common cause of genu valgum in children is rickets.

GENU VARUM (BOW-LEGS)

- Knee are abnormally divergent and ankles approximated. Bilateral bow legs can be estimated by measuring the **distance between the medial malleoli when heels are touching; it should be < 6 cm to label as Genu Varum. Normally 8 cm.**
- A normal children show maximum varus at 6 months to **1 year** of age, neutral alignment by 1-1/2 to 2 years of age, maximum genu valgum (8°) at 4 years of age, and a gradual decrease in genu valgum to 6 degrees by 11 years of age.
- The presence of genu varum after 2 years of age can be considered abnormal, as spontaneous resolution of the varus to neutral tibio femoral alignment by 2 years of age and to adult valgus alignment after 3 years of age is well documented.
- The causes of genu varum are similar to genu valgum except that the defective growth is on the medial side.

Two Important Causes are Discussed Below

- **Physiological genu varum,** which remains the most common etiology, even in a deformity that is slow to resolve and appears to be pathological. It is a deformity with tibio femoral angle of at least 10 degrees of varus, a radiologically normal appearing growth plate, medial bowing of the proximal tibia and often of the distal femur. The legs of most newborns are bowed, with 10–15 degrees of varus angulation. When the infant begins to stand and walk the bowing may appear more prominent and often appears to involve both the tibia and distal femur. Radiograph may be indicated if the varus deformity persists beyond 2 years of age or progresses.
- **Tibia vara** is defined as growth retardation at the medial aspect of proximal tibial epiphysis and physis usually resulting in progressive bow leg. Two forms of deformity are

  Blount distinguished, according to age at onset, two types of tibia vara: infantile, which begins before 8 years of age, and adolescent, which begins after 8 years of age but before skeletal maturity. **Nowadays following classification is followed:**

  1. **Infantile tibia vara (Blount's disease)** in which patient is <3 years old at the onset of condition (more common). It is characterized by abrupt angulation just below the proximal physis, an irregular physeal line, a wedge shaped epiphysis, and a beak like medial metaphysis. Apparent lateral subluxation of proximal tibia is often present. The triad of Blounts is Tibia vara, Genu Recurvatum (hyperextension), and internal tibial torsion (internal rotation of tibia). Siffert-Kartz Sign (Postero-medial Instability of Knee is seen)

     Metaphysio-diaphyseal angle is measured and angle more than 11 degrees require close observation

  2. **Late onset tibia vara** includes Juvenile form occurring between 4 and 10 years of age and adolescent form occurring after 10 years of age.

Non-physiological causes of genu varum, include skeletal dysplasia (e.g. metaphyseal chondrodysplasia, spondyloepiphyseal dysplasia, multiple epiphyseal dysplasia, achondroplasia), metabolic diseases (e.g. renal osteodystrophy, vit D resistant rickets), post traumatic deformity, post infectious sequelae, and proximal focal fibrocartilaginous dysplasia. In patients with familial hypophosphatemic rickets, the bone disease is active during early infancy, when physiological varus is present.

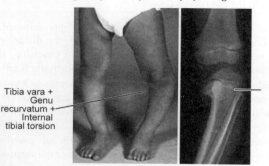

Fig. 18.19: Blount's disease

Siffert—Kartz Sign

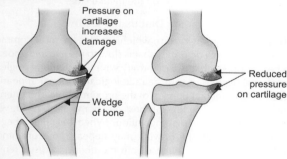

Fig. 18.20: Osteotomy to correct varus in Blount's

- If the child is between 3–4 years of age HKAFOs, i.e. hip knee ankle foot orthosis, medial upright elastic Blount's brace especially if there is only unilateral involvement. Full time orthotic treatment (i.e. 23 hours a day) is traditional, so that the knee is fully protected during the day.
- Surgical overcorrection of mechanical axis to at least 5 degrees valgus, with lateral translation of distal osteotomy fragment achieved by 4 years of age is believed to be optimal. The risk of delaying corrective osteotomy (even few months) past the critical age of 4 years can result in failure to achieve permanent reversal of the inhibition of proximal medial physis.
- High tibial osteotomy just distal to the patellar tendon insertion with fibular osteotomy in proximal third diaphysis is recommended.

MULTIPLE CHOICE QUESTIONS

1. **Characteristic of blounts disease:** (DNB June 2017)
   A. Genu valgum
   B. Genu varus
   C. Coxa vara
   D. Coxa valgus
   Ans. is 'B' Genu varus

2. **Blount's diseases in a bowleg deformity due to:** (TN 2011, 2014)
   A. Defect in posteromedial part of upper tibial epiphysis
   B. Endocrinopathy
   C. Recovery stage of rickets
   D. Deformity in proximal tibia
   Ans. is 'A' Defect in posteromedial part of upper tibial epiphysis

3. **Varus is:** (NEET Pattern 2012)
   A. Distal part towards midline
   B. Distal part away from the midline
   C. Proximal part towards midline
   D. Proximal part away from midline
   Ans. is 'A' Distal part towards midline

4. **Charlie chaplin gait is seen in:** (NEET Pattern 2012)
   A. CDH
   B. Congenital coxa vara
   C. Genu valgum
   D. External tibial torsion
   Ans. is 'D' External tibial torsion

5. **Blount's disease is:** (AIPG 2011, AIIMS Nov 2010, PGI June 2K)
   A. Genu valgus   B. Tibia vara
   C. Flat foot   D. Genu recurvatum
   Ans. is 'B > D' Tibia vara > Genu recurvatum

6. **Which statement is true regarding genu varum (bowleg)?** (PGI Dec 01)
   A. In infants, it may be considered normal
   B. Occurs due to epiphyseal dysplasia
   C. Seldom associated with tibial angulation
   D. Affects only tibia but never femur
   Ans. is 'A' In infants, it may be considered normal; 'B' Occurs due to epiphyseal dysplasia and 'C' Seldom associated with tibial angulation

7. **Critical age of osteotomy for genu varum is:** (JIPMER 98, AMU 97)
   A. 4 years   B. 6 years
   C. 8 years   D. 10 years
   Ans. is 'A' 4 years

8. **True regarding genu varum is:** (JIPMER 95, PGI 94)
   A. Orthosis is a must only during weight bearing
   B. Orthosis is recommended during day time
   C. Orthosis is recommended during night time
   D. Orthosis is recommended full time
   Ans. is 'D' Orthosis is recommended full time

ROCKER BOTTOM FOOT

Rocker bottom foot, is a foot with a **convex plantar surface** with a apex of convexity at the talar head. **Talus is vertical** so that its head forms the most prominent part of the sole. The fore foot is deviated outward and dorsally. It may be produced by Congenital vertical talus (congenital convex pes valgus or teratological dorsolateral dislocation of talocalcaneonavicular joint) which may be present alone or more commonly associated with myelomeningocele, arthrogryposis, prune belly syndrome, spinal muscular atrophy, neurofibromatosis, CDH, and with trisomy 13–15 and 18.

Pediatric Orthopedics

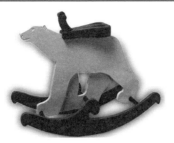

Fig. 18.21: Rocker bottom

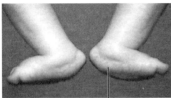

Fig. 18.22: Rocker bottom foot

Causes

1. **Oblique/Vertical talus**
2. **Improper correction of CTEV**, i.e. forceful correction of equinus by dorsiflexion before adduction, varus and inversion may actually cause movement at mid tarsal joint (not at ankle joint) producing rocker bottom foot.

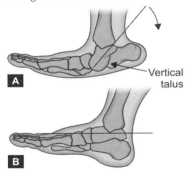

Figs. 18.23A and B: (A) Vertical talus; (B) Normal talus

Rx* Grice procedure is extra-articular arthrodesis of subtalar (talocalcaneal) joint, done for Congenital Vertical Talus.

MULTIPLE CHOICE QUESTIONS

1. Rocker bottom foot is due to: *(NEET Pattern 2013)*
   A. Over treatment of CTEV
   B. Malunited fracture calcaneum
   C. Horizontal talus
   D. Neural tube defect
   Ans. is 'A' Over treatment of CTEV

2. Rocker bottom foot is seen in: *(PGI Dec 2008)*
   A. Congenital vertical talus
   B. Excessive correction of Grice procedure
   C. Arthrogryposis
   D. Holding club foot in too long corrected position
   E. Force dorsiflexion against equinus varus
   Ans. is 'A' Congenital vertical talus; 'C' Arthrogryposis; 'D' Holding club foot in too long corrected position and 'E' Force dorsiflexion against equinus varus

3. Nail patella syndrome the patella is: *NEET Pattern 2012)*
   A. Small or absent   B. Larger
   C. Square   D. Triangular
   Ans. is 'A' Small or absent

CLUB FOOT/CONGENITAL TALIPES EQUINOVARUS (CTEV)

Club is a stick to play golf CTEV foot resembles it so called as club foot. Talipes is a generic term for foot deformity that centers around the talus (Talipes = talus and pes = foot). In its most characteristic form there are usually said to be four elements of deformity Equinus of ankle, inversion of foot, adduction of fore foot and medial rotation of tibia. **In India the most common congenital anomaly is CTEV where as in western countries DDH is the commonest.**

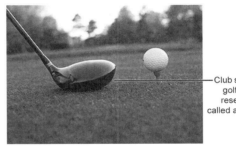

Fig. 18.24: Club

Etiology and Associated Anomalies

- Idiopathic (most common)
- Secondary club foot:
  1. Neurological disorders and neural tube defects, e.g. myelonieningocele and spinal dysraphism Paralytic disorder (muscular imbalance) as polio (does not present at birth), spina bifida, myelodysplasia, and Freidreich's ataxia.

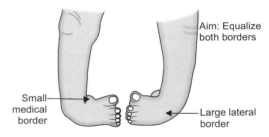

Fig. 18.25: CTEV

  2. Arthrogryposis multiplex congenita, Larsen syndrome, Sacral agenesis, tibial deficiency, constriction rings and amniotic bands
  3. Hip deformities are associated, e.g. DDH

Pathological Anatomy

- The club foot characteristically involves foot ankle and leg. Deformities of foot may be in the hind foot (ankle and subtalar joints), mid foot (mid tarsal, i.e. talonavicular and calcaneocuboid joints) and forefoot.
- **Talo calcaneo navicular joint complex** is area involved in pathomechanics of all hind foot and mid foot deformities.

- Clubfoot is always associated with a permanent decrease in calf circumference related to fibrosis of calf musculature.
- In a new born child it is possible to dorsiflex and evert the foot till the dorsum of foot touches anterior surface of tibia. This is not possible in CTEV. This is known as *'dorsiflexion test'* and can be used as a screening test.

Ankle (Tibio talar) Joint
Plantar flexion or Equinus

Subtalar (Talocalcaneal) Joint
Inversion

Mid tarsal (talonavicular and calcaneocuboid) Joint
- Adduction (medial subluxation) and inversion (supination) of mid and fore foot

Pirani/Dimeglio scoring is for CTEV

Pirani Scoring

Look	Feel	Move
Lateral border (0 to 1)	Talar head (0 to 1)	Equinus (0 to 1)
Medial crease (0 to 1)	Heel (0 to 1)	
Posterior crease (0 to 1)		0 (normal) → 6 (worse)

- Kites angle – AP view talocalcaneal angle.
- Normal value is 20–40 degrees (decreased in CTEV and may become parallel)

Atypical Clubfoot (Resistant clubfoot)

Short great toe/Sole Crease
  Hyperextended great toe/Heel crease
    Others (AMC, NF, Spina Bifida)
      Rigid feet
        Tight heel
SHORT-CALF

Conservative Management of CTEV

	Kites method –followed earlier	Ponsetti method now preferred
At birth	Manipulation by mother initial weeks	Manipulation and cast
Change of cast	Every 2 weeks	Weekly
Correction order	C-A-V-E	C-AV-E
Fulcrum while manipulating	Calcaneocuboid joint	Head of talus
Duration of treatment	6–9 months	6–8 weeks

Note: First cast in CTEV is applied in supination to correct **c**avus. Subsequently in kites one deformity is corrected at a time, **a**dduction first than **v**arus and then **e**quinus (CAVE).

In ponsetti method adduction and Varus are corrected simultaneously and Equinus is corrected at last.

Thus in Kites method one deformity is corrected at a time but in ponsetti adduction and varus are corrected simultaneously, *equinus is corrected at end in both*.

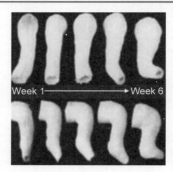

Fig. 18.26: Sequential correction

Cavus increased plantar arch
  Adduction (Adduction of forefoot and mid foot.)
    Varus or Inversion (Inversion of fore, mid and hind foot.)
      Equinus (Equinus (plantar flexion) of ankle)
        (Most Resistant)
CAVE (Order of Correction of CTEV)

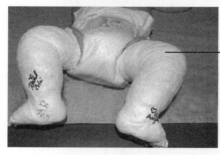

Fig. 18.27: Above knee CTEV cast

Above knee cast: As rule of splintage immobilize one joint above one joint below and to correct ankle equinus knee has to be immobilized thus above knee cast.

Above knee cast: As rule of splintage immobilize one joint above one joint below and to correct ankle equinus knee has to be immobilized thus above knee cast.

If this order of correction is not followed and the equinus is corrected before adduction and inversion by forcefully dorsiflexing the foot, it may actually move at mid tarsal joints (not at ankle joint) producing rocker bottom deformity.

Even if the correction is achieved maintenance of foot in **Dennis Brown splint** is required whole time up to 1 year and after 1 year day time CTEV shoes and night time Dennis brown splint is used up to 7 years of age. (as recurrence after 7 years of age is not known).

The objective is to achieve (ideally) overcorrection. Sometimes it may be necessary to perform percutaneous TendoAchilles lengthening (Tenotomy) in order to overcome equinus (Ponsetti method).

Operative Treatment

The results of early operation, in particular neonatal surgery, have not been shown to be better than those of late surgery. Delaying surgery until the child is near walking age has the advantage of operating of larger foot (making surgery easier).

Posteromedial soft tissue release, (Turcos) is best done at young age (1–3 years).

Posterior release or complete subtalar release can also be performed.

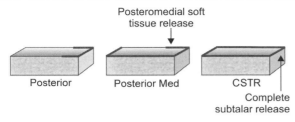

Fig. 18.28: Soft tissue releases

But in children older than 3 years of age lateral column shortening procedures are often performed in conjunction with posteromedial soft tissue release.

3–8 years

Soft tissue release together with shortening of lateral side of foot by

Lichtblau's Procedure (i.e. Shortening of calcaneal neck proximal to calcaneocuboid joint). Preferred in <6 years of age as calcaneocuboid fusion is more difficult to achieve in this age.

Evan-Dillwyn Procedure (i.e. resection and fusion of calcaneocuboid joint).

In 3–8 years of age (esp> 6 years) is ideal procedure.

Dwyer's osteotomy of calcaneum is done to **correct calcaneal varus in >5 years.**

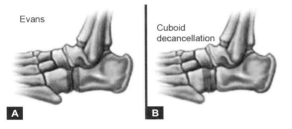

Figs. 18.29A and B: Lateral column shortening

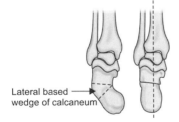

Fig. 18.30: Dwyers osteotomy to correct heel varus (>5 yrs)

8–10 years

Wedge Tarsectomy is done as deformity is more and requires multiple bones to be removed.

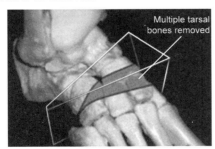

Fig. 18.31: Wedge tarsectomy (8–10 yrs)

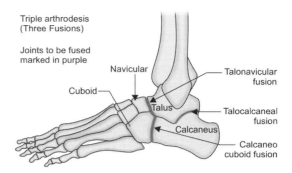

Fig. 18.32: Triple arthrodesis (>10 yrs)

> 10 years

Triple arthrodesis is necessary for recurrent **or** persistent clubfoot deformity in older children (chronic cases). It is best done at > 10 years of age when foot growth is complete and the bones are ossified to achieve good fusion.

It involves fusion of three joints: **TN: Talonavicular; TC: Talocalcaneal; CC: Calcaneo-Cuboid**

- Pseudoarthrosis (most commonly of talonavicular joint) is commonest complication, which can be reduced by performing surgery after skeletal maturity and doing internal fixation.
- JESS and Ilizarov external fixators also can be used to correct deformity after skeletal maturity.
- **CTEV shoes has outer shoe raise, straight medial border and no heel it was designed by thomas.**

Note: CTEV has high chances of recurrence till 7 years of age, hence recurrence is prevented by use of Dennis Brown splint at night and CTEV shoes during day time in a walking child.

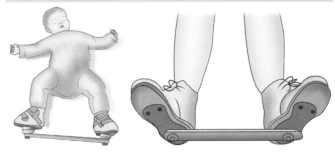

Fig. 18.33: Dennis Brown splint

MULTIPLE CHOICE QUESTIONS

1. The following muscles cause inversion of foot except:
   (AIIMS Nov 2018)
   - A. Tibialis Anterior
   - B. Tibialis Posterior
   - C. Peroneus Longus
   - D. EHL

   Ans. is 'C' Peroneus Longus

2. Pirani scoring includes all except:
   (PGI May 2017, PGI Nov 2016)
   - A. Medial crease
   - B. Protrusion of cuboid bone
   - C. Lateral crease border
   - D. Curvature of lateral
   - E. Concavity of sole

   Ans. is 'B' Protrusion of cuboid bone; 'C' Lateral crease; 'E' Concavity of sole

3. Talocalcaneonavicular joint is which type of synovial joint? *(AIIMS Nov 2017)*
   A. Ellipsoid
   B. Saddle
   C. Ball and Socket
   D. Plane

Ans. is 'C' Ball and Socket

Type of Joint	Axis	Movements	Examples
Plane/Gliding joint	Uniaxial	Gliding	Intercarpal joints, Intertarsal joints, Between articular processes of vertebrae
Hinge Joints	Uniaxial	Flexion, Extension	Elbow joints, Ankle joints, Interphalangeal joints
Pivot Joints	Uniaxial	Rotation	Median atlantoaxial joint, Superior and inferior radioulnar joints
Condylar Joints	Biaxial	Flexion, Extension, Limited rotation	Knee joints, Joints between condyles of mandible and temporal bone
Ellipsoid joints	Biaxial	Flexion, Extension, Abduction, adduction, Circumduction	Wrist joint, Metacarpophalangeal joint, Atlantoaxial joints (lateral)
Saddle joints	Multiaxial	Flexion, Extension, Abduction, adduction, Conjunct rotation	Sternoclavicular joint, First carpometacarpal joint, Calcaneocuboid joint
Ball & socket joints	Multiaxial	Flexion, Extension, Abduction, adduction, Circumduction, Rotation	Shoulder joint, Hip joint, Talocalcaneonavicular joint

4. Ponsetti technique failure in children should be managed with: *(DNB June 2017)*
   A. Posteromedial soft tissue release
   B. Anterolateral soft tissue release
   C. Triple arthrodesis
   D. Lateral closing wedge osteotomy of calcaneum

Ans. is 'A' Posteromedial soft tissue release

5. Ideal age for PMSTR is: *(DNB June 2017)*
   A. <1 year
   B. 1-3 years
   C. 3-6 years
   D. 6-9 years

Ans. is 'B' 1-3 years

6. In Ponseti technique last deformity into get corrected in CTEV: *(PGI May 2017)*
   A. Equinus
   B. Talipus
   C. Varus
   D. Cavus
   E. All deformity corrected simultaneously

Ans. is 'A' Equinus

7. CTEV shoe true is: *(NEET Dec 2016)*
   A. It is the same as normal shoe
   B. It has straight medial border
   C. It has medical shoe raise
   D. It has heel with extra length

Ans. is 'B' It has straight medial border

8. Treatment of fresh case of CTEV in newborn is usually done by: *(NEET Dec 2016)*
   A. Ponseti technique
   B. Kites technique
   C. Kochers technique
   D. Wilsons technique

Ans. is 'A' Ponseti technique

9. Dennis brown splint is used for: *(NEET Dec 2016)*
   A. CTEV
   B. Rocker bottom foot
   C. Manus valgus
   D. Manus varus

Ans. is 'A' CTEV

10. Which of the following is true about CTEV? *(NEET Dec 2016)*
    A. It is more common in females
    B. Right foot is usually more affected than the left
    C. Talus is displaced medial and plantar wards
    D. Tibia usually shows lateral torsion

Ans. is 'C' Talus is displaced medial and plantar wards

11. Which of the following is not true about the manipulation methods to correct CTEV? *(NEET Dec 2016)*
    A. Involves serial casting and below knee plaster casting
    B. In kites method deformities are corrected sequentially adduction → inversion → equinus
    C. Ponseti's technique has success rate of 90-98%
    D. Ponseti's method of correction involves cavus → adduction → heel varus → equinus

Ans. is 'A' Involves serial casting and below knee plaster casting

12. Which of the following is the management for neglected case of CTEV in a patient >10 years of age? *(NEET Dec 2016)*
    A. Triple arthrodesis
    B. Ankle arthrodesis
    C. Jess fixation
    D. Ponseti casting

Ans. is 'A' Triple arthrodesis

13. Who devised correction of CTEV by serial casting? *(AI Dec 15)*
    A. Ignacio Ponseti
    B. Gerhard Kuntscher
    C. Gavriil Ilizarov
    D. Hugh Owen Thomas

Ans. is 'A' Ignacio Ponseti

14. Club foot clinically present as what deformity? *(AI Dec 15)*
    A. Calcaneovalgus
    B. Equinovarus
    C. Equino Cavovarus
    D. Calcaneovarus

Ans. is 'C' Equino Cavovarus

15. Overcorrection of CTEV may lead to which of the following deformity? *(CET Nov 15)*
    A. Rocker bottom foot
    B. Calcaneovalgus
    C. Metatarsus Adductus
    D. Hammer toe

Ans. is 'A' Rocker bottom foot

16. All of the following are described procedures for CTEV except: *(CET Nov 15)*
    A. Dwyer's osteotomy
    B. Posteromedial soft tissue release
    C. Triple Arthrodesis
    D. Salter's osteotomy

Ans. is 'D' Salter's osteotomy

17. All of the following are done for management of clubfoot at birth except: *(CET Nov 15)*
    A. Manipulation
    B. Serial Casting
    C. Recording the deformity to see improvements serially
    D. Posteromedial soft tissue release

Ans. is 'D' Posteromedial soft tissue release

Pediatric Orthopedics

18. The last deformity to be corrected by Ponsetti method for CTEV is: *(CET July 16)*
    A. Heel Varus
    B. Equinus
    C. Foot Adduction
    D. Cavus
Ans. is 'B' Equinus

19. The typical deformity in CTEV is: *(NEET 2015)*
    A. Ankle equinus
    B. Subtalar inversion
    C. Forefoot adduction
    D. All of the above
Ans. is 'D' All of the above

20. True about Atypical CTEV:
    (PGI May 2015) (add mnemonic from FB)
    A. Foot is flexed downward
    B. Sole crease are not found
    C. Difficult to treat than typical variety
    D. May occur due to neurological disorder
    E. May be associated with Meningomyelocele
Ans. is 'A' Foot is flexed downward; 'C' Difficult to treat than typical variety; 'D' May occur due to neurological disorder; and 'E' May be associated with Meningomyelocele

21. What is the best management of CTEV in newborn?
    A. Manipulation alone *(JIPMER 2014)*
    B. Manipulation and corrective splint
    C. Corrective surgery
    D. Wait and watch
Ans. is 'B' Manipulation and corrective splint

22. In correction of CTEV, which one of the following deformities resists?
    A. Equinus
    B. Varus
    C. Adduction
    D. Cavus
Ans. is 'A' Equinus.

23. True about Clubfoot: *(PGI Nov 2014)*
    A. Abduction of forefoot
    B. Associated with breech presentation
    C. Dennis-Brown splint used
    D. Adduction of forefoot
    E. Associated with spina bifida
Ans. is 'C' Dennis-Brown splint used; 'D' Adduction of forefoot; and 'E' Associated with spina bifida

24. Causes of secondary clubfoot at birth are all except:
    A. Idiopathic *(AIIMS Nov 2013)*
    B. Arthrogryposis Multiplex Congenita
    C. Poliomyelitis
    D. Spina bifida
Ans. is 'C' Poliomyelitis
   – Poliomyelitis does not cause clubfoot at birth.

25. Splint used in CTEV after correction: *NEET Pattern 2013)*
    A. Bohler-Brown splint
    B. Thomas splint
    C. Dennis Brown splint
    D. None of the above
Ans. is 'C' Dennis Brown splint

26. In neglected cases of CTEV, joint fused are:
    (NEET Pattern 2012)
    A. Calcaneocuboid, talonavicular and talocalcaneal
    B. Tibiotalar, calcaneocuboid and talonavicular
    C. Ankle joint, calcaneocuboid and talonavicular
    D. None of the above
Ans. is 'A' Calcaneocuboid, talonavicular and talocalcaneal

27. Most common cause of CTEV: *(NEET Pattern 2013)*
    A. Arthrogryposis multiplex congenita
    B. Spina bifida
    C. Idiopathic
    D. Neural tube defect
Ans. is 'C' Idiopathic

28. Most common congenital anamoly in India:
    A. CTEV
    B. DDH *(NEET Pattern 2012)*
    C. Genu Valgum
    D. Hallux valgus
Ans. is 'A' CTEV

29. Single step Posteromedial release is: *(NEET Pattern 2012)*
    A. Ponsetti
    B. Kites
    C. Turcos
    D. Cincinnati
Ans. is 'C' Turcos

30. CTEV shoe was designed by: *(NEET Pattern 2012)*
    A. Kites
    B. Ponsetti
    C. Turcos
    D. Thomas
Ans. is 'D' Thomas

31. CTEV surgery at 2 years of age: *(NEET Pattern 2012)*
    A. No surgery
    B. Soft tissue release
    C. Arthrodesis
    D. Bone osteotomy
Ans. is 'B' Soft tissue release

32. A newborn child presents with inverted foot and the dorsum of the foot can not touch the anterior tibia. The most probable diagnosis: *(AIIMS May 2012, Nov 2010)*
    A. Congenital vertical talus
    B. Arthrogryposis multiplex congenita
    C. Congenital talipes equino varus
    D. PES planus
Ans. is 'C' Congenital talipes equino varus

33. The ideal treatment of bilateral idiopathic Clubfoot in a newborn is:
    (AI 2006, UP 99, AIIMS Dec 95, Nov 93, Andhra 93, BHU 87)
    A. Manipulation by mother
    B. Manipulation and dennis brown splint
    C. Manipulation and casts
    D. Surgical release
Ans. is 'C' Manipulation and casts

34. Triple arthrodesis involves: *(AI 2001)*
    A. Calcaneocuboid, talonavicular and talocalcaneal
    B. Tibiotalar, calcaneocuboid and talonavicular
    C. Ankle joint, calcaneocuboid and talonavicular
    D. None of the above
Ans. is 'A' Calcaneocuboid, talonavicular and talocalcaneal

35. CTEV is caused by: *(PGI Dec 01, PGI June 01)*
    A. Neurological disorder
    B. Idiopathic
    C. Spina fibida
    D. Cubitus varus
    E. Arthrogryposis multiplex
Ans. is 'A' Neurological disorder; 'B' Idiopathic; 'C' Spina fibida and 'E' Arthrogryposis multiplex

36. The club foot characteristically involves: *(Bihar 1999)*
    A. Foot and ankle
    B. Foot, ankle and leg
    C. Foot only
    D. Foot, ankle, leg and knee joint
Ans. is 'B' Foot, ankle and leg

37. Most important pathology in club foot is:
    (Bihar 1999, 88, TN 90)
    A. Congenital talonavicular dislocation
    B. Tightening of Tendoachilles
    C. Calcaneal fracture
    D. Lateral derangement
Ans. is 'A' Congenital talonavicular dislocation

38. A Child 3 years of age is treated for CTEV by: (TN 97)
    A. Triple arthrodesis
    B. Posteromedial soft tissue release
    C. Lateral wedge resection
    D. Tendo achilles lengthening and posterior capsulatomy
Ans. is 'B' Posteromedial soft tissue release

39. Treatment for chronic cases of club foot is:
    (JIPMER 95, PGI 78, 83)
    A. Triple arthrodesis
    B. Dorso medial release
    C. Amputation
    D. None
Ans. is 'A' Triple arthrodesis

40. In correction of clubfoot by manipulation which deformity should be corrected first? (AMU 95)
    A. Forefoot adduction
    B. Varus
    C. Upper end tibia
    D. Calcaneum
Ans. is 'A' Forefoot adduction

41. Triple arthrodesis is NOT done before-skeletal maturation because of: (AIIMS 94)
    A. Shortening of foot
    B. Recurrence of deformity
    C. Inadequate fusion
    D. Complete correction not possible
Ans. is 'C' Inadequate fusion
    – Triple arthrodesis is usually done after 10–12 years as the growth of foot is complete and the bones of foot are completely ossified. Before this age bones are not completely ossified and cartilaginous, therefore fusion (arthrodesis) may not be adequate.

42. The most common congenital anomaly among the following is encountered in our country: (TN 94)
    A. Congenital Pseudoartosis of tibia
    B. Congenital dislocation of hip
    C. Congenital talipes equino varus
    D. Multiple congenital contractures
Ans. is 'C' Congenital talipes equino varus
    CTEV is the commonest and most important congenital deformity of the foot in India.

43. 'Pseudoarthrosis' in Triple fusion is seen at the joint of:
    (Delhi 1990)
    A. Calcaneocuboid
    B. Calcaneonavicular
    C. Naviculocuboid
    D. Talonavicular
Ans. is 'D' Talonavicular

RADIAL CLUB HAND

Absent or deficiency in Radius and associated with inadequately developed Thumb also called as Radial Club Hand

Absent Radius or thumb is associated with
- Trisomy 13,18
- Fanconis syndrome
- **Tar syndrome (thrombocytopenia absent radius)**
- Vater syndrome (vertebral anomalies, anorectal malformation/ Tracheo-oesophageal fistula/esophageal atresia/radial club hand/renal agenesis).
- **Holt oram syndrome (cardiac defects with absent radius)**
- Ectodermal dysplasia
- Very rarely leukemias
- Order of investigations in a patient with absent radius is Echocardiography> platelets count >karyotyping>bone marrow.

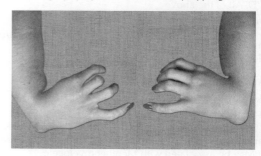

Fig. 18.34: Bilateral Radial Club hand

Treatment
1. Centralization of ulna
2. Pollicization is transposition of finger to replace (reconstruct) absent thumb
   This reconstruction of thumb is usually done by migrating index finger to the position of thumb in a patient with congenital absence or marked hypoplasia of thumb.

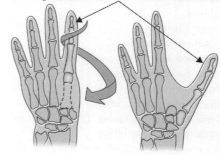

Fig. 18.35: Pollicization

3. Tendon transfers.

MULTIPLE CHOICE QUESTION

1. Pollicization is: (AI 08)
    A. Amputation of thumb
    B. Equalization of fingers
    C. Toe to thumb transplantation
    D. Reconstruction of thumb
Ans. is 'D' Reconstruction of thumb

FRACTURES IN CHILDREN

The immature skeleton has several unique properties that affect the management of injuries in children. These properties include thicker periosteum, soft bones, an increased resiliency to stress, an increased potential to remodel, shorter healing times, and the

presence of a physis. This can lead to some characteristic fracture patterns in pediatric population.
- **Distal radius and ulna** is the most common site of fracture in children accounting for nearly a quarter of fracture.
- 2nd in frequency is **Hand injury**
- 3rd in frequency are **elbow injuries** amongst them supracondylar fracture humerus are most common and
- 4th common is **clavicle fracture**
- Please remember that clavicle is the most common fractured bone in adults and during birth.
  * Dislocations and comminuted fractures are rare in children.

Remember most common joint to dislocate in adults is shoulder but in children is Elbow.

Plastic Deformation

- Immature bone is weaker in bending strength but absorbs more energy prior to fracture. This may result in permanent deformation of bone **(without fracture)** known as plastic deformation.
- It is most common in forearm particularly ulna.
- Reduction (correction of deformity) is recommended, if there is (1) >20 degrees of angulation, if a child is >4 years old and has either a (2) clinically evident deformity or (3) limitation of pronation and supination.

Buckle (Torus) Fracture

- It is so called, because of its resemblance to the base of an architectural column.
- Most commonly occurs at the **transition between metaphysis and diaphysis where buckling of cortex takes place.**

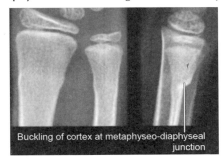

Fig. 18.36: Torus fracture

Greenstick Fractures

- The **cortex in tension fractures completely** while the **cortex in compression remain intact** but frequently undergo plastic deformation.

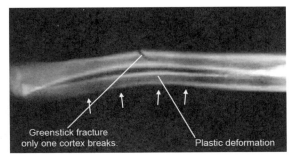

Fig. 18.37: Greenstick fracture and plastic deformation

So it is an incomplete fracture and it is necessary to complete the fracture on the intact compression side for reduction and POP application.

Toddler's Fracture

It is a fracture in ambulatory child (9 months –3 years).
It is spiral or oblique fracture of lower 2/3 of tibia (Undisplaced). Fibula and periosteum is intact. The mode of trauma is twisting injury.

Remodeling Potential in Children

Remodeling of bone is best (maximum) for metaphyseal angulation deformity and least (worst) for diaphyseal rotation deformity.

Amount of Growth Remaining

Skeletal age is most important factor. Lesser the age, more the ability.

Growth Potential of that Physis

80% of humerus growth comes from the proximal physis. So deformity associated with proximal humerus fracture is much likely to remodel than the deformity associated with distal humerus fractures.

Battered Baby Syndrome/Shaken Infant Syndrome/Infantile Whiplash Syndrome

- It is a term used to define a clinical condition in young children usually under 3 years of age who have received **non accidental violence or injury,** on one or more occasions at the hands of an adult responsible for child's welfare.
- This syndrome must be considered in any child
  i. **In whom degree** and type **of injury is at variance with the history given.**
  ii. When injuries of different ages and in different stages of healing are found.
  iii. **When there is purposeful delay in seeking medical attention despite serious injury.**
  iv. *Who exhibits evidence of fracture of any bone, subdural hematoma, failure to thrive, soft tissue swelling or skin bruising (ecchymosis).*

Fractures Characteristics

1. **A classic finding is a chip fracture in which a corner of the metaphysis of a long bone is torn off with damage to epiphysis and periosteum.**
2. **Metaphyseal bucket handle fractures are seen.**
   1 and 2 are the most characteristic fractures
3. Inflicted fractures of the shaft are more likely to *be spiral* rather than transverse they are seen in this frequency — femur > humerus . tibia.
4. Subepiphyseal microfractures are seen (not seen on X-rays—seen on MRI).
5. Nobbing fractures are seen in the ribs due to shaking of the child.
6. Skull has egg shell fractures, occipital impression fractures and fractures crossing the suture line.
7. The imaging in this syndrome involves good quality skeletal survey most importantly involving X-rays of skull, chest and extremities. Babygram is not preferred

MULTIPLE CHOICE QUESTIONS

1. Common fractures in children are all except:
   (NEET Pattern 2013)
   A. Lateral condyle humerus   B. Supracondylar humerus
   C. Fracture of hand   D. Radius-ulna fracture
   Ans. is 'A' Lateral condyle humerus
   Order of fracture in children are
   – Distal forearm (23.3%)
   – Hand (20.1%)
   – Elbow 12% (Supracondylar humerus > Lateral Condyle Humerus)
   – Clavicle 6.4%

2. Which of the following statement is/are correct about fracture management in children?   (PGI MAY 2018)
   A. Supracondylar fracture of humerus can be managed by closed reduction
   B. Lateral condylar fracture of humerus is known as fracture of necessity
   C. Lateral condylar fracture of humerus is managed by open reduction and screwing
   D. Forearm fracture in children can be managed by closed reduction and casting
   E. Femoral neck fracture in adults is managed by surgery and 3 screws
   Ans. 'A' Supracondylar fracture of humerus can be managed by closed reduction; 'B' Lateral condylar fracture of humerus is known as fracture of necessity; 'C' Lateral condylar fracture of humerus is managed by open reduction and screwing; 'D' Forearm fracture in children can be managed by closed reduction and casting; & 'E' Femoral neck fracture in adults is managed by surgery and 3 screws

3. A child falls from a chair. Complains of pain in the mid leg. No visible deformity. He is unable to bear his weight on standing. What is the diagnosis?
   (JIPMER 2015)
   A. Oblique fracture   B. Spiral fracture
   C. Comminuted fracture   D. Fracture of epiphysis
   Ans. 'B' Spiral fracture

4. All are incomplete fracture in children except:
   (JIPMER Dec 2016)
   A. Greenstick fracture   B. Incremental
   C. Torus fracture   D. Plastic
   Ans. is 'B' Incremental

5. Common fractures in childhood are all except:
   (NEET Dec 2016)
   A. Forearm bone fracture
   B. Fracture supracondylar humerus
   C. Spiral fracture of shaft tibia
   D. Fracture of hand bones
   Ans. is 'C' Spiral fracture of shaft tibia

6. Child abuse all the following are X-ray feature except:
   A. Metaphyseal Corner fracture   (AIIMS Nov 16)
   B. Metaphyseal bucket handle fracture
   C. Metaphyseal fragment displacement
   D. Subepiphyseal microfractures
   Ans. is 'D' Subepiphyseal microfractures
   These are seen on MRI not X-rays.

7. A 6-year-child is brought to emergency with complete of severe pain in aim after a fall, immediate X-ray done shows fracture distal radius and ulna. Which of the following term best describes the fracture?
   (AI 2016)

   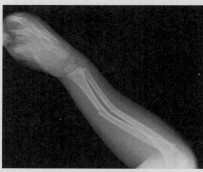

   A. Torus   B. Greenstick
   C. Barton's   D. Colles
   Ans. is 'B' Greenstick

8. A 4-year-old child presented to the clinic with a history off all on outstretched hand Radiographs revealed a broken anterior cortex with an intact posterior cortex of the radius with an exaggerated bowing of the radius. The fracture sustained is known as: (AI Dec 15)
   A. Torus Fracture
   B. Greenstick fracture
   C. Galeazzi fracture
   D. Monteggia fracture dislocation
   Ans. is 'B' Greenstick fracture

9. Greenstick fractures are seen in: (AI Dec 15)
   A. Children   B. Elderly
   C. Young adults   D. Common in all age groups
   Ans. is 'A' Children

10. Which of the following is true about fracture in children?
    A. Brittle bone   (JIPMER 2015)
    B. Angulation and rotation not tolerated
    C. Immobilization leads to fixity of adjacent joints
    D. Complete fracture is more common than greenstick
    Ans. is 'B' Angulation and rotation not tolerated

11. Most common bone to be fractured in children is:
    A. Distal radius   B. Clavicle   (NEET 2015)
    C. Supracondylar humerus   D. Radius/ulna
    Ans. is 'D' Radius/ulna

12. Madelung's deformity involves: (NEET Pattern 2013)
    A. Humerus   B. Proximal ulna
    C. Distal radius   D. Carpals
    Ans. is 'C' Distal radius

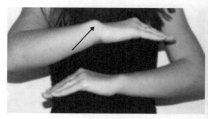 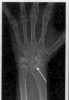 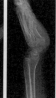

Distal radius joint surface is inclined anteriorly and towards ulna. There is deficiency of volar and ulnar part of distal radius. The ulnar head becomes prominent. The deformity is more common in females and is often bilateral. The functions are good and usually don't require intervention.

In case there is a requirement radial osteotomy and excision of ulnar head can be done.

13. Green stick fracture is: (NEET Pattern 2012)
    A. Fracture in adults
    B. Complete fracture
    C. Incomplete fracture
    D. Fracture spine

Ans. is 'C' Incomplete fracture

14. A 6-year-old child falls in right-sided forearm region and develops fracture in dorsal surface of mid region of radius. The best treatment is: (UP 08)
    A. Antibiotics and sedative
    B. Bone plating and external fixation
    C. Slab with wait for bone imperfect
    D. Break the cortex other side and immobilization by POP

Ans. is 'D' Break the cortex other side and immobilization by POP

15. An 8-year-old child is brought by parents to the casualty with a spiral fracture of Femur and varying degree of Ecchymosis all over body. The etiology is: (AIIMS Nov 2005, AI 2000)
    A. Hit and run accident
    B. Battered baby syndrome
    C. Hockey stick injury
    D. Osteogenesis imperfect

Ans. is 'B' Battered baby syndrome

16. In children, all are true except: (AI 2000)
    A. Dislocations are rare
    B. Comminuted fractures are common
    C. Thick periosteum
    D. Soft bones

Ans. is 'B' Comminuted fractures are common

17. Which statements pertaining to green stick fracture is correct? (Andhra 1999, AI 93, AIIMS 96)
    A. Any fracture in child
    B. Is generally incomplete
    C. Fracture only in rickets children
    D. All of the above

Ans. is 'B' Is generally incomplete

18. In children best remodelling is seen in fracture with: (AIIMS Feb 1997)
    A. Angulation in diaphysis
    B. Angulation in metaphysis
    C. Rotation in diaphysis
    D. Rotation in metaphysic

Ans. is 'B' Angulation in metaphysis

19. Which is the commonest fracture in children?
    A. Fracture clavicle (PGI 96, AI 95)
    B. Supracondylar fracture
    C. Green stick fracture of lower end of radius
    D. All of the above

Ans. is 'C' Green stick fracture of lower end of radius

EPIPHYSEAL INJURY

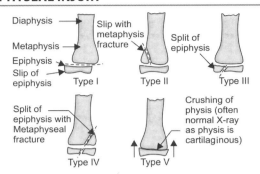

Fig. 18.38: Salter-Harris classification for epiphyseal injury

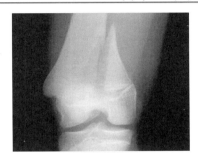

Fig. 18.39: Salter-Harris type 2

Salter-Harris types	Feature
I	Fracture line is entirely with in Physis causing epiphyseal slip
II	Fracture line extends from physis into the Metaphysis (Thurston-Holland's fragment sign)
III	Fracture line extends from physis into the Epiphysis causing epiphyseal split
IV	Fracture line extends across the Epiphysis, (articular surface), Physis, and metaphysis
V	Crush injury of physis with initially normal X-rays

Traumatic conditions that heal and subsequently have secondary presentation

- Physeal injury–progressive deformity with delayed appearance. (Deformity Appearing shortly (within months) after trauma- Malunited fracture).
- Sudecks dystrophy–Fracture heals and subsequently presents with causalgia
- Tardy ulnar nerve palsy with increasing deformity at elbow, e.g. cubitus valgus
- Avascular necrosis appearing 3–6 months after trauma
- Secondary osteoarthritis after trauma may take years to manifest.

EPIPHYSEAL APPEARANCE ON RADIOLOGY FOR DIAGNOSIS

Epiphyseal Enlargement

Most common causes of epiphyseal enlargement are chronic inflammation (e.g. JRA) due to chronic increase in blood flow. Causes of Epiphyseal enlargement are:

a. **Solitary**
   i. *Post inflammatory (JRA, Septic arthritis)*
   ii. *Perthes disease (in repair stage)*

iii. **Hemophilia (Hemophilic arthropathy)**
iv. *Turner syndrome*
v. *Trevor disease (Dysplasia epiphysealis hemimelica)*
b. **Generalized**
   i. Hyperthyroidism
   ii. Acromegaly or cerebral gigantism
   iii. Spondyloepiphyseal dysplasia
   iv. Rickets
   v. McCune-Albright syndrome

Epipyseal dysgenesis/Fragmented/punctate epiphysis Hypothyroidism.

MULTIPLE CHOICE QUESTIONS

1. Which of the following is false regarding Salter Harris classification? *(NEET Dec 2016)*
   A. Classifies epiphyseal injuries
   B. Type II is the most common type of epiphyseal injury
   C. Type IV classifies injury through epiphysis, physis, metaphysis
   D. Type V is the perichondrial ring injury

Ans. is 'D' Type V is the perichondrial ring injury

2. Salter-Harris classification is used for: *(AI Dec 15)*
   A. Supracondylar humerus fractures in children
   B. Estimation of growth of the physes
   C. Physeal injuries
   D. Severity of degloving injuries to the limb

Ans. is 'C' Physeal injuries

3. A 4 year-old-child suffered from a fall on outstretched band. X-rays revealed a fracture with the fracture line at the physes with a small metaphyseal fragment. There was no epiphyseal fracture. What type of injury by Salter Harris Classification is this? *(CET Nov 15)*
   A. I   B. II
   C. III   D. IV

Ans. is 'B' II

4. Metaphyseal fracture touching physis but not crossing it, comes under which type of Salter-Harris physeal injury?
   A. I   B. II   *(NEET 2015)*
   C. III   D. IV

Ans. is 'B' II

5. Thurston Holland sign is seen in: *(NEET Pattern 2013)*
   A. Type I   B. Type II
   C. Types III D. Type IV

Ans. is 'B' Type II

6. Salter-Harris classification is for: *(NEET Pattern 2012)*
   A. Fracture supracondylar humerus
   B. Fracture epiphysis in children
   C. Fracture lateral condyle humerus
   D. Fracture shaft femur

Ans. is 'B' Fracture epiphysis in children

7. Perichondrial ring is: *(PGI June 2008)*
   A. Seen around foramen magnum
   B. Seen around epiphyseal plate
   C. More prominent in adults
   D. Shear strength increases with age

Ans. is 'B' Seen around epiphyseal plate

   – *The perichondrial ring* surrounds the growth plate circumferentially, similar to perichondrial groove. Perichondrial ring extends towards metaphysis and become continuous with periosteum of metaphysis. *With increasing age, perichondrial ring is thinned and its shear resistance (strength) is decreased.*
   – Rang's type VI is Injury to PeriChondrial ring.
   – Peterson type I fracture is a transverse fracture of metaphysis with extension longitudinally into the physis (commonly seen in distal radius). **Paterson type VI** injury is an open injury associated with loss of physis.

8. Type VI Rang's injury includes: *(PGI Dec 08)*
   A. Transverse fracture of metaphysic with longitudinal extension into physis.
   B. Open injury with loss of physis
   C. Thurston Holland's sign
   D. Perichondrial ring injury

Ans. is 'D' Perichondrial ring injury
   – *Rang's type VI is perichondrial ring injury.*

9. An 8-year-old boy with a history of fall from 10 feet height complains of pain in the right ankle. X-ray taken at that time are normal without any fracture line. But after 2 years, he developed a calcaneovalgus deformity. The diagnosis is: *(AIIMS May 2001)*
   A. Undiagnosed malunited fracture
   B. Avascular nercrosis talus
   C. Tibial epiphyseal injury
   D. Ligamentous injury of ankle joint

Ans. is 'C' Tibial epiphyseal injury

Epiphyseal injuries can have normal X-rays as cartilage is not seen on X-rays and there can be deformities subsequently due to damage to growth plate.

10. Epiphyseal enlargement occurs in: *(AIIMS May 2001)*
    A. Paget's disease
    B. Sheurmann's disease
    C. Epiphyseal dysplasia
    D. Juvenile Rheumatoid Arthritis

Ans. is 'D' Juvenile Rheumatoid Arthritis

11. Epiphyseal dysgenesis is a feature of: *(AIIMS May 1993)*
    A. Hyperparathyroidism
    B. Hypoparathyroidism
    C. Hypothyroidism
    D. Hyperthyroidism

Ans. is 'C' Hypothyroidism

12. All of the following are features of pyle disease except: *(DNB JULY 2016)*
    A. It is an autosomal recessive disease
    B. It is an epiphyseal dysplasia
    C. Mental retardation is uncommon
    D. Dental caries and mandibular prognathism

Ans. is 'B' It is an epiphyseal dysplasia

Metaphyseal Dysplasia (Pyle's Disease)
- A.R
- Mental retardation (intellectual disability)
- Genu Valgum
- Widening of Bones (e.g. Femur)
- Dental carries, Mandibular prognathism

Pediatric Orthopedics

PAEDIATRIC SPINAL PROBLEM

Klippel-Feil Syndrome

Klippel-Feil Syndrome is **congenital fusion of one or more cervical vertebrae presenting with classical triad of low hair line, short 'web' neck** (prominence of trapezius muscle), **and limited neck motion** seen in 50% cases.

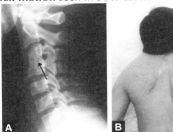

Figs. 18.40A and B: Klippel-Feil Syndrome (A) Synostosis and (B) Short webbed neck with low posterior hair line

Abnormal head position, true torticollis, and restricted range of motion, without an obvious SCM (sternocleido mastoid) contracture, is an indication for X-rays of cervical spine for evidence of cervical fusion.

It is associated with congenital osseous fusions (synostosis) and **failure of segmentation of the cervical spine,** involving two or more vertebrae. Such fusions can involve the craniocervical junction (occiput to C2), the subaxial cervical spine or both; and results from a failure of the normal division of the cervical somites during the 3rd to 8th week of embryogenesis.

Associated Feature

Musculoskeletal System

- **Scoliosis** (~60%) due to fusion of cervical and cervicothoracic junction.
- **Sprengel's deformity** (~50%) it is congenitally elevated or undescended scapula.
  (Omovertebral bone bridges the cervical spine to the scapula and limits the neck and shoulder motion.)
- Webbing of neck, facial asymmetry and torticollis.
- Radiographic findings of congenital cervical vertebral fusion are diagnostic.
- Neurological sequelae due to involvement of brain stem or cervical cord may be present.
- Syndactyly and diffuse or focal upper extremity hypoplasia.
- Secondary osteoarthritis, disc degeneration, spinal stenosis.

Other Findings

- Genito renal anomalies (~35%, so USG is recommended)
- Congenital heart defects (~15%, so ECHO is recommended)

Congenital High Scapula (Sprengel's deformity)

- It consists of permanent elevation of the shoulder girdle due to developmental defect.
- **The scapula is smaller in its vertical diameter and appears broad. It lies high in position.**
- Para scapular muscles are composed of imperfectly developed muscle fibers or fibrous tissue.
- From the superior angle of scapula a sheet or band like structure composed of fibrous tissue cartilage or bone extends upwards to attach to the transverse process of several cervical vertebrae **known as Omovertebral bar.**

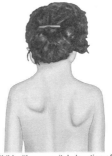
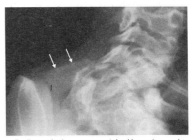

Child with congenital elevation of left scapula. Note Shortness of neck on that side tendency to torticollis

Radiograph shows omovertebral bone (arrows) connection scapula to spinous processes of cervical vertebrae via osteochondral joint (J)

Fig. 18.41: Sprengel shoulder

C/F: Shoulder and the scapula at a higher level than the opposite one, Restriction of shoulder movement.

Treatment: There is no definitive treatment available: Surgery (Woodward procedure) is done for cosmetic reasons only.

MULTIPLE CHOICE QUESTIONS

1. Sprengel's deformity associated with all except: *(AIIMS Nov 2017)*
   A. Congenital scoliosis
   B. Dextrocardia
   C. Diastematomyelia
   D. Klippel-Feil syndrome

   Ans. is 'B' Dextrocardia

2. Which of the following is/are feature/s of sprengel's deformity? *(NEET Dec 2016)*
   A. Elevated shoulder on affected side
   B. smaller than usual scapula
   C. Short neck
   D. All of the above

   Ans. is 'D' All of the above

3. The characteristic triad of Klippel-Feil syndrome includes all the following, except: *(AI 2010)*
   A. Short neck
   B. Low hair line
   C. Limited neck movements
   D. Elevated scapula

   Ans. is 'D' Elevated scapula

   - Scapula (Sprengel deformity) may be associated with Klippel-Feil syndrome, but does not form part of the characteristic triad.
   - The characteristic triad of Klippel-Feil syndrome includes a short neck, low hair line and restriction of neck motion.

4. In Klippel-Feil syndrome, the patient has all of the following clinical features except: *(AI 2005)*
   A. Low hair line
   B. Bilateral Neck webbing
   C. Bilateral shortness of sternomastoid muscles
   D. Gross limitations of neck movements.

   Ans. is 'C' Bilateral shortness of sternomastoid muscles

5. Sprengel's shoulder is due to deformity: *(TN 2002, UP 2K, AIIMS 84, 80)*
   A. Scapula
   B. Humerus
   C. Clavicle
   D. Vertebra

   Ans. is 'A' Scapula

CONGENITAL (INFANTILE) MUSCULAR TORTICOLLIS OR WRY NECK

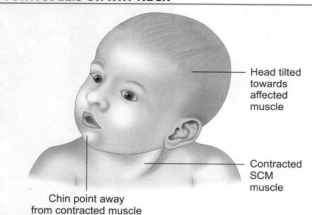

Fig. 18.42: Torticollis

Torticollis or twisted neck is a symptom of cervical spine abnormality. It may be of two types congenital and secondary. Congenital or infantile torticollis is commonest form of wry neck. It is due to fibrosis of sternocleidomastoid (SCM) muscle on one side that fails to elongate as child grows. The cause is muscle ischemia from a distorted position in utero (breech) or birth injury. A history of difficult labour followed by lump over SCM (sternomastoid tumor) in first few weeks of life, which disappears in few months is present. Then there is neither deformity nor obvious limitation of movements. Deformity does not become apparent until the child is 1–2 years old.

- It is associated with breech delivery, shoulder dystocia, birth injury and SCM ischemia/tumor.
- The head is tilted toward the involved SCM and the chin is rotated towards the contralateral shoulder, producing the 'Cock robin' appearance. SCM on involved side may feel tight and hard and a mass or knot can be detected in the body of SCM in first 3 months of life.
- It can disappear spontaneously
- There may be asymmetrical development of face (plagiocephaly).

Treatment: Unipolar (one head of SCM) or bipolar (two heads of SCM) release, Optimum age: 1–4 years.

MULTIPLE CHOICE QUESTIONS

1. Not true about sternocleidomastoid (SCM) tumour: *(JIPMER May 2016)*
   A. It is present at upper 2-3rd and lower 1-3 junction of SCM
   B. It is always present at birth
   C. It is associated with oligohydramnios and limb defects
   D. It undergoes spontaneous resolution

Ans. is 'B' It is always present at birth

2. The muscle affected in congenital torticollis is: *(PGM-CET 2015)*
   A. Trapezius   B. Rhomboideus Major
   C. Rhomboideus Minor   D. Sternocleidomastoid

Ans. is 'D' Sternocleidomastoid

3. Which of the following is not true in case of congenital torticollis? *(AIIMS May 10, 07, All India 2007)*
   A. Seen only in cases of breech vaginal delivery
   B. It can disappear spontaneously
   C. It is also known as sternomastoid tumour
   D. Untreated, neglected cases can result in plagiocephaly

Ans. is 'A' Seen only in cases of breech vaginal delivery

4. All the following are true in infantile torticollis, except:
   A. It arises before birth *(PGI 97)*
   B. There is facial asymmetry
   C. Commonest form of wryneck
   D. Infarction of sterno-cleidomastoid muscle

Ans. is 'A' It arises before birth

VERTEBRA PLANA

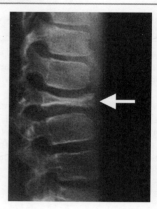

Fig. 18.43: Vertebra plana

Vertebra plana is collapse and increased density of one vertebral body, with normal or increased disc space. Causes are Eosinophilic granuloma (histiocytosis), Ewings's sarcoma, metastasis, leukemia, tuberculosis (very rare) and Calves' disease (osteochondritis of vertebral body).

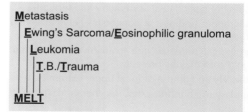

MULTIPLE CHOICE QUESTIONS

1. Vertebra Plana is seen in all except: *(AI Dec 15)*
   A. Histiocytosis X   B. Leukemia
   C. Excessive use of systemic steroids
   D. Scheuermann's disease

Ans. is 'D' Scheuermann's disease

2. Vertebra plana seen in: *(PGI June 2006)*
   A. Eosinophilia granuloma   B. Trauma disease
   C. Paget's disease   D. Malignancy
   E. Ewing's sarcoma

Ans. is 'A' Eosinophilia granuloma; 'B' Trauma disease; 'D' Malignancy and 'E' Ewing's sarcoma

SCOLIOSIS

Test for Scoliosis

Scoliosis is lateral curvature of spine. Most of the time, the cause of scoliosis is unknown. This is called idiopathic scoliosis. It is the most common type. It is grouped by age.
- In children age 3 and younger, it is called infantile scoliosis.
- In age 4–10, it is called juvenile scoliosis.
- In age >10, it is called adolescent scoliosis.

Types of Scoliosis

Structural Scoliosis	Non-Structure Scoliosis
Structural curve becomes more prominent on forward bending (Adams test) as opposed to postural scoliosis.	i. Compensatory: due to limb length discrepancy or sciatic list (due to disc prolapsed) – They disappear on sitting.
	ii. Postural scoliosis: Disappears on forward bending.

Scoliosis Most Often Affects Girls

Cobbs angle is used to measure scoliosis
- *Congenital scoliosis:* This type of scoliosis is present at birth and is associated with vertebral anomalies.
- Congenital vertebral anomalies that lead to scoliosis
- Risk of progression of common vertebral anomalies.
- Unsegmented bar with hemivertebra. This carries the worst prognosis and greatest risk of progression (5–10 degrees per year).
- Block Vertebra This carries the best prognosis and lowest risk of progression (Stable or minimal progression) (<1 degree to 1 degree per year).

A	B	C
Failure of formation	**Failure of segmentation**	**Combination**
• Hemivertebra	• Unsegmented bar	Unsegmented bar with hemivertebra
• Wedge vertebra	• Block vertebra	

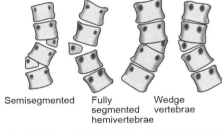
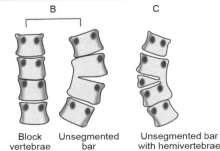

Figs. 18.44A to C: Types of scoliosis

- *Neuromuscular scoliosis:* This type is caused by a nervous system problem such as **cerebral palsy, muscular dystrophy,** spina bifida, and **polio.**

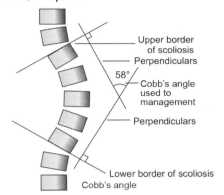

Fig. 18.45: Cobb's angle

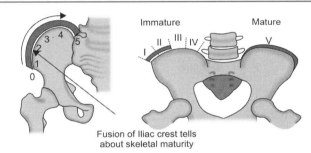

Fig. 18.46: Risser's sign

Skeletal maturity can be assessed by the Risser sign. A radiograph is employed to see how far the patient's iliac apophysis has progressed from the anterior superior iliac spine. During development, the iliac apophysis first appears laterally and grows medially. The stages are Risser I through Risser V, where Risser V denotes that the apophysis has completely fused with the iliac crest and therefore skeletal maturity can be assumed hence further progress of curve of scoliosis will not take place.

Treatment

Brace treatment is restricted to immature children in an attempt to prevent curve progression during further skeletal growth. So it is indicated in Growing adolescents (Risser 0, 1 or 2) who, on presentation, have curves in range of 30–45 degrees or who have had documented progression exceeding 5 degrees in curve that initially measured 20–30 degrees.

TLSOs are the most commonly used orthoses today, but their use is restricted to patients whose curve apex is at or below T7. Fortunately, this is the case in most idiopathic scoliosis.

These patient should have deformities that are considered cosmetically acceptable. Patient should be realistically willing to wear the brace the prescribed amount of time.

Contraindication

- Large curves (**>45 degrees**) in growing adolescents (need surgical treatment). However, there is an exception to this rule. Very immature adolescents who have not yet reached their peak height velocity and who have large curves (~50º) may benefit from brace in an effort to delay progression until maturity is reached.
- Extreme thoracic hypokyphosis (as normal positioning of pads could exacerbate rib deformity).

- Skeletally mature adolescent (Riser 4 or 5, and in females 2 years post-menarchial).
- High thoracic or cervico thoracic curve (relative contraindication).

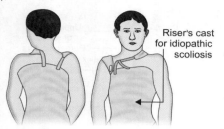

Fig. 18.47: Riser's cast

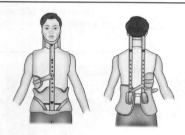

Fig. 18.48: Milwaukee brace

Treatment Plan of Idiopathic Scoliosis

Curve Magnitude (degree)		Risser Sign Grade	
< 25	Observation	1 or 2	Observation
30–45	Brace	3	Observation
> 45	Surgery	4 or 5	Surgery (when curve >50 degree)

Suspensory plaster cast of sayre, Rissers cast hinge or turnbuckle cast of Hibbs and Kisser, Milwaukee brace, Boston brace, Charleston night-time bending brace, Wilmington brace and thoraco-lumbo-sacral orthoses (TLSOs) are used to treat idiopathic scoliosis. (Lower Dorsal scoliosis > Lumbar Scoliosis).

Surgical treatment consists of corrective osteotomies and fusion.

MULTIPLE CHOICE QUESTIONS

1. Idiopathic scoliosis can be treated by: (AI 2016)
   A. Minerva cast   B. Milwaukee brace
   C. Crutchfield traction   D. PTB cast
Ans. is 'B' Milwaukee brace

2. Cobb's angle is used to measure the degree:
   A. Kyphoscoliosis   (CET Nov 15)
   B. Angular deformity of the knee
   C. Extent of depression in calcaneal fracture
   D. Extent of spondylolisthesis
Ans. is 'A' Kyphoscoliosis

3. Vertebral rotation in scoliosis is checked in: (NEET 2015)
   A. Forward bending   B. Backward bending
   C. Sideways   D. Without bending
Ans. is 'A' Forward bending

4. Turn-buckle cast is used for: (NEET Pattern 2013)
   A. Fracture shaft humerus   B. Fracture shaft femur
   C. Scoliosis   D. Cervical spine injury
Ans. is 'C' Scoliosis

5. In scoliosis degree of deformity is calculated by: (NEET Pattern 2012)
   A. Cobbs method   B. Hamburger method
   C. Haldane method   D. Milwaukee method
Ans. is 'A' Cobbs method

6. Angle measured for measurement of scoliosis:
   A. Cobbs   B. Bohlers (NEET Pattern 2012)
   C. Kites   D. Baumanns
Ans. is 'A' Cobbs

7. Risers sign is for: (NEET Pattern 2012)
   A. Kyphosis   B. Scoliosis
   C. Shortening   D. Lengthening
Ans. is 'B' Scoliosis

8. Progression of congenital scoliosis is least likely in which of the following vertebra anomalies? (AI 2010)
   A. Fully segmented hemivertebra
   B. Wedge vertebra
   C. Block vertebra
   D. Unilateral unsegmented bar with Hemivertebra
Ans. is 'C' Block vertebra
   - Unsegmented bar - with hemivertebra> unsegmented bar> hemivertebra> wedge vertebra> block vertebra.

9. Risser Localizer cast is used in the management of: (AIIMS Nov 2008)
   A. Kyphosis   B. Spondylolysthesis
   C. Idiopathic scoliosis   D. Lordosis
Ans. is 'C' Idiopathic scoliosis

NEUROFIBROMATOSIS (NF)

It is hereditary, hamartomatous disorder, that affects central and peripheral nervous system, skeletal, skin and deeper soft tissue. It is one of the commonest single gene disorder affecting the skeletal system.

NF - 1/Von Recklinghausen's Disease

- Most common single gene disorder affecting human nervous system.
- Also called as peripheral neurofibromatosis, is due to defect in chromosome 17.
- AD inheritance, and 50% patients result from new mutation. 100% penetrance, i.e. individual with abnormal chromosome 17 will show same clinical feature.
- Clinical presentation includes-cafe au lait spots (most common feature) axillary, and inguinal freckling (2nd m.c), cutaneous neurofibromas, plexiform neurofibromas (~5% are premalignant), Lisch nodule on iris, veruccous hyperplasia (thickened overgrown valvety soft skin), elephantiasis (pachydermatocele), optic glioma, skeletal abnormalities (scoliosis, congenital pseudoarthrosis of tibia, hemihypertrophy) and cognitive deficits (learning disability).
- Complications include epilepsy, hydrocephalus, cognitive deficits, intracranial tumor, optic glioma, short stature, precocious puberty, hypothalamic dysfunction, renal artery stenosis and hypertension.

Diagnostic criteria for NF-1 are met if Two or More criteria are found

- > 6 cafe au-lait spots, at least 15 mm in greatest diameter in adults and 5 mm in children.
- Neurofibromas of any type or one plexiform neurofibroma
- Axillary or inguinal freckling (crowe's sign)
- Lisch nodule (iris hamartomas)

- Optic glioma
- Musculoskeletal lesion such as scoliosis, sphenoid dysplasia, or thinning of cortex of long bone, with or with out pseudoarthrosis.
- A first degree relative (parent, sibling, or offspring) with NF-1 by above criteria.

NF-2

- Also known as central neurofibromatosis or bilateral acoustic neurofibromatosis and is due to defect in long arm of chromosome 22.
- Less common type, AD inheritance, and 50% cases are due to new mutation.
- Musculoskeletal deformities encountered in NF–1 are generally absent in NF–2.
- 8th nerve vestibular schwannomas occur in nearly every individual with NF2 (not seen in NFl).
- Meningioma occur in 50% cases.

Diagnostic criteria for NF-2 are met if a person has either of the following:

- Bilateral 8th nerve masses seen on MRI
- A first degree relative with NF2 and either a unilateral 8th nerve mass or two of the following
- Neurofibroma
- Meningioma
- Glioma
- Schwannoma
- Juvenile posterior subscapsular lenticular opacity.

Note: Usually Skeletal disorders are Autosomal Dominant and Inborn errors of metabolism are autosomal recessive.

MULTIPLE CHOICE QUESTIONS

1. Neurofibromatosis inheritance:
   - A. Autosomal dominant
   - B. Autosomal recessive
   - C. X linked dominant
   - D. X linked recessive

   Ans. is 'A' Autosomal dominant

2. Musculoskeletal abnormalities in neurofibromatosis is:
   - A. Hypertrophy of limb
   - B. Scoliosis *(UP 2001)*
   - C. Pseudo arthrosis
   - D. All of the above

   Ans. is 'D' All of the above

   Musculoskeletal abnormalities in neurofibromatosis
   - *Pseudoarthrosis of tibia*
   - Short stature
   - *Scoliosis (Most common)*
   - *Limb hypertrophy* due to multiple neurofibromas
   - Distinctive osseous lesion: sphenoid dysplasia or cortical thinning of long bones.

3. The common features of Neurofibromatosis include all, except: *(TN 99)*
   - A. Optic glioma
   - B. Dumbbell neurofibroma
   - C. Scoliosis
   - D. Periventricular calcifications

   Ans. is 'D' Periventricular calcifications

CONGENITAL PSEUDOARTHROSIS

Pseudoarthrosis

It is a false joint that may develop after a fracture that has not united properly due to inadequate immobilization. If a nonunion allows for too much motion along the fracture gap, the central portion of the callus undergoes cystic degeneration and the luminal surface can actually become lined by synovial like cells, creating a false joint filled with clear fluid- known as pseudoarthrosis.

Most Common Cause of Pseudoarthrosis

Idiopathic> Neurofibromatosis (NF-1) – (Actually an association, not a cause)

Causes of Pseudoarthrosis are

1. Neurofibromatosis (50% patients of pseudoarthrosis have NF)
2. Nonunion of fracture (including pathological fractures)
3. Congenital (mostly in lower to middle third of tibia with cupping of proximal bone end and pointing of distal bone end)
4. Osteogenesis imperfecta
5. Fibrous dysplasia
6. Cleidocranial dysplasia
7. Ankylosing spondylitis (in fused bamboo spine)
8. Post-surgical, e.g. Triple arthrodesis, spinal fusion as a complication.
   - Tibia is most commonly involved bone. Five forms of congenital pseudoarthrosis of tibia are—dysplastic, cystic, sclerotic, fibular and clubfoot or congenital band type.
   - The most common dysplastic type is tapered at defective site; an hour glass Constriction, it is associated with neurofibromatosis.
   - Poor fracture healing and recurrent fracture is common even if union is achieved.
   - Cast immobilization is generally unsuccessful.
   - **Initial treatment is nailing and bone grafting or Ilizarov fixator.**
   - Vascularized Fibular graft is done if multiple failed surgeries.

MULTIPLE CHOICE QUESTIONS

1. The following deformity is seen in a child. What is the likely cause? *(AIIMS May 2016)*

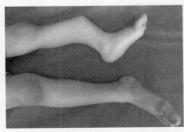

   - A. Tibial Hemimelia
   - B. Fibula Hemimelia
   - C. Congenital pseudoarthrosis of Tibia
   - D. Congenital posteromedial angulation of Tibia

   Ans. is 'C' Congenital pseudoarthrosis of Tibia

2. In some old fractures, cartilaginous tissue forms over the fractured bone ends with a cavity in between containing clear fluid. This condition is called as: *(AI 2004)*
   A. Delayed union   B. Slow union
   C. Non-union   D. Pseudoarthrosis

Ans. is 'D' Pseudoarthrosis

3. Pseudoarthrosis may be seen in all of the following conditions except: *(AI 1998)*
   A. Fracture   B. Idiopathic
   C. Neurofibromatosis D. Osteomyelitis

Ans. is 'D' Osteomyelitis

4. Pseudoarthrosis can be due to all except:
   (All India 1998, PGI 1993)
   A. Congenital   B. Post-inflammatory
   C. Trauma   D. None of the above

Ans. is 'B' Post-inflammatory

5. Pseudoarthrosis of tibia is best treated by: *(Delhi 96)*
   A. Internal fixation
   B. Internal fixation and bone grafting
   C. Above knee POP cast
   D. Below knee POP cast

Ans. is 'B' Internal fixation and bone grafting
   Treatment of choice is fixation and bone grafting

6. Cause of congenital pseudoarthrosis is: *(Andhra 1994)*
   A. Intrauterine fracture
   B. Neurofibromatosis
   C. Fibrous dysplasia
   D. Unknown

Ans. is 'D' Unknown
   Neurofibromatosis is an association it is not a cause

7. Congenital pseudo arthrosis is seen in the following:
   (Tamil Nadu 1993)
   A. Hip joint   B. Femur
   C. Radius - ulna   D. Tibia

Ans. is 'D' Tibia
   Tibia is the commonest affected bone in pseudoarthrossis.

DUCHENNE MUSCULAR DYSTROPHY

1. **X-linked Recessive (Xp 21)**
2. **Dystrophin gene mutation is seen**
3. **Boys** (more common)
4. **Average age of presentation is 4 years**
5. Patient is Unable to walk by 12 years of age
6. Average life span is 26 years
7. Proximal muscle weakness is seen
8. Contractures of Achilles and Hamstring is seen
9. **Pseudohypertrophy of calf** and tongue is seen
10. Gait—patient is usually a toe walker
11. There is increase in Lumbar Lordosis
12. Scoliosis is seen
13. **Gower's sign (patient climbs on himself)**

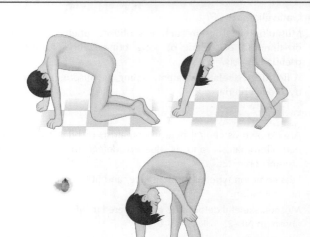

Fig. 18.49: Gower's Sign

14. Cardiomyopathy and congestive heart failure is seen
15. There is increase in Creatine Kinase and EMG shows Muscle damage. Definitive diagnosis is by muscle biopsy and genetic testing.

Fascio Scapulohumeral Dystrophy

* Face (facial muscle weakness) + Scapula (Winging) + Humerus (Limitation of overhead activity) defects are seen
* AD (Chromosome 4)
* Progressive disease.

MULTIPLE CHOICE QUESTIONS

1. The child with the following clinical presentation will most probably have the underlying diagnosis:
   (AIIMS Nov 16)

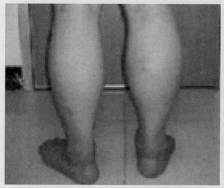

   A. Dystrophy   B. Neuropathy
   C. Metaphyseal dysplasia   D. NF

Ans. is 'A' Dystrophy

2. Mutation seen in Marfan syndrome: *(AI 2016)*
   A. Fibrillin-1 gene   B. FGFR-3 gene
   C. COLA-1   D. Fibrillin-2

Ans. is 'A' Fibrilliin-1 gene

Pediatric Orthopedics

Marfan Syndrome: Fibrillin 1 defect
1. There is increase in the height (Disproportionate)
2. The limbs are long and there is arachnodactyly (fingers and hand are long and have spider like appearance)
3. Scoliosis is seen
4. Pectus excavatum/Pectus carinatum
5. Hyperlaxity
6. High-arched palate
7. Pes planus
8. Hammer toes
9. Early OA is a features
10. Ghent criterion is used for diagnosis of Marfan syndrome

Hemimelia (absence of one axis of the limb) involves either the preaxial border (radial border in upper limb and medial border in lower limb) or the post axial border (Ulnar border in upper limb and lateral border in lower limb). The frequency of hemimelia is fibular > radial.

The defect in tibia or fibula

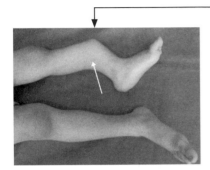
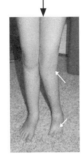
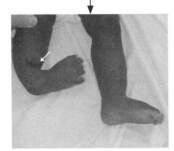
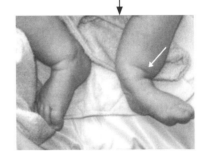

Congenital pseudoarthrosis of tibia | Fibular hemimelia | Tibial hemimelia | Posteromedial bowing of tibia

Congenital pseudoarthrosis of tibia there is anterolateral bowing.

Fibular hemimelia—this is the most common hemimelia the patient presents with limb length discrepancies, valgus at knee, hypoplastic lateral structures, ankle deformity (equinovalgus) and absent or hypoplastic fourth or fifth toe

Tibial hemimelia—this is a very rare hemimelia the patient presents with limb length discrepancies, varus at knee, hypoplastic medial structures, ankle deformity (equinovarus) and absent or hypoplastic first to third toe

Posteromedial bowing of tibia. This condition is the least severe of the four conditions. The deformity is often self resolving.

Crawford Classification:
- Type 1:
  - Anterolateral bowing of tibia
- Type 2:
  - Anterolateral bowing
  - Increased cortical thickness
  - Narrow medullary canal
  - Tubular defect
- Type 3:
  - Cystic lesion
- Type 4:
  - Presence of fracture, a cyst or frank pseudoarthosis

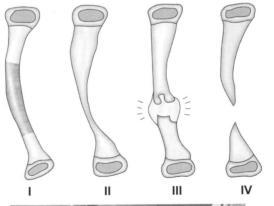

I II III IV

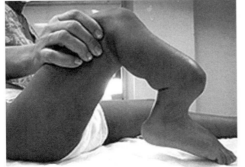
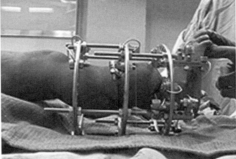

Treatment of Congenital pseudoarthrosis of tibia by Ilizarov fixator.

Chapter 19: Osteochondritis and Avascular Necrosis

It is ischemic necrosis of osteoarticular fragment of bone leading to compression, fragmentation or separation of a small segment of a articular cartilage and underlying bone. This occurs mainly in adolescent and young adults, often during phases of increased physical activity, and may be initiated by trauma or repetitive stress. It can be of three types:

1. **Crushing Osteochondritis**—due to increased pressure, e.g. Kohlers/Kienbocks/Perthes/Scheuermann's/Calves/Friebergs/Iselene.
2. **Splitting Osteochondritis**—due to increased wear during movement and than ischemic changes, e.g. Osteochondritis Dissecans, e.g. Knee (Lateral part of medial femoral condyle) or Elbow.
3. **Pulling/traction osteochondritis**—pull of tendon or ligament causes separation of fragment, e.g. Osgood Schlatters/Severs/Johansson Larsens.

Types of osteochondritis	Bones affected
Kienbock	Lunate
Kohler	Navicular
Perthes	Femur head
Scheuermann	Ring epiphysis of vertebrae
Calves	Central bony nucleus of vertebrae

Contd...

Types of osteochondritis	Bones affected
Frieberg	2nd metatarsal head
Islene	5th metatarsal base
Osgood shattler	Tibial tuberosity
Sever's	Calcaneum
Johanson-Larsens	Lower pole of patella
Blounts	Tibia
Panner's	Capitulum of elbow
Preiser's	Scaphoid
Schmier's	Pisiform
Witt's	Triquetrum
Agati	Trapezoid
Haglund	Calcaneus
Fleischner Thiemann	Phalanges
Haas	Head of humerus
Konig's	Tubular bones
Wegner	Osteochondritis with epiphyseal separation
Mouclaire's	Metacarpal head

Contd...

Scheuermann – **R**ing epiphysis of vertebrae
Lateral part of **M**edial femoral condyle *
Osteochondritis **D**issecans
Severe 's- **C**alcaneum
Panner's – **C**apitulum of elbow
Osgood Shattler's – **T**ibial tuberocity
Frieberg- 2nd **M**etatarsal head
Kienbock**L**unate
Perthes – **F**emur head

S R Ki La**M**bi **MOD**ern Se**C**retary **P C** **O**o**T**y Mein **FM** Pe Ko**L**avari **P**er**F**orm
Kar**N**e ke Baad Is**M**ile Karke **C**a**v**e mein **J**a **P**achunchi

Johanson – Larsens – lower pole of **P**atella

Calves – central bony nucleus of **V**ertebrae

Islene – 5th **M**etatarsal base

Kohler - **N**avicular

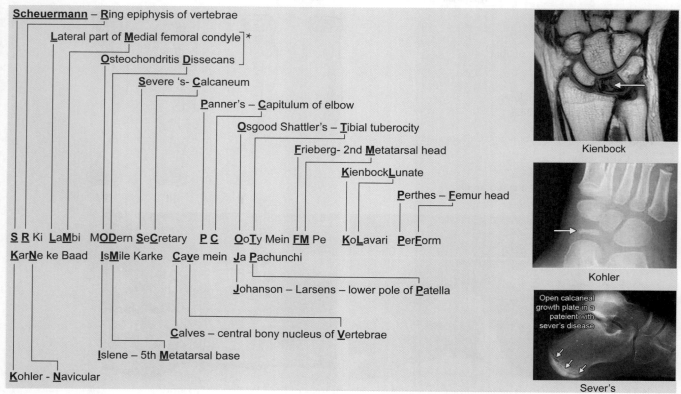

Kienbock

Kohler

Sever's

MULTIPLE CHOICE QUESTIONS

1. Osteochondritis in Kohler's Disease affects which bone? *(JIPMER NOV 2017)*
   A. Lunate
   B. Patella
   C. Navicular
   D. Femur head
Ans. is 'C' Navicular

2. Kienbock Osteonecrosis, all are true except: *(PGI Nov 2017)*
   A. Tenderness over base of 5th metatarsal is present
   B. Pain is more on wrist flexion than wrist extension
   C. Is the osteochondritis of lunate
   D. Is associated with positive ulnar variance
   E. More common in elderly
Ans. is 'A' Tenderness over base of 5th metatarsal is present; 'B' Pain is more on wrist flexion than wrist extension; 'D' Is associated with positive ulnar variance; 'E' More common in elderly

Kienbock disease
Age: 20-40 years
Osteochondritis of lunate
Dominant side
Finesterer's sign: Tenderness at base of 3rd metacarpal on making a fist.
Negative ulnar variance (ulnar articular surface short of radial surface)
Pain on wrist dorsiflexion
Treatment:
Early stage correct negative ulnar variance and vascularized pronator quadratus graft.
Advanced stage with collapse wrist arthrodesis or arthroplasty.

3. Haglunds deformity is seen in which joint? *(AIIMS May 2017)*
   A. Elbow
   B. Knee
   C. Wrist
   D. Ankle
Ans. is 'D' Ankle
Haglund deformity is prominent Calcaneal tuberosity and overlying bursitis (retro-calcaneal)

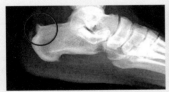
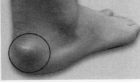

4. Kienbock's disease is osteochondritis of: *(NEET 2015)*
   A. Scaphoid
   B. Lunate
   C. Calcaneum
   D. Tibial tuberosity
Ans. is 'B' Lunate

5. Scheuermann's disease occurs in: *(APPG 2015)*
   A. Adults
   B. Elderly
   C. Infants
   D. Adolescents
Ans. is 'D' Adolescents

6. Sever disease involves: *(NEET Pattern 2013)*
   A. Lunate
   B. Tibial tubercle
   C. Calcaneum
   D. Navicular
Ans. is 'C' Calcaneum

7. Most common site of osteochondritis dissecans: *(NEET Pattern 2013)*
   A. Lateral part of the medial femoral condyle
   B. Medial part of the medial femoral condyle
   C. Lateral part of the lateral femoral condyle
   D. Medial part of the lateral femoral condyle
Ans. is 'A' Lateral part of the medial femoral condyle

8. Osteonecrosis is not seen in: *(NEET Pattern 2012)*
   A. Ollier's disease
   B. Kienboch
   C. Kohler's disease
   D. Perthe's disease
Ans. is 'A' Olliers disease

9. Perthes disease is: *(NEET Pattern 2012)*
   A. Fracture of femoral shaft
   B. Osteochondritis of femoral epiphysis
   C. Infarction of femoral head
   D. Fracture dislocation of femoral neck
Ans. is 'B' Osteochondritis of femoral epiphysis

10. In elbow, osteochondritis usually involves: *(NEET Pattern 2012)*
    A. Olecranon
    B. Trochlea
    C. Radial head
    D. Capitulum
Ans. is 'D' Capitulum

11. Infarction of the distal epiphysis of the second metatarsal bone is: *(NEET Pattern 2012)*
    A. Kienbock's disease
    B. Kohler's disease
    C. Freiberg's disease
    D. Perthes disease
Ans. is 'C' Freiberg's disease

12. Osgood Schlatter disease: *(PGI June 07, Dec 01)*
    A. Involve the knee joint
    B. Pelvis
    C. Wrist joint
    D. Cervical spine
Ans. is 'A' Involve the knee joint

13. Islene's disease is osteochondritis of: *(JIPMER 99)*
    A. 2nd Metacarpal
    B. 5th Metacarpal
    C. 2nd Metatarsal
    D. 5th Metatarsal
Ans. is 'D' 5th Metatarsal

14. Osteochondritis is not seen in—disease: *(Delhi 1999)*
    A. Slipped capital femoral epiphysis
    B. Panner's disease
    C. Calve's disease
    D. Kohler's disease
Ans. is 'A' Slipped capital femoral epiphysis

15. Osteochondritis in Osgood Schlatter disease affect which bone? *(UP 93)*
    A. Capitulum's bone
    B. Metacarpal
    C. Navicular
    D. Tibial tuberosity
Ans. is 'D' Tibial tuberosity

16. Freiberg's osteochondritis is: (AI 90)
    A. 2nd Metatarsal head
    B. 5th Metatarsal head
    C. 2nd Metatarsal base
    D. 5th Metatarsal base

Ans. is 'A' 2nd Metatarsal head

OSTEOCHONDRITIS DISSECANS

- It is a poorly understood disorder, which leads to softening and separation of a portion of joint surface; resulting in development of small segment of necrotic bone in joint.
- Knee (lower-lateral part of medial femoral condyle) is the most commonly affected joint. Elbow (capitulum) is 2nd common.
- The cause is trauma either a single impact with the edge of patella or repeated microtrauma.
- Patient is usually adolescent male, presents with intermittent ache and swelling, localized tenderness and **Wilson's sign** (i.e. pain is felt in extension of flexed knee in medial rotation, but not in lateral rotation).
- The best X-ray view is intercondylar (tunnel view-30 degrees knee flexion).

MRI can make early diagnosis of cartilaginous lesions.

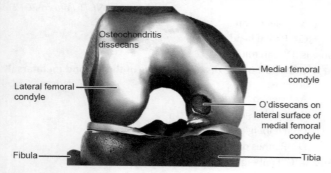

Fig. 19.1: Knee – osteochondritis dissecans

Treatment Options

O'Driscoll '4R' for treatment

1. Relief by physiotherapy and pain control modalities few lesions can resolve over time
2. **Resect**
   Excision if small fragment
3. **Replace the joint surface**
4. **Restore the cartilage lesion**
   Fixation with headless screws (Herbert Screw) and protected weight bearing till union.

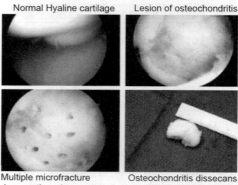

Fig. 19.2: Microfracture technique

If lesion < 2 cm² — Autologous Chondrocyte Transplantation that is cartilage cells are grown in artificial media and then transplanted into cartilage defect.

Microfracture technique or abrasion arthroplasty — Making drill holes at the base of lesion causing regeneration of fibrocartilage and filling the defect of hyaline cartilage (in normal joint). Thus it is substituting for hyaline cartilage by fibrocartilage.

MULTIPLE CHOICE QUESTIONS

1. Microfracture technique is carried out for:
   (NEET Pattern 2012)
   A. Non-union   B. Osteochondral defects
   C. Tumors   D. Osteopetrosis

Ans. is 'B' Osteochondral defects

2. Most common site of osteochondritis dissecans:
   (AIIMS June 1998)
   A. Lateral part of the medial femoral condyle
   B. Medial part of the medial femoral condyle
   C. Lateral part of the lateral femoral condyle
   D. Medial part of the lateral femoral condyle

Ans. is 'A' Lateral part of the medial femoral condyle

3. Which joint is commonly involved in osteochondritis dissecans? (AI 1995)
   A. Ankle joint   B. Knee joint
   C. Wrist joint   D. Elbow joint

Ans. is 'B' Knee joint

Knee is the most commonly affected joint. Other joints such as hip, ankle, elbow (capitulum) and shoulder can also be involved.

Avascular Necrosis

AVASCULAR NECROSIS OF BONE

Common site of avascular necrosis	Cause
Head of femur	Fracture neck femur Posterior dislocation hip (>12 hours dislocation)
Proximal pole of scaphoid	Fracture through waist of scaphoid
Body of talus	Fracture neck of talus
Proximal pole of lunate	Dislocation
Capitulum	
Head of Humerus	
Distal Femoral Condyles	

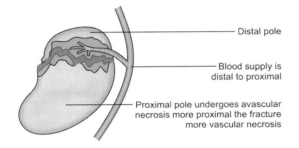

Fig. 19.3: Scaphoid blood supply

Main blood supply to proximal pole of scaphoid is through the intraosseous channels from distal to proximal as shown in diagram above.

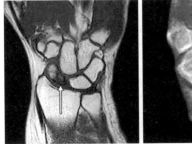 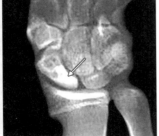

Fig. 19.4: Avascular necrosis of scaphoid

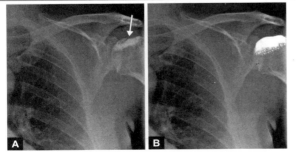

Figs. 19.5A and B: Avascular Necrosis of humeral head—Snow Cap Sign

BLOOD SUPPLY TO FEMORAL HEAD

Blood Supply to Femoral Head

Crock described the blood supply to the proximal end of the femur, dividing it into three major groups: (1) an extracapsular arterial ring located at the base of the femoral neck, (2) ascending cervical branches of the arterial ring on the surface of the femoral neck, and (3) arteries of the ligamentum teres.

The extracapsular arterial ring is formed **posteriorly by a large branch of the medial femoral circumflex artery and anteriorly by a branch from the lateral femoral circumflex artery.** The ascending cervical branches or retinacular vessels ascend on the surface of the femoral neck in anterior, posterior, medial, and lateral groups; the lateral vessels are the most important. Their proximity to the surface of the femoral neck makes them vulnerable to injury in femoral neck fractures. As the articular margin of the femoral head is approached by the ascending cervical vessels, a second, less distinct ring of vessels is formed, referred to by Chung as the *subsynovial intra-articular arterial ring*. It is from ring of vessels that vessels penetrate the head and are referred to as the epiphyseal arteries, the most important being the lateral epiphyseal arterial group supplying the lateral weight bearing portion of the femoral head. These epiphyseal vessels are joined by inferior metaphyseal vessels and vessels from the ligamentum teres.

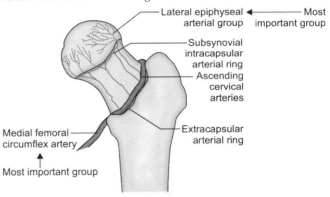

Fig. 19.6: Blood supply to femur head (Posterior aspect)

Intraosseous Blood Supply

Cartilaginous growth plate—starts appearing at 4 years age so metaphyseal arteries do not enter after 4 years of age. When growth plate disappears in adolescence, metaphyseal arteries enter epiphysis again. Foveal artery appears at 8 years of age. So most precarious blood supply is at age 4–8 years (Truetas hypothesis). Hence this is the age in which AVN of femoral epiphysis is seen in children called as Perthes disease.

In fracture neck femur the more proximal the lesion, more are the chances of avascular necrosis. So subcapital fracture neck femur has maximum chances of AVN (worst prognosis). Subcapital > transcervical > basicervical fracture is order of risk of development of Avascular necrosis.

Age-wise Blood Supply of Neck Femur	
Age	Supply
<4 years	Metaphyseal artery, Retinacular arteries
4–8 years	Single arterial supply- Retinacular artery
>8 years	Retinacular artery, Foveal artery
Adolescent	Retinacular artery, Foveal artery, Metaphyseal artery

AVASCULAR NECROSIS/OSTEONECROSIS

Avascular necrosis is the cellular death of components of bone due to impaired blood supply.

Affects Anterolateral Aspect of Femoral Head

Etiopathogenesis

- Idiopathic (most common)—Called as Chandeliers Disease
  Causes of AVN of femoral head
  - *Trauma:* Neck femur fracture, Posterior dislocation of hip. (>12-hour duration)
  - **Substance:** Alcohol, steroid use.
  - *Infection:* Septic arthritis, osteomyelitis
  - *Storage disorders:* Gaucher's disease
  - **Caisson disease: Dysbaric osteonecrosis (Nitrogen accumulates)**
  - *Hemoglobinopathy and Coagulation disorder:* Sickel cell disease, Familial thrombophilia A. Hypofibrinolysis, Hypolipoproteinemia.

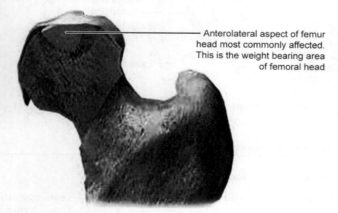

Fig. 19.7: Region of femoral head affected in AVN

  - *Congenital disorders:* Perthes disease, Slipped capital femoral epiphysis.
  - *Hematological malignancies:* Leukemia, lymphoma, polycythemia.
  - *Hyperlipedemia:* Nephrotic syndrome
  - *Other:* SLE, ionising radiation, Pregnancy, pancreatitis, Amyloid, Renal failure **and** dialysis, Hyperparathyroidism.

Clinical Features

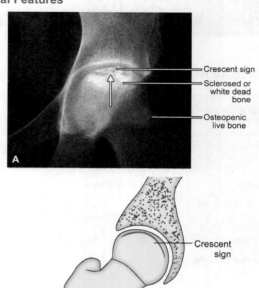

Figs. 19.8A and B: X-ray hip of a patient with avascular necrosis

Age 20–50 years with slight male preponderance (**Young Male**)

Bilateral in 50% of idiopathic cases, and 80% of steroid induced cases.

Decreased range of motion especially internal rotation followed by abduction.

This is a characteristic feature of any disease in which femoral head shape is altered–abduction and internal rotation is reduced. (Also seen in Perthes, Slipped Capital Femoral Epiphysis).

A characteristic sign is a tendency for hip to twist into external rotation during passive flexion; this corresponds to the 'Sectoral sign' in which, with the hip extended, internal rotation is almost full but with hip flexed it is grossly restricted, it is due to a sector of femoral head being involved in AVN.

X-rays Sclerosed area—area of necrosis and Crescent sign- Crescentic defect in subchondral area.

MRI is the investigation of choice double line sign is seen

T1–AVN: Reduced intensity or irregular outline of head

T2–high signal intensity called as double line sign

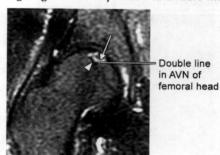

Fig. 19.9: MRI hip in AVN

Classification systems
1. Ficat and Arlet staging
2. University at Pennsylvania system:
   Mild AVN < 15% of Femoral head involved
   Moderate AVN 15–30% of Femoral head involved
   Severe AVN >30% of Femoral head involved

Treatment
1. Early stages protected weight bearing.
2. Pre collapse stage–core decompression to decrease intraosseous pressure in femoral head (**Intraosseous Pressure Normal 10–20 mm Hg it is 3–4 times in AVN**) drill holes are made in femoral head this procedure also opens the channels for vascular ingrowths and it is also supplemented with bone grafting (vascular or non-vascular) or electrical stimulation or Bone Morphogenic Proteins.

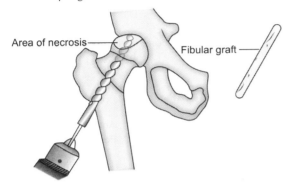

Fig. 19.10: Core decompression to decrease intra-osseous pressure

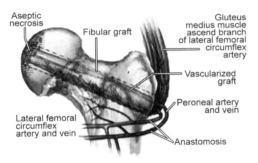

Fig. 19.11: Core decompression and vascularised fibular graft

3. Muscle Pedicle graft–Quadratus femoris (Meyers graft)/Tensor fascia lata graft (Joshi's graft) can be fixed in femoral head to augment vascularity.

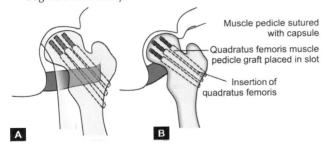

Figs. 19.12A and B: Muscle pedicle graft

4. Rotational osteotomy—To get the intact part of femoral head in acetabulum weight bearing area (anterolateral aspect of femur head) this is an extensive procedure requiring vascular repair alongwith it.

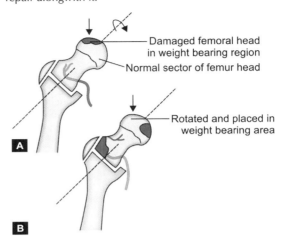

Figs. 19.13A and B: Rotational osteotomy

5. Arthritis/Collapse of femoral head—Total hip replacement one of the very commonly done procedure as most patients present at stage of arthritis.

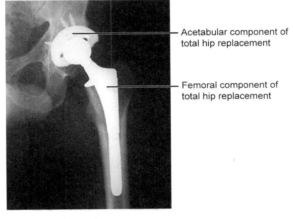

Fig. 19.14: Total hip replacement

MULTIPLE CHOICE QUESTIONS

1. Meyer pedicle graft used for: *(DNB Pattern 2018)*
   A. Fracture through neck of the talus
   B. Non-union fracture neck of femur
   C. Fracture through the waist of the scaphoid
   D. Inter-trochanteric fracture femur

   Ans. is 'B' Non-union fracture neck of femur

2. A patient who used to work out regularly at the gym gradually developed pain in the hip which is aggravated while squatting. He gives history of regular steroid and creatine use over last six months. There is flattening of femoral head and subchondral cysts were seen on X-ray. What is the likely diagnosis? *(AIIMS Nov 2017)*
   A. AVN of hip   B. TB
   C. Fracture neck of femur   D. Osteomalacia

   Ans. is 'A' AVN of hip

3. **True about avascular necrosis of femur:** *(PGI May 2017)*
   A. Affected side hip is kept non-weight bearing
   B. Asymptomatic cases may occur
   C. Radionuclide scan show increased uptake due to new bone formation in the area around the infarct
   D. Trendelenburg sign is negative
   E. MRI is investigation of choice

   Ans. is 'A' Affected side hip is kept non-weight bearing; 'B' Asymptomatic cases may occur; 'C' Radionuclide scan show increased uptake due to new bone formation in the area around the infarct; 'E' MRI is investigation of choice
   - MRI is investigation of choice.
   - Trendelenburg test is positive in AVN

4. **Potential causes of AVN include:** *(PGI Nov 2016)*
   A. Prolonged intake of steroids
   B. Caisson's disease
   C. Sickle cell anemia
   D. Posterior dislocation hip
   E. Intracapsular fracture femur neck

   Ans. is 'A' Prolonged intake of steroids; 'B' Caisson's disease; 'C' Sickle cell anemia; 'D' Posterior dislocation hip; 'E' Intracapsular fracture femur neck

5. **AVN of the hip may occur following which following fractures?** *(AI Dec 15)*
   A. Intertrochanteric fracture of the hip
   B. Subtrochanteric fracture
   C. Transcervical fracture of the neck of femur
   D. Fracture of posterior lip of the acetabulum

   Ans. is 'C' Transcervical fracture of the neck of femur

6. **AVN following transcervical neck femur fracture occurs due to damage to which of the following vessels?** *(AI Dec 15)*
   A. Lateral retinacular branch of lateral circumflex femoral artery
   B. Lateral retinacular branch of medial circumflex femoral artery
   C. Medial retinacular branch of lateral circumflex femoral artery
   D. Obturator artery

   Ans. is 'B' Lateral retinacular branch of medial circumflex femoral artery

7. **Most common cause of AVN of the hip is:** *(CET Nov 15)*
   A. Idiopathic
   B. Alcoholism
   C. Caissons disease
   D. Fracture neck of femur (post-traumatic)

   Ans. is 'A' Idiopathic

8. **Which of the following part of the bone is not prone for AVN?** *(TN 2014)*
   A. Proximal scaphoid   B. Body of talus
   C. Femoral neck   D. Femoral head

   Ans. 'C' Femoral neck

9. **Sectoral sign is positive in:** *(NEET 2015)*
   A. Avascular necrosis of femur head
   B. Osteoarthritis of hip
   C. Protrusio acetabuli
   D. Slipped capital femoral epiphyses

   Ans. is 'A' Avascular necrosis of femur head

10. **After chronic use of steroids severe pain in right hip with immobility is due to:** *(NEET Pattern 2012)*
    A. Avascular necrosis   B. Perthes disease
    C. Hip dislocation   D. Osteoarthritis

    Ans. is 'A' Avascular necrosis

11. **Avascular necrosis investigation of choice is:**
    A. X-ray   B. CT scan
    C. Bone scan   D. MRI *(NEET Pattern 2012)*

    Ans. is 'D' MRI

12. **Osteonecrosis is seen in all except:** *(NEET Pattern 2012)*
    A. Fracture neck femur   B. Sickle cell anemia
    C. Perthes disease   D. Paget's disease

    Ans. is 'D' Paget's disease

13. **AVN affects all except:** *(NEET Pattern 2012)*
    A. Femur   B. Scaphoid
    C. Talus   D. Iliac crest

    Ans. is 'D' Iliac crest

14. **Avascular necrosis of bone investigation of choice:**
    A. CT scan   B. MRI *(NEET Pattern 2012)*
    C. Bone scan   D. USG

    Ans. is 'B' MRI

15. **Avascular necrosis affects which part of femoral head?** *(NEET Pattern 2012)*
    A. Anteromedial   B. Anterolateral
    C. Posteromedial   D. Posterolateral

    Ans. is 'B' Anterolateral

16. **Femur head avascular necrosis is due to damage to:**
    A. Medial circumflex arteries *(NEET Pattern 2012)*
    B. Lateral circumflex arteries
    C. Artery to ligamentum teres
    D. Obturator artery

    Ans. is 'A' Medial circumflex arteries

17. **Avascular necrosis is seen at proximal pole of scaphoid because:** *(AI 2012)*
    A. Blood supply enters proximal pole
    B. Blood supply enters through the waist
    C. Blood supply enters through the distal pole
    D. Proximal pole is intra-articular

    Ans. is 'C' Blood supply enters through the distal pole

18. **Post-traumatic avascular necrosis commonly occurs in which fracture?** *(PGI June 09, 2K, PGI Dec 07)*
    A. Neck femur   B. Surgical neck humerus
    C. Neck of talus   D. Waist of scaphoid
    E. Neck radius

    Ans. is 'A' Neck of femur; 'C' Neck of talus; and 'D' Waist of scaphoid

19. **A vascular necrosis can be a possible sequelae of fracture of all of the following bones, except:** *(PGI June 04, AI 2003, AI 1999)*
    A. Femur neck   B. Scaphoid
    C. Talus   D. Calcaneum

    Ans. is 'D' Calcaneum

20. **AVN can occur at all except:**
    A. Femur neck   B. Body of talus
    C. Proximal scaphoid   D. None

    Ans. is 'A' Femur neck
    - These types of questions are to see your reflex please remember that femur neck fracture causes AVN at head of femur not the neck of femur so answer is neck femur as all other sites have avascular necrosis.

21. An elderly woman was admitted with a fracture of the neck of right femur which failed to unite. On examination an avascular necrosis of the head of femur was noted. The condition would have resulted most probably from the damage to: *(AIIMS Nov 2003)*
    A. Superior gluteal artery
    B. Inferior gluteal artery
    C. Acetabular branch of obturator
    D. Retinacular branches of circumflex femoral arteries

Ans. is 'D' Retinacular braches of circumflex femoral arteries
  – The major blood supply of femoral head is by lateral (superior) retinacular branch of medial circumflex artery.

22. Avascular necrosis of head of the femur is most common in: *(AIIMS Feb 1997, AI 1996, DNB 2000, AMU 97, CSE 2000)*
    A. Subcapital fracture
    B. Basal fracture
    C. Fracture intertrochanteric
    D. Transcervical fracture

Ans. is 'A' Subcapital fracture

23. Caissons disease the pain in joints and muscle is because of:
    A. N_2
    B. O_2
    C. N_2O
    D. NO_2

Ans. is 'A' N_2

24. Avascular necrosis of head of femur can occur in:
    A. Sickle cell anaemia *(PGI Dec 09, 08, 04, 02 and June 05)*
    B. Caisson's disease
    C. Intracapsular fracture neck
    D. Trochanteric fracture

Ans. is 'A' Sickle cell anaemia; 'B' Caisson's disease; and 'C' Intracapsular fracture neck

25. A 30-year-old HIV positive male who is on antiretroviral therapy (protease inhibitors) has pain in the right hip joint for 2 months. He has difficulty in abduction and internal rotation. Which of the following is most likely diagnosis? *(All India 2008)*
    A. Septic arthritis
    B. Osteoarthritis
    C. Avascular necrosis
    D. Tubercular arthritis

Ans. is 'C' Avascular necrosis
  – Limitation of abduction and internal rotation is a characteristic clinical feature of altered shape of femoral head. It is seen in AVN and can be seen in Perthes or Slipped capital femoral epiphysis. Use of Protease inhibitor in HIV patients is associated with an increased risk of avascular necrosis of femoral head (AVN) or Osteonecrosis.
  – In this question if it is asked that patient has Flexion Abduction and External rotation deformity then Tuberculosis will be a better answer because this is seen in Stage 1 of Tuberculosis of hip and is usually not seen in AVN.

	TB hip in HIV	AVN in HIV
Incidence	More common, usually unilateral	Less common, usually bilateral
Deformity	Faber-stage of synovitis may be prolonged on treatment than subsequently stage of arthritis (FADIR)	Limitation of abduction and internal rotation so initially position is adduction and external rotation (opposite to movements limited) and than subsequently with onset of arthritis FADIR

  – Thus if it is given restriction of abduction and internal rotation mark the answer as avascular necrosis and if it is mentioned flexion, abduction and external rotation deformity than answer is tuberculosis.

26. A patient is using oral steroids for a period of 5 years and patient complaints of pain in the both hip regions. Which one of the following is a diagnostic modality for confirmation of diagnosis? *(AI 2005, AIIMS Nov 2003, WB, NIMS 2000)*
    A. Plain X-ray
    B. CT scan
    C. MRI
    D. Isotope Bone scan

Ans. is 'C' MRI

Steroid intake think of AVN

27. A 50-year-old man sustained posterior dislocation of left hip in an accident. Dislocation was reduced after 3 days. He started complaining of pain in left hip after 6 months. X-ray of the pelvis was normal. The most relevant investigation at this stage will be: *(AIIMS Nov 2004)*
    A. CRP Levels in blood
    B. Ultrasonography of hip
    C. Arthrography of hip
    D. MRI of hip

Ans. is 'D' MRI of hip
  – MRI shows characteristic increased intensity in the marrow long before the appearance of X-ray signs. Therefore MRI is the most reliable way of diagnosing Avascular necrosis.
  – MRI is the investigation of choice double line sign is seen.

28. A woman of 45, a known cause of pemphigus vulgaris on a regular treatment with controlled primary disease presented with pain in the right hip and knee. Examination revealed no limb length discrepancy but the patient has tenderness in the Scarpa's triangle and limitation of abduction and internal rotation of the right hip joint as compared to the other side. The most probable diagnosis is: *(AIIMS May 2004 and Nov 2001)*
    A. Stress fracture of neck of femur
    B. Avascular necrosis of femoral head
    C. Perthes disease
    D. Transient synovitis of hip

Ans. is 'B' Avascular necrosis of femoral head
  – This patient is on steroids indirectly indicated by pemphigus vulgaris taking treatment (steroid is the preferred drug). Pain in hip and knee (pain of hip can refer to knee because of common nerve—obturator giving a twig to both joints). Limitation of abduction and internal rotation, indicates altered shape of femoral head so indicates Avascular necrosis of femoral head.
  – Stress fracture there is no limitation of abduction and internal rotation.
  – Perthes (4–8 years) and transient synovitis (6–12 years) will not be considered in this age group.

29. Pathological changes in Caisson's disease is due to: *(AIIMS 91)*
    A. N_2
    B. O_2
    C. CO_2
    D. CO

Ans. is 'A' N_2

20 CHAPTER

DNB CET Questions

DNB QUESTIONS FROM 2017 TO 2012

1. Martels sign seen in which of the following condition?
   A. Rheumatoid arthritis
   B. Osteoarthritis
   C. Gouty arthritis
   D. Ochronosis
   Ans. is 'C' Gouty arthritis

2. Most specific antibody seen in RA:
   A. Anti CCP
   B. Rheumatoid factor
   C. ANA
   D. Anti dsDNA
   Ans. is 'A' Anti CCP

3. Compartment syndrome is commonly seen in:
   A. Fracture of proximal tibia
   B. Fracture shaft humerus
   C. Fracture of femur shaft
   D. Fracture distal end radius
   Ans. is 'A' Fracture of proximal tibia

4. In surgical anterolateral approach to tibia, incision is taken over the tibialis anterior muscle mass rather than over the shaft. What is/are the advantages?
   A. Medially based flap
   B. Less chances of wound dehiscence
   C. Can be converted to an extensile approach
   D. All of the above
   Ans. is 'D' All of the above

5. Unna boot is used for treatment of:
   A. Diabetic foot ulcer
   B. Varicose ulcers
   C. Ankle instability
   D. Calcaneum fracture
   Ans. is 'B' Varicose ulcer

6. Which of the following is true about DDH:
   A. Male gender is risk factor
   B. Limbs are in adduction, internal rotation and flexion in old children
   C. Femur neck is retroverted
   D. Ligamentum teres is atrophied
   Ans. is 'B' Limbs are in adduction, internal rotation and flexion in old children

7. A patient presents with normal babinsky reflex with ankle areflexia with presence of saddle anesthesia and difficulty in micturition. What is the most probable diagnosis?
   A. Cauda equina syndrome
   B. Brown Sequard syndrome
   C. Leriche syndrome
   D. Williams syndrome
   Ans. is 'A' Cauda equina syndrome

8. Most common site of metastases in case of osteosarcoma is:
   A. Brain
   B. Lungs
   C. Liver
   D. Bladder
   Ans. is 'B' Lungs

9. Paprika sign during debridement is crucial in management which of the following condition?
   A. Chronic osteomyelitis
   B. Osteosarcoma
   C. Osteoid osteoma
   D. Brodies abscess
   Ans. is 'A' Chronic osteomyelitis

10. A 40-year-old female presents with urine darkening on standing, joint and stiffness, and pigment deposition in joints. What is the probable diagnosis?
    A. Phenylketonuria
    B. Tyrosinemia
    C. Alkaptonuria
    D. Tyrosinemia
    Ans. is 'C' Alkaptonuria

11. What suggests segmental demyelination on NCV?
    A. Decreased CMAP amplitudes
    B. Uniform slowing of nerve conduction
    C. Decreased area under CMAP curve
    D. No evidence of distal conduction
    Ans. is 'A' Decreased CMAP amplitudes

12. Negative pressure wound therapy false:
    A. Necrotic tissue with eschar in wound is a contraindication to its use
    B. Pressure is 30 mm Hg
    C. Give good granulation tissue
    D. Used intermittently or continuously
    Ans. is 'B' Pressure is 30 mm Hg

13. What is the age of tendon transfer in post polio residual paralysis:
    A. <6 months
    B. 1 year
    C. 2 years
    D. >5 years
    Ans. is 'D' >5 years

14. Which of the following is seen in popliteal entrapment syndrome?
    A. Evidence of atherosclerosis
    B. Exercise induced calf claudication
    C. Abnormal relation between popliteal artery and lateral head of gastrocnemius
    D. Decreased ankle pulses with ankle extension
    Ans. is 'B' Exercise induced calf claudication

15. Denis classification is used to assess:
    A. Stability of spine
    B. Degree of calcium content
    C. Degree of tumor invasion
    D. Amount of femur head subluxation in dysplastic hips
Ans. is 'A' Stability of spine

16. Ponseti technique failure in children should be managed with:
    A. Posteromedial soft tissue release
    B. Anterolateral soft tissue release
    C. Triple arthrodesis
    D. Lateral closing wedge osteotomy of calcaneum
Ans. is 'A' Posteromedial soft tissue release

17. Which of the following is not true about Klumpke's paralysis?
    A. Involves lower trunk of brachial plexus
    B. Intrinsic muscles of hand are paralysed
    C. Claw hand is a feature
    D. Horner's syndrome can never be associated
Ans. is 'D' Horner's syndrome can never be associated

18. Acute flaccid complete paralysis with areflexia and loss of perianal reflexes, below the level of spinal cord injury is due to:
    A. Spinal shock   B. Denervation
    C. Malingering   D. UMN paralysis
Ans. is 'A' Spinal shock

19. Bakers cyst is a type of:
    A. Pulsion diverticulum of knee joint
    B. Retention cyst
    C. Bursistis
    D. Benign tumor
Ans. is 'A' Pulsion diverticulum of knee joint

20. Tenderness in anatomical snuff box is characteristic of which carpal bone fractures?
    A. Scaphoid   B. Capitate
    C. Lunate   D. Triquetral
Ans. is 'A' Scaphoid

21. Which of the following is not true about osteoid osteoma?
    A. Most common true benign tumor of bone
    B. Occurs between 10-30 years of age
    C. Lesion appears ill defined on X-ray with permeative margins
    D. Bone scan shows increased uptakes in the lesion
Ans. is 'C' Lesion appears ill defined on X-ray with permeative margins

22. Fasciotomy -all of the following are cut except:
    A. Skin   B. Superficial fascia
    C. Deep fascia   D. Muscles
Ans. is 'D' Muscles

23. High crural index is seen in:
    A. Jumping athletes
    B. Gymnasts
    C. Weight lifters
    D. Long distance runners
Ans. is 'A' Jumping athletes

24. Brachial plexus injury with Horner's syndrome, nerve root level involved is:
    A. C5   B. C6
    C. C7   D. T1
Ans. is 'D' T1

25. Positive Adson's test is seen in:
    A. Thoracic outlet syndrome
    B. Burger disease
    C. Varicose veins
    D. Radial nerve injury
Ans. is 'A' Thoracic outlet syndrome

26. Tendon used for repair of flexor tendon injury in hand requiring reconstruction from forearm to fingertip is:
    A. Palmaris
    B. Plantaris
    C. Extensor digitorum communis
    D. Extensor digiti minimi
Ans. is 'B' Plantaris

27. Which of the following is not a type I geographic lesion of bone?
    A. Fibrous dysplasia
    B. Brodies abscess
    C. Giant cell tumor
    D. Ewing's sarcoma
Ans. is 'D' Ewing's sarcoma

28. Transverse carpal ligament is: *(DNB CET July 2015)*
    A. Flexor retinaculum of hand
    B. Extensor retinaculum of hand
    C. Radial collateral ligament
    D. Intercarpal ligament
Ans. is 'A' Flexor retinaculum of hand

29. Physiological interruption of transmission is: *(DNB CET July 2015)*
    A. Neuropraxia   B. Neurotmesis
    C. Axonotmesis   D. None of the above
Ans. is 'A' Neuropraxia

30. MC organism in acute osteomyelitis: *(DNB CET July 2015)*
    A. Staphylococcus aureus
    B. Salmonella
    C. Pseudomonas aeruginosae
    D. Streptococcus pneumonia
Ans. is 'A' Staphylococcus aureus

31. Breech presentation is a risk factor for the following condition: *(DNB CET July 2015)*
    A. CTEV   B. SCFE
    C. DDH   D. Perthes disease
Ans. is 'C' DDH

32. Most common cause of chronic osteomyelitis: *(DNB CET July 2015)*
    A. Staphylococcus aureus
    B. Streptococcus pyogenes
    C. Mycobacterium tuberculosis
    D. Staphylococcus epidermidis
Ans. is 'A' Staphylococcus aureus

33. Following is true about spinal injuries except: *(DNB CET July 2015)*
    A. Forms 6% of all trauma cases
    B. Neurodeficit is present in 50% of all the cases
    C. Traumatic injuries most commonly affect the cervical spine
    D. Cervical spine is more prone to fracture than dislocation
Ans. is 'D' Cervical spine is more prone to fracture than dislocation

34. Tennis elbow is characterized by: *(DNB CET July 2015)*
    A. Tenderness over the medial epicondyle
    B. Tendinitis of common extensor origin
    C. Tendinitis of common flexor origin
    D. Painful flexion and extension
Ans. is 'B' Tendinitis of common extensor origin

35. Distal interphalangeal joints are involved in all except: *(DNB CET July 2015)*
    A. Psoriatic arthritis
    B. Rheumatoid arthritis
    C. Reactive arthritis
    D. Osteoarthritis
Ans. is 'B' Rheumatoid arthritis

36. Froment's test is used in: *(DNB CET July 2015)*
    A. Ulnar nerve injury
    B. Median nerve injury
    C. Radial nerve injury
    D. Axillary nerve injury
Ans. is 'A' Ulnar nerve injury

37. Barton's fracture: *(DNB CET July 2015)*
    A. Volar fracture of distal end radius
    B. Dorsal fracture of distal end radius
    C. Radial styloid fracture
    D. Ulnar styloid fracture
Ans. is 'A' Volar fracture of distal end radius
    (A>B according to incidence)

38. Which of the following is the marker of bone formation: *(DNB CET July 2015)*
    A. Procollagen type I
    B. Urine N telopeptide
    C. Urine hydroxyproline
    D. Osteonectin
Ans. is 'A' Procollagen type I

39. Holstein-Lewis sign is related which nerve: *(DNB CET July 2015)*
    A. Median
    B. Radial
    C. Ulnar
    D. Axillary
Ans. is 'B' Radial

40. A 24 years old woman walking up experiences pain in heel which decreases on walking down. X-ray shows bone spur. Diagnosis: *(DNB CET July 2015)*
    A. Plantar fasciitis
    B. Calcaneal exostosis
    C. Osteomyelitis of calcaneum
    D. Achilles tendonitis
Ans. is 'D' Achilles tendonitis

41. Genu valgum deformity is seen in all except: *(DNB CET July 2015)*
    A. Rickets
    B. Bone dysplasia
    C. Rheumatoid arthritis
    D. Medial compartment osteoarthritis
Ans. is 'D' Medial compartment osteoarthritis

42. Crystal of pseudogout is made up of: *(DNB CET July 2015)*
    A. CPPD
    B. Urate
    C. Calcium carbonate
    D. Xanthine
Ans. is 'A' CPPD

43. Green extra-articular arthrodesis done for: *(DNB CET July 2015)*
    A. Genu Valgum
    B. Coxa vara
    C. Congenital vertical talus
    D. Cubitus varus
Ans. is 'C' Congenital vertical talus

44. Galeazzi fracture is: *(DNB CET July 2015)*
    A. Fracture distal 1/3 radius with DRUJ subluxation
    B. Fracture proximal 1/3 radius with DRUJ subluxation
    C. Fracture distal 1/3 radius without DRUJ subluxation
    D. Fracture proximal 1/3 radius without DRUJ subluxation
Ans. is 'A' Fracture distal 1/3 radius with DRUJ subluxation

45. Which nerve is compressed in carpal tunnel syndrome? *(DNB CET July 2015)*
    A. Median nerve
    B. Ulnar nerve
    C. Radial nerve
    D. Axillary nerve
Ans. is 'A' Median nerve

46. What is the treatment for a newborn child with CTEV? *(DNB CET July 2015)*
    A. Jess fixation
    B. Manipulation and strapping or serial cast
    C. Posteromedial soft tissue release
    D. Triple arthrodesis
Ans. is 'B' Manipulation and strapping or serial cast

47. Which is the nerve involved in case of ape thumb deformity? *(DNB CET July 2015)*
    A. Median
    B. Radial
    C. Ulnar
    D. Axillary
Ans. is 'A' Median

48. Median nerve lesion at the wrist causes all of the following except: *(DNB CET July 2015)*
    A. Thenar atrophy
    B. Weakness of Adductor pollicis
    C. Weakness of 1 and 2 lumbricals
    D. Weakness of Flexor pollicis brevis
Ans. is 'B' Weakness of Adductor pollicis

49. Finkelstein test used for: *(DNB CET July 2015)*
    A. Carpal tunnel syndrome
    B. Cubital tunnel syndrome
    C. De Quervain's tenovaginitis
    D. Median nerve injury
Ans. is 'C' De Quervain's tenovaginitis

50. False about osteoarthritis is: *(DNB CET July 2015)*
    A. Involves synovial joints
    B. Progressive softening of the articular cartilage
    C. It is an inflammatory arthritis
    D. Marginal osteophytes are produced
Ans. is 'C' It is an inflammatory arthritis

51. Bisphosphonates are used for all except:
    (DNB CET July 2015)
    A. Osteolytic bone metastases
    B. Osteoporosis
    C. Osteosclerosis
    D. Paget's disease
Ans. is 'C' Osteosclerosis

52. French osteotomy is used in treatment of:
    (DNB CET July 2015)
    A. Cubitus varus   B. Cubitus valgus
    C. Coxa vara   D. Coxa valga
Ans. is 'A' Cubitus varus

53. Ewing's sarcoma clinically mimics: *(DNB CET July 2015)*
    A. Osteomyelitis   B. Osteochondroses
    C. Osteosclerosis   D. Heterotopic ossification
Ans. is 'A' Osteomyelitis

54. Milwaukee brace is used in treatment of:
    (DNB CET July 2015)
    A. Scoliosis   B. Kyphosis
    C. Cubitus varus   D. Genu varum
Ans. is 'A' Scoliosis

55. Tardy ulnar nerve palsy is seen in: *(DNB CET July 2015)*
    A. Medial condyle fracture humerus
    B. Lateral condyle fracture humerus
    C. Humerus shaft fracture
    D. Fracture shaft radius
Ans. is 'B' Lateral condyle fracture humerus

56. Following are the clinical tests used in diagnosis of CDH:
    (DNB CET July 2015)
    A. Barlow test   B. Ortolani test
    C. Both of the above D. None of the above
Ans. is 'C' Both of the above

57. Gustilo Anderson classification is used for:
    (DNB CET July 2015)
    A. Compound fractures
    B. Closed fractures
    C. Distal end radius fractures
    D. Femur head fractures
Ans. is 'A' Compound fractures

58. Genu valgum deformity is seen in all except:
    (DNB CET July 2015)
    A. Rickets
    B. Bone Dysplasia
    C. Rheumatoid arthritis
    D. Medial compartment osteoarthritis
Ans. is 'D' Medial compartment osteoarthritis

59. Wormian bones are seen in all except:
    (DNB CET July 2015)
    A. Fibrous dysplasia   B. Osteogenesis imperfecta
    C. Cretinism   D. Rickets
Ans. is 'A' Fibrous dysplasia

60. Which of the following fracture needs a violent force?
    (DNB CET July 2015)
    A. Fracture Neck of femur   B. Intertrochanteric fracture
    C. Clavicle fracture   D. Colles fracture
Ans. is 'C' Clavicle fracture

61. A person comes with fracture tibia with swelling of lower leg pulse feeble but palpable. Intracompartmental pressure is raised. What is the next step in management?
    (DNB CET July 2015)
    A. Fasciotomy
    B. External fixation
    C. Lower limb venography
    D. Interlock nail
Ans. is 'A' Fasciotomy

62. A football player came with twisting injury to left leg with pain, X-ray was normal, but on clinical examination anterior drawer test, lachman test positive diagnosis:
    (DNB CET July 2015)
    A. Medial meniscus tear
    B. ACL tear
    C. PCL tear
    D. Proximal tibia fracture
Ans. is 'B' ACL tear

63. Ankylosing spondylitis is associated with:
    (DNB CET July 2015)
    A. HLA-B27   B. HLA-B8
    C. HLA - DW4/DR4   D. HLA - DR3
Ans. is 'A' HLA-B27

64. Osgood-Schlatter disease is osteochondritis of:
    (DNB CET July 2015)
    A. Tibial tuberosity   B. Lunate
    C. Calcaneum   D. Navicular
Ans. is 'A' Tibial tuberosity

65. Pen test is done for which nerve injury:
    (DNB CET July 2015)
    A. Median   B. Ulnar
    C. Radial   D. Axillary
Ans. is 'A' Median

66. Antalgic hip gait is related to which of the following?
    (DNB CET July 2015)
    A. Waddling gait   B. Painful hip gait
    C. Trendelenburg gait D. Short leg gait
Ans. is 'B' Painful hip gait

67. Injury to popliteal artery in fracture lower end of femur can be caused by: *(DNB CET July 2015)*
    A. Proximal fragment   B. Muscle haematoma
    C. Distal fragment   D. Tissue swelling
Ans. is 'C' Distal fragment

68. Osteoarthritis involves all except: *(DNB CET July 2015)*
    A. Hip   B. Knee
    C. PIP   D. Wrist
Ans. is 'D' Wrist

69. Which nerve mostly damaged in post dislocation of hip?
    (DNB CET July 2015)
    A. Sciatic nerve   B. Femoral nerve
    C. Obturator nerve   D. Superior gluteal nerve
Ans. is 'A' Sciatic nerve

70. Bouchard's nodes are seen in: *(DNB CET July 2015)*
    A. Proximal IP joints   B. Distal IP joints
    C. Sternoclavicular joints   D. Knee joint
Ans. is 'A' Proximal IP joints

71. Entrapment neuropathy at the arcade of Frohse involves which nerve? (DNB CET July 2015)
    A. Median nerve
    B. Posterior interosseous nerve
    C. Ulnar nerve
    D. Axillary nerve
Ans. is 'B' Posterior interosseous nerve

72. Golfers elbow: (DNB CET July 2015)
    A. Medial epicondylitis
    B. Lateral epicondylitis
    C. Posterior elbow dislocation
    D. Lateral collateral ligament injury
Ans. is 'A' Medial epicondylitis

73. Congenital elevation of scapula is called: (DNB CET July 2015)
    A. Sprengel shoulder
    B. Bouchard
    C. Boutonniere
    D. None of the above
Ans. is 'A' Sprengel shoulder

74. Ramesh Singh, a 40 years old man, was admitted with fracture shaft femur following a road traffic accident. Three days after trauma he was tachypnoeic, and had conjunctival petechiae. Most likely diagnosis is: (DNB CET July 2015)
    A. Pulmonary embolism
    B. Sepsis syndrome
    C. Fat embolism
    D. Hemothorax
Ans. is 'C' Fat embolism

75. Triple deformity of knee includes following except: (DNB CET July 2015)
    A. Flexion of knee
    B. External rotation of tibia
    C. Posterior subluxation of tibia
    D. Extension of knee
Ans. is 'D' Extension of knee

76. All are the features of rheumatoid arthritis except: (DNB CET July 2015)
    A. Osteosclerosis of joint
    B. Soft tissue swelling
    C. Narrowing of joint space
    D. Periarticular osteoporosis
Ans. is 'A' Osteosclerosis of joint

77. Boxer's fracture is: (DNB CET July 2015)
    A. Fracture base of 5th metacarpal
    B. Fracture neck of 5th metacarpal
    C. Fracture base of first metacarpal
    D. Fracture neck of first metacarpal
Ans. is 'B' Fracture neck of 5th metacarpal

78. Common sites of fracture non union are the following except: (DNB CET July 2015)
    A. Waist of scaphoid
    B. Neck of femur
    C. Distal 1/3 tibia fibula
    D. Distal end radius
Ans. is 'D' Distal end radius

79. Column concept of spine stability was given by: (DNB CET July 2015)
    A. Denis
    B. Frenkel
    C. Wilson
    D. Todd
Ans. is 'A' Denis

80. All of the following are diaphyseal tumors except: (DNB CET July 2015)
    A. Ewings sarcoma
    B. Histiocytosis
    C. Fibrosarcoma
    D. Aneurysmal bone cyst
Ans. is 'D' Aneurysmal bone cyst

81. Which of the following is an epiphyseal lesion? (DNB CET July 2015)
    A. Chondroblastoma
    B. Chondrosarcoma
    C. Fibrosarcoma
    D. Non ossifying fibroma
Ans. is 'A' Chondroblastoma

82. Diaphyseal aclasis is: (DNB CET July 2015)
    A. Multiple exostosis
    B. Multiple enchondromatosis
    C. Multiple hemangioma
    D. Multiple osteoid osteoma
Ans. is 'A' Multiple exostosis

83. Which nerve is damaged in fracture surgical neck humerus? (DNB CET July 2015)
    A. Axillary
    B. Radial
    C. Ulnar
    D. Median
Ans. is 'A' Axillary

84. Anterolateral avulsion fracture of the distal tibial physis is known as: (DNB CET July 2015)
    A. Potts fracture
    B. Tillaux fracture
    C. Chopart fracture
    D. Jones fracture
Ans. is 'B' Tillaux fracture

85. Involvement of the joints of hand is relatively uncommon in which of the following arthritis? (DNB CET July 2015)
    A. Ankylosing spondylitis
    B. Reactive arthritis
    C. Psoriatic arthritis
    D. Rheumatoid arthritis
Ans. is 'A' Ankylosing spondylitis

86. Most common site for vertebral cancer is: (DNB CET July 2015)
    A. Cervical
    B. Lumbosacral
    C. Thoracic
    D. Cervicodorsal
Ans. is 'C' Thoracic

87. Bohler's angle is used in fracture of: (DNB CET July 2015)
    A. Scaphoid
    B. Talus
    C. Calcaneum
    D. Navicular
Ans. is 'C' Calcaneum

88. Posada's fracture is: *(DNB CET July 2015)*
    A. Transcondylar fracture of humerus
    B. Fracture lateral condyle of humerus
    C. Fracture medial condyle of humerus
    D. Fracture anatomical neck of humerus
Ans. is 'A' Transcondylar fracture of humerus

89. Most sensitive test for carpal tunnel syndrome:
    (DNB CET July 2015)
    A. Phalen's test   B. Tinel's sign
    C. Tourniquet test D. None
Ans. is 'A' Phalen's test

90. Nerve roots involved in Klumpke's paralysis:
    (DNB CET July 2015)
    A. C_{4-5} B. C_{5-6}
    C. C_{6-7} D. C_8T_1
Ans. is 'D' C_8T_1

91. Limbs elevated against gravity but not against force is which power: *(DNB CET July 2015)*
    A. Grade I   B. Grade II
    C. Grade III   D. Grade IV
Ans. is 'C' Grade III

MRC Grading
Grade 5 Normal power
Grade 4 Active movement against gravity with resistance
Grade 3 Active movement against gravity without resistance
Grade 2 Active movement with gravity eliminated
Grade 1 Only a trace or flicker of movement
Grade 0 No movement

92. Feature of osteoarthritis is: *(DNB CET July 2015)*
    A. Heberden node   B. Increased ESR
    C. Onycholysis   D. Z deformity
Ans. is 'A' Heberden node

93. Meralgia paraesthetica is: *(DNB CET July 2015)*
    A. Medial cutaneous nerve of thigh
    B. Lateral cutaneous nerve of thigh
    C. Lateral cutaneous nerve of hand
    D. Medial cutaneous nerve of hand
Ans. is 'B' Lateral cutaneous nerve of thigh

94. Which of the following nerves has the best prognosis for repair after injury? *(DNB CET July 2015)*
    A. Ulnar   B. Radial
    C. Median   D. Lateral popliteal
Ans. is 'B' Radial

95. Osteoclasts remove bone at which of the following sites?
    (DNB CET July 2015)
    A. Howships lacunae   B. Resorption bays
    C. Both of the above   D. None of the above
Ans. is 'C' Both of the above

96. Clubfoot features are all except: *(DNB CET Nov 2014)*
    A. Forefoot adduction
    B. Eversion at subtalar joint
    C. Forefoot adduction at mid-tarsal joint
    D. Plantar flexion of ankle
Ans. is 'B' Eversion at subtalar joint

97. Which of the following is true about skeletal tuberculosis in children? *(DNB CET Nov 2014)*
    A. Most common sites are hip (40%), Spine (20%), Knee (10%)
    B. Most common site is upper limb
    C. Dorsolumbar junction is most commonly affected
    D. Progression to kyphosis deformity is least with lumbar lesions
Ans. is 'D' Progression to kyphosis deformity is least with lumbar lesions

98. Pulp space infection painful due to: *(DNB CET Nov 2014)*
    A. Dense fibrous septae   B. Small phalanx
    C. Rich blood supply   D. Rich nerve supply
Ans. is 'A' Dense fibrous septae

99. Tinel sign is seen in: *(DNB CET Nov 2014)*
    A. Nerve degeneration   B. Nerve regeneration
    C. Muscle degeneration   D. Muscle regeneration
Ans. is 'B' Nerve regeneration

100. Cause of Dupuytren's contracture is: *(DNB CET Nov 2014)*
    A. DM   B. Alcohol
    C. Smoking D. All of the above
Ans. is 'D' All of the above

101. CPPD crystals are seen in which disease?
    (DNB CET Nov 2014)
    A. Hypothyroidism
    B. Primary hyperparathyroidism
    C. Hemochromatosis
    D. All of the above
Ans. is 'D' All of the above

102. Commonest shoulder dislocation: *(DNB CET Nov 2014)*
    A. Preglenoid   B. Subcoracoid
    C. Posterior   D. Subclavicular
Ans. is 'B' Subcoracoid

103. Winging of scapula which muscle is affected?
    (DNB CET Nov 2014)
    A. Teres minor   B. Latissimus dorsi
    C. Subscapularis   D. Serratus anterior
Ans. is 'D' Serratus anterior

104. Most commonly involved bone in Paget's disease:
    (DNB CET Nov 2014)
    A. Skull   B. Femur
    C. Pelvis   D. Vertebrae
Ans. is 'C' Pelvis

105. Most common bone involved in haemangioma:
    (DNB CET Nov 2014)
    A. Femur   B. Tibia
    C. Pelvis   D. Vertebrae
Ans. is 'D' Vertebrae

106. Not a feature of TB spine: *(DNB CET Nov 2014)*
    A. Back pain earliest symptom
    B. Stiffness of back
    C. Exaggerated lumbar lordosis
    D. Cold abscess
Ans. is 'C' Exaggerated lumbar lordosis

107. Golden hour of fracture femur is: *(DNB CET Nov 2014)*
    A. 1 hr after injury
    B. 1 hr prior to injury
    C. 1 hr after reaching the hospital
    D. 1 hr after surgical procedure
Ans. is 'A' 1 hr after injury

108. Perthes disease etiology is: *(DNB CET Nov 2014)*
    A. Pyogenic   B. Tubercular
    C. Traumatic   D. Unknown
Ans. is 'D' Unknown

109. Congenital dislocation of hip in older child most common sign appreciated is: *(DNB CET Nov 2014)*
    A. Barlow test
    B. Ortolani test
    C. Painful ROM
    D. Limited abduction of Lower Limb
Ans. is 'D' Limited abduction of Lower Limb

110. Dinner fork deformity is seen in: *(DNB CET Nov 2014)*
    A. Colle's fracture
    B. March fracture
    C. Lateral condyle fracture
    D. Supracondylar fracture
Ans. is 'A' Colle's fracture

111. Undertaker's fracture is: *(DNB CET Nov 2014)*
    A. C23   B. C34
    C. C56   D. C67
Ans. is 'D' C67

112. A 34 years old male with femur shaft fracture develops petechiae over chest 4 days after the injury. What is the most probable diagnosis? *(DNB CET Nov 2014)*
    A. Fat embolism   B. Air embolism
    C. Thrombocytopenia   D. Hypocomplementemia
Ans. is 'A' Fat embolism

113. Perthes affects age group: *(DNB CET Nov 2014)*
    A. <4 yrs   B. 4–8 yrs
    C. 10–25 yrs   D. >25 yrs
Ans. is 'B' 4–8 yrs

114. Reflex sympathetic dystrophy true is: *(DNB CET Nov 2014)*
    A. Osteoporosis   B. Increased skin temp
    C. Common in athletes D. Vasoconstriction
Ans. is 'A' Osteoporosis

115. Investigation of choice for spinal TB: *(DNB CET Nov 2014)*
    A. X-ray   B. CT Scan
    C. MRI   D. PET Scan
Ans. is 'C' MRI

116. Most common site of TB: *(DNB CET Nov 2014)*
    A. Spine   B. Knee
    C. Hip   D. Shoulder
Ans. is 'A' Spine

117. Trabeculae are aligned in which stage of fracture neck femur? *(DNB CET Nov 2014)*
    A. Stage 1   B. Stage 2
    C. Stage 3   D. Stage 4
Ans. is 'B' Stage 2

118. Trendelenburg test is positive in palsy of: *(DNB CET Nov 2014)*
    A. Gluteus maximus   B. Gluteus medius
    C. Rectus femoris   D. Vastus medialis
Ans. is 'B' Gluteus medius

119. Charlie Chaplin gait is seen in: *(DNB CET Nov 2014)*
    A. Congenital coxa vara   B. Tibial torsion
    C. DDH   D. Genu valgus
Ans. is 'B' Tibial torsion

120. Patients with bilateral CDH walk with the following gait: *(DNB CET Nov 2014)*
    A. Waddling   B. Stumbling
    C. Knock knee   D. Antalgic
Ans. is 'A' Waddling

121. Index finger infection spreads to: *(DNB CET Nov 2014)*
    A. Thenar space   B. Mid palmar space
    C. Hypothenar space   D. Flexion space
Ans. is 'A' Thenar space

122. Winging of scapula is seen in paralysis of which muscle: *(DNB CET Nov 2014)*
    A. Serratus anterior B. Supraspinatus
    C. Pectoralis major   D. Infraspinatus
Ans. is 'A' Serratus anterior

123. Treatment of partially corrected CTEV with cavus deformity is: *(DNB CET Nov 2014)*
    A. Posteromedial release B. Lateral release
    C. Plantar release   D. Medial release
Ans. is 'C' Plantar release

124. Pseudofracture occurs in: *(DNB CET Nov 2014)*
    A. Osteomalacia   B. Osteoporosis
    C. Osteopetrosis D. Osteosclerosis
Ans. is 'A' Osteomalacia

125. Earliest site of bone involvement in hematogenous osteomyelitis is: *(DNB CET Nov 2014)*
    A. Metaphysis   B. Epiphysis
    C. Diaphysis   D. Apophysis
Ans. is 'A' Metaphysis

126. Clergyman's knee involves: *(DNB CET Nov 2014)*
    A. Olecranon bursa   B. Suprapatellar bursa
    C. Infrapatellar bursa D. Prepatellar bursa
Ans. is 'C' Infrapatellar bursa

127. 'Ulnar paradox' is seen in: *(DNB CET Nov 2014)*
    A. High ulnar lesion   B. Low ulnar lesion
    C. Triple nerve disease D. PIN Palsy
Ans. is 'A' High ulnar lesion

128. Deforming force on proximal fragment in Bennett's fracture: *(DNB CET Nov 2014)*
    A. APL   B. APB
    C. EPL   D. EPB
Ans. is 'A' APL

129. Age group affected of following lesion: *(DNB CET Nov 2014)*

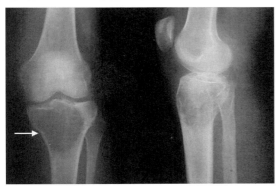

    A. 5–10 years   B. 10–20 years
    C. 20–40 years   D. >50 years

Ans. is 'C' 20–40 years

130. Chronic discharging sinus with bone particle is seen in: *(DNB CET Nov 2014)*
    A. Chronic osteomyelitis
    B. Acute osteomyelitis
    C. Subacute osteomyelitis
    D. Gaffe's osteomyelitis

Ans. is 'A' Chronic osteomyelitis

131. Osgood-Schlatter disease: *(DNB CET Nov 2014)*
    A. Tibial tuberosity
    B. Femur head
    C. Navicular
    D. Calcaneum

Ans. is 'A' Tibial tuberosity

132. Deformity of hip joint in case of tubercular synovitis of hip joint is: *(DNB CET Nov 2014)*
    A. Flexion abduction external rotation
    B. Flexion adduction external rotation
    C. Flexion abduction internal rotation
    D. Flexion adduction internal rotation

Ans. is 'A' Flexion abduction external rotation

133. A patient presents with pain in the thigh, relieved by aspirin. X-ray shows a radiolucent mass surrounded by sclerosis. Diagnosis is: *(DNB CET Nov 2014)*
    A. Osteoma
    B. Osteoid osteoma
    C. Osteoblastoma
    D. Osteoclastoma

Ans. is 'B' Osteoid osteoma

134. Nerve involved in Arcade of Frohse: *(DNB CET Nov 2014)*
    A. Median   B. Ulnar
    C. PIN   D. Radial

Ans. is 'C' PIN

135. What is seen in Maffucci syndrome?
    A. Enchondromas with hemangioma
    B. Hemangiomas and limb hyperplasia
    C. Hemangioma and capillary malformation
    D. Hemangiomas and precocious puberty

Ans. is 'A' Enchondromas with hemangioma

136. Holdsworth classification of thoracolumbar spine fracture is based on how many columns of spine?
    A. Two   B. Three
    C. Four   D. Five

Ans. is 'A' Two

137. Bone tumor arising from epiphysis is:
    A. Osteoid osteoma   B. Chondrosarcoma
    C. Ewing's sarcoma   D. Chondroblastoma

Ans. is 'D' Chondroblastoma

138. Meralgia paresthetica involves:
    A. Lateral cutaneous nerve of thigh
    B. Forearm
    C. Radial nerve
    D. Cutaneous branches of obturator nerve

Ans. is 'A' Lateral cutaneous nerve of thigh

139. Swan neck deformity seen in:
    A. Osteoarthritis   B. Rheumatoid arthritis
    C. Pyogenic arthritis   D. Gout

Ans. is 'B' Rheumatoid arthritis

140. Which carpal is prone for avascular necrosis?
    A. Talus   B. Scaphoid
    C. Pisiform   D. Navicular

Ans. is 'B' Scaphoid

141. Phalen's test is done for?
    A. De Quervain's tenosynovitis
    B. Carpal tunnel syndrome
    C. Tennis elbow
    D. Rotator cuff injury

Ans. is 'B' Carpal tunnel syndrome

142. Most common cause of CTEV is:
    A. Neural   B. Muscular
    C. Osseus   D. Idiopathic

Ans. is 'D' Idiopathic

143. Ponseti method is used for:
    A. Rickets   B. Blount's disease
    C. CTEV   D. Congenital vertical talus

Ans. is 'C' CTEV

144. Essex lopresti is a fracture of:
    A. Radial head with ulnar styloid
    B. Radial head with interosseous membrane
    C. Radial head with ulnar head
    D. Radial head alone

Ans. is 'B' Radial head with interosseous membrane

145. Fall on foot causes:
    A. Pond fracture
    B. Gutter fracture
    C. Cerebral hemisphere divided into half
    D. Compression fracture

Ans. is 'D' Compression fracture

146. Unhappy triad doesn't include injury to:
    A. ACL   B. MCL
    C. LCL   D. Medial meniscus

Ans. is 'C' LCL

147. Clergyman's knee is:
    A. Pre-patellar bursitis
    B. Infrapatellar bursitis
    C. Suprapatellar bursitis
    D. Pre-anserine bursitis
Ans. is 'B' Infrapatellar bursitis

148. Hill-Sachs lesion is seen in:
    A. Anterolateral part of humeral head
    B. Anterioposterior part of humerus head
    C. Posterolateral part of humeral head
    D. Posterioanterior part of humerus head
Ans. is 'C' Posterolateral part of humeral head

149. Fracture of distal tibial epiphysis with anterolateral displacement is called as?
    A. Pott's fracture
    B. Cotton's fracture
    C. Triplane fracture
    D. Tillaux fracture
Ans. is 'D' Tillaux fracture
    - Tillaux fracture is seen in adolescent due to fusion of medial part of tibial physis but unfused anterolateral part causing its avulsion in ankle injuries

150. Positive Trendelenburg's sign is seen in paralysis of:
    A. Gluteus maximus
    B. Gluteus medius
    C. Calf muscles
    D. Hamstrings
Ans. is 'B' Gluteus medius

151. Motor cyslist's fracture is:
    A. The base of skull break in two halves—left lateral and right lateral
    B. Skull base breaks into two halves—anterior and posterior
    C. Comminuted fracture of skull
    D. Ring fracture of skull base
Ans. is 'B' Skull base breaks into two halves—anterior and posterior

152. Most common primary malignancy of bone is:
    A. Multiple myeloma
    B. Osteoid osteoma
    C. Osteosarcoma
    D. PNET
Ans. is 'A' Multiple myeloma

153. Idiopathic scoliosis is most commonly:
    A. Dextroscoliosis of thoracic spine
    B. Levoscoliosis of thoracic spine
    C. Dextroscoliosis of lumbar spine
    D. Levoscoliosis of lumbar spine
Ans. is 'A' Dextroscoliosis of thoracic spine

154. Snowstorm appearance of knee joint with multiple loose bodies is seen in:
    A. Chondromalacia patellae
    B. Ewing's sarcoma of knee joint
    C. Fracture involving articular surface
    D. Synovial chondromatosis
Ans. is 'D' Synovial chondromatosis

155. O'Donoghue triad includes injury to which ligaments of the knee:
    A. Medial collateral ligament + Posterior cruciate ligament + medial meniscus
    B. Medial collateral ligament + Anterior cruciate ligament + medial meniscus
    C. Medical collateral ligament + Anterior cruciate ligament + lateral meniscus
    D. Medial collateral ligament + Posterior cruciate ligament + lateral meniscus
Ans. is 'B' Medial collateral ligament + Anterior cruciate ligament + medial meniscus

156. Tibial collateral ligament is formed by:
    A. Adductor magnus
    B. Adductor longus
    C. Semimembranosus
    D. Semitendinosus
Ans. is 'A' Adductor magnus

157. Agnes Hunt traction is used for:
    A. Supracondylar fracture of humerus
    B. Fracture shaft of femur
    C. Correction of hip deformity
    D. Trochanteric traction
Ans. is 'C' Correction of hip deformity

158. Axillary nerve damage is caused by damage to:
    A. Shaft of humerus
    B. Surgical neck humerus
    C. Medial epicondyle
    D. Lateral epicondyle
Ans. is 'B' Surgical neck humerus

159. Osgood-Schlatters disease involves:
    A. Tibial tuberosity
    B. Femoral condyle
    C. Lateral malleolus
    D. Medial malleolus
Ans. is 'A' Tibial tuberosity

160. Jones operation is done for:
    A. CTEV
    B. Hallus valgus correction
    C. Cavus deformity of foot
    D. Claw hallux
Ans. is 'D' Claw hallux

161. A crickets player sustained injury while catching the ball, his hand is as shown Mallet finger, this condition is better known as:

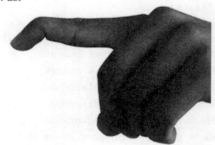

    A. Trigger finger
    B. Mallet finger
    C. Benediction hand
    D. Claw hand
Ans. is 'B' Mallet finger

162. After injury at wrist a patient is asked to extend the hand as shown he has Claw hand. This is due to:

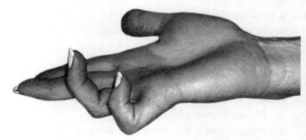

    A. Medial nerve injury
    B. Ulnar nerve injury
    C. Radial nerve injury
    D. Dupuytren's contracture
Ans. is 'B' Ulnar nerve injury (Ulnar Claw hand is shown)

163. C6-C7 cervical spine fracture is seen in:
    A. Chance fracture
    B. Clay-Shoveler's fracture
    C. Hangman's fracture
    D. Jefferson fracture

Ans. is 'B' Clay-Shoveler's fracture

164. Bone cement setting time is:
    A. 30 seconds
    B. 1–2 min
    C. 8–10 min
    D. > 30 min

Ans. is 'C' 8–10 min

165. In a case of partial amputation with heavy contamination, first step in management should be:
    A. Wound closure and suturing
    B. Wound irrigation and debridement
    C. Anti-gas gangrene serum
    D. Antibiotics

Ans. is 'B' Wound irrigation and debridement

166. An old lady presented with long standing arthritis of both hands and feet. X-ray feature which suggests rheumatoid arthritis rather than seronegative spondyloarthropathies is:
    A. Loss of joint space
    B. Periarticular erosions
    C. Juxtaarticular erosions
    D. Periosteal reaction

Ans. is 'B' Periarticular erosions

167. A 65-year-old male has been diagnosed with osteoarthritis, feature or deformity seen is:
    A. Swan neck deformity
    B. Boutonniere deformity
    C. Heberden's nodes
    D. Opera glass deformity

Ans. is 'C' Heberden's nodes

168. Most common deformity seen in Osteoarthritis is:
    A. Genu valgum
    B. Genu varum
    C. Genu recurvatum
    D. Triple knee deformity

Ans. is 'B' Genu varum

169. Synovial sarcoma most commonly arises from:
    A. Synovial lining
    B. Capsule of joint
    C. Bursa around the joint
    D. None

Ans. is 'C' Bursa around the joint

170. Most common site of fracture of mandible is:
    A. Neck of condyle
    B. Angle of mandible
    C. Symphysis
    D. Ramus

Ans. is 'A' Neck of condyle

171. Hawkins sign denotes:
    A. Retained vascularity
    B. Non-union
    C. Decrease vascularity
    D. Avascular necrosis

Ans. is 'A' Retained vascularity

172. Phalen test is done for:
    A. De Quervain's tenosynovitis
    B. Carpal tunnel syndrome
    C. Rotator cuff injury
    D. Tennis elbow

Ans. is 'B' Carpal tunnel syndrome

173. Finkelstein test is used for diagnosis of:
    A. Thoracic outlet syndrome
    B. Carpal tunnel syndrome
    C. Tarsal tunnel syndrome
    D. De Quervain tenosynovitis

Ans. is 'D' De Quervain tenosynovitis

174. Keller's operation is done for:
    A. Hallux valgus
    B. Hallux valgus
    C. Genu varus
    D. CTEV

Ans. is 'A' Hallux valgus

175. Immediate treatment of a patient with multiple fracture and fluid loss is best done by:
    A. Blood
    B. Dextran
    C. Normal saline
    D. Ringer lactate

Ans. is 'D' Ringer lactate

176. An elderly falls on an outstretched hand and sustained injury of right forearm. X-ray film is shown. What is this injury:

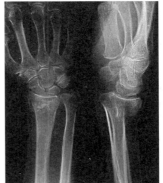

   A. Colle's fracture
   B. Galeazzi fracture
   C. Barton's fracture
   D. Chauffeur's fracture

Ans. is 'A' Colle's fracture

177. Charlie Chaplin gait is seen in:
    A. Congenital coxa vara
    B. Tibial torsion
    C. Genu valgus
    D. CDH

Ans. is 'B' Tibial torsion

   Charlie Chaplin gait is due to external tibial torsion

178. Allen's test is for integrity of palmar arch and it tests which of the following:
    A. Radial artery
    B. Ulnar artery
    C. Both
    D. None

Ans. is 'C' Both
   – Allens test is for both radial and ulnar artery
   – Modified allens test is for ulnar artery

179. Myositis ossificans is:
    A. Worm calcification
    B. Callus formation
    C. Regeneration
    D. Post-traumatic ossification

Ans. is 'D' Post-traumatic ossification

180. Which isotope is used for treating bone cancer?
    A. Sr
    B. Ga
    C. I 123
    D. Tc

Ans. is 'A' Sr

181. Attachments at styloid process of Radius:
    A. Pronation teres
    B. Brachioradialis
    C. Supination
    D. Pronator quadritus
Ans. is 'B' Brachioradialis

182. Cause of osteomalacia:
    A. Deficiency of Vitamin A
    B. Deficiency of Vitamin D
    C. Deficiency of Vitamin E
    D. Deficiency of Vitamin K
Ans. is 'B' Deficiency of Vitamin D

183. Which of the following is a dangerous cast?
    A. Collis cast
    B. Above knee cast
    C. Above elbow cast
    D. Below knee cast
Ans. is 'C' Above elbow cast

184. Hangman's fracture:
    A. C2–C3
    B. C3–C4
    C. C4–C5
    D. C5–C6
Ans. is 'A' C2–C3

185. Green stick fracture:
    A. Break in one cortex in children
    B. Break in both cortex in children
    C. Undisplaced fracture in adult
    D. Displaced fracture in adult
Ans. is 'A' Break in one cortex in children

186. In CTEV manipulation is required at:
    A. As patients requirements
    B. In adolescent
    C. After 25 years
    D. From birth
Ans. is 'D' From birth

187. Fallen leaf sign is seen in:
    A. Aneurysmal bone cyst
    B. Simple bone cyst
    C. Osteosarcoma
    D. Osteoclastoma
Ans. is 'B' Simple bone cyst

188. Most common patellar bursitis is:
    A. Prepatellar bursitis
    B. Suprapatellar bursitis
    C. Infrapatellar bursitis
    D. Pes anserinus bursitis
Ans. is 'A' Prepatellar bursitis

189. Most common site of tuberculosis of spine is:
    A. Thoracolumbar
    B. Sacral
    C. Cervical
    D. Lumbosacral
Ans. is 'A' Thoracolumbar

190. Which of the following is biphasic tumor?
    A. Rhabdomyosarcoma
    B. Synovial sarcoma
    C. Osteosarcoma
    D. Osteoblastoma
Ans. is 'B' Synovial sarcoma
    – Synovial sarcomas are morphologically biphasic as they have dual lines of differentiation (Epithelial and Mesenchymal).

191. Bechterew disease is:
    A. Ankylosing spondylitis
    B. Behcet's disease
    C. Sjögren's syndrome
    D. Psoriasis
Ans. is 'A' Ankylosing spondylitis

192. Fair bank's triangle is seen in:
    A. Tibia vara
    B. Genu valgum
    C. Hip fracture
    D. Coxa vara
Ans. is 'D' Coxa vara

193. Terry Thomas sign is seen in:
    A. Kienbock's disease
    B. Carpal instability
    C. Calcaneal disorders
    D. Hip trauma
Ans. is 'B' Carpal instability

194. All are true about CTEV except:
    A. Talus is only bone involved
    B. Posterior and medial tendons are involved
    C. Tibialis posterior acts like a guy rope
    D. Inversion and equinus is seen
Ans. is 'A' Talus is only bone involved

195. RA not seen in:
    A. Heberden's node
    B. Cervical instability
    C. PIP involvement
    D. Vasculitis
Ans. is 'A' Heberden's node

196. Patient is unable to extend elbow and Triceps reflex negative, cervical disc prolapse involved:
    A. C6–C7
    B. C7–T1
    C. C4–C5
    D. C5–C6
Ans. is 'A' C6–C7

197. Vitamin D resistant rickets:
    A. X-dominant
    B. X-recessive
    C. AD
    D. AR
Ans. is 'A' X-dominant

198. Tissue release in CTEV one at a time was given by:
    A. Kite
    B. Ponseti
    C. Turcos
    D. Thomas
Ans. is 'C' Turcos

199. Poncet's disease is:
    A. TB + polyarthritis
    B. TB + monoarthritis
    C. Rheumatoid arthritis with neutropenia
    D. Rheumatoid arthritis with leucopenia
Ans. is 'A' TB + polyarthritis

200. CD markers of Langerhans histiocytosis
    A. CD1a
    B. CD99
    C. CD34
    D. CD5
Ans. is 'A' CD1a

201. Carpal tunnel syndrome nerve involved:
    A. Ulnar
    B. Radial
    C. Median
    D. Sciatic
Ans. is 'C' Median

202. Adductor pollicis – Nerve supply is:
    A. Ulnar
    B. Radial
    C. Median
    D. Sciatic
Ans. is 'A' Ulnar

203. **Pulled elbow is:**
    A. Subluxation of radial head
    B. Tear of medial collateral ligament
    C. Tear of lateral collateral ligament
    D. Tear interosseous membrane
Ans. is 'A' Subluxation of radial head

204. **Sacrococcygeal tumor – Origin is:**
    A. Totipotent cell   B. Epithelial cell
    C. Columanar cell   D. Muscle
Ans. is 'A' Totipotent cell

205. **Unlocking of knee is caused by:**
    A. Quadriceps   B. Popliteus
    C. Hamstrings   D. ACL
Ans. is 'B' Popliteus

206. **Lengthening is seen in which stage of TB hip:**
    A. Stage I   B. Stage II
    C. Stage III   D. Stage IV
Ans. is 'A' Stage I

207. **Syndesmosis is seen between:**
    A. Tibia and fibula   B. Radius and carpal bones
    C. Femur and tibia   D. Humerus and ulna
Ans. is 'A' Tibia and fibula

208. **Modified Allen's test:**
    A. Radial artery   B. Ulnar artery
    C. Radial and ulnar artery D. Brachial artery
Ans. is 'B' Ulnar artery

209. **Complex condylar joint amongst the following is:**
    A. Hip   B. Shoulder
    C. Knee   D. Elbow
Ans. is 'C' Knee

210. **Lateral malleolus is:**
    A. Lower end fibula   B. Upper end fibula
    C. Lower end tibia   D. Upper end tibia
Ans. is 'A' Lower end Fibula

211. **Nutrient artery rule is:**
    A. Goes towards the growing end usually
    B. Goes away from the growing end usually
    C. Variable
    D. Every bone does not have its own blood supply
Ans. is 'B' Goes away from the growing end usually

212. **Maximum blood supply of bone:**
    A. Epiphysis   B. Metaphysis
    C. Diaphysis   D. Joints
Ans. is 'B' Metaphysis

213. **Vertebra with constant number:**
    A. Cervical   B. Thoracic
    C. Lumbar   D. Sacral
Ans. is 'A' Cervical

214. **Bone with no muscle attachment:**
    A. 5th Metatarsal   B. 1st Metatarsal
    C. Talus   D. Calcaneum
Ans. is 'C' Talus

215. **Medullary cavity is absent in:**
    A. Clavicle   B. Humerus
    C. Fibula   D. Ulna
Ans. is 'A' Clavicle

216. **Epiphyseal closure is mediated by:**
    A. Thyroxine   B. Sex steroids
    C. Calcitonin   D. Growth hormone
Ans. is 'B' Sex steroids

217. **Isotope used in bone scans:**
    A. Technetium   B. Gallium
    C. Selenium   D. Chromium
Ans. is 'A' Technetium

218. **Prominent spine is:**
    A. C2   B. C7
    C. L2   D. T10
Ans. is 'B' C7

219. **Example of syndesmosis joint is:**
    A. Elbow joint   B. Tibiofibular
    C. Hip   D. Knee
Ans. is 'B' Tibiofibular

220. **Ivory osteoma is also called as:**
    A. Campanacci disease
    B. Codman's tumor
    C. Compact or eburnated osteoma
    D. Maffucci syndrome
Ans. is 'C' Compact or eburnated osteoma
    – Ivory osteoma is called as compact or eburnated osteoma, Codman's tumor is chondroblastoma, campanacci disease is ossifying fibroma and Maffucci syndrome is enchondroma, Hemangioma 4 phlebolith.

221. **Purely epiphyseal lesion before skeletal maturity is:**
    A. Giant cell tumor   B. Chondroblastoma
    C. Osteoblastoma   D. Osteosarcoma
Ans. is 'B' Chondroblastoma is purely epiphyseal lesion before skeletal maturity.

222. **Fracture clavicle all the following are used for treatment except:**
    A. Figure of eight bandage B. Plating
    C. K-wire fixation   D. Bone grafting
Ans. is 'D' Bone grafting
    – Treatment for fracture clavicle is usually non-operative but can be operated and fixation method can be plating or K-wire fixation. Bone graft is usually not required for fracture clavicle.

223. **Most common tendon used as tendon graft is:**
    A. Palmaris longus   B. Flexor digitorum profundus
    C. Biceps brachi   D. Gluteus medius
Ans. is 'A' Palmaris longus is commonest tendon used as a graft

224. **Thomas test is for:**
    A. Hip deformity
    B. Knee deformity
    C. Tendoachilles tear
    D. Impingement syndrome of shoulder
Ans. is 'A' Hip deformity
    – Tendoachilles tear is tested by Thompson test and impingement syndrome of shoulder is tested by Neer's test and Hawkins-Kennedy test.

225. Slipped Capital Femoral Epiphysis what is relation to the femoral metaphysis after slip:
    A. Anterolateral   B. Posterolateral
    C. Anteromedial   D. Posteromedial
Ans. is 'D' The slipped epiphysis is related to the posteromedial part of femoral metaphysis in case of SCFE.

226. Medial arch most important muscle is:
    A. Tendoachilles   B. Tibialis posterior tendon
    C. Extensor hallucis longus   D. Adductor pollicis
Ans. is 'B' Tibialis posterior tendon
    – Medial longitudinal arch most important muscles for maintaining the arch are Tibialis posterior and Tibialis anterior in this order and most important bones are Talus and Navicular.

227. Terry Thomas sign is seen in:
    A. Scaphoid fracture
    B. Scapholunate dissociation
    C. Fracture acetabulum
    D. Meniscus cyst
Ans. is 'B' Terry Thomas sign refers to gap seen between scaphoid and lunate in scapholunate dissociation seen as below compared to space between teeth of Terry Thomas.

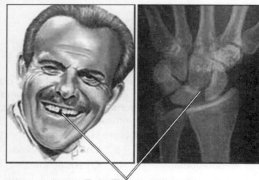

Terry Thomas sign

228. Rheumatoid arthritis most common part of spine affected: (DNB CET 2012)
    A. Upper cervical spine   B. Lower cervical spine
    C. Dorsal spine   D. Lumbar spine
Ans. is 'A' Upper cervical spine. Rheumatoid arthritis is a disease of appendicular spine and when it involves axial skeleton it involves upper cervical spine.

229. Anatomical snuff box tenderness indicates fracture of:
    A. Scaphoid fracture   B. Lunate fracture
    C. Talus fracture   D. Navicular fracture
Ans. is 'A' Scaphoid fracture. Anatomical snuff box refers to space bound by Anteriorly by Abductor pollicis longus and extensor pollicis brevis and posteriorly by extensor pollicis longus and the floor contains scaphoid and trapezium.

230. Varus or Valgus deformity is seen in which plane of body:
    A. Sagittal plane   B. Coronal plane
    C. Transverse plane   D. Oblique plane
Ans. is 'B' Coronal plane
    – Varus deformity refers to movement of distal part towards midline and valgus refers to movement of distal part away from midline and they are seen in coronal plane.

231. Posterior Scalloping of vertebra is seen in all except: (DNB CET)
    A. Aneurysm   B. Tumor
    C. Acromegaly   D. Neurofibromatosis
Ans. is 'A' Aneurysm

232. Flail chest there is: (DNB CET)
    A. Single rib fracture both sides
    B. Multiple rib fracture with paradoxical movement
    C. Congenital
    D. Tuberculosis of ribs
Ans. is 'B' Multiple rib fracture with paradoxical movement

233. What is the type of joint seen in the growth plate:
    A. Fibrous
    B. Primary cartilaginous
    C. Secondary cartilaginous
    D. Plane synovial
Ans. is 'B' Primary cartilaginous

234. The first costochondral joint is a:
    A. Fibrous joint   B. Synovial joint
    C. Syndesmosis   D. Synchondrosis
Ans. is 'D' Synchondrosis

235. Primary curvatures of vertebral column are:
    A. Cervical and lumbar   B. Thoracic and sacral
    C. Cervical and thoracic   D. Thoracic and lumbar
Ans. is 'B' Thoracic and sacral

236. A 38-year-old woman comes to her physician complaining of lower back pain. X-ray films of her back show a lordosis of the vertebral column. This increased curvature of the vertebral column is best described by which of the following terms:
    A. Concave anteriorly   B. Concave posteriorly
    C. Convex anteriorly   D. Convex posteriorly
Ans. is 'C' Convex anteriorly

237. A 22-year-old male suffers a whiplash injury during an automobile accident. There is a posterolateral herniation of the nucleus pulposus of the intervertebral disc between vertebrae C4 and C5. What neural structure is most likely to be injured:
    A. Anterior ramus C5   B. Posterior ramus C4
    C. Spinal nerve C4   D. Spinal nerve C5
Ans. is 'D' Spinal nerve C5

238. Shoulder abduction all happens except:
    A. Humerus elevation
    B. Clavicle rotation
    C. Medial rotation of scapula
    D. Acromio-clavicular joint movement
Ans. is 'C' Medial rotation of scapula

239. Which of the following ligaments prevent hyperextension of hip?
    A. Iliofemoral ligament   B. Pubo-femoral ligament
    C. Ischiofemoral ligament   D. Ligamentum teres femoralis
Ans. is 'A' Iliofemoral ligament

240. Coronary ligament of knee is situated between:
    A. Menisci and synovium
    B. Two posterior horns of menisci
    C. Meniscus and tibial condyle
    D. Meniscus and femoral condyle
Ans. is 'C' Meniscus and tibial condyle

241. Transverse arch of foot is maintained by:
    A. Flexor digitorum brevis
    B. Adductor hallucis
    C. Abductor hallucis brevis
    D. Peroneus brevis

Ans. is 'B' Adductor hallucis

242. A patient presents with the condition known as flat foot. The foot is displaced laterally and everted, and the head of the talus is no longer supported. Which of the following ligaments probably is stretched:
    A. Plantar calcaneonavicular (spring)
    B. Calcaneofibular
    C. Plantar calcaneocuboid (short plantar)
    D. Anterior tibiotalar

Ans. is 'A' Plantar calcaneonavicular (spring)

DNB CET QUESTIONS FROM 2011-1992

243. In genu valgus, the deformity is tibia and fibula: *(DNB CET 2011)*
    A. Tilted laterally in relation to long-axis of femur
    B. Titled medially in relation to femur
    C. Rotated medially in relation to femur
    D. Rotated laterally in relation to femur

Ans. is 'A' Titled laterally in relation to long-axis of femur
    – Varus distal part goes towards midline and valgus distal part away from midline

244. Felon is seen in: *(DNB CET 2011)*
    A. Index finger
    B. Thumb
    C. Great toe
    D. Ring finger

Ans. is 'B' Thumb
    – Felon is infection of pulp space of finger and is seen in Thumb > index finger

245. Spina ventosa is: *(DNB CET 2011)*
    A. TB spine   B. TB hip
    C. TB dactylitis   D. TB knee joint

Ans. is 'C' TB dactylitis

246. MC malignant bone tumor: *(DNB CET 2011)*
    A. Osteosarcoma   B. Ewing's sarcoma
    C. Osteochondroma D. Metastasis

Ans. is 'D' Metastasis
    – Metastases>multiple myeloma>osteosarcoma is order of bone malignancy

247. Most common cause of tardy ulnar nerve palsy is: *(DNB CET 2011, 1996)*
    A. Supracondylar fracture
    B. Fracture of lateral condyle
    C. Posterior elbow dislocation
    D. Olecranon fracture

Ans. is 'B' Fracture of lateral condyle
    – Tardy ulnar nerve palsy is seen due to cubitus valgus most commonly and most common cause is non-union lateral condyle fracture.

248. Allen's test is for the patency of: *(DNB CET 2011)*
    A. Radial and ulnar artery
    B. Subclavian artery
    C. Vertebral artery
    D. Internal carotid artery

Ans. is 'A' Radial and ulnar artery

249. OA commonly affects: *(DNB CET 2011)*
    A. MP joints   B. DIP
    C. Ankle joint   D. All of the above

Ans. is 'B' DIP
    – MCP and ankle are usually not affected in OA

250. Position in post-dislocation hip: *(DNB CET 2011)*
    A. Flexion, abduction, external rotation
    B. Flexion, adduction, external rotation
    C. Flexion, abduction, internal rotation
    D. Flexion, adduction, internal rotation

Ans. is 'D' Flexion, adduction, internal rotation

251. Child comes with pronated forearm and X-ray is normal, diagnosis: *(DNB CET 2011)*
    A. Supracondylar fracture
    B. Dislocation of elbow
    C. Pulled elbow
    D. Fracture lateral epicondyle

Ans. is 'C' Pulled elbow
    – Pronated forearm in a child with normal X-rays goes towards pulled elbow

252. Klumpke's paralysis involves: *(DNB CET 2011)*
    A. C8 – T1   B. C5 – C6
    C. L5 – S1   D. C3 – C4

Ans. is 'A' C8 – T1
    – Erbs palsy involves C5–C6 and Klumpke's palsy involves C8 and T1

253. Most common site of osteoma in paranasal sinuses: *(DNB CET 2011)*
    A. Maxillary   B. Frontal
    C. Ethmoid   D. Sphenoid

Ans. is 'B' Frontal
    – Ivory Osteomas most commonly involve frontal sinus

254. Distal interphalangeal joint involvement is seen in: *(DNB CET 2011)*
    A. Osteoarthritis   B. Rheumatoid arthritis
    C. Rheumatic fever   D. Reiter's disease

Ans. is 'A' Osteoarthritis
    – DIP is one of the most common involved joint in OA

255. Osteoarthritis does not involve: *(DNB CET 2011)*
    A. Hip   B. Ankle
    C. Cervical spine D. Knees

Ans. is 'B' Ankle
    – DIP is most commonly involved joint and knee and hip are also commonly involved. Ankle involvement is rare.

256. Most common malignant tumor of bone: *(DNB CET 2011)*
    A. Osteosarcoma
    B. Multiple myeloma
    C. Ewing's tumor
    D. Osteochondroma

Ans. is 'B' Multiple myeloma
- Metastases>multiple myeloma>osteosarcoma

257. Not a site of gouty tophi deposition: *(DNB CET 2011)*
    A. Shoulder
    B. Muscle
    C. Synovial membrane of knee
    D. Achilles tendon

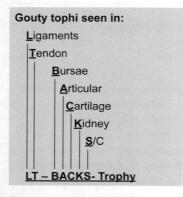

Gouty tophi seen in:
Ligaments
Tendon
Bursae
Articular
Cartilage
Kidney
S/C

LT – BACKS- Trophy

Ans. is 'B' Muscle

258. Multiple loose bodies in knee with snow storm appearance: *(DNB CET 2011)*
    A. Rheumatoid arthritis
    B. Synovial chondromatosis
    C. SLE
    D. Reiter's syndrome

Ans. is 'B' Synovial chondromatosis

259. CRP is not increased in: *(DNB CET 2011)*
    A. Osteoarthritis
    B. Rheumatoid arthritis
    C. Rheumatic fever
    D. SLE

Ans. is 'A' Osteoarthritis
- Non-inflammatory arthritis like OA does not have elevation of ESR or CRP

260. Arthritis mutilans is seen in: *(DNB CET 2011)*
    A. SLE
    B. Psoriatic arthropathy
    C. Osteoarthritis
    D. Gout

Ans. is 'B' Psoriatic arthropathy

Arthritis Mutilans

A destructive arthritis of the hands and feet with resorption of bone ends and telescoping joints (main – en – lorgnette).
1. Rheumatoid arthritis
2. Juvenile chronic arthritis
3. Psoriatic arthropathy
4. Diabetes
5. Leprosy
6. Neuropathic arthropathy
7. Reiter's syndrome – in the feet.

261. ESR is not increased in: *(DNB CET 2011)*
    A. RA
    B. OA
    C. SLE
    D. Multiple myeloma

Ans. is 'B' OA
- Non-inflammatory arthritis like OA does not have elevation of ESR or CRP

262. Tension band wiring is used for: *(DNB CET 2011)*
    A. Ulna
    B. Patella
    C. Clavicle
    D. Radius

Ans. is 'B' Patella
- Tension band wiring is for olecranon, patella and medial malleolus

263. Bone tumor arising from epiphysis and recurs till epiphysis fuse: *(DNB CET 2011)*
    A. Osteoclastoma
    B. Chondroblastoma
    C. Osteoid and stage
    D. Osteoblastoma

Ans. is 'A' Osteoclastoma
- Osteoclastoma is after skeletal maturity and chondroblastoma is before skeletal maturity.

264. Joint involved in rheumatoid arthritis includes all except: *(DNB CET December 2011)*
    A. PIP
    B. DIP
    C. MCP
    D. Cervical spine

Ans. is 'B' DIP
- DIP is not involved usually in case of rheumatoid arthritis.
- 14 Joints involved are Right and Left PIP, MCP, Wrist, Elbow, Knee, Ankle and MTP.

265. Renal osteodystrophy skeletal abnormality is because of: *(DNB CET 2011)*
    A. Impaired synthesis of D3
    B. Hypocalcemia
    C. Hyperphosphatemia
    D. Loss of Vitamin D and calcium through dialysis

Ans. is 'C' Hyperphosphatemia
- Hyperphosphatemia is the principal regulator of increased serum parathyroid hormone levels in CRF that in turn causes the skeletal manifestations of renal osteodystrophy.

266. Klippel-Feil syndrome includes all except: *(DNB CET 2011)*
    A. Bilateral neck webbing
    B. Bilateral SCM shortening
    C. Low hairline
    D. Restriction of neck movements

Ans. is 'B' Bilateral SCM shortening
- Short webbed neck, low posterior hairline and restricted neck movements is triad of Klippel-Feil Syndrome

267. Characteristic subperiosteal bone resorption in Hyperparathyroidism is best seen at: *(DNB CET 2011)*
    A. Rib margins
    B. Medial margin of proximal humerus
    C. Radial border of middle phalanx
    D. Lamina dura

Ans. is 'C' Radial border of middle phalanx
- Radial border of middle phalanx resorption is characteristic for hyperparathyroidism
- Other features are Osteopenia, loss of lamina dura, Brown tumor, Salt and pepper skull and basket weave appearance of cortex.

268. Which is not a fibrous joint? *(DNB CET 2011)*
    A. Skull sutures
    B. First costochondral joint
    C. Tooth socket
    D. Inferior tibiofibular syndesmosis
Ans. is 'B' First costochondral joint

Classification of joints
1. Synarthroses (bone-solid connective tissue—bone)
    A. Fibrous joints
        1. Sutures (Bone-Collagenous sutural ligament—Bone) e.g., Sutures of the skull
        2. Syndesmoses (Bone-Collagenous interosseous ligament, membrane or cord—Bone) e.g., Inferior tibiofibular joints
        3. Gomphoses—(Bone—Complex collagenous periodontium—Dental cement) e.g., Tooth in its socket
    B. Cartilaginous joints
        1. Synchondrosis/Primary cartilaginous joints—(Bone Hyaline cartilage—Bone) e.g:
            A. Joints between epiphysis and diaphysis of a growing long bone
            B. First chondrosternal joint
            C. Costochondral joints
            D. Spheno-occipital joints
        2. Symphysis/Secondary cartilaginous joints—(Bone-Hyaline cartilage—Fibrocartilaginous disc—Hyaline cartilage—Bone) Typically occur in the Median Plane of the body e.g.:
            A. Symphysis pubis
            B. Manubriosternal joint
            C. Intervertebral joints between vertebral bodies

Synovial joints:

Type of joint	Axis	Movements	Examples
Plane/Gliding joint	Uniaxial	Gliding	Intercarpal joints, Intertarsal joints, Between articular processes of vertebrae
Hinge joints	Uniaxial	Flexion, Extension	Elbow joints, Ankle joints, Interphalangeal joints
Pivot joints	Uniaxial	Rotation	Median atlantoaxial joint, Superior and inferior radioulnar joints
Condylar joints	Biaxial	Flexion, Extension, Limited rotation	Knee joints, Joints between condyles of mandible and temporal bone
Ellipsoid joints	Biaxial	Flexion, Extension, Abduction, Adduction, Circumduction	Wrist joint, Metacarpophalangeal joint, Atlantoaxial joints (lateral)
Saddle joints	Multiaxial	Flexion, Extension, Abduction, Adduction, Conjunct rotation	Sternoclavicular joint, First carpometacarpal joint, Calcaneocuboid joint
Ball & Socket Joints	Multiaxial	Flexion, Extension, Abduction, Adduction, Circumduction, Rotation	Shoulder joint, Hip joint, Talocalcaneonavicular joint

269. Cozen test is for: *(DNB CET 2011)*
    A. Golfers elbow
    B. Tennis elbow
    C. Little leaguers elbow
    D. Frozen shoulder
Ans. is 'B' Tennis elbow
    – Cozen test is for tennis elbow (Lateral epicondylitis)
    – Golfers elbow—Medial epicondylitis
    – Frozen shoulder—Adhesive capsulitis
    – Little leaguers elbow-avulsion of tip of medial epicondyle

270. Pott's spine is commonest at: *(DNB CET 2010)*
    A. Thoracolumbar   B. Sacral
    C. Cervical   D. Lumbosacral
Ans. is 'A' Thoracolumbar region

271. In Froment's sign which muscle is tested?
    (DNB CET 2010, 09, 08, 07, 03, 1996)
    A. Adductor pollicis
    B. Opponens pollicis brevis
    C. Flexor pollicis brevis
    D. Abductor pollicis
Ans. is 'A' Adductor pollicis
    – Book test is testing of adductor pollicis supplied by ulnar nerve and in adductor pollicis palsy Froment sign is seen.

272. Fenestrated hip prosthesis is: *(DNB CET 2010)*
    A. Bipolar prosthesis   B. Austin Moore
    C. Thompson prosthesis   D. All
Ans. is 'B' Austin Moore
    – Austin Moore and Thompson are unipolar prosthesis

	Austin moore	Thompson
Parts	Head, Neck, Collar, Shoulder, Stem	Head, Neck, Collar, Stem (no shoulder)
Fixation	Without bone cement	With bone cement
Extraction	Easier	Very difficult
Stem fenestrations	Two in number	Nil
Used when	Calcar femorale > 1.25 cm	Calcar femorale < 1.25 cm

273. Thomas test is for: *(DNB CET 2010)*
    A. Hip flexion   B. Knee flexion
    C. Hip abduction   D. Hip rotation
Ans. is 'A' Hip flexion

274. Salmonella osteomyelitis is common in: *(DNB CET 2010)*
    A. Sickle cell disease   B. HIV
    C. IV drug abusers   D. Pregnancy
Ans. is 'A' Sickle cell disease

275. Intranasal calcitonin is most commonly used for:
(DNB CET 2010)
A. Paget's disease
B. Osteoporosis
C. Hypercalcemia
D. Osteopetrosis

Ans. is 'B' Osteoporosis
- Most common indication amongst the mentioned is for osteoporosis

276. Most common type of elbow dislocation is:
(DNB CET 2010)
A. Posterior
B. Posterolateral
C. Posteromedial
D. Lateral

Ans. is 'A' Posterior

277. Indication for surgical compartment release in compartment syndrome in any compartment is absolute pressure greater than: (DNB CET 2010)
A. 15 mm Hg
B. 20 mm Hg
C. 30 mm Hg
D. 40 mm Hg

Ans. is 'C' 30 mm Hg
- The normal pressure is <11 mm Hg and pressure more than
- 30 mm Hg is taken as value for fasciotomy.

278. True about Slipped Capital Femoral Epiphysis is:
A. Seen in thin children (DNB CET 2010)
B. Trethowan sign is seen
C. Major traumatic condition
D. Seen in adults

Ans. is 'B' Trethowan sign is seen
- SCFE is seen in adolescents, seen in obese overweight individuals and seen as a result of minor trauma. Trethowan sign is seen.

279. Shepherd crook deformity is seen in: (DNB CET 2010)
A. Fibrous dysplasia
B. Adamantinoma
C. Non-ossifying fibroma
D. Fibrous cortical defect

Ans. is 'A' Fibrous dysplasia

280. Diastatic fractures involve: (DNB CET 2010)
A. Skull bones
B. Long bones
C. Sternum
D. Ribs

Ans. is 'A' Skull bones

281. Fracture shaft humerus nerve involved: (DNB CET 2010)
A. Median nerve
B. Radial nerve
C. Axillary nerve
D. Ulnar nerve

Ans. is 'B' Radial nerve

282. Marble bone disease is also known as: (DNB CET 2010)
A. Osteoporosis
B. Osteochondritis
C. Osteopetrosis
D. Osteogenesis imperfecta

Ans. is 'C' Osteopetrosis

283. Non-traumatic amputation is seen in: (DNB CET 2010)
A. Sickle cell disease
B. Diabetes mellitus
C. Leprosy
D. All of the above

Ans. is 'D' All of the above
- Amputations are divided into Traumatic Amputations (those involving loss of a body part caused by an injury) and Non-traumatic Amputations. The later often occurs secondary to diabetes, poor circulation, or infection.
- Diabetes is the most common cause of non-traumatic amputation of the lower limb. This is primarily a result of peripheral neuropathy. 60% of non-traumatic lower-limb amputations occur among diabetics in the US.

Causes of non-traumatic amputation:
- Diabetes mellitus
- Osteomyelitis
- Peripheral neuropathy
- Sickle cell anemia
- Leprosy
- Peripheral vascular disease
- Acro-osteolysis neurogenic
- Charcot-Marie-Tooth disease, Type 2B
- Compartment syndrome
- Frostbite
- Gangrene
- Mycetoma
- Sensory neuropathy

284. Siffert-katz sign is seen in: (DNB CET 2010)
A. Perthes sign
B. Blounts disease
C. Osteogenesis imperfecta
D. Pulled elbow

Ans. is 'B' Blounts disease
- In infantile form of Blount's disease varus deformity is usually accompanied by medial tibial torsion, a limp and posteromedial subluxation of knee when held in partial flexion (Siffert-katz sign).

285. Ewing's sarcoma is believed to arise from:
(DNB CET 2010)
A. Aberrant cartilage rests
B. Endothelial cells in the bone marrow
C. Mesothelial cells
D. Periosteocytes

Ans. is 'B' Endothelial cells in bone marrow.
- Ewings arises from marrow

286. Osteochondritis known as Sever's disease involves:
A. Talus
B. Lunate (DNB CET 2010)
C. Tarsal navicular
D. Calcaneus

Ans. is 'D' Calcaneus

287. A small boy is brought to the emergency department by his parents if found to have a spiral fracture of the femur, with a variety of ecchymoses. Likely cause is:
(DNB CET 2010)
A. Automobile hit and run accident
B. Fall from a tree
C. Child abuse
D. Fall from a bicycle

Ans. is 'C' Child abuse
- Child with ecchymosis with spiral fractures is battered baby syndrome or child abuse.

288. Regarding pseudogout, wrong statement is:
(DNB CET 2010)
A. It does not affect large joints
B. It does not affect small joints
C. Chondrocalcinosis
D. Deposition of calcium pyrophosphate

Ans. is 'A' It does not affect large joints
- Pseudogout most commonly involves knee, largest joint in body.

289. Normal bone remodelling in response to stress was described by: *(DNB CET 2009)*
    A. Pauwels
    B. Kuntscar
    C. Wolff
    D. Hugh Owen Thomas

Ans. is 'C' Wolff
    – Remodelling takes place according to wolffs law.

290. The following are true of multiple exostoses except: *(DNB CET 2009)*
    A. Hereditary transmission (Autosomal dominant)
    B. Presence of multiple exostoses
    C. Osteopenia
    D. Growth defects

Ans. is 'C' Osteopenia
    – Osteopenia is not associated with osteochondroma. Hereditary transmission, growth defects are seen with multiple osteochondromas.

291. The commonest donor site for autologous bone graft is: *(DNB CET 2009)*
    A. Fibula
    B. Rib
    C. Greater trochanter
    D. Iliac crest

Ans. is 'D' Iliac crest
    – Iliac crest is most common donor site for bone grafting.

292. The following biological factors causing delayed union are true, except: *(DNB CET 2009)*
    A. Inadequate blood supply
    B. Severe soft tissue damage
    C. Periosteal stripping
    D. None

Ans. is 'D' None
    – ALL the factors mentioned above cause delayed or non-union.

293. The following sites are most commonly affected in a traumatic osteonecrosis, except: *(DNB CET 2009)*
    A. The head of the femur
    B. The proximal part of scaphoid
    C. The posterior half of the talus
    D. The head of the radius.

Ans. is 'D' The head of the radius
    – AVN is not known to involve radial head.

294. The most common cause for anterior knee pain: *(DNB CET 2009)*
    A. Prepatellar bursitis
    B. Congenital discoid meniscus
    C. Plica syndrome
    D. Chondromalacia patellae

Ans. is 'D' Chondromalacia patellae
    – Chondromalacia patellae is most common cause of anterior knee pain. Theatre sign is seen.

295. The most common type of spondylolisthesis: *(DNB CET 2009, 10)*
    A. Congenital dysplastic
    B. Isthmic spondylolytic
    C. Degenerative
    D. Traumatic

Ans. is 'B' Isthmic spondylolytic
    – Spondylolisthesis most commonly is isthmic type and involves L5 – S1.

296. The following are associated with fibular hemimelia except: *(DNB CET 2009)*
    A. Short tibia
    B. Anterior bowing of legs
    C. Equinovalgus deformity of the foot and ankle
    D. Presence of polydactyly

Ans. is 'D' Presence of polydactyly
    – There is hypoplasia or less development in fibular hemimelia causing failure to develop post axial part of the limb. It has short tibia, equinovalgus deformity and bowing of leg.

297. De Quervain's disease classically affects the: *(DNB CET 2009)*
    A. Flexor pollicis longus and brevis
    B. Extensor carpi radialis and extensor pollicis longus
    C. Abductor pollicis longus and brevis
    D. Extensor pollicis brevis and abductor pollicis longus

Ans. is 'D' Extensor pollicis brevis and abductor pollicis longus

298. Heberden's nodes are found in: *(DNB CET 2009)*
    A. PIP joints in osteoarthritis
    B. DIP joints in osteoarthritis
    C. PIP joints in rheumatoid arthritis
    D. DIP joints in rheumatoid arthritis

Ans. is 'B' DIP joints in osteoarthritis
    – DIP involvement cause Heberden's nodes and PIP cause Bouchard's nodes

299. Meralgia paresthetica is due to involvement of: *(DNB CET 2009)*
    A. Medical cutaneous nerve of thigh
    B. Lateral cutaneous nerve of thigh
    C. Sural nerve
    D. Femoral nerve

Ans. is 'B' Lateral cutaneous nerve of thigh

300. Bankart's lesion involves which of the following part of the glenoid labrum: *(DNB CET 2009)*
    A. Anterior part
    B. Superior part
    C. Anterosuperior part
    D. Anteroinferior part

Ans. is 'A' Anterior part
    – Bankart lesion involves anterior part.

301. Which of the following tumors arise from epiphysis: *(DNB CET 2009)*
    A. Ewing's sarcoma
    B. Osteoclastoma (GCT)
    C. Chondromyxoid fibroma
    D. Osteosarcoma

Ans. is 'B' Osteoclastoma (GCT)
    – Chondroblastoma and GCT are 2 important epiphyseal tumors.

302. Bohler's angle is decreased in fracture of: *(DNB CET 2009)*
    A. Calcaneum
    B. Talus
    C. Navicular
    D. Cuboid

Ans. is 'A' Calcaneum
    – Bohler's angle and angle of Gissane are measured for calcaneum.

303. Most common site of osteosarcoma is: *(DNB CET 2009)*
   A. Upper end of femur   B. Lower end of femur
   C. Lower end of humerus   D. Lower end of tibia

Ans. is 'B' Lower end of femur
   – Osteosarcoma and GCT both involves lower end femur most commonly.

304. Surgical staging of bone tumors is by: *(DNB CET 2009)*
   A. Edmonton   B. Manchester
   C. Enneking   D. TNM

Ans. is 'C' Enneking
   – Bone tumors staging is Enneking.

305. Kanavel sign is seen in: *(DNB CET 2009)*
   A. Tenosynovitis   B. Trigger finger
   C. Dupuytren's contracture   D. Carpal tunnel syndrome

Ans. is 'A' Tenosynovitis
   Kanavel sign is seen in tenosynovitis they include flexion of finger, uniform swelling, pain on extension and uniform percussion tenderness.

306. Best prognosis after nerve repair: *(DNB CET 2009)*
   A. Radial   B. Median
   C. Sciatic   D. Ulnar

Ans. is 'A' Radial

307. Velpeau bandage and sling and swathe splint are used in: *(DNB CET 2009)*
   A. Shoulder dislocation
   B. Fracture scapula
   C. Acromioclavicular dislocation
   D. Fracture clavicle

Ans. is 'C' Acromioclavicular dislocation

308. Watson Jones approach is done for: *(DNB CET 2009)*
   A. Neglected club foot   B. Muscle paralysis
   C. Valgus deformity   D. Hip replacement

Ans. is 'D' Hip replacement
   – Watson Jones procedure is for ankle instability and approach is anterolateral approach to hip joint.

309. Riser localiser cast is used in the management of: *(DNB CET 2009)*
   A. Kyphosis   B. Spondylolisthesis
   C. Idiopathic scoliosis   D. Lordosis

Ans. is 'C' Idiopathic scoliosis
   – Riser cast is used for idiopathic scoliosis

310. Most common cause of insertional tendonitis of tendo achilles is: *(DNB CET 2009)*
   A. Overuse   B. Improper shoe wear
   C. Runners and jumpers   D. Steroid injections

Ans. is 'A' Overuse
   – Most common cause of insertional tendonitis is overuse and of non-insertional tendonitis is runners and jumpers.

311. Tarsal tunnel syndrome is caused with which arthritis? *(DNB CET 2009)*
   A. Ankylosing spondylitis   B. Osteoarthritis
   C. Rheumatoid arthritis   D. Psoriatic arthritis

Ans. is 'B' Osteoarthritis
   – Most common cause of Tarsal tunnel syndrome is idiopathic>O.A>R.A

312. Osteosclerotic bone metastasis is found most commonly in which carcinoma? *(DNB CET 2009)*
   A. Kidney   B. Thyroid
   C. Lung   D. Prostate

Ans. is 'D' Prostate
   – Osteoblastic secondaries are seen in prostate, carcinoid and medulloblastoma.

313. Earliest site of bone involvement in hematogenous osteomyelitis: *(DNB CET 2009)*
   A. Metaphysis
   B. Diaphysis
   C. Epiphysis
   D. Point of entry of the nutrient artery

Ans. is 'A' Metaphysis
   – Osteomyelitis is most commonly transmitted through hematogenous route and seeds in metaphysis.

314. Posterior glenohumeral instability can be tested by: *(DNB CET 2009)*
   A. Jerk test   B. Crank test
   C. Fulcrum test   D. Sulcus test

Ans. is 'A' Jerk test
   – Jerk test is for posterior glenohumeral instability and lift off test is for subscapularis tear.

315. Kocher Langenbeck approach for emergency acetabular fixation is done in all except: *(DNB CET 2009)*
   A. Open fracture
   B. Progressive sciatic nerve injury
   C. Recurrence dislocation in spite of closed reduction and traction
   D. None of the above

Ans. is 'D' None of the above
   – Emergency acetabular fixation is done for open fractures, vascular injury, joint instability and progressive nerve injury.

316. About congenital torticollis all are true except: *(DNB CET 2009)*
   A. Always associated with breech extraction
   B. Spontaneous resolution in most cases
   C. Two-third have palpable mass
   D. Uncorrected cases develop plagiocephaly

Ans. is 'A' Always associated with breech extraction
   – All the cases of torticollis are not associated with breech delivery

317. TB Spine most commonly affects: *(DNB CET June 2009)*
   A. Lumbar vertebra   B. Cervical
   C. Thoracic   D. Sacral

Ans. is 'C' Thoracic
   – Most common location of pott's spine is dorsal

318. Avascular necrosis for patients can be retarded by?
   A. 500 mg Ca daily   *(DNB CET June 2009)*
   B. 1000 mg Ca daily
   C. 1500 mg Ca daily
   D. 2000 mg Ca daily

Ans. is 'C' 1500 mg Ca daily
   – Adequate calcium intake is 1500 mg/day to decrease the chances of avascular necrosis

319. The deformity of tibia in triple deformity of the knee is: *(DNB CET June 2009)*
   A. Extension, Posterior subluxation and external rotation
   B. Flexion, Posterior subluxation and external rotation
   C. Flexion, Posterior subluxation and internal rotation
   D. Extension, Anterior subluxation and internal rotation
Ans. is 'B' Flexion, Posterior subluxation and external rotation

320. Pseudoflexion deformity of hip is seen in? *(DNB CET June 2009)*
   A. Iliopsoas abscess
   B. Tom smith arthritis
   C. Anterior dislocation of hip
   D. Central dislocation of hip
Ans. is 'A' Iliopsoas abscess
   – Pseudoflexion deformity rotations are free in position of deformity.

321. Vascular sign of narath is seen in? *(DNB CET June 2009)*
   A. Posterior dislocation of hip
   B. Sub trochanteric fracture of hip
   C. Anterior dislocation of hip
   D. Central dislocation of hip
Ans. is 'A' Posterior dislocation of hip
   – Vascular sign of narath is positive in case posterior dislocation due to absence of ground resistance to femoral artery pulsations in dislocated head.

322. Fracture shaft of humerus damages which nerve? *(DNB CET June 2009)*
   A. Radial nerve   B. Median nerve
   C. Axillary nerve   D. Ulnar nerve
Ans. is 'A' Radial nerve
   – Radial nerve is involved in fracture humerus

323. Gun stock deformity is seen in? *(DNB CET June 2009)*
   A. Supracondylar fracture humerus
   B. Lateral condylar fracture of humerus
   C. Medial condylar fracture of humerus
   D. All of the above
Ans. is 'A' Supracondylar fracture humerus
   – Cubitus varus or gun stock deformity most common cause is malunited supracondylar fracture humerus.

324. Forced inversion in plantar flexed foot injuries? *(DNB CET June 2009)*
   A. Talofibular ligament
   B. Deltoid ligament
   C. Medial collateral ligament
   D. All of the above
Ans. is 'A' Talofibular ligament
   – Plantar flexion of ankle is weakest position of ankle and causes damage to lateral structures most commonly anterior talofibular ligament.

325. Which is not true about CTEV shoe? *(DNB CET June 2009)*
   A. Used only from the age the child starts walking
   B. Straight outer border
   C. No heel
   D. Raise outer portion
Ans. is 'B' Straight outer border
   – CTEV shoes has straight inner border, outer shoe raise and no heel and is used after walking age.

326. Jones fracture is: *(DNB CET June 2009)*
   A. Avulsion fracture of base of fifth metatarsal
   B. Bimalleolar fracture of the ankle
   C. Burst fracture of 1st cervical vertebra
   D. Avulsion fracture of the medial femoral condyle
Ans. is 'A' Avulsion fracture of base of fifth metatarsal

327. Adventitious bursa is: *(DNB CET 2008, 04, 1999, 1994)*
   A. Normal
   B. Abnormal over friction site
   C. An infected defect
   D. A congenital cyst
Ans. is 'B' Abnormal over friction site
   – Adventitious bursae are seen at the areas of friction due to overuse.

328. Which of the line of management for congenital pseudarthrosis of Tibia? *(2008, 02)*
   A. Amputation   B. Charnley implant
   C. Immobilization   D. Vascularized fibular graft
Ans. is 'D' Vascularized fibular graft
   – Congenital pseudarthrosis of tibia the treatment option is fixation and bone grafting in cases of failure vascularised fibular graft is advised.

329. Linear striations are typically seen in: *(DNB CET 2008)*
   A. Vertebral myeloma   B. Vertebral lymphangiomas
   C. Vertebral metastasis   D. Vertebral hemangiomas
Ans. is 'D' Vertebral hemangiomas
   – Linear striations or corduroy appearance is characteristically seen in hemangiomas

330. Most common medial meniscal tear is: *(DNB CET 2008)*
   A. Longitudinal tear   B. Oblique tear
   C. Radial tear   D. Horizontal tear
Ans. is 'A' Longitudinal tear
   – Most common medial meniscus tear is longitudinal tear

331. Dupuytren's contracture most often involves: *(DNB CET 2007, 06, 05, 01, 1999, 1995)*
   A. Little finger   B. Ring finger
   C. Thumb   D. Any of the above
Ans. is 'B' Ring finger
   – Dupuytren's contracture involves ring finger>little finger
   – Most common joint involved is MCP>PIP>DIP

332. The commonest site of March fracture is: *(DNB CET 2007, 1995)*
   A. Metatarsals   B. Ankle
   C. Tibia   D. Fibula
Ans. is 'A' Metatarsals
   – Stress fracture is most common at 2nd metatarsal neck >3rd metatarsal neck

333. Most common cause of neuropathic joints is: *(DNB CET 2007, 05, 03, 01, 1999, 97)*
   A. Leprosy   B. Diabetes
   C. Rheumatoid arthritis D. Syphilis
Ans. is 'B' Diabetes
   – Diabetes is most common cause of neuropathic joints causing involvement of midtarsal joints most commonly.

Orthopedics Quick Review

334. Radiosensitive tumors is: *(DNB CET 2007, 04, 01)*
- A. Ewing's sarcoma
- B. Osteosarcoma
- C. Osteoclastoma
- D. Synovial sarcoma

Ans. is 'A' Ewing's sarcoma
- Ewing's is highly radiosensitive tumor it melts like snow with radiotherapy even then preferred treatment places chemotherapy at the top.

335. Chemotherapeutic agents of choice for osteogenic sarcoma: *(DNB CET 2007, 02)*
- A. Doxorubicin
- B. Methotrexate
- C. Cyclophosphamide
- D. 5-FU

Ans. is 'B' Methotrexate is most important for osteosarcoma.

336. Card test detect the function of: *(DNB CET 2007)*
- A. Median nerve
- B. Ulnar nerve
- C. Axillary nerve
- D. Radial nerve

Ans. is 'B' Ulnar nerve
- Card test is for ulnar nerve to test palmar interossei.

337. Sequestrum is a: *(DNB CET 2007)*
- A. Infected bone
- B. New bone
- C. Dead bone
- D. Woven bone

Ans. is 'C' Dead bone
- Sequestrum is avascular piece of bone surrounded by granulation tissue it is pathognomonic of chronic osteomyelitis

338. One of the following is a disease caused by osteoclast dysfunction: *(DNB CET 2007)*
- A. Osteopetrosis
- B. Rickets
- C. Renal osteodystrophy
- D. Osteogenesis imperfect

Ans. is 'A' Osteopetrosis
- Pagets and osteopetrosis are 2 diseases due to osteoclast defect.

339. Fibrosis is commonest in: *(DNB CET 2007)*
- A. Tendo calcaneus
- B. Sternocleidomastoid
- C. Trapezius
- D. Serratus anterior

Ans. is 'B' Sternocleidomastoid
- Congenital muscular torticollis or wry neck involves sternocleidomastoid and in it fibrosis is seen.

340. Which group of muscles is most commonly affected in poliomyelitis? *(DNB CET 2007)*
- A. Dorsiflexion of the ankle
- B. Flexors of the knee
- C. Flexors of the hip
- D. Extensors of the hip

Ans. is 'A' Dorsiflexion of the ankle
- Most commonly affected muscle in lower limb is quadriceps>tibialis anterior (ankle dorsiflexor).

341. Myositis ossificans is commonly seen at the: *(DNB CET 2006, 03, 2K, 1994)*
- A. Knee
- B. Elbow
- C. Shoulder
- D. Hip

Ans. is 'B' Elbow
- Most common location of myositis ossificans is elbow > Hip.

342. The complication of Colles fracture is: *(DNB CET 2006, 2K, 1995)*
- A. Stiffness of finger
- B. Ulnar nerve palsy
- C. Radial nerve palsy
- D. None of the above

Ans. is 'A' Stiffness of finger
- Most common complication for Colles is finger stiffness > malunion

343. Claw hand is seen in: *(DNB CET 2006, 04, 01, 1999, 1995)*
- A. Ulnar nerve injury
- B. Carpal tunnel syndrome
- C. Multiple sclerosis
- D. Cervical rib

Ans. is 'A' Ulnar nerve injury
- Claw hand is seen in ulnar nerve injury, median nerve injury or combined nerve injury.

344. Avascular necrosis of head of femur occurs commonly at: *(DNB CET 2006, 04, 03, 02, 1997)*
- A. Subcapital region
- B. Transcervical region
- C. Subchondral region
- D. Trochanteric region

Ans. is 'A' Subcapital region
- Subcapital > transcervical > basicervical is the order of involvement of Avascular necrosis in fracture neck femur

345. The first sign of Volkmann's ischemia is: *(DNB CET 2006, 05, 02)*
- A. Pain on passive movements
- B. Absence of arterial pulsation
- C. Development of contracture
- D. Pain out of proportion

Ans. is 'A' Pain on passive movements
- 1st sign of volkmann's ischemia is pain on passive stretch at the distal most joint of the extremity.

346. A 10-year-old child sustained an elbow injury about four years ago. He now complains of deformity at the elbow and numbness of ulnar two fingers of the ipsilateral hand. Most probably the bony injury sustained was: *(DNB CET 2006)*
- A. Supracondylar fracture of humerus
- B. Fracture of olecranon
- C. Fracture of lateral condyle of humerus
- D. Ulnar nerve injury

Ans. is 'C' Fracture of lateral condyle of humerus
- The case mentioned here is a case of tardy ulnar nerve palsy seen most commonly due to cubitus valgus due to lateral condyle fracture humerus.

347. March fracture usually occurs in the: *(DNB CET 2006)*
- A. 1st metatarsal
- B. 2nd metatarsal
- C. 4th metatarsal
- D. Head of the talus

Ans. is 'B' 2nd metatarsal
- March fracture involves 2nd metatarsal neck>3rd metatarsal neck.

348. In congenital dislocation of hip, clinical sign which shows that the affected thigh is at a lower level when the knees and hips are flexed to 90 degrees is known as: *(DNB CET 2006)*
- A. Ortolani's sign
- B. Barlow's sign
- C. Von Rosen's sign
- D. Galeazzi's sign

Ans. is 'D' Galeazzi's sign
- Galeazzi sign or Allis sign is done for DDH in which on hip flexion and knee flexion the knee on affected side is at lower levels.

349. Trigger finger is: *(DNB CET 2005, 04, 02, 1998)*
    A. Injury to fingers while operating a gun
    B. Stenosis tendovaginitis of flexor tendon of affected finger
    C. A feature of carpal tunnel syndrome
    D. Any of the above.

Ans. is 'B' Stenosis tendovaginitis of flexor tendon of affected finger
    – Trigger finger is stenosing tenosynovitis of flexor tendon with constriction at A1 pulley and nodule at MCP

350. Which of the following arises in the medullary canal? *(DNB CET 2005, 01)*
    A. Osteosarcoma
    B. Ewing's sarcoma
    C. Synovial sarcoma
    D. Osteoclastoma

Ans. is 'B' Ewing's sarcoma
    – Ewing sarcoma arises from the marrow

351. Froment's sign is diagnostic of the following nerve injury: *(DNB CET 2005)*
    A. Median
    B. Ulnar
    C. Radial
    D. Musculocutaneous

Ans. is 'B' Ulnar
    – Froment sign is seen in ulnar nerve palsy. Other test for ulnar nerve palsy are Igawa test, Wartenbergs test and Card test.

352. Cubitus varus is the commonest complication of: *(DNB CET 2005)*
    A. Supracondylar fracture of humerus
    B. Fracture of olecranon
    C. Fracture head of radius
    D. Posterior dislocation of elbow

Ans. is 'A' Supracondylar fracture of humerus
    – Cubitus varus is most commonly due to malunited supracondylar fracture humerus.

353. Commonly performed procedure of triple arthrodesis of foot includes fusion of the: *(DNB CET 2005)*
    A. Tibiotalar, talocalcaneal and talonavicular joints
    B. Talocalcaneal, talonavicular and calcaneocuboid joints
    C. Talonavicular, calcaneocuboid and ankle joints
    D. Ankle, subtalar and midtarsal joints

Ans. is 'B' Talocalcaneal, talonavicular and calcaneocuboid joints
    – Triple arthrodesis is done in CTEV after 10 years of age and involves fusion of talonavicular, talocalcaneal and calcaneocuboid joints.

354. Bone growth is influenced maximum by: *(DNB CET 2004, 1996)*
    A. Thyroxine
    B. Growth hormone
    C. Parathormone
    D. Estrogen

Ans. is 'B' Growth hormone
    – Maximum growth of bone is regulated by growth hormone

355. When the L4 – L5 intervertebral disc prolapses, the nerve root that is usually compressed is: *(DNB CET 2004)*
    A. L4
    B. L5
    C. S1
    D. S2

Ans. is 'B' L5
    – Most common disc prolapse is L4-L5>L5-S1 and most common type is paracentral causing compression of lower nerve root.

356. The ideal treatment of a 3-day-old fracture neck of femur in a 50-year-old male would be: *(DNB CET 2004)*
    A. Compression screw fixation
    B. POP hip spica
    C. Hemi replacement arthroplasty
    D. Total hip replacement

Ans. is 'A' Compression screw fixation
    – Age <65 <3 weeks fracture is treated by reduction + screw fixation
    – >3 weeks fracture-fixation +bone grafting or osteotomy
    – >65 years – hemiarthroplasty and any age arthritis. Total hip replacement is advised.

357. Abduction and external rotation deformity at the hip may be seen in all of the following conditions except: *(DNB CET 2004)*
    A. Tuberculosis
    B. Posterior dislocation
    C. Poliomyelitis
    D. Fracture neck of femur

Ans. is 'B' Posterior dislocation
    – Posterior dislocation causes FADIR that is flexion, adduction and internal rotation.

358. A compartment syndrome in a leg can result from all of the following except: *(DNB CET 2004)*
    A. Edema of muscles due to injury
    B. Fracture hematoma within the compartment
    C. Edema of muscles due to ischemia
    D. Compound fracture

Ans. is 'D' Compound fracture
    – Compartment syndrome is rare in open fracture rest all the mentioned conditions it is possible.

359. Commonest site for acute osteomyelitis is: *(DNB CET 2003, 1999, 1994)*
    A. Hip joint
    B. Tibia
    C. Femur
    D. Radial

Ans. is 'C' Femur
    – Most common cause of acute osteomyelitis is *Staphylococcus aureus* infection through hematogenous route and most common location is lower end femur.

360. Which of the following is not useful in the treatment of osteoporosis? *(DNB CET 2003, 1992)*
    A. Vitamin C
    B. Vitamin D
    C. Calcium
    D. Bisphosphonates

Ans. is 'A' Vitamin C

Drug used in osteoporosis:
1. Inhibit resorption: Bisphosphonates, Denosumab, calcitonin, estrogen, SERMS, gallium nitrate.
2. Stimulate formation: Teriparatide (PTH analogue), calcium, calcitriol, fluorides.
3. Both actions: Strontium ranelate.

361. Looser's zone is characteristic of: *(DNB CET 2003, 1992)*
    A. Scurvy
    B. Osteomalacia
    C. Hyperparathyroidism
    D. Paget's disease

Ans. is 'B' Osteomalacia
    – Looser zones are characteristic for osteomalacia or any bone softening disorder and most common site is femur neck.

362. Which of the following nerve injuries producing the deformities is incorrect? *(DNB CET 2003, 1993)*
   A. Upper trunk Porter's tip hand
   B. Ulnar nerve Claw hand
   C. Axillary nerve Wrist drop
   D. Radial nerve Wrist drop

Ans. is 'C' Axillary nerve Wrist drop
   – Axillary nerve palsy causes shoulder flattening and wrist drop is seen in radial nerve palsy.

363. Lachman sign is positive in: *(DNB CET 2003, 1993)*
   A. Anterior cruciate ligament injury
   B. Posterior cruciate ligament injury
   C. Medial meniscus injury
   D. Lateral meniscus injury

Ans. is 'A' Anterior cruciate ligament injury
   – Lachman test is most sensitive and specific test for acute or chronic injuries of ACL.

364. Sun-ray appearance is seen in: *(DNB CET 2003, 1998, 1993)*
   A. Osteosarcoma   B. Osteoclastoma
   C. Osteochondroma   D. Ewing's tumor

Ans. is 'A' Osteosarcoma
   – No periosteal reaction is specific for any tumor but sun ray appearance is most commonly seen with osteosarcoma.

365. Which nerve is closely related shoulder joint capsule? *(DNB CET 2002)*
   A. Axillary nerve   B. Radial nerve
   C. Median nerve   D. Musculocutaneous nerve

Ans. is 'A' Axillary nerve is closely related to shoulder and is the most common nerve involved in anterior or inferior dislocation of shoulder.

366. The attitude of lower-limb in case of posterior dislocation of hip is: *(2002)*
   A. Flexion, adduction, internal rotation
   B. Extension, abduction, external rotation
   C. Flexion, abduction, internal rotation
   D. Extension, adduction, internal rotation

Ans. is 'A' Flexion, adduction, internal rotation
   – Posterior dislocation attitude is FADIR-Flexion, adduction and internal rotation and anterior dislocation is Faber-Flexion, abduction and external rotation.

367. Which of the following is first to ossify in foetal life? *(DNB CET 2001, 1999, 96)*
   A. Vertebra   B. Rib
   C. Skull   D. None of the above

Ans. is 'D' None of the above
   – Clavicle is the first bone to ossify in body.

368. Mallet finger is avulsion of: *(DNB CET 2000, 1995)*
   A. Terminal slip of extensor tendon to distal phalanx
   B. Terminal slip of flexor tendon to distal phalanx
   C. Terminal slip of flexor tendon to proximal phalanx
   D. Terminal slip of extensor tendon to proximal phalanx

Ans. is 'A' Terminal slip of extensor tendon to distal phalanx
   – Avulsion of extensor tendon from distal phalanx is mallet finger.

369. Volkmann's ischemia most commonly involves:
   A. Pronator teres   *(DNB CET 2000, 1996)*
   B. Flexor carpi radialis longus
   C. Flexor digitorum profundus
   D. Flexor digitorum superficialis

Ans. is 'C' Flexor digitorum profundus
   – Most common muscle involved is Flexor digitorum profundus > Flexor pollicis longus.

370. Treatment of club foot should begin:
   A. As soon as possible after birth *(DNB CET 2000, 1997)*
   B. 1 month after birth
   C. 1 year after birth
   D. None of the above

Ans. is 'A' As soon as possible after birth
   – Ponseti method is the one followed worldwide now and its principles are manipulation and cast at birth and weekly change of cast.

371. Commonest cause of Compartment syndrome is: *(DNB CET 2000, 1998)*
   A. Fractures
   B. Gas gangrene
   C. Superficial injury to muscles
   D. Operative trauma

Ans. is 'A' Fractures
   – Commonest cause of compartment syndrome is fracture.

372. Monteggia fracture is fracture of: *(DNB CET 1999, 97)*
   A. Upper 1/3rd of ulna   B. Lower 1/3rd of ulna
   C. Upper 1/3rd of radius D. Lower 1/3rd of radius

Ans. is 'A' Upper 1/3rd of Ulna
   – Monteggia fracture is fracture of upper 1/3rd ulna with dislocation of radial head.

373. Match the following: *(DNB CET 1999, 1998)*
   A. (I) Erb's paralysis (i) Lower trunk injury
   B. (II) Klumpke's paralysis (ii) Axillary nerve injury
   C. (III) Crutch paralysis (iii) Radial nerve injury
   D. (IV) Fracture surgical neck – (iv) Upper trunk injury
   A. I (iv) II (iii) III (ii) IV (i)
   B. I (iii) II (ii) III (iv) IV (i)
   C. I (iv) II (i) III (iii) IV (ii)
   D. I (i) II (iii) III (iv) IV (ii)

Ans. is 'C' I (iv) II (i) III (iii) IV (ii)
   – Erb's palsy involves upper trunk
   – Klumpke's palsy involves lower trunk
   – Crutch palsy involves radial nerve
   – Fracture surgical neck involves axillary nerve

374. Commonest benign bone tumor is: *(DNB CET 1999, 1998)*
   A. Bone cyst   B. Blastoma
   C. Chordoma   D. Osteoma

Ans. is 'D' Osteoma
   – Osteoid osteoma is the most common true benign bone tumor.

375. Von Rosen splint is used in the treatment of: *(DNB CET 1998)*
   A. Club foot   B. Congenital coxa vara
   C. Congenital dislocation   D. Legg-Calve-Perthes disease

Ans. is 'C' Congenital dislocation

- Von Rosen splint is used for DDH
- Dennis brown splint is used for CTEV
- Petrie's cast is used for Perthes disease

376. Deformity in hammer toe is flexion at: *(DNB CET 1998)*
   A. DIP
   B. PIP
   C. Metatarsophalangeal
   D. Calcaneonavicular

Ans. is 'B' PIP
- Deformity in hammer toe is flexion at PIP and in claw toe is hyperextension at MCP and flexion at PIP and DIP.

377. Compound palmar ganglion is: *(DNB CET 1998)*
   A. Tuberculosis affection of ulnar bursa
   B. Pyogenic affection of ulnar bursa
   C. Non-specific affection of ulnar bursa
   D. Ulnar bursitis due to compound

Ans. is 'A' Tuberculosis affection of ulnar bursa
- Compound palmar ganglion is tubercular infection of ulnar bursa

378. Paraplegia due to T.B. spine most commonly occurs at: *(DNB CET 1997)*
   A. Cervical spine
   B. Upper thoracic spine
   C. Lower thoracic spine
   D. Lumbar spine

Ans. is 'B' Upper thoracic spine
- Paraplegia is most commonly seen at upper dorsal spine because of narrow space in central canal at this space causing compromise of neural structures.

379. The nerve most commonly involved in fracture of surgical neck of humerus: *(DNB CET 1997)*
   A. Axillary nerve
   B. Median nerve
   C. Radial nerve
   D. Ulna nerve

Ans. is 'A' Axillary nerve
- Nerve most commonly involved in fractures of surgical neck humerus is axillary nerve.

380. In a newborn child, abduction and internal rotation produces a click sound. It is: *(DNB CET 1997)*
   A. Ortolani's sign
   B. Telescoping sign
   C. McMurray's sign
   D. Lachmans sign

Ans. is 'A' Ortolani's sign
- Ortolani is test of reduction of hip by abduction of hip
- Barlow's is test of dislocation of hip by adduction

381. Most common cause of kyphosis in a male in India is: *(DNB CET 1997)*
   A. Congenital
   B. T.B.
   C. Trauma
   D. Secondaries

Ans. is 'B' T.B.
- Most common cause of kyphosis in males is Tuberculosis and in females is osteoporosis.

382. Which of the following enzymes differentiates osteoclast from osteoblast? *(DNB CET 1996)*
   A. Alkaline phosphatase
   B. Acid phosphatase
   C. Deoxyribonuclease
   D. None of the above

Ans. is 'B' Acid phosphatase
- Osteoclast has acid phosphatase that differentiates it from osteoblast.

383. Epiphyseal dysgenesis is seen in: *(DNB CET 1996)*
   A. Rheumatoid arthritis
   B. Still's disease
   C. Down's syndrome
   D. Hypothyroidism

Ans. is 'D' Hypothyroidism
- Epiphyseal enlargement is seen in Juvenile rheumatoid arthritis and epiphyseal dysgenesis is seen in hypothyroidism.

384. The most common cause of osteomyelitis are: *(DNB CET 1995)*
   A. Staphylococci
   B. Streptococci
   C. H. influenzae
   D. Gonococci

Ans. is 'A' Staphylococci
- The most common organism causing osteomyelitis is staphylococci.

385. Match the following: *(DNB CET 1995)*
   I. Ewing's tumour   (i) Flat bones
   II. Chondrosarcoma   (ii) Diaphysis
   III. Osteosarcoma   (iii) Metaphysis
   IV. Giant cell tumor   (iv) Epiphysis
   A. I (i) II (ii) III (iii) IV (iv)
   B. I (ii) II (i) III (iii) IV (iv)
   C. I (ii) II (i) III (iv) IV (iii)
   D. I (ii) II (iii) III (iv) IV (i)

Ans. is 'B' I (ii) II (i) III (iii) IV (iv)
- Ewings and multiple myeloma are diaphyseal tumor
- GCT and Chondroblastoma are epiphyseal
- Osteosarcoma and ABC are metaphyseal
- Chondrosarcoma involves flat bones

386. The compression fracture is commonest in: *(DNB CET 1994)*
   A. Cervical
   B. Upper thoracic
   C. Thoracolumbar
   D. Lumbosacral

Ans. is 'C' Thoracolumbar
- Compression fractures are most common at dorsolumbar junction lower dorsal >upper lumbar.

387. The fracture of tibia in adults heals in: *(DNB CET 1994)*
   A. 4 weeks
   B. 6 weeks
   C. 12 weeks
   D. 20 weeks

Ans. is 'C' 12 weeks
- Apley's rule of union is 3 weeks for upper limbs and six weeks for lower limb fracture in children and in adults this time is double, so adult tibial fracture will unite in about 12 weeks.

388. Find incorrect match: *(DNB CET 1994)*
   A. Hyperparathyroidism—Subperiosteal erosion of phalanges
   B. Rickets—Triradiate pelvis
   C. Osteosarcoma—Multiple calcified secondaries in brain are commonest
   D. Osteoclastoma—Soap-bubble appearance

Ans. is 'C' Osteosarcoma—Multiple calcified secondaries in brain are commonest
- Triradiate pelvis is a feature of Osteomalacia but can be seen in rickets and calcified mets in osteosarcoma are rare in brain they are most commonly in lungs.

389. **Medial epicondyle fracture results in injury to _____ nerve:** *(DNB CET 1993)*
    A. Radial B. Median
    C. Ulnar D. Axillary

Ans. is 'C' Ulnar
- Ulnar nerve is related to medial epicondyle hence it is involved in these fracture.

390. **Calcaneal lengthening is done in:** *(DNB CET 1993)*
    A. Equinus deformity
    B. Cuboid deformity
    C. Flat deformity
    D. Foot drop

Ans. is 'A' Equinus deformity
- Equinus deformity has tightening of tendoachilles and its lengthening is carried out in equinus deformity in cerebral palsy and polio.

391. **Non-union is common in fracture of:** *(DNB CET 1993)*
    A. Lower tibia B. Ulna
    C. Supracondylar humerus D. Coracoid process

Ans. is 'A' Lower tibia

> **F**emur neck
> **L**ateral condyle of humerus
> **U**lna lower 1/3rd
> **B**ody of **T**alus, Lower 1/3rd of Tibia
> **S**caphoid
>
> **F-L-U-T-S** (Fracture involved in Non-union)

392. **Find the incorrect answer from the choice given for question below:** *(DNB CET 1992)*
    A. Smith Peterson nail is used for subtrochanteric fracture
    B. Kutschner's nail is used for Shaft femur
    C. Nail is used for Tibial shaft.
    D. Rush nail is used for Shaft ulna

Ans. is 'A' Smith Peterson nail is used for subtrochanteric fracture
- Smith-Peterson nail was used for fracture neck femur earlier but is not used now due to poor results it was never a treatment option for subtrochanteric fracture femur.
- Subtrochanteric fractures are treated by BLADE PLATE or cephalomedullary nails.

Complete Summary of Orthopedics

1. IMAGING FOR ORTHOPEDICS

1. **Father of Orthopedics—Nicolas Andry**
2. **Father of Modern Orthopedics—Robert Jones**
3. X-rays is done for screening (Cartilage not seen) Glass pieces are visualized on X-rays due to presence of lead in them.
4. CT Scan is done for bone Cortex and Calcification.
5. Calcification of Ligament–CT Scan.
6. MRI is done for Soft tissues/Cartilage/Bone Marrow/Unilateral stress fractures (Investigation of choice)/Single Metastatic lesion
7. MRI is done for occult fracture neck femur (Marrow edema).
8. Sunray appearance is a periosteal reaction.
9. Perthes (AVN of Femoral epiphysis) Investigation of choice is MRI
10. Bone scan is done for bilateral stress fractures. (Investigation of choice) and metastasis.
11. Multiple Metastasis–PET CT scan > Bone Scan (better for Osteoblastic metastasis).
12. Arthroscopy is done for joints (knee > Shoulder).
13. Tumors and infection can mimic each other.
14. Differentiated by tissue diagnosis.
15. Periosteum does not contain dense regular connective tissue as seen in tendon, ligament and aponeurosis.
16. Periosteal reactions.
    a. Sunray appearance/Sunburst/Spiculated appearance – Calcification along the Sharpey's fibres can be seen in any malignant lesion but usually osteosarcoma.
    b. Codmans triangle is usually seen in Osteosarcoma.
    c. Onion peel appearance is usually seen in Ewing's sarcoma
17. Culture is best investigation for infection, TB Spine CT guided biopsy gold standard
18. Histopathology is the best investigation for tumors
19. MRI > USG is investigation of choice for DDH
20. Obese Limping child with hip pain the possible investigation required are X-rays, USG (aspiration) and MRI (CT scan not done).
21. Rim sign is seen in MRI in chronic Osteomyelitis
22. Order of investigation
    Note: **Order of investigation done in case of osteomyelitis is X-ray→MRI→Bone scan. CT scan least preferred**
    In osteomyelitis order of investigation that show **positive changes are in the following order MRI→Bone scan→X-ray**
23. Intra-osseous skeletal tumor is best detected by MRI.

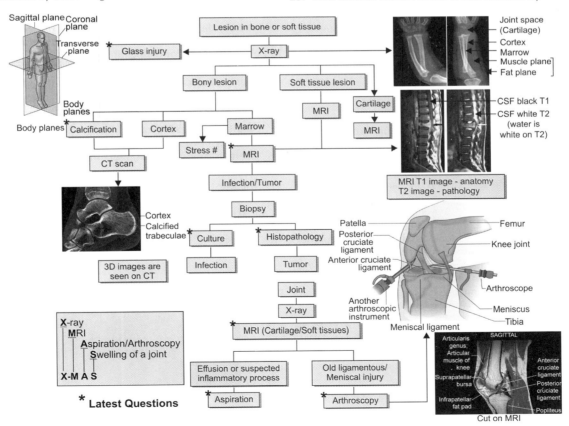

* Latest Questions

STUDENTS DOUBTS

1. Sir, please tell important view son X-rays.

Ans.
i. Brodens view : Subtalar joint
ii. Von Rosen view : DDH
iii. Swimmers view : Cervicothoracic junction
iv. Oblique view : Scaphoid
v. Judet view : Acetabulum (Pelvis)
vi. Open Mouth view : Odontoid
vii. Shentons Arch : Pelvis

2. Best diagnostic test for calcification of ligaments MRI or CT?

Ans. Calcification of any tissue in body CT Scan is the investigation of choice.

Remember C for CT scan C for Cortex and C for Calcification. M for MRI, M for Marrow. MRI is also the best radiological investigation for soft tissues and cartilage.

3. Stress fracture, investigation of choice:

   A. X-ray   B. CT
   C. MRI   D. Bone scan

Ans. Classical teaching is fracture is breach in cortex. But in cases of stress fracture there is marrow compression which is appreciated much early than a cortical breach and for marrow MRI is the investigation remembered as M for MRI, M for Marrow. Bilateral stress fracture Bone Scan is preferred as it can identify multiple sites in one investigation and the uptake in Bone scan is dependent on osteoblastic activity. Remember B for Bone Scan, B for Blastic (Osteoblastic activity).

Thus stress fracture – if Unilateral than MRI is done, for bilateral Bone scan is done and if not mentioned anything than MRI is the best.

4. Sir, A young girl presented with history of trauma 2 months back, now she presents with swelling at mid shaft of femur and low grade fever. ESR is mildly raised. X-ray shows a lamellated periosteal reaction. Next line of investigation:

   A. MRI   B. Biopsy
   C. Bone scan   D. Blood

Ans. This is clinical presentation of some chronic or aggressive lesion of femur the probabilities are Ewing's Sarcoma or chronic osteomyelitis as both can have same presentation (Please remember most common presentation of Ewings is pain, swelling and fever which are same as infection or osteomyelitis) and periosteal reaction (Lamellated reaction or Onion peel reaction is seen in both malignant bone tumors like Ewings and Chronic osteomyelitis), thus the next investigation will be MRI to look at the extent of lesion, its soft tissue component. Further we need to obtain the tissue for confirmation of diagnosis (culture for infection and histopathology for tumors) and in this regards MRI can help us localize the margin of lesion for localizing the site of biopsy on the basis of last extent of marrow edema.

5. Sir, What will be the order of investigations for DDH.

Ans. If the question is asked about Investigation of choice for DDH than MRI > USG will be the order as MRI will be more useful for assessment of complete disease spectrum, management and complications of DDH.

But if the question is asked for screening of neonatal hip or hip instability than USG is investigation of choice.

2. INFECTIVE DISEASES OF BONE AND JOINT

1. X-rays in Osteomyelitis: After 24–48 hours loss of soft tissue planes and on day 7–10 periosteal reaction is seen. (Periosteal reaction is usually absent in tuberculosis)
2. Best radiological investigation for bone infection is MRI > Bone Scan
3. Bone and joint infections gold standard is always culture and sensitivity
4. Inflammatory Joint swellings order of investigations is:

   X-ray
   MRI
   Aspiration/Arthroscopy
   Swelling of a joint
   X-**M A S**

Knee is the most common joint involved in septic arthritis
Joint infection is an orthopedic emergency.

Acute Osteomyelitis

- Metaphysis is commonest and first affected
- Lower femur metaphysis commonest site, in adults thoracolumbar spine is commonest site.
- *Staphylococcus aureus* most common organism overall and also in posttraumatic and postsurgical osteomyelitis.
- Sickle cell anemia—*Salmonella* (Diaphyseal)
- Intravenous drug abusers—*Pseudomonas*
- In patients with prosthetic material-Coagulase negative staph > Propionibacterium
- Open injuries—*Staphylococcus*
- Foot injuries—*Pseudomonas*
- Loss of movement of limb clinical indicator

FABER-Flexion Abduction and External rotation at Hip is seen in Infection, Synovitis, Iliotibial Band Contracture (seen in Polio) and Anterior dislocation of Hip.

FADIR-Flexion, Adduction and Internal Rotation of Hip is seen in Posterior Dislocation of hip and Arthritis (Due to any cause).

Osteomyelitis in Newborn

- S. aureus > Group B Strep > Gram Negative.
- Multifocal (> 50% cases)
- Paucity of Clinical Signs
- Hematogenous spread, metaphyseal
- Poor prognosis

- The most common bone affected in congenital syphilis—Tibia

Subacute Osteomyelitis-Brodies Abscess
(Swelling with rim of reactive bone)

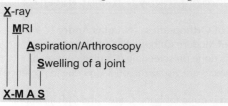

Lytic cavity with sclerotic margins

Chronic Osteomyelitis

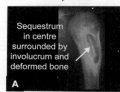
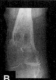
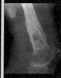

Sequestrum in centre surrounded by involucrum and deformed bone

Fig. 21.2.1: Chronic osteomyelitis (A) Upper end humerus (B) Lower end femur

Complete Summary of Orthopedics

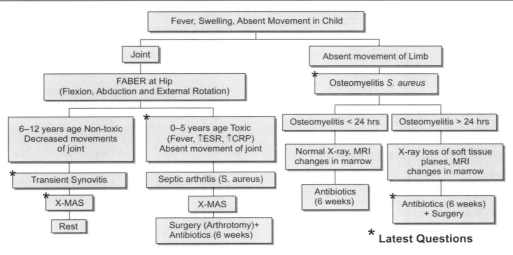

Causative organism; *Staphylococcus aureus*

Sequestrum: Avascular piece of bone surrounded by granulation tissue-pathognomic of chronic osteomyelitis. It is radiodense fragment.

Involucrum is reactive bone around the sequestrum

Cloacae are draining sinuses in the involucrum

Paprika sign is appearance of live bone after removal of dead bone in chronic osteomyelitis.

Negative Pressure Wound therapy is to heal chronic wounds. The pressure is between –75 to –125 mm Hg.

The most common joint affected in Brucellosis–Hip joint.

- Tom Smith Arthritis is pyogenic infection of hip in infancy. There is resorption of capital femoral Epiphysis

Swelling with Multiple Discharging Sinus

- **Over mandible (or head - neck region)** – Actinomycosis
- **On Foot** – Madura foot/Maduromycosis

1. Multiple discharging sinuses
2. Discharge of granules   } Triad
3. Swelling (painless)

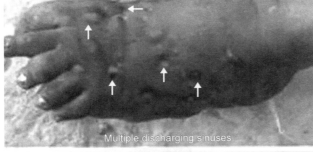

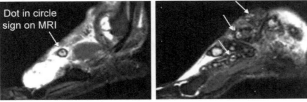

Fig. 21.2.2: Mycetoma (Dot in circle sign on MRI)

Multifocal Osteomyelitis is associated with SAPHO Syndrome

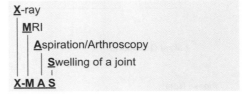

Synovitis
 Acne
  Pustulosis palmo-plantar
   Hyperostosis
    Osteitis
SAPHO

Sickle cell anemia can have multifocal Osteomyelitis organism is salmonella

Paronychia (Most common infection of hand) – infection of nail bed, organism is *Staph. aureus*

Felon—infection of pulp space, Staph Aureus, most commonly affects thumb > Index finger

Treatment is longitudinal incision and complications are osteomyelitis > tenosynovitis

Infectious Tenosynovitis (Kanavel sign are seen)—Staph aureus. Infection of little finger can spread to thumb.

- Infection of little finger can spread to thumb. **Index finger infection spreads to Thenar space**

STUDENTS DOUBTS

1. Sir, A 7-year-old boy with abrupt onset of pain in hip with hip held in abduction. Hemogram is normal. ESR is raised. What is the next line of management: *(AIIMS May 09)*
   A. Hospitalize and observe   B. Ambulatory observation
   C. Intravenous antibiotics   D. USG guided aspiration of hip

Ans. Remember the rule X-MAS for order of investigations for joint swellings

X-ray
 MRI
  Aspiration/Arthroscopy
   Swelling of a joint
X-M A S

In this question we do not have MRI as an option so we will choose aspiration as the answer also remember aspiration of fluid then sending for investigations can help us differentiate between infections and non-infectious conditions.

3. TUBERCULOSIS OF BONE AND JOINTS

- Hematogenous spread Paucibacillary lesions.
- Spine (50%) > hip (15%) > knee (10%) of all musculoskeletal cases. (Bursal involvement is rarest)
- Spina Ventosa is Tuberculosis of short bones of hand.
- Tuberculosis of shoulder is dry (no effusion) – caries sicca (dry)
- Tuberculosis with polyarthritis is called as Poncet's disease.
- Pott's spine – Tuberculosis of spine [Involves bone (vertebra) and Cartilage (Disc)].
- TB Spine is anterior disease (Involves bone and disc)

Note: Involvement of Posterior elements and single vertebra is relatively rare in TB.

- Paradiscal region commonest, rarest is synovitis of facet joints, Second Rarest is spinous process.
- Most commonly affects Dorsolumbar area > Dorsal > lumbar> dorsolumbar junction.
- 1st Neurological Sign: Increased deep tendon reflexes or Clonus, Twitching of muscles maybe even earlier.
- Most common cause of paraplegia is compression by granulation tissue and pus.

Investigations

- **X-ray: Loss of Curvature of spine due to muscle spasm > Paradiscal Lesion**
- **MRI: Best Radiological Investigation**
- **CT Guided Biopsy or tissue diagnosis – Best Investigation**
- Earliest radiological sign of healing in tuberculosis – sharpening of fuzzy paradiscal margins
- Middle Path Regimen is used for T.B Spine.

- Hong Kong operation is for Tuberculosis of spine.
- Anterior decompression + ATT is used in patients with bowel bladder involvement, non-improving neural deficit and worsening neural status.

Prognostic Factor

Feature	Better prognosis	Poor prognosis
Degree of cord involvement	Partial	Complete (grade IV)
Duration of cord involvement	Shorter	Longer (>12 months)
Speed onset	Slow	Rapid
Type	Early onset	Late onset
Age	Younger	Older
General condition	Good	Poor
Vertebral disease	Active	Healed
Kyphotic deformity	<60 degree	>60 degree
Cord on MRI	Normal	Myelomalacia/syrinx (cord damaged)
Preoperative	Wet lesion	Dry lesion

- TB Hip: Acetabulum is commonest site. Babcocks triangle femur metaphysis also is a common site.
- Painful limp is the earliest and most common symptom of tuberculosis of hip joint.
- **The earliest X-ray feature of TB hip is juxta-articular osteopenia > joint space reduction.**

TB hip in HIV Positive patient is more common than AVN of Hip. TB Hip the clinical presentation is usually FABER (Stage 1-Synovitis-Apparent Lengthening) and then FADIR with arthritis.

TB hip and Knee sequelae is fibrous ankylosis and TB spine there is bony ankylosis.

Girdlestone excision arthroplasty is carried out for Tuberculosis of hip.

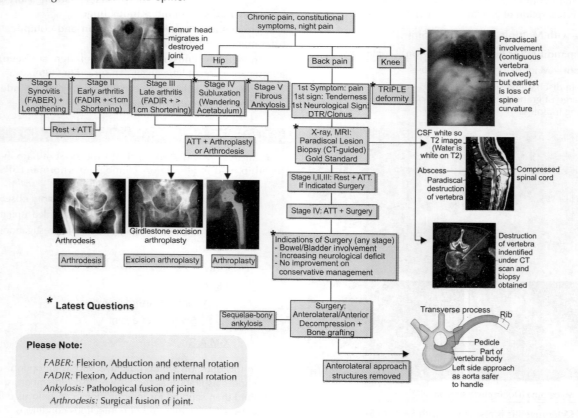

Please Note:
FABER: Flexion, Abduction and external rotation
FADIR: Flexion, Adduction and internal rotation
Ankylosis: Pathological fusion of joint
Arthrodesis: Surgical fusion of joint.

TB in children
1. 1/3 case of TB in children will have extrapulmonary TB
2. Order of involvement is Spine > Hip > Knee
3. MC presentation is Kyphus of dorsal spine.
4. Dorsal spine is most commonly involved.
5. Dorsal Lesions have chances to Worsen during active growth.
6. Lumbar Lordosis is obliterated in TB Spine. The deformity in this area decreases with growth.

Triple deformity:
- Posterior subluxation of tibia
- External rotation of leg
- Flexion of knee.

Triple deformity of knee is seen in TB/RA

STUDENTS DOUBTS

1. Sir, What is the most common cause of bony ankylosis septic or tuberculosis?

Ans. Most common cause of bony ankylosis is septic arthritis. The distribution is as follows:
   1. *Peripheral joints: Bony ankylosis. Septic arthritis commonest case*
   2. *Peripheral joints: Fibrous ankylosis—Tuberculosis is commonest cause*
   3. *Spine: Bony ankylosis—Tuberculosis commonest cause.*

2. A 30-years-old HIV patient on antiretroviral therapy complains pain in right hip since 2 months he has deformity of flexion, abduction and External Rotation. Most likely diagnosis:
   A. Septic arthritis B. OA
   C. Avascular necrosis D. TB Hip

Ans. is 'D' TB Hip

	TB hip in HIV	AVN hip in HIV
Incidence	More Common	Less Common
Deformity	FABER-stage of synovitis maybe prolonged on treatment than subsequently with onset of arthritis – FADIR	Limitation of abduction and internal rotation so initially position is adduction and external rotation (opposite to movements limited) and then subsequently with onset of arthritis FADIR develops.
Side affected	Unilateral usually	Bilateral usually can be unilateral

3. Sir, For TB Spine what is better for diagnosis MRI or CT guided biopsy?

Ans. Always remember growth of organism is most valuable for diagnosis of infection or TB hence CT guided biopsy is better.

4. Sir, What is order of involvement of neural structures in Potts Spine?

Ans. **M**otor than **S**ensory than **U**rinary (MSU)

5. Sir, Tuberculosis of the spine commonly affects all of the following parts of the vertebra except:
   A. Body B. Lamina
   C. Spinous process D. Pedicle

Ans. The paradiscal type is most common > central type (central part of vertebral body) > anterior type (anterior surface of vertebral body) > appendiceal type (involving pedicle, lamina, and less commonly transverse process, 2nd least common is spinous process and rarest variety is synovitis of facet joints).

6. Sir, When do we operate in Pott's spine.

Ans. In any disease of spine Disc prolapse, Trauma, Tumor or Tuberculosis the indications of surgery are the same:
   Bowel bladder involvement.
   No improvement on conservative treatment.
   Worsening on conservative treatment.

4. ORTHOPEDICS ONCOLOGY

Important Points to be Remembered
- Most common bone tumors – Secondaries
- Most common cause of secondaries in children—Neuroblastoma
- Most common primary malignant bone tumor – Multiple Myeloma
- Second most common primary malignant bone tumor – Osteosarcoma
- Commonest malignant bone tumor of flat bone – Chondrosarcoma
- Commonest tumor of skull vault ivory Osteoma or compact osteoma or eburnated osteoma (latest 2012)
- Commonest true benign tumor – Osteoid osteoma
- Most common benign tumor of spine – Hemangioma (Striated vertebra are seen)
- Benign bone tumor have well defined margin, uniform consistency on feel and narrow zone of activity.
- Malignant tumor have ill defined margins, variable consistency and wide zone of activity. (AIIMS May 2011)

Differential Diagnosis of Bone Tumors
- Osteomyelitis has same clinical presentation as Ewing's sarcoma and osteosarcoma.
- Myositis ossificans mimics Osteosarcoma but Myositis has dense peripheral calcification and osteosarcoma has central calcification.
- **Bone infarct ~ Enchondroma**
- **Bone islands ~ Osteoid osteoma**
- **Fibrous dysplasia ~ Giant cell tumor**

Polyostotic bone lesions
- Fibrous dysplasia
- Enchondroma
- Osteochondroma
- Ewing's sarcoma
- Giant cell tumor (Goltz syndrome)

Important Ages and Location
- 1st decade usually Ewing's sarcoma (Can Be 5–20 Years), unicameral Bone Cyst.
- 2nd decade usually osteosarcoma, Aneurysmal Bone Cyst.
- After skeletal maturity Giant cell tumor (Epiphysiometaphyseal > epiphyseal).
- Epiphyseal before skeletal maturity (chondroblastoma) – Purely Epiphyseal.
- After 40 metastases or Multiple myeloma.

Please note that Ewing's Sarcoma most common age group is 2nd decade but it is the most common bone tumor of 1st decade.

Remember usually the questions are asked in this combination

1st decade Diaphyseal—Ewing's Sarcoma

2nd decade Metaphyseal—Osteosarcoma

Classical Radiological Features*

• Sun ray appearance*/Codman's triangle	Osteosarcoma but can be seen in any malignant lesion
• Onion peel appearance*	Ewing sarcoma but can be seen in any malignant lesion or chronic osteomyelitis
• Soap bubble appearance*	Osteoclastoma, adamantinoma
• Ground glass appearance	Fibrous dysplasia
• Patchy calcification*	Chondrogenic tumors
• Homogenous calcification	Osteogenic tumors

While Marking Answers on Calcifications Choose Cartilaginous Tumors Before Osteogenic and Amongst Cartilaginous Prefer Malignant More Than Benign

- I Geographic lesions:
  - IA: Well defined with sclerotic margins: Simple Bone Cyst (SBC), Fibrous dysplasia
  - IB: Well defined without sclerotic rim: Aneurysmal Bone Cyst (ABC) Giant Cell Tumor (GCT)
  - IC: Ill defined margins: Chondrosarcoma
- II Moth Eaten: Multiple Lytic lesions: Myeloma metastasis
- III Permeative: Poorly demarcated, numerous lytic lesions: Ewings sarcoma, Myeloma, metastasis

Winking owl Sign: One pedicle destroyed due to metastasis
Blind Bat Sign: Both pedicle of vertebra destroyed due to metastasis

Order of investigations of bone tumors is usually X-rays than MRI and then biopsy.

Biopsy is the ultimate diagnostic technique.

Enneking's Classification System is used for bone tumors.

Most of the benign tumors and cartilaginous tumors are treated by surgery.

Osteosarcoma and cartilaginous tumors are radioresistant.

Unicameral bone cyst is seen at upper end of humerus, is single cavity, central cyst and has fallen leaf sign or trap door sign. The treatment option is curettage and bone grafting, steroid or sclerosant injection. Radiotherapy is not used.

Aneurysmal bone cyst is seen in lower limbs (Tibia) eccentric cavity, multiloculated. Treatment is extended curettage.

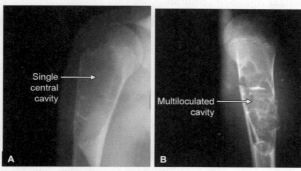

Figs. 21.4.1A and B: (A) Unicameral or simple bone cyst; (B) Aneurysmal bone cyst

Eccentric Expansile Cysts

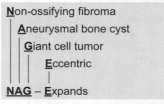

Non-ossifying fibroma
Aneurysmal bone cyst
Giant cell tumor
Eccentric

NAG – **E**xpands

Central Cysts

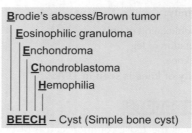

Brodie's abscess/Brown tumor
Eosinophilic granuloma
Enchondroma
Chondroblastoma
Hemophilia

BEECH – Cyst (Simple bone cyst)

OSTEOCHONDROMA–BONY GROWTH WITH CARTILAGE CAP

- Diaphyseal aclasia (Exostosis) is developmental malformation
- Masada syndrome: Multiple osteochondromatosis in forearm
- *Treatment:* Extraperiosteal resection.
- Malignant transformation into chondrosarcoma—In these cases, the cartilage cap usually is more than 2 cm thick. (Best evaluated by MRI).
- Nora's lesion is parosteal Osteochondromatosis lesion seen in phalanx/metacarpals.

OSTEOID OSTEOMA – MC FEMUR DIAPHYSIS

- It is commonest benign true bone tumor, exceeded in incidence only by osteochondroma and non-ossifying fibroma.
- The typical patient with an osteoid osteoma has pain that is worse at night and is relieved by aspirin or other nonsteroidal anti-inflammatory medications.
- CT is the best study to identify the nidus (lytic lesion in the cortex surrounded by sclerosis) and confirm the diagnosis.
- Osteosarcoma > Osteoid osteoma for Bone tumor with Bone matrix.
- Osteoid osteoma has both Osteoclast and Osteoblast
- Surgical management involves removal of the entire nidus burr-down technique.
- Radiofrequency ablation is used for osteoid osteoma.

ENCHONDROMA

- Enchondroma-most common tumor of bones of hand.
- Multiple enchondromatosis is also known as Ollier disease.
- Maffuccis syndrome is enchondroma, subcutaneous hemangioma and phlebolith.
- Treatment is extended Curettage

CHONDROBLASTOMA/CODMAN'S TUMOR

Classic **"chicken wire"** calcification

Epiphysis + calcification + upper end humerus = Chondroblastoma.

LANGERHANS CELL HISTIOCYTOSIS (LCH): DESTRUCTION DUE TO HISTIOCYTES, IDIOPATHIC

1. Letterer: Siwe disease: a fulminant systemic disease, age group < 3 years, fatal
2. Hand-Schuller Christian disease: Triad of lytic skull lesions, Exophthalmos and diabetes insipidus.
3. Eosinophilic Granuloma: Solitary lesion of bone or lung (Pulmonary histrocytosis X) 1st decade of life. Skull is the most common site in skeletal system – Bevelled edge lytic lesion is seen in skull (double contour).

Biopsy: Gold standard (cells with Birbeck's granules (tennis racket appearance) under election microscopy)

Treatment

Spontaneous resolution. Highly radiosensitive and Excision + Curettage for resistant cases.

GIANT CELL TUMOR GCT

Most Common Site is Distal Femur but Distal end Radius Tumor is GCT Till Proved Otherwise

- Although these tumors typically are benign, pulmonary metastases occur in approximately 3% of patients.
- Malignant giant cell tumors represent less than 5% of total GCT.
- GCT malignant component is mononuclear cells.
- Closest giant cell variant ABC (Closest) and Non-ossifying fibroma (Commonest).

Treatment of GCT at common sites*:

Lower end of femur	Excision with Turn-o plasty*
Upper end of tibia	Excision with Turn-o plasty*
Lower end of radius	Excision with fibular grafting
Lower end of ulna	Excision*
Upper end of fibula	Excision*

Note: Chemotherapy is not used in GCT.

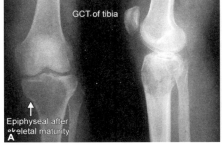
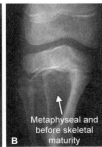

Figs. 21.4.2A and B: (A) GCT upper end tibia (B) ABC upper end tibia

	Giant Cell Tumor	Aneurysmal Bone Cyst
Category of tumor	Aggressive tumor	Active tumor
Age	After skeletal maturity	Before skeletal maturity
Region	Epiphyseal tumor (next to the joint surface) and extending to the metaphyseal region	Metaphyseal tumor rarely goes to the epiphyseal (if after skeletal maturity)
Radiological appearance	Soap bubble appearance-free septations	Air fluid levels-irregular septations separating blood filled sinusoids (seen on MRI)
Bones affected	1. Lower end femur >2. Upper end tibia 3. Lower end radius (characteristic site)	Lower limbs (tibia)

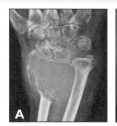
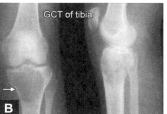
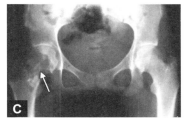

Figs. 21.4.3A to C: (A) GCT lower end radius (B) GCT of tibia (C) GCT upper end femur

Adamantinoma: Most common long bone affected tibia
Ameloblastoma: Most commonly affects mandible
- Please note that most common tumor of mandible is squamous cell carcinoma.

FIBROUS DYSPLASIA

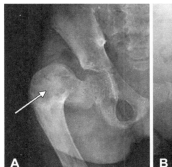
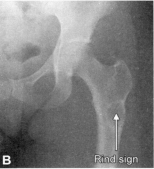

Figs. 21.4.4A and B: (A) Shepherd crook deformity (B) Rind sign

- McCune-Albright syndrome refers to polyostotic fibrous dysplasia, cutaneous pigmentation (café au lait spots), and endocrine abnormalities. (Precocious puberty).
- Mazabraud syndrome is polyostotic fibrous dysplasia with intramuscular myxomas.
- Fibrous dysplasia of proximal femur has shepherd crook deformity.
- Ground glass appearance and Rind sign (sclerotic margin) is seen on X-rays.
- **Fibrous Dysplasia is Developmental anomaly of bone formation.**

OSTEOSARCOMA-MATRIX FORMING TUMOR CAUSE OF CALCIFICATION

- Osteosarcoma is Cancer of young (10–20 years).
- Characteristic histological feature is malignant cells with osteoid formation.
- Osteosarcoma may be more common in patients with the hereditary form of retinoblastoma and Li-Fraumeni syndrome. Osteosarcoma is associated with FBJ murine virus.
- Osteosarcoma is the most common radiation induced sarcoma
- Osteosarcoma occurs in Paget's disease (<1% cases).
- Pulsatile bone tumors in following order answer must be preferred.

Osteosarcoma > ABC > Angioendothelioma of bone > GCT
(Amongst metastasis RENAL and thyroid pulsatile metastasis.)

- *Most commonly involves Femur lower end and shows codmans triangle or sunray appearance of periosteal reactions.*

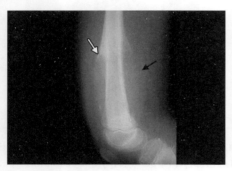

Fig. 21.4.5: Codman's triangle

- *Chemotherapy + Limb Salvage Surgery + Chemotherapy (Methotrexate is most important)*
- *Etoposide is not included in the 'T-10' protocol for osteosarcoma*
- **Osteosarcoma is radioresistant.**
- Osteosarcoma most common Metastasis is to lung.

EWING'S SARCOMA – PRESENTATION LIKE OSTEOMYELITIS

Classically, Ewing sarcoma appears radiographically as a *destructive lesion in the diaphysis* of a long bone (Femur) with an "onion skin" periosteal reaction.

Ewing sarcoma more often originates in the metaphysis of a long bone, but frequently extends for a considerable distance into the diaphysis. **Origin is from marrow cells.**

MIC 2 (CD 99) positive cells, glycogen positive cells are seen in Biopsy.

The t(11; 22) (q24; q12) is the most common translocation of Ewing sarcoma and is present in greater than 90% of cases. Other diagnostic translocations, including t(21; 22), t(17,22), t(7;22) trisomy 8, trisomy 12 and del 1.

Poor prognostic Factors are: Males age > 12, Fever, anemia, Increased TLC, platelets, LDH, Proximal lesion, **chemoresistance, relapse and distant metastasis. (Last 3 are worst prognostic factors.)**

- Treatment of Ewing's sarcoma – Chemotherapy followed by surgery followed by chemotherapy.

ABCD (Actinomycin D/Bleomycin /Cyclophosphamide/ Doxorubicin) is chemotherapy.

(Ewing sarcoma is the most radiosensitive and chemosensitive bone tumor).

Chondrosarcoma is most common tumor associated with **Hyperglycemia**

Treatment of Chondrosarcoma is surgical excision.

Chordoma

- *Chordoma is rare malignant tumor originating from the remnants of primitive notochord. It commonly occurs in the sacrococcygeal or in the spheno-occipital regions. Sacrum is the most common site—Sacrum 50% clivus (35%), cervical thoracic/lumbar (15%).*
  On Biopsy: **Physaliferous cells** are seen.

> 40 multiple lesions in bone diagnosis is metastasis > multiple myeloma (KAHLER'S DISEASE).

- Elderly with multiple bone pains, increased ESR and hypercalcemia is multiple myeloma till proved otherwise.
- Moth eaten bone is seen.
  Features of Multiple Myeloma with more than 20% Plasma Cells in Peripheral Smear—Plasma Cell Leukemia

Causes of Lytic Lesions in Skull
- Metastasis
- Eosinophilic granuloma and epidermoid
- Lymphoma/Langerhans cell histiocytosis
- Tuberculosis
- Hyperparathyroidism
- Osteomyelitis
- Radiation
- Multiple myeloma

Metastatic Bone Disease

- Most common primary is Breast (Also into Orbit) > Prostate overall.
- **Most common sites of primary for bone metastasis.**
  - In males – Prostate > Lung
  - In Female – Breast > Lung
  - In Children – Neuroblastoma
- **Skeletal sites most frequently involved**
  Spine (Dorsal)
- **Lytic expansile metastasis seen in**
  - Renal Cancer
  - Thyroid carcinomas
- Purely Osteoblastic secondaries
  - **Prostate/Carcinoid/Medulloblastoma**
- **Metastasis distal to knee and elbow is rare and usually arises from a primary tumors of the**
  - Bronchus, Bladder and Colon (BBC)

"BBC Can Go Anywhere even distal to Elbow and Knee"

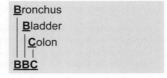

Metastasis from Bone to Bone – 'BONE'

> **B**one to Bone
> **O**steosarcoma
> **N**euroblastoma
> **E**wing's Sarcoma
> **BONE**

Sarcomas of soft tissue origin do not frequently involve bone, the ones involving are 'SARLA'

> **S**ynovial Cell Sarcoma
> **A**ngiosarcoma
> **R**habdomyosarcoma
> **L**iposarcoma
> **A**ngiosarcoma
> **SARLA**

- Rhabdomyosarcoma is the most common soft tissue tumor in child.
- Liposarcoma is the most common soft tissue tumor in adult.
  Sarcomas metastasizing through lymphatic and causing lymph node involvement are:

> **C**lear cell sarcoma
> **L**ymphosarcoma
> **E**pithelial sarcoma
> **A**ngiosarcoma
> **R**habdomyosarcoma
> **M**alignant fibrous histiocytoma
> **S**ynovial cell sarcoma
> **CLEAR-MS**

The term 'synovial cell sarcoma' is a misnomer as synovial cell sarcomas do not arise from synovium. Synovial sarcomas are biphasic tumors and gene affected is SYT-SSX.

Oncogenic Osteomalacia

Hypophosphatemic Vitamin D resistant rickets or osteomalacia can be associated with

- Hemangiopericytomas
- **Fibrosarcoma**
- GCT
- Osteosarcoma
- Pigmented Villo Nodular synovitis
  The mediator is phosphatonin; FGF-23
  It is a reversible condition along with malignancy.

STUDENTS DOUBTS

1. X-ray of Tibia of an adolescent boy is shown. Probable diagnosis: *(JIPMER May 2018)*

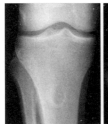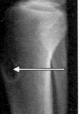

A. Chondromyxoid fibroma B. Osteosarcoma
C. Bone cyst with fracture D. Fibrosis cystica

Ans. is 'A' Chondromyxoid fibroma

2. Sir, A 45-year-old female came with complaints of pain in the lower limb around knee joint (upper part of tibia and lower part of femur). There is increased globulin and decreased albumin, osteolytic lesions are seen on X-ray. Blood investigations reveal hypercalcemia, hypophosphatemia. The diagnosis might be?
(JIPMER May 2016)

A. Multiple myeloma   B. Hyperparathyroidism
C. GCT   D. Bone cyst

Ans. is 'A' Multiple myeloma

3. Sir, Most common bone tumor.

Ans. Tumor like Fibrous Cortical Defect (Non-ossifying fibroma) > Osteochondroma

4. MC true benign Bone tumor-osteoid osteoma.

Ans. Yes

5. MC tumor of jaw-SCC.

Ans. Yes

6. MC tumor of mandible

Ans. Squamous cell carcinoma.
Jaw or mandible both Squamous cell carcinoma.
Ameloblastoma – most common site mandible
Ameloblastoma of long bones – now called adamantinoma and is most common in tibial diaphysis.

7. MC primary malignant bone tumor-multiple myeloma.

Ans. Yes

8. MC malignant bone tumor-osteosarcoma or metastasis.

Ans. Metastasis

9. Sir, Tissue most sensitive to radiation.
A. Diaphysis   B. Epiphysis
C. Metaphysis   D. Cartilage.

Ans. Growing cartilage physis is most sensitive part of bone.

10. Sir, A question comes that, a 8-year-old boy presented with pain in the arm. On X-ray his upper end of humerus has an expansile lesion in the metaphysis with breech of overlying cortex. Diagnosis is Aneurysmal bone cyst or unicameral bone cyst.

Ans. **1st decade upper end of humerus an expansile lesion the first choice will be unicameral bone cyst. Please remember that both the cysts are expansile.**
I understand few books have taken this answer as aneurysmal bone cyst and ruled out unicameral cyst on the basis that it is non expansile and that's not appropriate as both the cysts are expansile but ABC is more expansile. So in combination with other factors, age and upper humerus—UBC will be preferred. Also remember ABC is more common in lower limbs (Tibia).

11. Sir, Which is the tumor that is purely epiphyseal and is seen before skeletal maturity?

Ans. Chondroblastoma also remember that GCT is seen after skeletal maturity and is epiphyseometaphyseal.

12. Sir, Can GCT occur before skeletal maturity?

Ans. Yes, very rarely and in that case it is metaphyseal.

13. Sir, If in PGI if it comes GCT is seen at should we mark both Epiphysis and Metaphysis?

Ans. Yes

14. Sir, A 8-year-male progressive swelling upper end tibia – irregular, local temperature raised, variable consistency and ill-defined margins: *(DPG 2009)*
    A. Giant cell tumor   B. Ewing's sarcoma
    C. Osteogenic sarcoma   D. Secondary metastasis
Ans. is 'C' Osteogenic sarcoma
    The clinical presentation in question can occur both in Ewing's sarcoma and osteosarcoma. However, swelling is around the knee joint at upper end of tibia, which favours the diagnosis of osteosarcoma (metaphyseal lesion).
    Ewing's sarcoma usually occurs in the diaphysis of the bone (middle of the shaft). Also remember that in case of conflict between age and part of bone affected part is given preference as in this question age goes towards Ewing's sarcoma (**1st decade**) **and part towards osteosarcoma so answer is osteosarcoma.**

15. Sir, Than part of bone affected should be the basis of decision for diagnosis.
Ans. No the basis of diagnosis of any bone tumor is biopsy and for any infection is culture.

16. Sir, Can you please tell the pulsatile bone tumors?
Ans. Osteosarcoma, ABC, Angioendothelioma of bone and GCT
    Amongst metastasis Renal and Thyroid have pulsatile metastasis.

17. Sir, Hyperglycemia is associated with
    A. Multiple myeloma   B. Ewing sarcoma
    C. Osteosarcoma   D. Chondrosarcoma
Ans. Chondrosarcoma has highest rates (85%) of hyperglycemia although all other tumors can also cause it but in them the frequency is not that high.

18. Sir, According to a newer hypothesis Ewing's sarcoma arises from
    A. Epiphysis   B. Diaphysis
    C. Medullary cavity   D. Cortex
Ans. This is one of the most frequently asked questions please remember that Ewings is a round cell tumor that belongs to the family of primitive neuroectodermal tumors and it arises from medullary cavity and from **metaphysis**.

19. Sir, Metaphysis but Ewings is diaphyseal tumor.
Ans. Yes, Ewing's is diaphyseal tumor with origin from metaphysis.

20. Sir, 60-year-male with bone pain and vertebral collapse and fracture pelvis diagnosis is—Metastasis, Multiple Myeloma, TB, Hemangioma.
Ans. More than 40 years you must always remember metastasis is the most important consideration if they additionally mention High ESR and hypercalcemia than you must think of Multiple Myeloma. Here metastasis is preferred.

21. Sir, Radiotherapy above how much dose and time can cause secondary radiation sarcoma?
Ans. > 2500 cGy after a period of 10–15 years and above > 50 Gy the risk is very high. The incidence of radiation induced Sarcoma is Osteosarcoma > Fibrosarcoma > MFH

22. Sir, Closest to giant cell tumor is non-ossifying fibroma or chondroblastoma?
Ans. Closest differential to GCT is Aneurysmal Bone Cyst amongst, the two asked lets compare.

	Giant cell tumor	Non-ossifying fibroma	Chondroblastoma
1.	Lytic	Lytic	Calcifications
2.	After skeletal maturity if before skeletal maturity in metaphysis	Metaphysis	Epiphysis before skeletal maturity
3.	Eccentric	Eccentric	Central
4.	Lower limb	Lower limb	Upper limb

Thus characters of non-ossifying fibroma are closer than Chondroblastoma. Hence, non-ossifying fibroma is preferred here.

23. Sir, How do we differentiate between Ewing's and PNET (Primitive Neuroectodermal tumors).
Ans. Ewings is poorly differentiated and Neuroectodermal tumors are well differentiated.

Immuno-histo-chemistry	Ewing's Sarcoma	PNET
CD99, Vimentin	Positive	Positive
Neuron Specific Enolase (NSE), PGP 9.5, S100, Chromagranin, Leu 7	Negative	Positive

24. Sir, Ewings most common metastasis to Lung or Bone
Ans. Lung > Bone

25. Most common Primary Bone tumor causing pulmonary metastasis.
Ans. Osteosarcoma > Ewing's Sarcoma

26. Sir, Most common tumor of multicentric origin
Ans. Benign – GCT
    Malignant – Ewings
    Overall GCT > Ewings

27. Sir please tell about some biopsy findings in bone tumors
Ans. Important Biopsy Patterns
- Fibrous dysplasia: Chinese letter pattern
- Chondroblastoma: Chicken wire appearance
- Malignant fibrous histiocytoma: Storiform pattern
- Fibrosarcoma: Herringbone pattern

NEET PATTERN

1. Tumor from the epiphysis:
    A. Chondroblastoma   B. Osteosarcoma
    C. Ewing's Sarcoma   D. Adamantinoma
Ans. is 'A' Chondroblastoma

2. Ewing's sarcoma most commonly seen is:
    A. Codmans triangle   B. Sunray appearance
    C. Onion peel appearance   D. None of the above
Ans. is 'C' Onion peel appearance

3. Codman's triangle is most commonly associated with:
    A. Ewing's sarcoma   B. Osteosarcoma
    C. Chondrosarcoma   D. Fibrosarcoma
Ans. is 'B' Osteosarcoma

4. The following X-ray most likely is of:

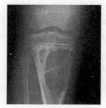

    A. Aneurysmal bone cyst   B. Unicameral bone cyst
    C. Ewing's sarcoma   D. Osteoid osteoma
Ans. is 'A' Aneurysmal bone cyst
    – Multiloculated eccentric cyst upper end tibia metaphysis will be most likely-ABC
    – UBC—single central cavity
    – Osteoid osteoma and Ewing's sarcoma are diaphyseal and not cystic.

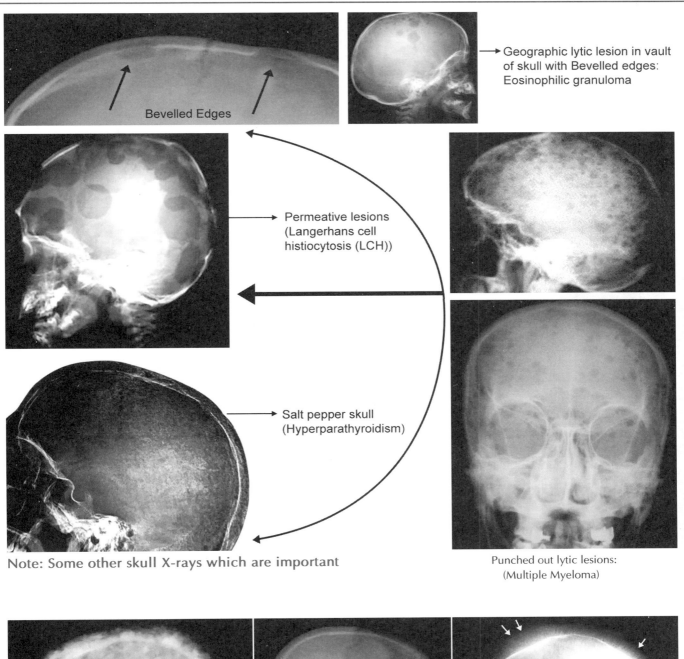

Note: Some other skull X-rays which are important

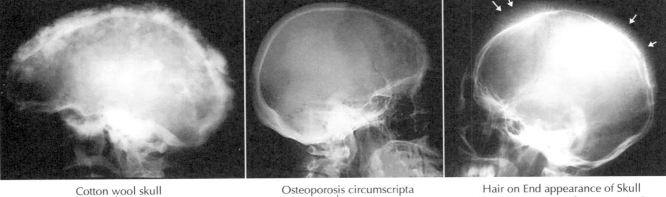

Cotton wool skull | Osteoporosis circumscripta | Hair on End appearance of Skull Thalassemia/Hemolytic Anemias/ Sickle cell anemia

Paget's disease

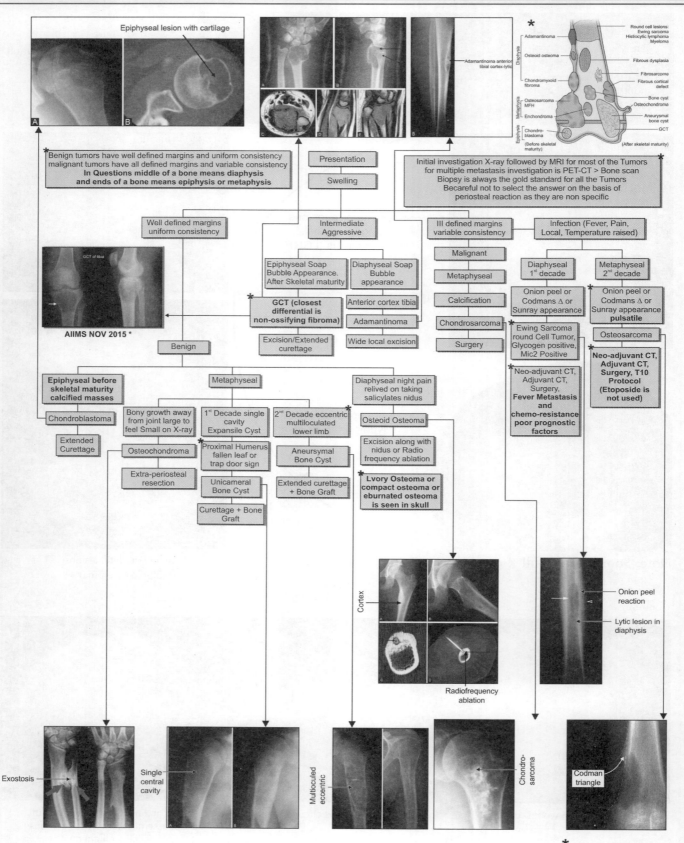

5. FRACTURE AND FRACTURE HEALING

- Tensile Strength of bone is due to collagen.
- Physis is the most active part of bone.
- **1st Centre of Primary ossification appears at end of 2nd month in intra-uterine life.**
- *Rate of mineralization of newly formed osteoid estimated by tetracycline labelling.*
- *Fracture, Partial or complete loss of continuity of cortex.*
- *Tenderness is the commonest sign of fracture.*
- *Abnormal mobility and Loss of transmitted movements surest sign of fracture*
- **Direct trauma – Transverse > Comminuted fracture**
- *Modelling – Growing skeleton*
- *Remodelling after Skeletal maturity – Resorption + Bone deposition (apposition)* **bone remodelling has both osteoclastic and osteoblastic activity at compression or tension site but the forces on bone decide where remodelling takes place compressile forces compression site and tensile forces tension site and in bone modelling there is osteoclastic activity at tension site and osteoblastic activity at compression site.**
- **Bone apposition is seen in**
  Howship's lacunae or cutting cones in normal adults (After resorption).
  Subperiosteal cambium layer In fractured bones (Best example of bone apposition) and after cancellous bone grafting. Bone apposition in these 2 examples does not require resorption.
- *Markers of Bone formation*
  Serum osteocalcin (very important marker)
  Serum bone specific alkaline phosphatase
- *Marker of Bone Resorption*
  Urine hydroxyproline
  Serum bone specific alkaline phosphatase
  Serum osteocalcin (very important marker)
- **Marker of Bone Resorption**
  Urine hydroxyproline
  Serum tartrate-resistant acid phosphatase (**TRAP**)
  High oxygen tension, high pH (aiding alkaline phosphate activity), compression at fracture site and stability (micromovement) predispose to osteoblasts hence enhances rate of union

Common sites of nonunion

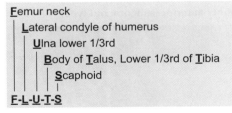

Common sites of malunion

```
Common Sites of Malunion
  Intertrochanteric fracture femur
    Supracondylar humerus
      Colle's fracture, Clavicle fracture
M-I-S-C
```

- Most common site of non union – Distal Tibia
- Most common cause of non-union – Inadequate immobilization

Note: Hypertrophic Nonunion is treated by stabilization of fracture ends.

Stress Fractures
- March fracture 2nd metatarsal neck > 3rd metatarsal neck
- Runners fracture-Fracture lower end fibula
- Tarsal bone to sustain stress fracture – Navicular

Vascular Repair is to be done in Gustilo Anderson Type-IIIC

Urgent Complications of Fracture
Vascular
Compartment syndrome
Nerve injury
Infection
Gas gangrene
Visceral
Hemarthrosis

Immediate Complications of Fracture
Hypovolemic Shock
Injury to Vessel or Nerve
Injury to Muscle & Tendon
Injury to Joints
Injury to Viscera

- Most common site of open fractures – Tibia
- Most common joint to be involved in open injuries – Knee

STUDENTS DOUBTS

1. MC cause of pathological fracture is osteoporosis or secondary deposits.

Ans. Osteoporosis > Metastases, But in India the most common cause is nutritional disorder

2. Stress fractures in metatarsals is most common at:
   A. Head
   B. Neck
   C. Shaft
   D. Any of the above

Ans. 2nd metatarsal neck

6. ADVANCED TRAUMA LIFE SUPPORT

Any trauma patient should be managed in following sequent of events (ABCDEF):

A. *Airway management with cervical spine stabilization (Cervical spine stabilization before Airway)*
B. *Breathing (ventilation)*
C. *Circulation*
D. *Disability (neurological status) assessment*
E. *Exposure and environmental control*
F. *Fracture splintage*

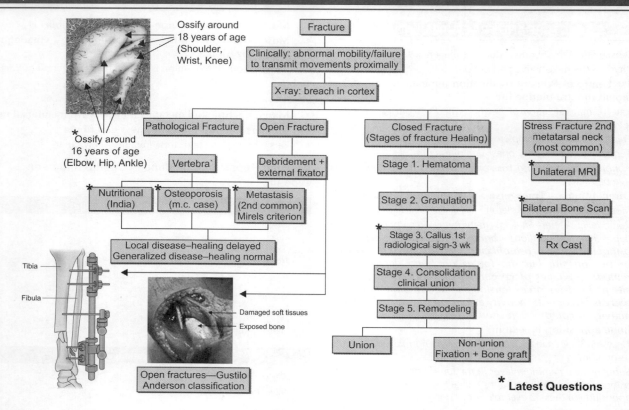

* Latest Questions

7. UPPER LIMB TRAUMATOLOGY

- Shoulder-Most commonly dislocates anteriorly.

1. Only one-fourth of the large humeral head articulates with the glenoid at any given time.
   Humeral head is rotated 15–20° posteriorly in relation to the shaft. (Retroversion)

2. Four rotator cuff muscles are – **supraspinatus (Most commonly damaged)**, infraspinatus, **subscapularis (Forgotten tendon of rotator cuff)** and teres minor. (They are dynamic stabilisers of shoulder. Their impingement causes painful arc syndrome).

3. The inferior part of shoulder joint capsule is the weakest area.

4. The tendon of the long head of biceps brachii muscle passes superiorly through the joint and restricts upward movement of humeral head on glenoid cavity.

5. Rotator interval is interval between leading edge of supraspinatus and superior edge of subscapularis. Coracohumeral ligament passes with in rotator interval.
   The Quadrangular space (Quadrilateral space, foramen of Velpeau) Contains axillary nerve and posterior circumflex humeral artery and vein.
   - 2 triangular spaces
   - Upper: Circumflex scapular vessels
   - Lower: Radial nerve and profunda brachii artery.

6. Lift Off Test (Gerber's test) is done to assess the strength of subscapularis muscle.

7. Rotator cuff tear in young patient is repaired
   Irreparable tear in young tendon transfer is done

8. Elderly patient with irreparable tear or arthritis: Reverse Shoulder replacement is carried out.

9. Sourcil sign: Massive retracted rotator cuff tear

10. Traumatic detachment of the ANTERIOR glenoid labrum has been called the *Bankart lesion. Excessive laxity of the shoulder capsule also causes instability of the shoulder joint.*

11. Hill-Sachs lesion is a defect in the posterolateral aspect of the humeral head-Anterior dislocation of shoulder.

12. (RAMP)—Reverse Hill-Sachs—Anteromedial humeral head -posterior dislocation of shoulder.
    Most common type of posterior shoulder dislocation – Subacromial
    Posterior dislocation of Shoulder light bulb sign is seen.

13. Recurrent dislocation is most common in shoulder joint, accounting for nearly 50% of all dislocations. Most commonly anterior (subcoracoid type).

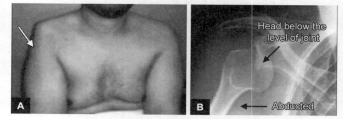

Figs. 21.7.1A and B: Shoulder Dislocation (A) Lost contour of shoulder (B) Abducted arm in anterior shoulder dislocation.

14. Recurrent Dislocation of Patella (2nd most common).

15. Rarest involved joint in Recurrent Dislocation – Ankle.

16. *Recurrent Anterior Dislocation -Abduction and External rotation force.*

17. Neglected shoulder dislocation at shoulder are treated by surgical management.
18. Puttiplat Surgery or Bristow latarjet procedure is done for recurrent shoulder dislocation.
- Most common early complication of anterior dislocation of shoulder is AXILLARY nerve injury.
- Most common complication of shoulder dislocation Recurrent dislocation (overall)
- **Inferior dislocation also axillary nerve is involved.**
- **Anterior instability test: Anterior apprehension test, Fulcrum test, Crank test surprise test.**
- **Jerk test is for posterior instability.**
- Sulcus test for inferior instability (multi-directional instability).
- X-ray shoulder highest bony landmark is lateral end clavicle > acromion.

Clavicle is the most common fractured bone (overall) in adults.
- Clavicle is the most common bone fractured during birth.
- The weakest point of midclavicle is the junction of middle and outer third (i.e. medial 2/3rd and lateral 1/3rd).
- Sling immobilization/Figure of eight bandage rarely plating or K-wire fixation.
- Malunion is the most common complication.

Order of Fracture in Children are:
- Distal forearm (23.3%)
- Hand (20.1%)
- Elbow 12% (Supracondylar Humerus > Lateral condyle fracture humerus)
- Clavicle 6.4%

Valpeau bandage (dressing) is used in acromioclavicular dislocation, fracture clavicle and shoulder dislocation but it is most effective in acromioclavicular dislocation. *(AIIMS Nov 2008)*

Fractures of Surgical Neck Humerus-4 part fractures can have AVN

Elderly osteoporotic females are usually involved (in such cases it is usually impacted).

Peripheral nerve injuries are common, especially involving the axillary nerve.

Analgesics with arm sling usual treatment

Injury	Common nerve involvement
Anterior or inferior shoulder dislocation	Axillary, (circumflex humeral) nerve
Fracture surgical neck humerus	Axillary nerve
Fracture shaft humerus	Radial nerve
Fracture supracondylar humerus	AIN > Median > Radial > Ulnar (amru)
Medial condyle/Epicondyle humerus	Ulnar nerve
Monteggia fracture dislocation	Posterior interosseous nerve
Volkman's ischemic contracture	Anterior interosseous nerve
Lunate dislocation	Median nerve
Hip dislocation	Sciatic nerve
Knee dislocation	C. Peroneal nerve

Humerus shaft fracture; The most common cause of delayed union or nonunion is distraction at fracture site due to gravity and weight of plaster. A spiral fracture of the distal third of the humerus is called a Holstein-Lewis fracture. It is frequently associated with radial nerve palsy. Hanging cast is used. Plating for treatment (usually).

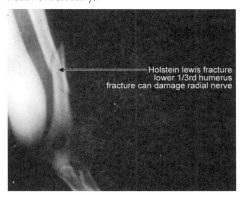
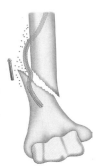

Fig. 21.7.2: Fracture humerus and Holstein-Lewis sign

Surgical Management of fracture shaft humerus is required for multiple fractures, Vascular Injuries, Pathological fractures and Radial Nerve involvement after manipulation.

Around Elbow 1st structure to ossify is capitellum

Three point bony relationship is not disturbed in fracture supracondylar humerus as the fracture occurs above the level of these bony landmarks and Classically Disturbed in dislocation of elbow.

Fractures of Necessity (Requiring Surgery)
1. *Lateral condyle fracture humerus*
2. *Displaced fracture olecranon and patella*
3. *Fracture neck femur*
4. *Galeazzi fracture dislocation*
5. *Monteggia fracture in adults*
6. *Articular fractures*

Fracture Lateral Condyle Humerus – Treatment is Open reduction + K-wire fixation

Complications of fracture lateral condyle humerus are:
- Nonunion—cubitus valgus (Treatment Milch osteotomy)
- Malunion cubitus varus (Treatment Modified French osteotomy)
- Tardy ulnar nerve palsy (Treatment Anterior Transposition of ulnar nerve)
- Growth disturbances
- Fracture Lower End Humerus (Jupiter fracture) can develop cubitus valgus and cubitus varus deformity.

Fracture Supracondylar Humerus Causes static cubitus varus

Supracondylar humeral fractures in children are most common elbow injuries, especially in children aged 5–8 years. Most common type of supracondylar fracture – Extension type (~98% of all supracondylar fracture).

Supracondylar humeral fractures are extra-articular with posterior displacement of the distal fragment.

<u>M</u>edial (Internal) rotation/<u>M</u>edial tilt/<u>M</u>edial or lateral shift
 <u>I</u>mpaction (proximal shift)
  <u>D</u>orsal displacement/<u>D</u>orsal tilt

<u>MID</u>-Position for supracondylar fracture humerus

Most commonly displacement is posteromedial

Associated nerve injuries most commonly involves anterior interosseous branch of median nerve

> **A**nterior interosseous nerve (Supplies FPL to Flex thumb)
> **M**edian nerve
> **R**adial nerve
> **U**lnar nerve
>
> **AMRU** (Order of Nerve Involved)

Nerve injuries are usually neuropraxia, hence transient.
- Nerve injury in Flexion type – Ulnar nerve
- Iatrogenic Nerve injury – Ulnar nerve

Treatment is closed reduction and cast if it fails or it fracture is displaced the fracture is fixed with K-wires.

Jones view is done to assess reduction.

Malunion – Cubitus varus (gun stock deformity) ~ Treatment modified French Osteotomy, (Lateral closing wedge osteotomy)

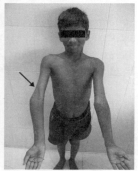

Fig. 21.7.3: Cubitus Varus

Baumans Angle-angle between the physis and long axis of humerus normal value 75–90°; it is increased in cubitus varus.

Fracture Supracondylar Humerus is:
- Most common fracture associated with vascular injury.
- Most common fracture to involve brachial artery. (10% cases)
- Vascular injury is an emergency.
- Supracondylar fracture hummers with pulselessness is treated by closed reduction and watched for reappearance of pulse.
- Most common cause of Volkman's ischemia and compartment syndrome in children.
- Most common cause of volkman's ischemic contracture

Articular Pain	Non-articular Pain
1. Infection, Arthritis, Trauma to Joint	Bursitis, Enthesitis, Polymyositis, Carpal Tunnel Syndrome
2. Limited movement on active and passive movement	Painful on active movement but not on passive movement
3. Deep Pain	Localized Pain

Side Swipe Injury-open fracture dislocation of elbow seen due to accidents involving side swipe over elbow.

Compartment syndrome-Tight cast think of compartment syndrome!

Compartment syndrome involves deep posterior compartment of leg > deep flexor compartment of forearm (commonest in children).

Clinical Feature
- The diagnosis of compartment syndrome is based on dramatically increasing pain (out of proportion to injury) after fracture/ any injury (1st symptom).
- Pain and resistance on passive extension of fingers (Distal most joint of extremity) (1st sign) "Stretch Pain".
- Pulse is not a reliable indicator as microcirculation is compromised.
- Deep flexor muscles are involved particularly flexor digitorum profundus > Flexor Pollicis Longus.
- *Fasciotomy is recommended for impending tissue ischemia when the tissue pressure reaches 30 mm Hg or the difference between diastolic blood pressure and compartment pressure is less than 30 mm Hg or neurovascular sign appear.*
- *Fasciotomy-Skin Superficial fascia, fat and deep fascia is incised.*

Note: Calf pressure during walking is 200–300 mm Hg.

Volkmann's Ischaemic Contracture (VIC) – Most commonly involve deep flexor compartment of forearm (FDP > FPL)

The earliest nerve involved is anterior interossei > median > ulnar.

Turn buckle splint is used

Max page muscle sliding operation is used

VIC is usually surgically treated when there is more than 30 degrees of deformity.

Myositis Ossificans/Heterotopic Ossification-History of Massage think of it!

Elbow > hip joint.

Parameter	Myositis Ossificans	Tumor Calcinosis
Side/Site	Unilateral-**Elbow**	Bilateral-Knee
Marker	ALP Levels Increased	PO_4 Levels Increased

ALP is marker of heterotopic Ossification.

In questions if they ask unilateral calcification then answer is myositis and if they ask bilateral calcification then answer is usually tumor calcinosis.

Treatment of Myositis Ossificans

In acute phase the treatment consist of limiting motion x 3 weeks.

Followed by only active exercises upto 1 year

Surgical excision > 1 year

Low dose irradiation, bisphosphonates and indomethacin may prevent heterotropic ossification, but the radiation should be avoided in children.

Elbow Dislocation: MC is Posterior
- Most common joint to dislocate in children
- Coronoid process is posterior to humerus
- Most prominent part is olecranon in dislocated elbow.
- Myositis ossificans is late complication

Terrible triad of elbow injury (Hotchkiss): Fracture of head of radius, fracture of coronoid and elbow dislocation.
- Monteggia fracture involves upper end ulna fracture with dislocation of Radial Head. Bados type 1-Anterior (or Extension) is most common type. PIN palsy may occur.
- Galeazzi fracture dislocation is fracture of radius with dislocation of distal radio-ulnar joint and triangular fibro cartilage complex injury and interosseous membrane injury.

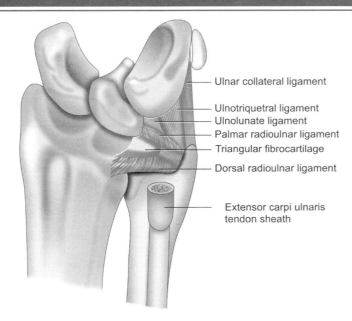

Fig. 21.7.4: Triangular fibrocartilage complex

■ **Pulled Elbow/Nurse Maid's Elbow/Malgaignes subluxation**
– "Age 1 to 4 yrs and forearm is pronated"
It is subluxation of radial head or more accurately subluxation of the annular (orbicular) ligament which slips up over the head of radius and is reduced by forceful supination.

■ Fracture Olecranon treatment is Tension Band wiring or rarely excision which is contraindicated if Fracture is extending to coronoid process

■ Essex lopresti fracture involves radial head and interosseous membrane

■ Proximal forearm fracture the forearm in cast is in supination.

■ **Colle's Fracture – (Extra-articular)**
Colle's fracture is fracture of lower end of radius at its cortico cancellous junction.

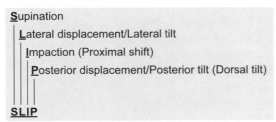

Most Colle's fractures can be successfully treated non-operatively and cast is applied on opposite forces to displacement- That is why position of immobilization in Colle's fracture is

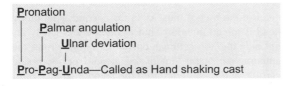

Complications of Colles
Finger stiffness is most common complication.
Malunion is the 2nd most common complication and it leads to dinner fork deformity.

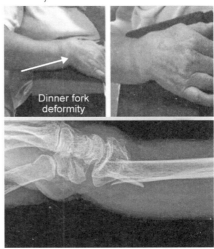

Fig. 21.7.5: Colle's fracture

Fernandez osteotomy is done for Malunited Colle's fracture.

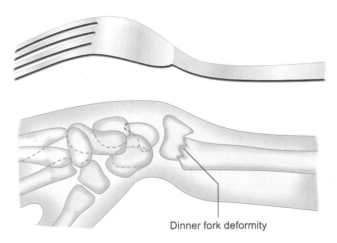

Fig. 21.7.6: Dinner fork deformity

■ **Sudeck's Osteoneuro Dystrophy/Reflex Sympathetic Dystrophy/Causalgia/Algodystrophy/Complex Regional Pain Syndrome. Red hot skinny skin, severe pain and patchy osteopenia.**

• CRPS type I is a regional pain syndrome that usually develops after tissue trauma, e.g. Colle's.
• CRPS type II is a regional pain syndrome that develops after injury to a peripheral nerve, Median > Sciatic (Tibial trunk)
• Treatment is usually physiotherapy and results are poor.
• Reflex Sympathetic Dystrophy—**Patchy Osteopenia**
• Hyperparathyroidism—**Generalised Osteopenia**
• Tuberculosis—**Disuse Osteopenia**

■ **Smith fracture** is reverse Colle's and there is garden spade deformity due to malunion

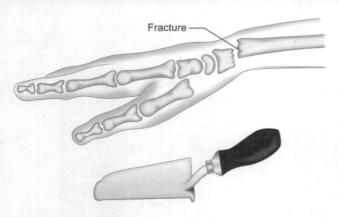

Fig. 21.7.7: Smith fracture

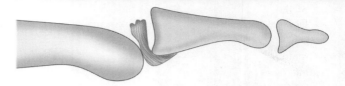

Fig. 21.7.8: Kaplan dislocation

Barton Fracture: Intra-articular fracture distal end radius with carpal bone subluxation

- Die Punch fracture: An impacted intraarticular fragment of distal radius.
- Modified Allen's test is done at Wrist
- Relative Incidence of Carpal Bone Fractures Scaphoid > Triquetral >Trapezium

Scaphoid: Middle third (Waist) fractures are most common. Distal pole avulsion type fracture is most common fracture type in children.

Sign – Tenderness in anatomical snuff box.

Watson test is done

Oblique view important for diagnosis.

MRI can diagnose occult fractures.

Treatment is glass holding cast if does not unite or markedly displaced fracture Headless screw is used.

Complication is nonunion > avascular necrosis.

Proximal 1/3rd fracture of scaphoid has maximum chances of AVN.

Scapholunate Dissociation

- Terry Thomas sign
- Ring sign
- David Letterman sign

- Spilled tea pot sign and pie sign Lunate dislocation
- Perilunate dislocation-lunate stays in place and carpal bones dislocate.
- Gilula lines: Congruent arcs of carpal bones in normal wrist X-ray.
- Scapholunate ligament is injured at wrist.

Bennett's Fracture—Fracture dislocation of 1st metacarpal base (Intraarticular)

Rolando Fracture—comminuted fracture of base of 1st metacarpal (Intra-articular).

Kaplan's dislocation: Dislocation of the MCP joint (classically of index finger)

Injuries with Characteristic Deformities

Deformity	Injury
Flattening of shoulder	Shoulder dislocation (anterior)
Dinner-fork deformity	Colle's fracture
Garden-Spade Deformity	Smith Fracture (Reverse Colle's fracture lower radius)
Mallet finger	Avulsion of the insertion of the extensor tendon from distal phalanx
Flexion, adduction and internal rotation of the hip	Posterior dislocation of the hip, arthritis
Flexion, abduction, external rotation of the hip	Anterior dislocation of the hip, septic hip synovitis of hip joint/Fluid in Hip joint and Iliotibial Band Contracture (Polio)
External rotation of the leg	Fracture neck of femur, **Trochanteric fracture (Lat border of foot touching bed)**

STUDENTS DOUBTS

1. Sir a patient had met with an accident and he can't abduct his right arm and can't lift it. On examination tenderness felt near right upper arm. X-ray showed fracture surgical neck of humerus. Muscle that was paralysed was?

   (JIPMER May 2016)

   A. Subscapularis B. Supraspinatus
   C. Infraspinatus D. Teres major

   Ans. is 'B' Supraspinatus

   The best answer here is deltoid (axillary nerve) since it is not mentioned than we chose supraspinatus (suprascapular nerve).

2. Sir what is lankford triad for

Ans. **Lankford described a triad for development of Reflex sympathetic dystrophy there should be:**
   1. Persistent painful stimulus
   2. Inherent sympathetic overactivity
   3. Abnormal sympathetic response

3. Bankart's lesion MC site:
   A. Anterior or
   B. Antero-inferior

Ans. Bankart's lesion is tearing in anterior part of glenoid labrum. In 1938, Bankart published his classic paper in which he recognized two types of acute dislocations. In the first type, the humeral head is forced through the capsule where it is the weakest, generally anteriorly and inferiorly in the interval between the lower border of the subscapularis and the long head of the triceps muscle. In the second type, the humeral head is forced anteriorly out of the glenoid cavity and tears not only the fibrocartilaginous labrum from almost the entire anterior half of the rim of the glenoid cavity, but also the capsule and periosteum from the anterior surface of the neck of the scapula. This traumatic detachment of the glenoid labrum has been called the **Bankart lesion.**

4. Sir, What is fat pad sign and malgaigne fracture?

Ans. Malgaignes fracture is used for two fractures one is in fracture pelvis causing fracture of pubic rami and ipsilateral sacroiliac area and second is supracondylar fracture humerus. In supracondylar fracture humerus the fat pad is normally seen at elbow it may be elevated due to swelling of fracture and here fracture is otherwise not evident on X-ray.

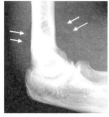

5. MC injury in child 7-year-old with fall on outstretched hand
   A. Colle's fracture   B. Supracondylar fracture humerus
   C. Clavicle fracture   D. Shoulder dislocation

Ans. is 'B' Supracondylar fracture humerus

"FOOSH" (Fracture due to fall on outstretched hand)
   – Fracture clavicle
   – Surgical neck of humerus fracture
   – Supracondylar fracture humerus and lateral condyle fracture humerus
   – Head and neck fracture of radius
   – Galeazzi fracture dislocation
   – Colle's fracture (Most common)
   – Radial styloid fracture
   – Fracture scaphoid

Colle's fracture is seen in elderly, dislocations are rare in children and amongst supracondylar and clavicle fracture supracondylar fracture is more common in children so it will be the preferred answer here.

6. Sir, Vascular Injuries in fracture or dislocation which one are priority?

Ans. Knee dislocation (Popliteal artery damage) > Elbow

7. Sir, Most common cause of Cubitus Varus or Cubitus Valgus

Ans. Cubitus varus is malunited supracondylar humerus
     Cubitus valgus is nonunion lateral condyle humerus

8. Sir, Lateral condyle humerus valgus or varus

Ans. In lateral condyle humerus
     1. Nonunion–Cubitus Valgus   2. Malunion–Cubitus Varus
     Nonunion is more common than malunion so Valgus > Varus

9. Sir, Is not Rolando extra-articular fracture!

Ans. No both Rolando and Bennetts are intra-articular fractures of base of **1st metacarpal but Bennetts is with dislocation and Rolando without dislocation.**

AIIMS/APPG/NEET PATTERN

1. AP & Lat. View of wrist is given. What is your diagnosis? *(AIIMS Nov 2015)*
   A. Galeazzi
   B. Monteggia
   C. Smith
   D. Colles

Ans. is 'A' Galeazzi

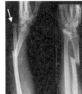

2. What is the diagnosis of this fracture? *(APPG 2015)*
   A. Monteggia fracture type I
   B. Side swipe fracture
   C. Galeazzi fracture
   D. Monteggia fracture type II

Ans. is 'A' Monteggia fracture type I

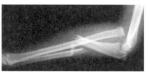

3. Which of the following is most common deformity in supracondylar fracture humerus?
   A. Cubitus valgus
   B. Cubitus varus
   C. Reversal of three point relationship at elbow
   D. Elbow recurvatum

Ans. is 'B' Cubitus varus

4. Supracondylar fracture humerus nerve injured
   A. Anterior interossei nerve   B. Posterior interossei nerve
   C. Median nerve   D. Ulnar nerve

Ans. is 'A' Anterior interossei nerve

5. Fracture proximal humerus most common nerve involved
   A. Anterior interossei nerve   B. Radial nerve
   C. Median nerve   D. Axillary nerve

Ans. is 'D' Axillary nerve

6. Essex lopresti injury involves
   A. Ulna   B. Interosseous membrane
   C. Scaphoid   D. Humerus

Ans. is 'B' Interosseous membrane.

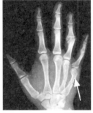 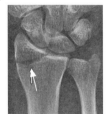

Boxer's Fracture (fracture neck of 5th metacarpal)   Chauffeur's fracture (Fracture of radial styloid)

Note: In boxers— Boxer's fracture is more common than Bennett's fracture

8. SPINAL INJURY

Dislocations are common in cervical spine

Cervical vertebrae have constant number and coccygeal vertebrae have maximum variation.

- **Vertebroplasty is percutaneous injection of bone cement (PMMA = polymethyl methacrylate) into vertebral body. It can be used for osteolytic spinal metastasis, multiple myeloma, aggressive hemangiomas, vertebral compression fractures (Osteoporotic). Its use is contraindicated in infections, Tuberculosis.**

Vertebroplasty prevents further collapse and kyphoplasty is correction of collapse of vertebra by using high pressures it is not preferred now.

- **Central Cord Syndrome-Motor weakness with arm weakness out of proportion to leg weakness**
   – Most common incomplete spinal cord injury syndrome: Central cord syndrome.
   – Incomplete spinal cord injury syndrome with worst prognosis: Anterior cord syndrome.

- Incomplete spinal cord injury syndrome with best prognosis: Brown-Sequard syndrome.
- **Areflexic bladder bower and lower limbs**
  - With symmetrical involvement – Conus medullaris Syndrome
  - Asymmetrical involvement – Cauda equina syndrome

Cervical spine injury has highest chances of dislocation without fracture.

Bulbocavernosus is the earliest reflex to reappear after spinal shock

- **Whiplash Injury**

Hyperextension of lower cervical spine.

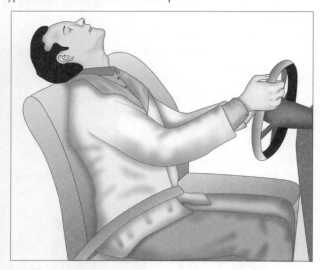

Fig. 21.8.1: Whiplash-injury

- **Jefferson's Fracture**

  Jefferson fracture is burst fracture of ring of atlas (Cl) vertebrae
  Burst fracture is a vertical compression fracture.

- **It is associated with injury in cervical spine in 50% cases**
- **Hangman's Fracture**

It occurs when a fracture line passes through the neural arch of the axis (C_2) vertebrae **traumatic spondylolisthesis of axis (C_2) vertebrae on C_3–H_2 (Hangmans involves 2nd Cervical Vertebra).**

Note: C_1 and C_2 injuries usually do not cause neural deficit because of wide spinal canal here.

Atlanto-occipital joint **Yes** movement occurs and atlanto-axial joint **No** movement (Left to Right) occurs.

Odontoid fracture: Most dangerous is Anderson and D'Alonzo type 2 and it is treated by screw fixation.

Fractures of Spine

1. Jefferson fracture: Burst fracture of C1 (vertical compression injury)
2. Hangman's fracture: Traumatic spondylolisthesis of C2(axis) over C3
3. Burst fracture: Vertical compression injuries
4. Whiplash injury: Sprained neck.
   Earlier were called as railroad spine/Erichsen's disease
   Hyperextension followed by flexion.
5. Flexion – Compression:
   – Wedge compression
   – Tear drop (may have bone fragment from antero-inferior part of vertebra).
6. Flexion – distraction: Facet dislocation
7. Clay-Shoveler's fracture: Avulsion fractures of spinous process of C7 > D1 Vertebra
8. Motor Cyclists fracture (Hinged fracture): Transverse fracture across base of skull leading to separation into anterior– posterior.
9. Undertakers fracture: Tearing of C6-7 disc space causing subluxation, caused by Undertaker's handling the dead body.
10. SCIWORA: Pediatric injury. X-rays are normal but there is neural deficit. This is due to lax ligaments permitting traction injury to cord. Cervical spine is most commonly affected.

Kissing spines: Baastrup's disease

- Flexion rotation injury is the most common spinal injury followed by compression extension injury (2nd most common).
  - *Translation injury is most severe*
- **Tear drop fracture is caused by combined axial compression and flexion injury.**
  - Patient with head injury, unexplained hypotension warrants evaluation of Lower cervical spine > Thoracic spine.
  - In axial load injuries (compression injuries), the most common site of trauma is at the thoracolumbar junction.
  - Most common type of Spina bifida – Spina bifida occulta
  - Most common site of Spina bifida – S1 > L5
  - Car seat belt injury causes chance fracture
  - Spine injury with no radiological abnormality is seen in –Children
  - Dennis has given 3 column theory for spine stability
  - Thumb and index finger sensory supply is by C6, C7 nerve
  - Block vertebra are seen in Klippel-Feil Syndrome.

Lordosis: Lordosis is inward curvature of spine causes are SOAP: (For increased Lordosis)

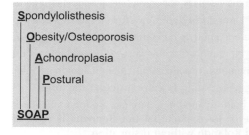

Lumbar and cervical region normally has Lordosis.

Complete Summary of Orthopedics

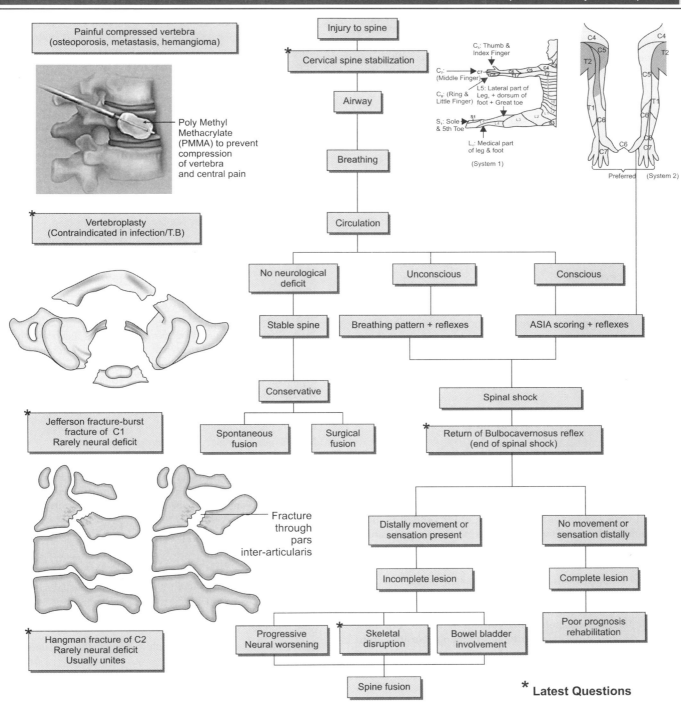

9. PELVIS AND HIP INJURY TRENDELENBURG SIGN

- Trendelenburg's test is done to assess the integrity of abductor mechanism. It is positive in the conditions in which any of the three—fulcrum (Femoral Head), lever arm (neck length) or power (muscles/nerve) is affected.

Causes of Positive Trendelenberg Test

Power-Paralysis of Abductor Muscles

- Superior gluteal nerve palsy (supply gluteus medius and minimus)

Note: Disc prolapse at L4–5 compresses L5 nerve root which supplies G.medius and minimus.

- Polio
- Iliotibial tract palsy
- **Abductors of hip are - Gluteus medius and minimus (main)**
- **Tensor fascia lata and sartorius (accessory)**

Decreased Lever Arm

- Fracture neck femur

   Absence of stable Fulcrum about which the abductor muscles can act dislocation of hip. Destruction of femoral head as in Perthes disease, AVN, late stages of TB hip (stage 4 and 5) and septic arthritis.

   Tuberculosis of Hip–Trendelenberg's test may be positive in TB hip only in late stages (stage 4 and 5) when the head of femur is destroyed.

   Patients walk with positive Trendelenburg sign on. **One hip**-Lurching/Trendelenburg Gait and **Both hip**–Wadding Gait

Thomas Test – to measure fixed flexion deformity of hip by neutralizing lumbar lordosis. Up to 30 degree flexion deformity of hip can be compensated by lumbar lordosis.

Shenton's line is an imaginary semicircular line joining the medial cortex of femoral neck to the lower border of superior pubic ramus. Its femoral part is of more significance. It is breeched in fracture neck femur, head femur, superior pubic rami and dislocation of hip.

- Bryant's triangle measures supra-trochanteric region.

Pelvic Fracture

In pelvis fracture intrapelvic hemorrhage is by far, the most serious complication. Hemorrhage frequently results from fracture surfaces. Amount of blood loss is around 4–8 units.
JUDET VIEW is done for Pelvis/Acetabulum

   The Spur Sign: Triangular fragment of bone. It is seen in both anterior and posterior column acetabular fractures. (Bicolumnar fracture)

CRITERION OF UNSTABLE PELVIS

Radiographic factors indicating unstable pelvis are:
- Posterior sacroiliac complex displacement >1cm
- Avulsion fracture of sacral or ischial end of the sacrospinous ligament.
- Avulsion fractures of the L5 transverse process
- Disruption of pubic symphysis with pubic diastasis of 2 cm with posterior pelvic injury or injury to anterior/ posterior sacroiliac ligament or sacrospinous ligaments.
- Presence of gap rather than impaction in the posterior pelvic ring.

Tiles Classification is for Fracture Pelvis

- **Crescent Fracture,** is a type II lateral compression injury that extends from posterior iliac crest, passing through iliac wing (just behind gluteal pillar), and may then exit in greater sciatic notch or more commonly may enter the sacroiliac (SI) joint. Treatment is operative.
- **Straddle fracture**

Bilateral fracture of both pubic rami.

- **Malgaigne fracture**

Fracture of pubis with a fracture of ilium near sacroiliac (SI) joint (Ipsilateral).

- Open book fracture: A pelvic fracture due to side-to-side compression of pelvis where the pubic symphysis is disrupted and pelvis opens up like a book.
- Bucket handle fracture: Fracture of pubic rami anteriorly and fracture of contralateral sacroiliac joint or ilium posteriorly.
- Wind swept pelvis: it is a lateral compression injury of ipsilateral hemipelvis and open book injury of contralateral hemipelvis.
- Duverney fracture: Isolated iliac wing fracture.
- Spur sign is seen in bicolumnar fracture of acetabulum
- Matta's roof arc angle: Acetabular fractures
- **Moral Lavallee lesion is seen in fracture acetabulum**
- **Kocher-Langenbeck (K-L) Approach** Posterolateral approach to hip has good posterior exposure but limited superior and anterior exposure. Incidence of sciatic nerve injury is 2–6%.

   Contraindicated in Morel – Lavallee lesion.

Deformity of Hip

- Flexion, abduction, external rotation, apparent lengthening—Synovitis.
- Flexion, adduction, internal rotation, true shortening—arthritis/posterior dislocation.
- Flexion, abduction, external rotation, true lengthening-anterior dislocation.
- External rotation, shortening-femoral neck fracture.
- Marked external rotation, shortening-intertrochanteric fracture femur.

Fracture around Hip

MRI is more sensitive (100% sensitivity) and specific for diagnosis of occult fracture neck femur.

Fracture neck femur is called as the unsolved fracture

Fracture neck femur has adduction and external rotation deformity.

- **Gardens Classification for Fracture Neck Femur**

   Garden 1—Valgus between head and neck trabeculae

   Garden 2—Undisplaced all trabeculae aligned

Garden 3—All trabeculae malaligned

Garden 4—Head & acetabulum aligned, neck not aligned

- Pauwel's angle is the angle formed by the line of fracture with the horizontal plane

Fracture neck femur cause of nonunion is high shearing force with precarious blood supply

Fracture Neck of Femur—Treatment

1. < 65 years, ≤ 3 week

    Closed reduction and internal fixation with multiple screw is the treatment of choice. In basicervical fracture Dynamic Hip Screw can be done.

    If closed reduction is not possible open reduction and screw fixation is indicated.

2. < 65 years, > 3 week fracture, osteotomy/bone grafting + fixation.

3. ≥ 65 years

    No pre-existing arthritis—hemiarthroplasty

4. Pre-existing arthritis (any age)—total hip replacement

McMurray osteotomy (Biomechanical osteotomy) used in case of non-union femur

Complication are Osteonecrosis > Nonunion > arthritis

Chances of AVN and nonunion in decreasing order is

- Subcapital > transcervical > basal > intertrochanteric
- Transphyseal > transcervical > cervicotrochanteric > intertrochanteric (in children)

Delbert Classification for Pediatric fracture neck femur

Type
1. Transepiphyseal
2. Transcervical
3. Cervicotrochanteric
4. Intertrochanteric

Incidence 2 > 3 > 4 > 1.

Intertrochanteric Fracture-Femur-Underwear Fracture

- Extra age, extra pain, extra shortening extra external rotation (as compared to Neck femur)
- Treatment of choice dynamic hip screw (undisplaced fracture)
- Displaced fracture: Proximal femoral nail (Cephallomedullary nail).
- Most common complication is malunion
- Most common dislocation of hip is posterior. (Sciatic nerve damaged)
- Most common acute complication of hip dislocation – Sciatic nerve damage
- Most common complication of hip dislocation – OA hip

    Posterior dislocation has maximum shortening in lower limb injuries.

    Associated fracture with dislocations do not have the classical deformities.

Femur head fractures are classified by Pipkins classification.

PIPKINS type IV is femur head fracture with acetabulum fracture

STUDENTS DOUBTS

1. Not true about Kocher Langenbach operation
    A. Adequate exposure of posterior segment
    B. Anterior segment exposure is inadequate
    C. Superior exposure adequate
    D. Sciatic nerve injury in 10% cases

Ans. is Kocher Langenbach approach is posterolateral approach to hip and has good exposure of posterior column but limited superior and anterior exposure, incidence of sciatic nerve palsy is 2–6%. This question is asked in two forms one is 3rd option has superior segment is adequately visualised in that case that option is incorrect and that will be the answer like in this question. Another form of this question is 3rd choice mentions superior segment exposure is limited in that case this option is correct and answer to the question becomes sciatic nerve palsy is seen in 10% cases as sciatic nerve injury is seen in 2–6% cases. So observe 3rd option and then decide.

NEET PATTERN

1. A 30-year-old man history of Road traffic accident presents with flexion adduction and Internal rotation of left lower limb most likely etiology is:
    A. Anterior hip dislocation
    B. Fracture neck femur
    C. Fracture subtrochanteric femur
    D. Posterior dislocation of hip

Ans. is 'D' Posterior dislocation of hip

10. LOWER LIMB TRAUMATOLOGY

Subtrochanteric Femoral Fractures

- Russell and Taylor classification.
    There is flexion, abduction and external rotation of proximal fragment.
- Treatment of choice is cephallomedullary nail.
- Smith Paterson triflanged nail was used for internal fixation of fracture neck femur (not subtrochanteric femur).

Diagnostic Criterion for Fat Embolism – Fracture shaft femur with breathlessness after 48 hours think of it:

Gurd's Major Criteria (4)
- Axillary or subconjunctival petechia
- PaO_2 below 60 mm Hg
- CNS depression
- Pulmonary edema

Gurd's Minor Criteria (8)
- Tachycardia
- Pyrexia
- ANEMIA
- Thrombocytopenia
- Fat globules present in sputum
- Fat present in urine (GURD TEST)
- Increasing ESR
- Emboli present in retina

1 major + 4 minor = fat embolism

- Treatment of fat embolism is oxygen and (IPPV)
- Waddells triad includes femur shaft fracture with intra-abdominal/intrathoracic injury and head injury

- Middle third of Femur is the most common location of femoral shaft fracture. (Children upper 1/3rd).
- Femoral shaft fractures: Most common associated injury involves the ligaments of knee and most commonly missed injury is fracture neck of femur

True Supracondylar fracture of femur is Type A
- Type A – Supracondylar fracture
- Type B – Intercondylar fracture
- Type C – Comminuted intercondylar fracture

Floating joint
Flail joint due to fracture of shafts of adjacent metaphysis of 2 ipsilateral bones e.g. floating knee = femur and tibia fracture.

Popliteal artery injury is common in anterior knee dislocation.

Insall-Salvati index is ratio of patellar tendon length to the length of patella (n) is between 0.8 to 1.2

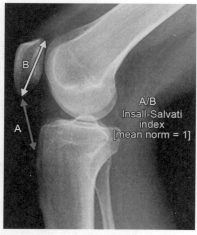

- < 0.8 – Patella baja (low lying patella)
- >1.2 – Patella atta (high lying patella)
- High crural index is seen in jumping athletes
- **Compartment syndrome of Leg – Test for toe dorsiflexion.**
- **Use of Single Crutch – In the opposite side for Fracture both bone leg and Hip Pathology.**
- **Mechanism of injury in lateral condylar fracture of proximal tibia—Strain of valgus knee with axial loading.**
- **Over 90% of ankle ligament injuries (twisted ankle or ankle sprain involve the lateral ligament complex usually the anterior talofibular ligament).**
- Deltoid ligament is injured around medial malleolus
- Ottawa ankle rule: used to avoid unneeded radiographs after ankle injury (i.e. which patient needs X-ray after ankle injury?). Ankle X-ray is required if there is pain in malleolar region plus bony tenderness along the distal posterior edge (or tip) of medial or lateral malleolus or inability to bear weight for four steps.
- Ottawa foot rule: X-ray foot is required if there is any pain in the midfoot zone plus bony tenderness at the base of the fifth metatarsal or at the navicular bone or inability to bear weight for four steps.
- Tibialis posterior attaches to navicular bone.
- Anterolateral approach to tibia can be converted to extensile approach, less chances of wound dehiscence are there and it has medially based vascular flap.

Tibial Pilon Fracture
The terms *tibial plafond fracture, pilon fracture,* and *distal tibial explosion fracture* all have been used to describe intraarticular fractures of the distal tibia.

- **Pronation of foot the joints that become parallel are—Talonavicular and calcaneocuboid**
- Toddler's fracture: A spiral fracture of the tibia seen in toddlers. (Twisting injury).
- Bosworth fracture: A fracture dislocation at ankle Fibula is trapped posterior to tibia.
- Tillaux fracture: This is avulsion of anterior tibial margin by the anterior tibiofibular ligament (Salter-Harris type III injury)
- LeForte-Wagstaffe fracture: This is fibular avulsion fracture of the anterior tibiofibular ligament (opposite of Tillaux fracture).
- Chalk stick fracture: in these fractures, the fracture line is transverse to the long axis of the bone. Seen in Osteopetrosis, Paget's Disease
- Growing fracture: These are skull fractures seen mainly in infancy and early childhood characterized by progressive diastatic enlargement of the fracture line

Fracture Talus-Complications—Osteoarthritis (Subtalar > ankle) > Avascular Necrosis

- Secondary Osteoarthritis of ankle and/or subtalar joint occurs some years after injury in over 50% of patients. There are several causes: articular damage because of initial trauma, malunion, distortion of articular surface and AVN.
- A vascular necrosis of body, incidence varies with the severity of displacement: in type 1 < 10%, in type II~40%, in type III > 90% and in type IV 100%.
- **Calcaneum (It is also called as Don Juan fracture) is the most commonly fractured tarsal bone-Tuber angle of Bohler (Tuber-joint angle)—Reduced in fracture calcaneum and Crucial angle of Gissaine-increases in intraarticular fractures.**
- Calcaneum in over 20% of these patients suffer associated injury of spine (most common), pelvis or hip, base of skull and talus.
- 5th metatarsal is the most commonly fractured metatarsal
- Jones fracture at the base of fifth metatarsal at the metaphysiodiaphyseal junction
- Pseudo-Jones/Dancer's fracture: Avulsion fracture of the tip of 5th metatarsal.
- Hammer toe is flexion deformity of PIP

Angles in Orthopedics
- Cobb's angle – Scoliosis
- Kite's angle – CTEV
- Meary's angle – Pes cavus
- Hilgenreiner's epiphyseal angle – Congenital coxa vara
- Baumann's angle-Supra condylar fracture
- Alpha angle and beta angles are for DDH.
- Coleman block test is done for pes cavus
- **Chronic ankle instability can be satisfactorily treated by Waston-Jones operation. In which reconstruction of ankle ligaments is carried out.**

Watson-Jones is also a lateral approach to the hip joint, which can be used for hip replacement (although rarely as more commonly used approaches are Moore's posterior and Hardinge's antero-lateral approach).

Complete Summary of Orthopedics

STUDENTS DOUBTS

1. Sir What is method of fixation of this #: (AIIMS Nov 16)
   A. Plating
   B. Nailing
   C. Screws
   D. Tension Band Wiring

   Ans. is 'D' Tension Band Wiring

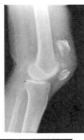

2. Sir, vertical fracture of medial malleolus is seen in which ankle injury.

Lauge Hansen Classification of Ankle Fracture

Supination adduction injury
- Avulsion of fibular tip
- Vertical fracture of medial malleolus

Supination external rotation (most common)
- Transverse fracture of medial malleolus/deltoid ligament injury
- Spiral fracture of fibula (anteroinferior to posterosuperior)

Pronation abduction
- Transverse fracture of medial malleolus/deltoid ligament injury
- Transverse fracture of fibula (above syndesmosis)

Pronation external rotation
- Transverse fracture of medial malleolus/deltoid ligament injury
- Spiral fracture of fibula (Antero-superior → Postero-inferior)

3. The classification for diaphyseal femoral fracture comminution was given by: (APPG 2014)
   A. Seinsheimer
   B. Evans
   C. Winquist and Hansen
   D. Frykman

   Ans. is 'C' Winquist and Hansen

4. Treatment of choice for fracture shaft femur in adults is: (AIIMS Nov 16)
   A. Locked intramedullary nail
   B. External fixation
   C. Closed reduction and cast immobilization
   D. Plate fixation

   Ans. is 'A' Locked intramedullary nail

5. Sir, Blunt injury to which region causes maximum vascular injury?
   A. Knee dislocation
   B. Elbow dislocation
   C. Tibial plateau fracture
   D. Inferior dislocation of clavicle

   Ans. is 'A' Knee dislocation in 40–66% cases can cause damage to popliteal artery of all the dislocations in body it is maximum associated with vascular injury

6. Sir, Watson Jones approach is for?
   A. Neglected club foot
   B. Muscle paralysis
   C. Hip replacement
   D. Valgus deformity

   Ans. is 'C' Watson Jones procedure is for ankle instability and Watson Jones surgical approach is anterolateral approach for hip joints. So, read the question before answering whether approach is asked or operation is asked.

11. FRACTURE MANAGEMENT

Plaster Casts and their uses:
- Plaster of Paris is $CaSO_4 \cdot 1/2 H_2O$
- Average setting time 7–10 minutes
- Drying time (time taken for the POP to convert from crystalline form to anhydrous form):
  - Arm cast—24–36 hours
  - Leg cast—48–60 hours
- Cold water will maximize the moulding time

Name of the cast	Use
Minerva cast	Cervical spine disease
Risser's cast	Scoliosis
Turn-buckle cast	Scoliosis
Shoulder spica*	Shoulder immobilization
U-Slab/hanging cast	Fracture of the humerus
Hip spica	Fracture of the femur
Cylinder cast/tube cast	Fracture of the patella
Patellar tendon bearing Cast (PTB cast)	Fracture of the tibia
Colle's cast	Fracture lower end radius
Glass holding cast	Fracture scaphoid^Q

Gallows Traction – Fracture shaft femur < 2 years of age.

Rush pin is used for fracture shaft femur not for traction
- Superficial heat therapy infrared therapy
- Skin traction maximum weight is 4–5 Kg
- Skeletal traction maximum weight is 20 Kg
- Thomas splint was described for TB Knee
- Halopelvic traction corrects spine deformities.

External Fixator is used for Open Fracture

Ilizarov fixator is used for Shortening with discharging sinus, nonunion and also for CTEV.

Surgical Excision Never done in growth plate injury, e.g. Lateral condyle fracture.

Most common bone for which nailing is done—Tibia.

Types of Plates

1. **Dynamic compression plates:** These are used to fix the diaphyseal region and can be used as neutralization Buttress mode or compression mode.
2. **LCDCP:** Limited contact–DCP It decreases the contact with bone surface hence preserving bone vascularity.
3. **Locking Compression plate**—The Screw locks in screw holes of the plates hence the name – locking plates.

   When do Locking Plates Work Best?
   - Osteopenic bone
   - Metaphyseal areas
   - Periprosthetic fractures
   - Failed fixation (nonunion)

Iliac crest is the ideal and most common site for harvesting bone graft.

Iliac crest is the site for 1st order bone grafting.

Cast Syndrome is due to hip spica or scoliosis cast superior mesenteric artery compressing 3rd part of duodenum.

Z plasty – relationship between angle of Z plasty and elongation
- 30 —25% elongation
- 45 —50% elongation
- 60 —75% elongation
- 75 —100% elongation
- 90 —125% elongation

Common Splints/Braces and their Uses:

Name	Use
Crammer-wire splint	Emergency immobilization
Aluminium splint	Immobilization of fingers
UPPER LIMB	
Cock-up splint	Radial nerve palsy
Knuckle bender splint	Ulnar nerve palsy/Median nerve palsy
Volkmann's splint or Turn Buckle splint	Volkmann's ischemic contracture (VIC)
Aeroplane splint	Brachial plexus injury
Dunlop traction	Supracondylar fracture of humerus
Smith's traction	Supracondylar fracture of humerus
Figure of eight bandage	Clavicle
Velpeau sling and swathe	Acromioclavicular dislocation > shoulder dislocation
Gutter splint	Phalangeal and metacarpal fractures
Thumb spica splint	Scaphoid fracture/ Metacarpal fracture/ Game keepers thumb
Sugar tong	Humeral fracture
Distal sugar tong/Reverse sugar tong	Distal forearm fracture
Double sugar tong	Elbow fracture
Buddy strapping	Phalangeal fracture
LOWER LIMB	
Thomas splint (Continuous Fixed Traction)	Fracture femur, knee immobilization
Böhler-Braun splint	Fracture femur, knee and tibia
Dennis Brown splint	CTEV
Toe-raising splint	Foot drop splint
Gallow's traction	Fracture shaft of femur in children below 2 years (or 12 kg body weight)
Bryant's traction	Fracture shaft of femur in children below 2 years

Contd...

Contd...

Russell's traction	Trochanteric fractures (described as skin traction)
Buck's traction	Conventional skin traction
Perkins traction	Fracture shaft femur in adults
90 degrees- 90 degrees traction	Fracture shaft of femur in children
Anges- Hunt traction	Correction of hip flexion deformity
well-leg traction	Correction of abduction deformity of hip
Pavlik harness, Von Rosen splint Ilfeld or Craig splint or Bachelor cast	Developmental Dysplasia of Hip
Broom stick (Petrie) cast	Legg Calve-Perthes Disease
SPINE	
Four- post collar	Neck immobilization
SOMI brace (Sternal occipital mandibular immobilization brace)	Cervical spine injury
ASHE (Anterior spinal hyper extension) brace	Dorso-lumbar spinal injury
Taylor's brace	Dorso-lumbar immobilization
Milwaukee brace	Scoliosis
Boston brace	Scoliosis
Lumbar corset	Backache
Goldthwaite brace	Lumbar Spine (T.B.)
•Head-halter traction	Cervical spine injuries
Crutchfield traction	Cervical spine injuries
Halo-pelvic traction	Scoliosis
Minerva cast, Halo device	Cervical spine
Risser's cast, Milwaukee brace, Boston brace	Scoliosis (usually Idiopathic or Dorsal)

- Unna boot is used for Varicose Ulcers

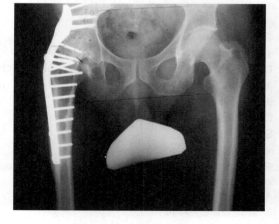

Fig. 21.11.1: Cobra plate for hip arthrodesis

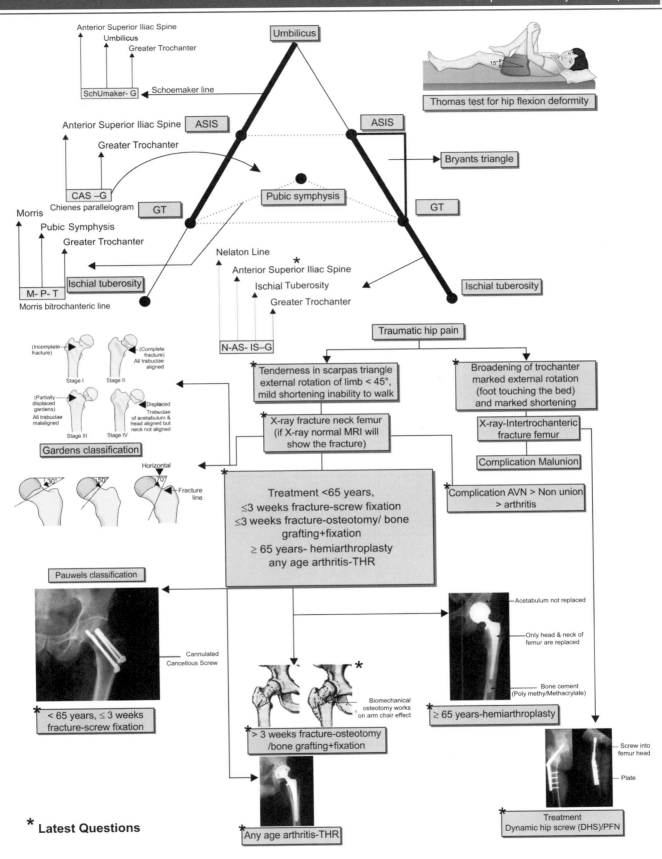

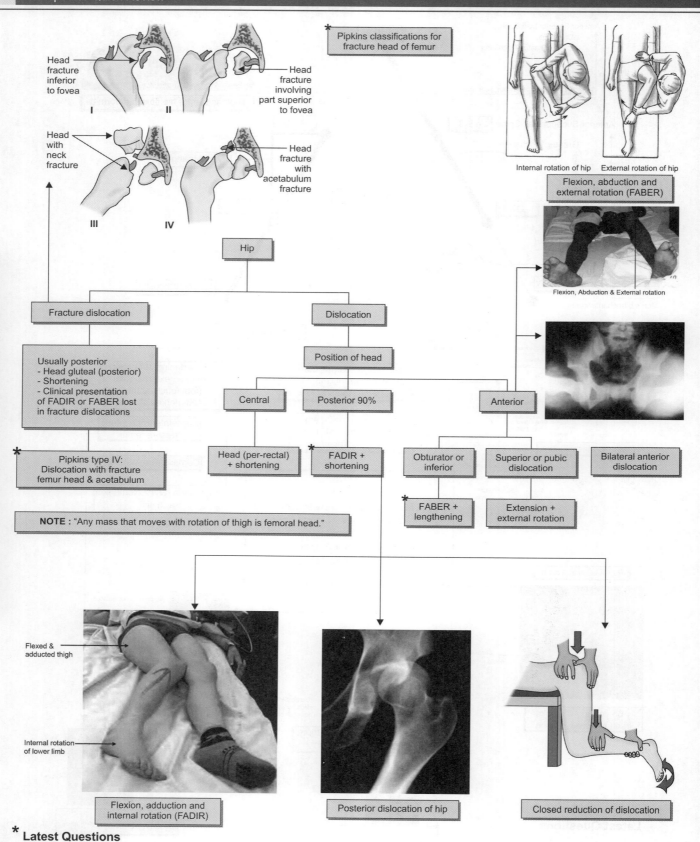

Complete Summary of Orthopedics

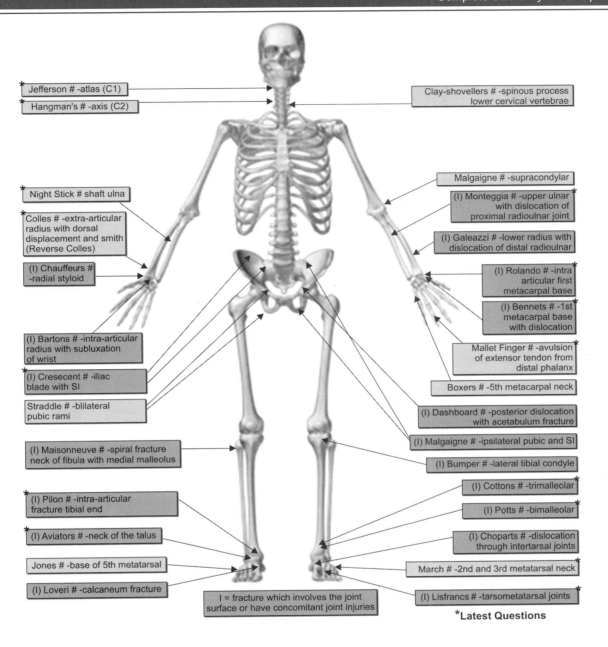

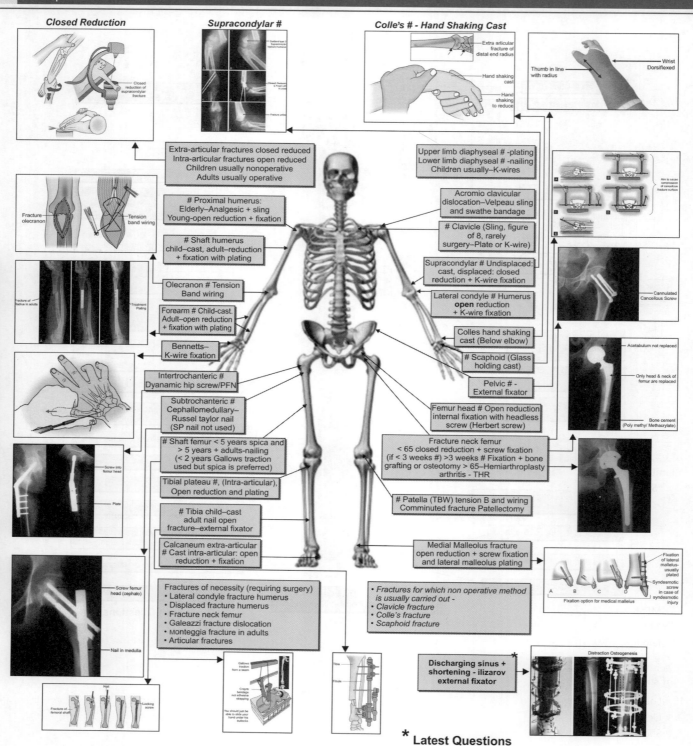

Complete Summary of Orthopedics

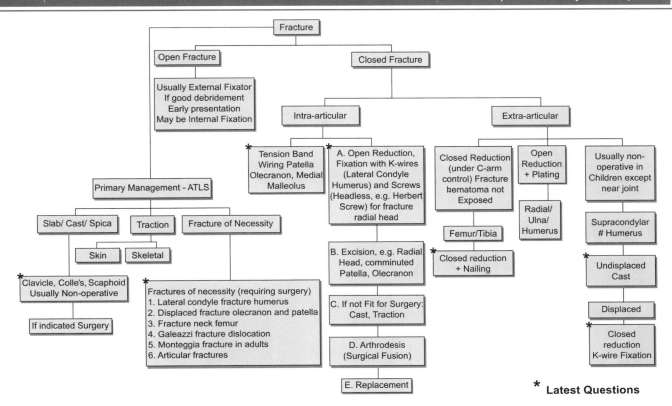

* **Latest Questions**

12. AMPUTATIONS

Mangled Extremity Severity Score (MESS): Predictor for Limb Survival after Crush injury

"SIVA"- the destroyer will decide survival.

Type	Point
Shock Group	0–2
Ischemia Group	1–4
Velocity of Trauma	1–4
Age Group	0–1
Total Score:	11

MESS score: Six or less consistent with a salvageable limb. Seven or greater amputation generally the eventual result.

Jaipur foot was designed by Dr P K Sethi

Reimplantation of Amputated Digit (Greens)-Order of repair of structures

1. Locate and tag vessels and nerves
2. Debride
3. Shorten and fix bone
4. Repair Extensor tendon
5. Repair flexor tendon
6. Repair arteries
7. Repair nerves
8. Repair Veins
9. Skin coverage.
   – But the skin is preserved the first as there has to be an adequate soft tissue coverage over deeper structures and sensation of palmar skin cannot be reproduced by any skin graft.

NEET PATTERN

1. Jaipur foot was designed by:
   A. Dr Dholakia B. Dr Joshi
   C. Dr P K Sethi D. Dr Ranawat
   Ans. is 'C' Dr P K Sethi

2. Mangled extremity Severity score is for:
   A. Survival of a victim
   B. Damage to nerve in a limb injury
   C. To predict survival of a limb in crushing injuries
   D. Scoring system for metastasis
   Ans. is 'C' To predict survival of a limb in crushing injuries

13. SPORTS INJURY

- Predominant collage in menisci/fibrocartilage – Type I collagen
- Predominant collagen in articular/hyaline cartilage – Type II collagen.
- Physiological locking is internal rotation of femur on tibia.
- If knee is extended from flexed position tibial tuberosity moves towards lateral border of patella.
- The twisting force (rotation) in a weight bearing flexed knee is the commonest mode of meniscal (semilunar cartilage) injury. Medial meniscus > Lateral meniscus. *(AIPG 2010)*
- *The commonest type of medial meniscal injury in a young adult is the bucket handle tear. This is vertical longitudinal tear that is complete.*

- **Smillie Classification – Meniscus Injury**

Meniscal Injury	Cruciate Injury/Collateral Ligament
1. Effusion	Hemarthrosis
2. Delayed Swelling	Immediate Swelling

- Bucket handle tear of meniscus - Double PCL sign on MRI
- Meniscal cysts- Lateral > Medial
  Menisci to tibial connection is by coronary ligaments
- Knee unlocking is by popliteus muscle
- Q angle provides a lateral vector to patella and is line between Quadriceps and Patellar tendon. Increase in Q angle predisposes patella to lateral overload and makes it prone to subluxate or dislocate laterally.

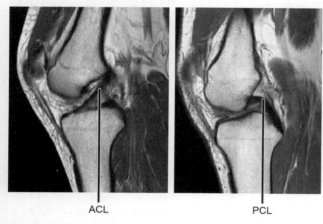

Fig. 21.13.1: Sagittal view of knee on MRI

| Anterior Cruciate Ligament (ACL) is most important for walking downhill |

- ACL prevents excess movement of femur on tibia in hyperextension injury.
- Lelli test is a new test for ACL
- ACL injury can have fractures in intercondylar areas of the tibia.
- ACL the anteromedial band is tight in flexion, providing the primary restraint, whereas the posterolateral bulky portion of this ligament is tight in extension providing the primary restraint.
- ACL tests are lachman (best), Anterior Drawer test, Pivot shift test, KT-1000 knee arthrometer to measure objectively.
- Segond Fracture: ACL tear plus avulsion of capsule from lateral tibial plateau
- Pellegrini Stieda Lesion: Calcification at femoral attachment site of MCL
- Tests for knee Effusion - Patellar tap/Bulge sign (About 10 ml)/ patellar Ballottement.

Recurrent dislocation Patella predisposing factors are:
1. Hyperlaxity
2. Genu Valgum
3. External tibial torsion
4. Patella too high or too low
5. Under developed lateral femoral Condyle
6. Weak medial ligaments/structures.

The patella dislocates almost always laterally.

| Celery stalk appearance of lower end femur is seen in degenerated ACL and Congenital rubella

| Anterolateral arthroscopy of knee is to see patella femoral articulation

- The etiology of Achilles insertional tendonitis is overuse
- Non-insertional Achilles tendonitis is more common and is seen in Atheletes. It is seen 2–6 cm above the insertion of Tendoachilles.
- Tendon rupture-supraspinatus, biceps, and Achilles tendons

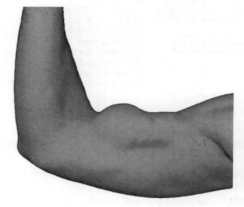

Fig. 21.13.2: Biceps tear -Popeye

Most TA tears occurs in left leg in the substance of TA, 2-6 cm above the calcaneal insertion (watershed zone). Test for TA rupture is Simmonds test or Thompson test.

- Most common ligament injured at ankle is anterior talofibular ligament.

Game Keeper's/Skier's Thumb: Injury to the thumb metacarpophalangeal joint ulnar collateral ligament. Due to forced radial deviatory of thumb. Steners lesion is associated. (Trapped adductor pollicis between torn ulnar collateral ligament) Treatment is cast for 4 weeks and if steners lesion is present then surgery.

- Mallet finger/baseball finger

It is avulsion of extensor tendon of the distal interphalangeal joint from its insertion at the base of distal phalanx. (Not the central slip as it attaches to middle phalanx) An acute mallet finger should be splinted and the DIP joint is kept in hyperextension for 6–8 weeks.

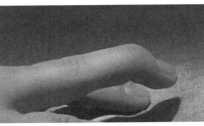
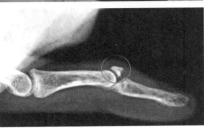

Fig. 21.13.3: Mallet finger

- Jersey finger is avulsion of Flexor Digitorum Profundus.
- Zone II (of flexor tendon injuries): Situated between the opening of the flexor sheath (the distal palmar crease) and insertion of flexor superficialis (flexor crease of proximal interphalangeal joint) is known as 'no man's land' or dangerous area of hand.
- Extensor tendon injuries are more common than flexor tendon injuries.
- Hand injuries are known to cause stiffness.

NEET PATTERN

1. Celery Stalk Appearance is seen in:
   A. Congenital syphilis
   B. Congenital rubella
   C. Both
   D. None

   Ans. is 'B' Congenital rubella

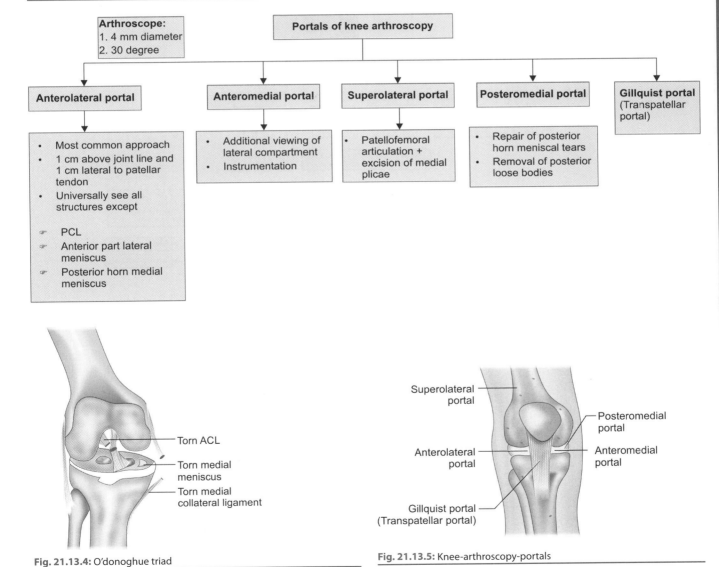

Fig. 21.13.4: O'donoghue triad

Fig. 21.13.5: Knee-arthroscopy-portals

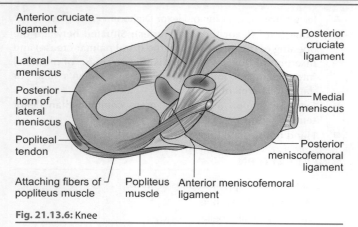

Fig. 21.13.6: Knee

Order of Structures (anterior to posterior) on Tibia upper Surface (MCL—Medical College Lucknow; LMC—Lucknow Medical College)

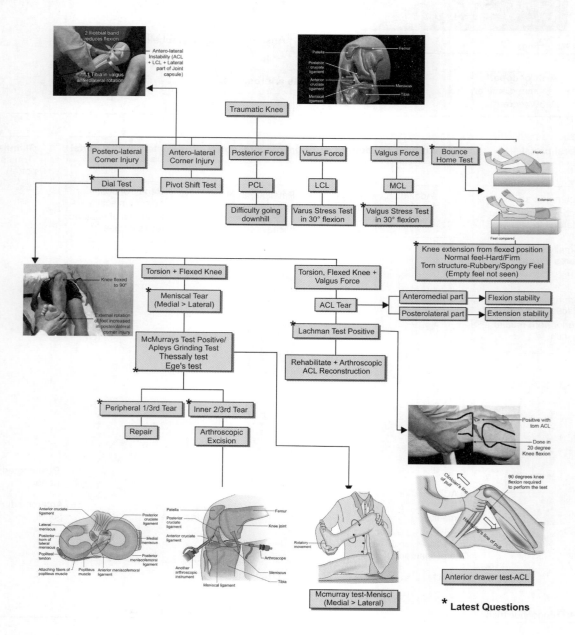

* Latest Questions

14. NEUROMUSCULAR DISEASE

Disc Degeneration and Prolapse

The commonest site of disc prolapse is lumbar spine due to less hydrated discs in this area. In more than 90% of cases lumbar disc herniation are localized at L4 – 5 (more common) and L5 – S1. The next commonest site of intervertebral disc prolapse is lower cervical spine (C5–6).

- Lower nerve root is affected usually like in L4 – 5 disc prolapse L5 nerve root is affected.
- L5 nerve root supplies Extensor Hallucis longus, thigh abductors, ankle dorsiflexion and sensory supply to lateral aspect of leg dorsum of foot and great toe. (It is most commonly involved in PIVD L4 – 5).
- S1 nerve root supplies Flexor hallucis longus, ankle plantar flexion, hip extension and sensation on sole of foot.
- Straight leg raising test, Bragard's sign, lasegue test are done to assess nerve root compression.

Investigations
- MRI is investigation of choice

Most common nerve used for nerve conduction study in H reflex is Tibial nerve (S1 radiculopathy)

Treatment
1. Rest with Antiinflammatory Medications
2. Indications for surgery:
   Bladder and bowel involvement (Cauda Equina Syndrome)
   Increasing neurological deficit
   Failure of conservative treatment (6 weeks)

Lumbar Canal Stenosis (Neurogenic Claudication) – Laminoplasty/Laminectomy is done

Anterolateral Corner: ACL + LCL + Lateral half of joint Capsule.
Posterolateral Corner: LCL + Popliteus (Most important)
ACL: Anterior Cruciate Ligament
PCL: Posterior Cruciate Ligament
LCL: Lateral Collateral Ligament
MCL: Medial Collateral Ligament

"Red Flag" and "Yellow Flag" Signs for Back Ache

Red flag (Requires further workup)	Yellow flag
Red flags are possible indicators of serious spinal pathology: Thoracic pain Radicular impingement Fever and unexplained weight loss Bladder or bowel dysfunction History of carcinoma Ill health or presence of other medical illness Progressive neurological deficit	Yellow flags are pyschosocial factors shown to be indicative of long term chronicity and disability: A negative attitude that back pain is harmful or potentially severely disabling Fear avoidance behaviour and reduced activity levels An expectation that passive, rather than active, treatment will be beneficial
Disturbed gait, saddle anesthesia Age of onset < 20 years or > 55 years Prolonged steroid intake	A tendency to depression, low morale, and social withdrawal Social or financial problems

Chronic backache prolonged bed rest is avoided

Spondylolysis (most common at L5) is characterized by presence of bony defect at pars interarticularis, which can result in spondylolisthesis.

Spondylolisthesis is the slippage forward of one vertebrae upon another. L5 and S1 (most common).

Oblique or lateral view in spondylolysis dog with a collar in neck and spondylolisthesis beheaded Scottish Terrier sign.

AP view is least useful except. In last stages on AP view inverted napolean hat sign is seen when complete slip occurs.
- CT SCAN can diagnose early defects and slips
- MRI can diagnose cord compression
- CT Scan and MRI are usually always done in spondylolisthesis

Spondyloptosis

A complete dislocation of one vertebra over the other is spondyloptosis (L_5 over S_1).

Frozen Shoulder or Adhesive Capsulitis

The cardinal feature is stubborn lack of active and passive movement in all directions, i.e. global restriction of movements in all planes. Often the first motion to be affected is internal rotation followed by abduction.

Rotator Cuff Syndrome Includes
i. Subacute tendonitis (Painful arc syndrome-painful abduction between 60º–120º)
ii. Chronic tendonitis (Impingement syndrome; Neer's test is used for it)
iii. Rotator cuff tears.
Treatment:
• Physiotherapy + NSAIDS
• Local injection of steroids
• Surgery if required for impingement syndrome or rotator cuff tears (especially in young individuals)

Painful arc Syndrome

It is anterior shoulder pain in **60–120° of glenohumeral abduction**. Most common cause is chronic supraspinatus tendinitis.

Cause of painful Arc Syndrome are
- Supraspinatus tendonitis (Most common cause)
- Subacromial bursitis
- Fracture of greater tuberosity

Shoulder Tests

1. **Subscapularis:**
   - Belly press test
   - Napoleon sign
   - Lift off test (Gerber)
   - Bear hug test
2. **Supraspinatus:**
   - Empty Can sign
   - Drop arm test
3. **Infraspinatus and teres minor**
   - External rotation resistance stress test
   - External rotation lag sign
   - Hornblower sign (mainly T. minor)
4. **SLAP tear (Superior labral tear anterior to posterior)**
   - O Briens test.

Tennis Elbow/lateral Epicondylitis

It is chronic tendonitis of common extensor origin (esp. extensor carpi radialis brevis) on lateral epicondyle. Cozen test/Mills maneuver and Maudsleys test are done.

Golfer's Elbow

Medial epicondylitis involving common flexor pronator origin.

De Quervain's Disease

The abductor pollicis longns and extensor pollicis brevis tendons may become inflamed beneath the retinacular pulley at the radial styloid with in the first extensor compartment. Finkelstein's test is positive.

Dupuytren's Contracture

This is nodular hyper trophy and contracture of superficial palmar fascia (palmar aponeurosis).

- Higher incidence in epileptics receiving phenytoin therapy, diabetics, alcoholic cirrhosis, AIDS, pulmonary tuberculosis.
- **Ectopic deposits may occur in dorsum of PIP joint (Garrod's/knuckle pads), sole of feet (Ledderhose's disease) and fibrosis of corpus cavernosum (Peyronie's disease).**
- **Flexion contracture most commonly occur at MP joint. > PIP joint > DIP joint.**
- **Ring finger is most commonly involved > little finger > thumb and index finger.**
- PIP contractures soon become irreversible.

Treatment

- Wait and watch
- Primary indication of surgery is fixed contracture of >30 degrees at MP joint or >15 degrees contracture at PIP joint. surgery is subtotal fasciectomy. Closure may be done by Z-plasty.

Stenosing Flexor Tenosynovitis (Trigger Finger)

Due to stenosing tenosynovitis the flexor tendon may become trapped at the entrance to its fibrous digital sheath. The usual cause is thickening of fibrous tendon sheath or constriction of mouth of fibrous digital sheath (mainly Al pulley) at the level of metacarpophalangeal joint. Most common cause is trauma.

Bursitis	Site
Student's Elbow/miner's elbow	Olecranon bursitis
Housemaid's knee	Prepatellar bursitis (commonest)
Clergyman's knee	Infrapatellar bursitis (superficial bursa)
Weaver's bottom	Ischial bursitis
Tailor's ankle	Lateral malleolus bursitis
Bunion	Medial side of great toe-1st metatarsal head bursitis
Bunionette	5th toe of foot-5th metatarsal head bursitis

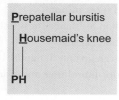

Prepatellar bursitis
Housemaid's knee
PH

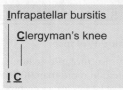

Infrapatellar bursitis
Clergyman's knee
I C

Athletic Pubalgia – The primary pathology in Athletic Pubalgia is: Abdominal muscle strain.

Chondromalacia patellae seen in adolescent females Patient has Anterior knee pain/Difficulty in climbing stairs/Movie Sign"/"Theater sign" increased pain on getting up after prolonged sitting.

Treatment of Ganglion

1. Usually unnecessary and it may resolve spontaneously.
2. Aspiration to reassure the patient.
3. Pressure symptoms (eg Nerve) – removal.

Meary's angle

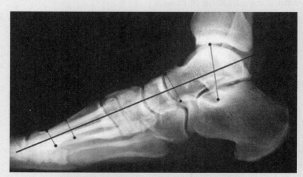

The longitudinal axis of 1st metatarsal and talus forms zero degree angle-Meary's angle

- Angle > 4 degrees (convex upward) pes cavus
- Angle > 4 degrees (convex downward) pes planus

Pes Planus (Flat foot)

- Flat foot refers to obliterated medial longitudinal arch
- Heel is often in valgus called as planovalgus
- Pes Planus is of 2 types: (Differentiated by Jack's test)

    Flexible: Disappears on non-weight bearing. Management is conservative

    Rigid: Due to Congenital Vertical talus or RA or Infection or tarsal coalition or tibialis posterior dysfunction. They often require surgical intervention

- Tarsal Coalition is autosomal dominant

    Fusion of tarsal bones [Talocalcaneal, calcaneonavicular (anteater nose sign) and talonavicular]

    Present at birth but becomes symptomatic later when fibrous connection becomes rigid bar

    Stiff flat foot (with spasm of peroneal spasm)

Diagnosis is by X-ray/CT Scan (better)

1. Initially conservative if fails
2. Surgery: Excision of coalition bar or arthrodesis

Tendon transfer in PPRP is >5 years.

1. Identify the abnormality shown in the following picture?
   (AIIMS Nov 2015)
   A. Hallux valgus
   B. Hallux varus
   C. Rheumatoid nodule
   D. Subcutaneous nodule

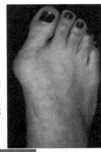

Ans. is 'A' Hallux valgus
- Keller's operation (excision arthroplasty): Hallux valgus
- Mitchell's & Chevron osteotomy: Hallux valgus
- Jone's operation: Claw toes

15. PERIPHERAL NERVE INJURY

SEDDONS order of nerve injury

Order of Nerve Injuries
Neuropraxia
 Axonotmesis
  Neurotmesis
NAN

- Neuropraxia 100% recovery and only wait and watch can apply splint till it recovers.
- Sunderland classification – type 1 to 5, Type 1—neuropraxia, type 2, 3, 4-axonotmesis, type 5 neurotmesis.
- Tinel sign (for nerve regeneration) is positive and progressive in axonotmesis and sunderland type 2 and 3.
- EMG is the best test for nerve recovery.
- Segmental Demyelination on NCV has decreased CMAP amplitudes.
- Autonomous zones-Median nerve tip of index finger/ulnar tip of little finger.
- Radial nerve autonomous zone is Dorsum of 1st web space.
- Closed nerve injuries are initially treated by wait and watch.
- Open nerve injuries are surgically managed.

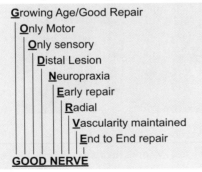

- Rate of nerve regeneration – 1 mm/day.
- Incidence of iatrogenic nerve injury is <3 percent.

Nerve	Trauma	Effect
Axillary nerve	Dislocation of the shoulder (Anterior and Inferior)	Deltoid palsy
Radial nerve	Fracture shaft of the humerus (lower 1/3rd)	Wrist drop
Ulnar nerve	Fracture medial epicondyle humerus	Claw hand

Nerve	Trauma	Effect
Sciatic nerve	Posterior dislocation of the hip	Foot drop
Common peroneal nerve	Knee dislocation/Fracture of neck of the fibula	Foot drop
Posterior Interosseous Nerve	Monteggia fracture	Finger drop
Anterior interosseous nerve	Supra condylar fracture Humerus	Kiloh nevin sign
Median nerve	Supracondylar fracture of humerus	Pointing index

Most common tendon for transfer is Palmaris Longus.

Brachial plexus most commonly—Erb's palsy (Policeman or waiters tip deformity).

Movements lost in EBRS palsy are

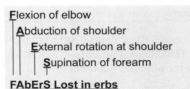

FAbErS Lost in erbs

Preganglionic injury poor prognosis and in them Histamine test is positive

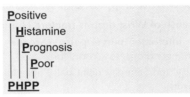

- Aeroplane splint is used for Brachial Plexus injuries
- Klumpkes paralysis C8-T1 nerve roots are involved
- Axillary Nerve Injury is associated with shoulder dislocation proximal humerus fracture and intramuscular injection (Improper use of Crutch is not a cause)
- Schaeffers test is for palmaris longus
- Most common combined nerve palsy is median and ulnar nerve

Median Nerve Palsy–Claw hand -pointing index (Flexors)/ Pen test (Abductor pollicis Brevis) and ape thumb deformity

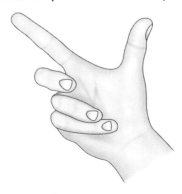

Fig. 21.15.1: Pointing index

Opposition is lost with median nerve palsy at wrist
Knuckle bender splint is used

Anterior Interosseous Nerve Palsy–KILOH NEVIN sign

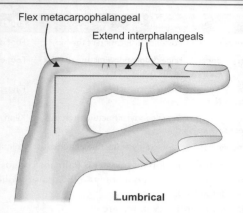

Fig. 21.15.2: Action of Lumbricals

Ulnar Nerve Palsy—Claw hand-CARD TEST (Palmar interossei)/IGAWA TEST (Dorsal interossei)/BOOK TEST/FROMENT SIGN (Adductor pollicis)/Wartenbergs sign

Ulnar paradox – High ulnar nerve Injury.
   Knuckle bender splint is used.

Radial Nerve – Wrist drop, Cock up splint is used

Commonest cause of Wrist drop is fracture Humerus.

   Posterior interossei nerve palsy (Arcade of Frohse) – Thumb drop or finger drop. No sensory loss.

- Crutch Palsy and Saturday night palsy are radial nerve palsy (Neuropraxias)
- Right lateral position maximum chances of injury are to Common Peroneal Nerve injury at the neck of fibula.

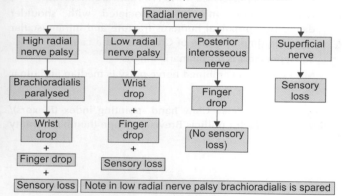

Jones Transfer

- Pronator Teres to Extensor carpi radialis longus/Extensor carpi radialis brevis—Wrist Extensors
- Flexor carpi ulnaris to Extensor digitorum communis— Finger Extensors
- Flexor carpi radialis to Extensor pollicis longus (Extensor pollicis brevis and Abductor pollicis longus)— Thumb function

Tendon Transfer

- Palmaris longus—Hand to fingertip
- Plantaris—Forearm to fingertip.
- Foot drop occurs in common peroneal nerve palsy.

Entrapment syndrome	Nerve involved
Carpal tunnel syndrome	Median nerve (at wrist) (Most Common)
Pronator syndrome	Median nerve (proximally compressed beneath - ligament of struthers, bicipital aponeurosis or origins of pronator teres or flexor digitorum superficialis).
Cubital tunnel syndrome	Ulnar nerve (between two heads of flexor carpi ulnaris)
Guyon's canal syndrome	Ulnar nerve (at wrist)
Thoracic outlet syndrome	Lower trunk of brachial plexus, (C8 and T1) and subclavian vessels (between clavicle and first rib)
Piriformis syndrome	Sciatic nerve
Meralgia paraesthetica	Lateral cutaneous nerve of thigh
Cheralgia paraesthetica	Superficial radial nerve
Tarsal tunnel syndrome	Posterior tibial nerve (behind and below medial malleolus)
Morton's metatarsalgia	Interdigital nerve compression (usually of 3rd, 4th toe)

Femoral nerve is usually not involved in nerve entrapment Syndrome

   Sensory symptoms can often be reproduced by percussing over the median nerve (Tinel's sign) or by holding the wrist fully flexed for a minute or two (Phalen's test) or tourniquet test or Durkan's direct compression over median nerve (most reliable clinical test for median nerve). Hand diagram is also highly specific for median nerve.

   Tests for thoracic outlet syndrome: Adsons test/wrights test/Roos test.

   Cervical rib can cause thoracic outlet syndrome

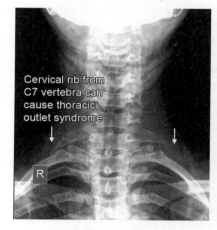

Fig. 21.15.3: Cervical rib

   Mulders click test -Mortons neuroma
   NCV investigation of choice.

   Tarsal tunnel syndrome – compression of posterior tibial nerve-Idiopathic > OA > RA

- **Popliteal Entrapment Syndrome has Exercise Induced Calf Claudications.**
- **Fracture unite slower with muscular or neural disorders, e.g. Polio.**
- **Contracture of iliotibial tract causes FABER (Flexion, abduction and External rotation) at hip and PERF (Posterior subluxation, External rotation and Flexion – TRIPLE Deformity) at knee.**

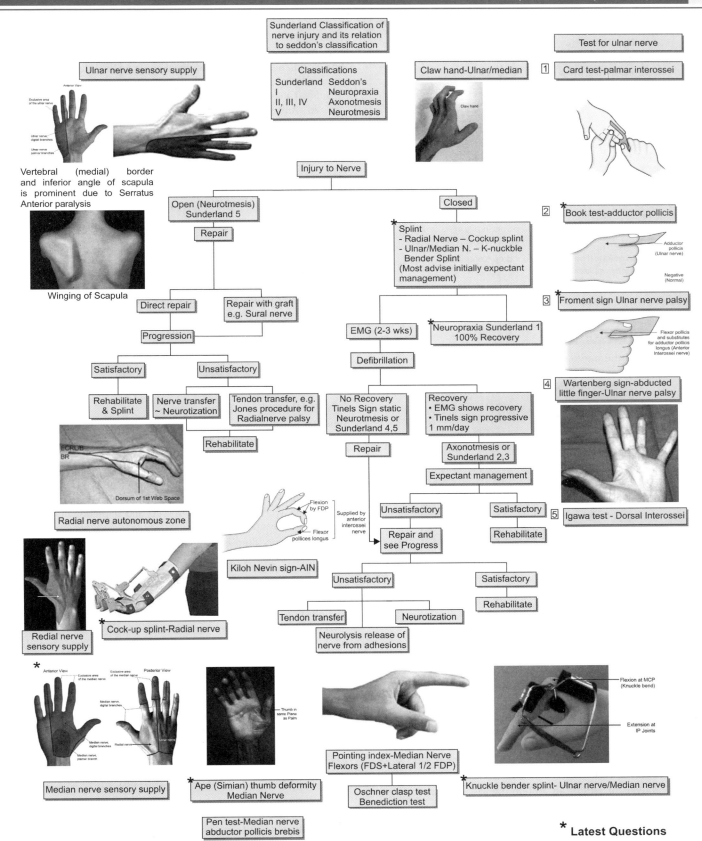

Nerve Palsy	Presentation
1. Erb's palsy	Policeman tip deformity (Porter's tip deformity)
2. Nerve of bell (Long thoracic nerve) palsy	Winging of scapula
3. Median Nerve Palsy (Labours nerve)	Pointing index Bendiction test Pen test (tests abductor pollicis brevis) Ochsner clasp test/Opposition of thumb lost/Ape thumb deformity
4. Ulnar nerve palsy (Musician nerve)	Book test (froment sign), Card test (PAD) – Palmar Interossei, Igawa's test (DAB) – Dorsal interossei
5. Radial nerve palsy	Wrist drop, (Finger drop and thumb drop Specifically in posterior interosseous nerve (PIN) injury)
6. Common peroneal nerve palsy (Lateral popliteal nerve palsy) or sciatic nerve palsy	Foot drop (complete)

Note: Winging of scapula—serratus anterior paralysis > trapezius paralysis

STUDENTS DOUBTS

1. Identify the nerve supply of the marked muscle:
(NEET Pattern 2019)

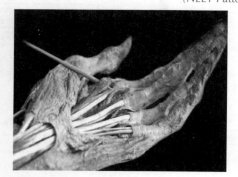

A. Radial Nerve
B. Median Nerve
C. Ulnar Nerve
D. Anterior Interosseous Nerve

Ans. is 'B' Median Nerve
The marked muscle is lumbrical (1st)
1st and 2nd lumbrical are supplied by median nerve.
3rd and 4th lumbrical are supplied by ulnar nerve.

2. Clawing of medial 2 fingers is seen more pronounced in
A. High ulnar nerve palsy
B. Median and ulnar nerve palsy combined
C. Low ulnar nerve palsy
D. Tardy ulnar nerve palsy

Ans. is 'C' Low ulnar nerve palsy

3. Paralysis of arm of an athlete the test with best recovery prognosis?
A. EMG-Electromyography B. Strength Duration curve

Ans. Electromyography is the best indicator of nerve recovery after injury or after nerve repair.

4. Sir, Worst prognosis in injury is of which of the two nerves?
A. Ulnar or   B. Lateral popliteal

Ans. Sciatic nerve > Lateral popliteal nerve > Ulnar nerve (worst to better)

5. Sir, Tarsal tunnel syndrome is caused with which arthritis?
A. Ankylosing spondylitis   B. Osteoarthritis
C. Rheumatoid arthritis   D. Psoriatic arthritis

Ans. Order of causes are Idiopathic > Osteoarthritis > Rheumatoid arthritis > Ankylosing Spondylitis.

NEET PATTERN

1. High stepping gait is seen in:
A. Common peroneal nerve palsy
B. T.B. hip
C. Hemiplegia
D. Cerebral palsy

Ans. is 'A' Common peroneal nerve palsy

2. Anterior interosseous nerve is a branch of:
A. Musculocutaneous nerve B. Median nerve
C. Radial nerve   D. Ulnar nerve

Ans. is 'B' Median nerve

16. JOINT DISORDERS

Synovial Fluid

Synovial Fluid: It is an ultradialysate of blood plasma transudated from synovial capillaries to which hyaluronic acid protein complex (mucin) has been added by synovial B cells.

Synovial fluid in different types of arthritis

1. Normal synovial fluid is clear, WBC count 200/μL
2. Non-inflammatory synovial fluid is clear, viscous, amber colored with a WBC 200-2000/μL and a predominance of mononuclear cell.
3. Inflammatory fluid is turbid, yellow, with an increased WBC count 2,000 to 50,000/μL and a polymorphonuclear leukocytic predominance.
3a. Inflammatory fluid has reduced viscosity, diminished hyaluronate.
3b. Infections (pyogenic) is purulent, WBC count > 50,000/μL, PMN > 90%
3c. Infections (Tuberculosis/granulomatous) is yellow, turbid, WBC count 10,000–20,000/μL, PMN 60% and presence of lymphocytes, plasma cells and histiocytes.

Normal aging vs osteoarthritic pathology of articular cartilage.

Cartilage property	Aging	Osteoarthritis
Total water content (Hydration)	Decreased	Increase (Decreased in advanced OA)
Proteolytic enzymes:	Normal	Increased
Proteoglycan content	Decreased	Decreased

There are 4 zones of articular cartilage from the articular surface to subchondral bone.

1. Superficial layer (zone 1) is a high H_2O content zone having progenitor cells of articular cartilage and chondrocytes (small in size, high in density)

2. Transitional zone (zone 2)
3. Middle zone (zone 3): zone with (a) Metabolically most active chondrocytes, (b) with highest proteoglycan (c) with least water content.
4. Calcified cartilage zone (zone 4): having hypertrophic chondrocytes, and is present only an joints
- New bone formation is a feature of noninflammatory arthritis, e.g. Osteoarthritis
- **The father of joint replacement surgery is Sir John Charnley**
- **Anterolateral approach of Hip after Splinting TFL Muscle seen is G. medius**

	Cemented arthroplasty	Uncemented arthroplasty
Interface	Implant cement bone	Implant bone
Weaklink	Cement bone interface	Strong construct

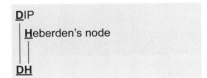

Fig. 21.16.1: Cemented verus uncemented arthroplasty

Complications of THR
- Infection
- *Dislocation*
- *Mortality-MI > cardiorespiratory arrest > pulmonary embolism*

Definite Management of Pulmonary Embolism is Thrombolysis

Contraindications of metal on metal bearing surfaces
- Patients with Renal Insufficiency (Chronic Renal Failure)
- Young females of child bearing age (Women who may potentially still have children)
- *Metal hypersensitivity*
- *They can also cause chromosomal changes*
- *Their role in carcinogenesis is under evaluation.*

Osteoarthritis

Osteoarthritis characteristically involves distal interphalangeal joint (Heberden's node), proximal interphalangeal joint (Bouchard's node) 1 carpometacarpal joint (base of thumb) of hand **with sparing of metacarpophalangeal joint and wrist joint.**
(ANKLE IS ALSO VERY RARELY INVOLVED)

```
DIP
Heberden's node

DH
```

- Seagull wing deformity is seen in Osteoarthritis of interphalangeal joints
- DIP involvement is seen in OA/ Psoriasis/Mallet finger/ Swan neck deformity/Boutonniere deformity
- Suprapatellar bursa communicates with the knee joint.

Due to decreased loading of painful extremity quadriceps weakness is common in patients of osteoarthritis of knee. Most importantly Vastus medialis is affected.

Classification system and stage wise management for OA knee
- Initial treatment is always conservative (Glucosamine are useful).
- Clinical picture is more significant than radiology or X-ray changes.
- If activities of daily living are affected surgery is advised.
- Surgery for young is HTO (if not contraindicated) if contraindicated TKR is performed.
- Surgery for elderly (> 60 years) is TKR.
- HTO-High Tibial Osteotomy.
- TKR-Total Knee Replacement.

Note: OA knee has subchondral sclerosis.

High Tibial Osteotomy (HTO)—More than 20 degrees correction needed is a contraindication

After knee replacement surgery proprioceptors of joints are altered. Effect is—Normal movement as better joint alignment and soft tissue balancing can improve joint proprioception.

PATELLAR CLUNK SYNDROME

It is Knee popping and catching due to fibrous nodule on superior pole of patella on knee extension in TKR patients. If symptoms are severe it requires resection of fibrous nodule (arthroscopic/open)

Rheumatoid Arthritis

Causes atlantoaxial instability which is assessed by flexion extension views.
- Anterolateral approach of Hip after Splinting TFL Muscle seen is G. medius
  Complications of THR
- Infection
- Dislocation
- Mortality-MI > cardiorespiratory arrest > pulmonary embolism

Causes atlantoaxial instability which is assessed by flexion extension views. (Cervical spine is the commonest area affected in spine in R.A.)

DIP is Usually Spared

Significance of Rheumatoid Factor (RF)
- If present in high titre, to designates patients at risk for severe systemic disease.
- 'Swan—neck deformity', i.e. hyperextension of PIP joints with compensatory flexion of the distal interphalangeal joints.
- Boutonniere deformity, i.e. flexion contracture of PIP joints and extension of DIP joints.

Orthopedics Quick Review

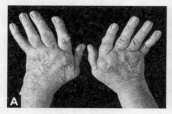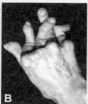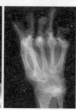

Figs. 21.16.2A and B: Deformities of hand in RA (A) Ulnar deviation of fingers (B) Arthritis Mutilans

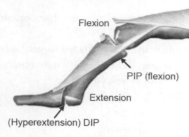
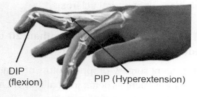

Fig. 21.16.3: Finger deformities in RA

- Earliest radiological change in RA—Periarticular osteopenia.
- Scleritis with autoimmune disease involving joints-Rheumatoid Arthritis.
- Uveitis is a feature of Ankylosing Spondylitis.
- RA patient with upper motor neuron sign requires evaluation of upper cervical spine which is assessed by spine flexion and extension views.
- Pannus is seen in RA.
- Windswept deformity of foot is seen in RA.
- Windswept deformity of knee is seen in Rickets > RA.

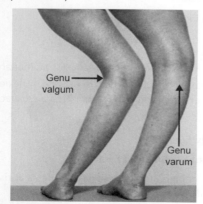

Fig. 21.16.4: Windswept deformity of knee

- Abatacept is used for its treatment.
- The first radiological sign of RA – Soft tissue swelling

- The most common cause of wrist arthritis – RA
- Most pathognomonic feature of RA – Rheumatoid nodules
- Most common site for rheumatoid nodules – Olecranon
- The DOC in RA – Methotrexate (DMARD)

Poor Prognostic Factors of RA

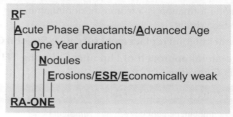

Pattern of Joint Involvement

	Osteoarthritis	Rheumatoid Arthritis	Psoriatic Arthritis
Involved	PIP, DIP and 1'CMC (corpometacarpal) joints	PIP, MCP, wrist	DIP, PIP and any joint
Spared	MCP (metacarpophalangeal) and wrist^Q	DIP joint usually	Sparing of any joint

Psoriasis-Pencil cup deformity and sausage digits are seen.

CASPAR CRITERION ARE USED FOR PSORIATIC ARTHRITIS

DOC: Methotrexate

HIV related arthritis: Cutaneous and mucosal lesions are rare.

Ankylosing Spondylitis (AS)/Marie-Strumpell or Bechtrew's Disease-HLA B27 Associated

Diagnostic Criteria – Modified New York Criterion

- Essential criteria is definite radiographic sacroiliitis.
- Supporting criteria: one of these three.
  - Inflammatory back pain.
  - Limited chest expansion (< 5 cm at 4th ICS) not a reliable criterion in elderly because of pulmonary disorders.
  - Limited lumbar spine motion in both sagittal and frontal plane (Schober test /Modified Schober test).

Never diagnose ankylosing spondylitis without sacroiliitis
Bamboo spine is seen

The first X-ray sign of AS – Haziness and Widening (Pseudo-widening) around SI joint

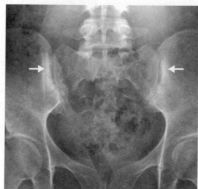

Fig. 21.16.5: Sacroiliitis

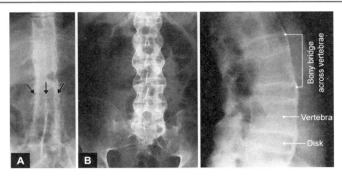

Figs. 21.16.6A and B: (A) Trolley track sign (Ossification along supraspinous ligaments and facet joints) (B) Bamboo Sign

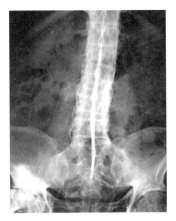

Fig. 21.16.7: Dagger sign (Ossification along supraspinous and interspinous ligaments)

Shiny corner sign and Anderson lesion (spinal pseudoarthrosis)—inflammatory involvement of I/V disc are seen in AS.

Spine fracture in AS occur around C5-C6/C6-C7

Extra–articular manifestation of AS
- Pulmonary fibrosis
- Ulcerative colitis
- Crohns disease
- Aortic incompetence

Elderly with backache with dorsolumbar tenderness with mild reduction in chest expansion—Ankylosing Hyperostosis.

Reactive arthritis/Reiter's syndrome
- Chlamydia and shigella are associated.
- HLA B27 positive
- Triad: Arthritis + Conjunctivitis + Urethritis/Cervicitis (In females)
- Mucocutaneous lesions: Circinate balanitis Keratoderma blennorrhagicum (Hyper-keratotic lesions on palms and soles)
- Enthesitis is seen; SI joint is commonly involved
- Anterior uveitis is seen.

Hemophiliac Arthropathy

Clotting factors
- < 1% – Spontaneous hemorrhage
- 1–5% – Hemorrhage on mild trauma
- > 5% – Hemorrhage on significant trauma

Joint Bleeding
- Weight bearing joints are most commonly involved, with the frequency of involvement in decreasing order, **knee > elbow > shoulder > ankle > wrist > hip.**
- Ankle most commonly involved in children.

There is periarticular osteopenia in hemophilia
- Arthroscopy is relatively contraindicated.

Intramuscular Bleeding
- In lower limbs most common sites of bleeding is **iliopsoas > quadriceps.**
- **In upper limb the most common site of bleeding is deltoid**
- Most hemophilic pseudotumors are caused by subperiosteal hemorrhage and the most common location is in thigh (50%). Next in frequency are abdomen, pelvis, and tibia.

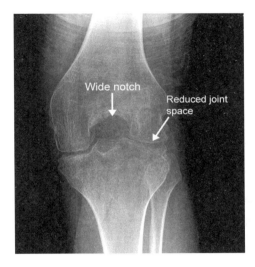

Fig. 21.16.8: Hemophiliac arthropathy

Knee is the most common joint to have loose bodies

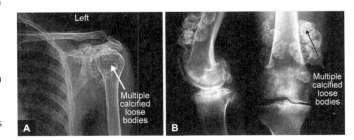

Figs. 21.16.9A and B: Synovial chondromatosis

Neuropathic Joint Disease/Charcot's Joint

It is progressive destructive arthritis arising from loss of pain sensation and proprioception (position sense). Diabetes mellitus (most common) cause. Joints involved are **Midtarsal (most common) >** tarsometatarsal metatarsophalangeal and ankle joint.

Disease	Joint Involvement
Diabetes	Midtarsal (most common) > tarsometatarsal, metatarsophalangeal and ankle joint > knee and spine
Tabes dorsalis	Knee (most common), hip, ankle and lumbar spine
Leprosy	Hand and foot joints
Syringomyelia	Shoulder (glenohumeral), elbow, wrist and cervical spine
Myelomeningocele	Ankle and foot
Congenital insensitivity to pain	Ankle and foot
Chronic Alcoholism	Foot
Amyloidosis	Peroneal Muscle atrophy (Charcot Marie tooth disease)

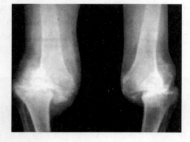

Fig. 21.16.10: Charcot's joint

- The appearance suggest that movements would be agonizing and yet it is often painless.
- The paradox is diagnostic the amount of pain experienced is less than would be anticipated based on degree of joint involvement.
- Usual treatment is bracing or arthrodesis, total ankle Replacement is contraindicated.

Congenital Syphilis

Clutton's joint is painless, symmetrical, sterile effusion mostly involving knee in 8–16 years of age. Spontaneous remission is usual in several weeks.

- Nonerosive arthritis: SLE
- Nondeforming arthritis: Behcets

Disease	Area involved
Septic	Knee
Syphilitic arthritis*	Knee
Gonococcal arthritis*	Knee
Gout*	MP joint of big toe
Pseudogout*	Knee
Rheumatoid arthritis	Metacarpophalangeal joint
Ankylosing spondylitis*	Sacro iliac joint
Diabetic charcot joint*	Foot joint (tarsals)
Senile osteoporosis*	Vertebra
Paget's disease*	Pelvic bones > femur > skull > tibia
Osteochondritis dissecans*	Knee
Actinomycosis*	Mandible
Haemophilic arthritis*	Knee
Disc prolapse*	Between L4 and L5
Acute osteomyelitis*	Lower end of femur (Metaphysis)
Brodies abscess*	Upper end of tibia

Feature	Gout (Protein Alcohol intake)	Pseudogout (Hpothyroidism associated)
Synovial fluid Analysis	Uric acid crystal, needle or rod shaped crystal, negatively birefringent crystals	Calcium pyrophosphate crystal, rhomboid shaped crystal, positive birefringent crystals
Associated with	ACTH, glucocorticoid withdrawal, hypouricemic therapy, Hyperuricaemia. **"Alcohol and Protein intake"**	Four 'H'S, i.e. hyperparathyroidism, hemochromatosis, hypophosphatasia, hypomagnesemia are associated. **Most common association is Hypothyroidism Chondrocalcinosis,** i.e. appearance of calcific material in articular cartilage and menisci is seen.
Clinical presentation	Intense pain	Moderate pain
Involved joint	Smaller joints (most commonly metatarsophalangeal joint of big toe)	Larger joints most commonly, knee

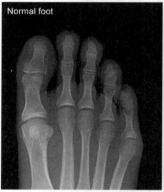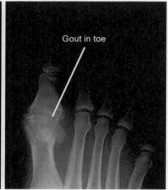

Fig. 21.16.11: Gout (Great toe) is called as podagra

Martel/G sign is seen in gout

Acute gout Colchicine is used if NSAIDs contraindicated

Arthritis with Soft–Tissue Nodules

1. Gout
2. Rheumatoid arthritis
3. Pigmented villonodular synovitis
4. Multicenteric reticulohistocytosis
5. Amyloidosis
6. Sarcoidosis

- Most common cause of anomaly of craniovertebral junctions is atlanto-occipital fusion. (C1+C2+ Occiput)
- Ankylosing spondylitis rarely involves craniovertebral junction and rheumatoid arthritis is a common cause of craniovertebral junction anomaly.

Alkaptonuria (Ochronosis) Calcification of Disc is Seen, Pigment Deposition in Joints and Urine Darkening on Standing is seen

Complete Summary of Orthopedics

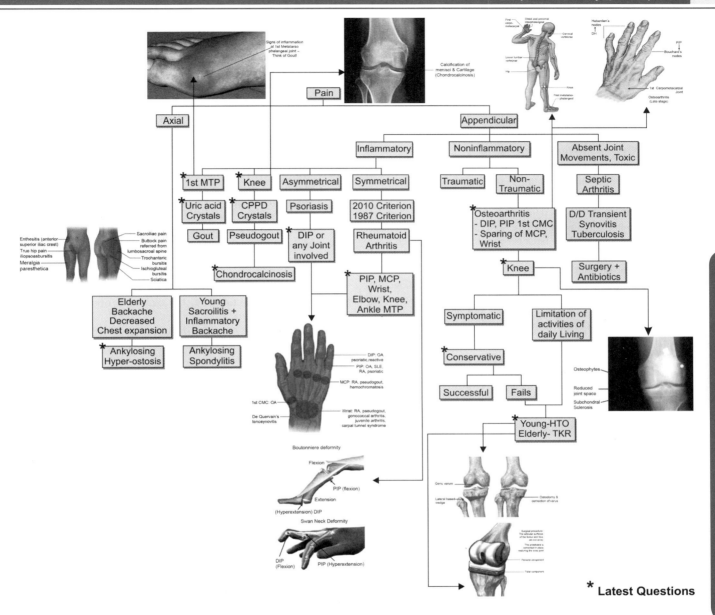

*Latest Questions

STUDENTS DOUBTS

1. True statement regarding Mseleni joint disease is:
   (JIPMER May 2018)
   A. Shoulder, elbow wrist involvement is characteristic
   B. Elderly males are commonly involved
   C. Height is unaffected
   D. Endemic to northern KwaZulu Natal area in South Africa

   Ans. is 'D' Endemic to northern KwaZulu Natal area in South Africa

   Mseleni joint disease: Epigenetic chondrodysplasia
   – This disease affects indigenous Bantu Population in Mseleni, KwaZulu Natal area, South Africa.
   – More common in females.
   – Hip is the commonest joint affected causing its arthritis.
   – The disease is often bilateral.
   – Severe short stature has been reported

2. Sir, What is the most common cause of loose bodies?

   Ans. A. Overall : OA
   B. Elderly : OA
   C. Young : Osteochondritis dissecans

3. Sir, A 65-year-old man with history of back pain since 3 months. ESR is raised. On Examination there is tenderness of dorsolumbar region and mild restriction of chest movements is found. On X-ray syndesmophytes are present in vertebrae. Diagnosis is:
   A. Ankylosing spondylitis
   B. Degenerative osteoarthritis of spine
   C. Ankylosing hyperosteosis
   D. Lumbar canal stenosis

   Ans. is 'C' Ankylosing hyperosteosis

	Ankylosing hyperostosis	Ankylosing spondylitis
Age	**Elderly**	Young
Sacroiliitis	**Absent**	Always present
Chest expansion	**Mild restriction**	Marked but not reliable in elderly
Tenderness	Dorsolumbar	Sacroiliac
ESR	Normal to mild rise	High
Syndesmophytes	Present	Present

4. Sir, Why not ankylosing spondylitis?

Ans. Diagnostic Criteria – Modified New York Criterion
- Essential criteria is definite radiographic sacroiliitis
- Supporting criteria: one of these three
- Inflammatory back pain
- Limited chest expansion (< 5 cm at 4th ICS) not a reliable criterion in elderly because of pulmonary disorders
- Limited lumbar spine motion in both sagittal and frontal plane (Schober test /Modified Schober test)

To diagnose Ankylosing Spondylitis we need radiographic sacroiliitis which is not mentioned in this case also age group for ankylosing spondylitis is young and not elderly which is the age group for Ankylosing hyperostosis.

5. Sir, Can you tell the latest criteria for axial spondyloarthritis?

Ans. ASAS criteria for classification of axial spondyloarthritis (Back pain > 3 months, age < 45 years) Sacroiliitis on Imaging + > 1 spondyloarthropathy (spA) feature or HLA B27 plus > 2 SPA features

SPA features: Inflammatory back pain
- Arthritis
- Enthesitis
- Anterior uveitis
- Dactylitis
- Psoriasis
- Crohns disease or Ulcerative colitis
- Good response to NSAIDS
- Family history of SPA
- HLA B27
- Elevated CRP

6. Sir, Most common site of pseudotumor like growth in hemophilic arthroplasty:
   A. Quadriceps   B. Hamsting
   C. Gastrocnemius   D. Iliopsoas

Ans. Iliopsoas > Quadriceps

7. Sir, Most common cause of Reiter's syndrome.

Ans. Chlamydia

8. Sir, Most common cause of Diarrhoea associated Reiter's syndrome.

Ans. Shigella

9. Sir, Most common cause of STD associated Reiter's syndrome.

Ans. Chlamydia

10. Sir, please tell few named prosthesis.

Ans:
- Charnley prosthesis: THR
- Bipolar (Talwalkar) prosthesis: Hemiarthroplasty
- Unipolar prosthesis: Hemiarthroplasty
  - Austin Moore porsthesis (Uncemented)
  - Thompson prosthesis (Cemented)
- Insall Burstein prosthesis: TKR
- Neer's prosthesis: Shoulder replacement
- Bakshi's prosthesis: Elbow replacement
- Swanson's prosthesis: Hand joints arthroplasty.

17. METABOLIC DISORDERS OF BONE

There are four types of metabolic bone diseases:

1. *Osteopenic diseases:* These diseases are characterized by a generalized decrease in bone mass (i.e. loss of bone matrix), though whatever bone is there, is normally mineralized (e.g. osteoporosis).
2. *Osteosclerotic diseases:* There are diseases characterized by an increase in bone mass (e.g. fluorosis).
3. *Osteomalacic diseases:* These are diseases characterized by an increase in the ratio of the organic fraction to the mineralized fraction, i.e. the available organic matter is undemineralized.
4. *Mixed diseases:* These are diseases that are a combination of osteopenia and osteomalacia (e.g. hyperparathyroidism).

Note:
- *Rickets:* Lack of adequate mineralization of growing bones.
- *Osteomalacia:* Lack of adequate mineralization of trabecular bone.
- *Osteoporosis:* Proportionate loss of bone volume and mineral.
- *Scurvy:* Defect in osteoid formation

- Biopsy is the gold standard investigation to make the diagnosis of osteomalacia

Rickets-Characteristic feature is widening near the joints- wrists or knees

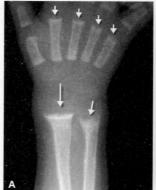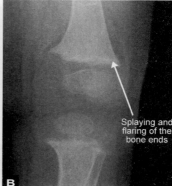

Figs. 21.17.1A and B: Rickets (A) Wrists (B) Knee

- Persistent hypocalcemia may cause secondary hyperparathyroidism.
- First clinical sign of rickets – Craniotabes
- Most common deformity in rickets – Genu varum

Rickets osteotomies to correct the deformities are carried out once radiological signs of healing are seen.

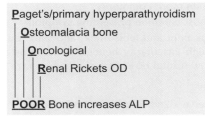

POOR Bone increases ALP

	Calcium	Phosphate	ALP	PTH
Osteoporosis	Normal	Normal	Normal	Normal
Rickets/osteomalacia	N or low	Low	High	High
Primary Hyperparathyroidism	High	Low	High	High
Paget's disease	Normal	Normal	High	Normal

Hypophosphatemic Rickets

X-linked dominant (commonest) it is due to PHEX gene mutation, autosomal dominant and autosomal recessive are 3 varieties of hypophosphatemic Rickets (Vitamin D resistant rickets)–increase incidence of skeletal deformities, no hypocalcemia, hypophosphatemia, phosphaturia, PTH is normal, Vitamin D is normal and ALP is high.

Hyperparathyroidism

	Primary (adenoma)	Secondary (usually due to osteomalacia)
Clinical Features	More	Less
Ca	High	Low or normal
PTH	Very high	High

Note: von Recklinghausen's disease of bone is also called as osteitis fibrosa cystica (it should not be confused with Von Recklinghausen's disease (Neurofibromatosis type 1): In Osteitis fibrosa cytica there is fibrosa that is bony trabeculae are replaced by fibrous tissue and there is cystica that is cystic cavity in bone filled with blood and blood degradation products gives it brown color.

- NF1 most common skeletal abnormality is scoliosis.

Radiological Features of Hyperparathyroidism

- Subperiosteal resorption of terminal tufts of phalanges, lateral end of clavicle and symphysis pubis.
- Loss of lamina dura (i.e. thin cortical bone of tooth socket surrounding teeth is seen as thin white line, is resorbed)
- Irregular, diffuse rarefaction of bones, i.e. generalized osteopenia, thinning of cortices, and indistinct bony trabeculae.
- Rotting fence post appearance of femur
- Brown tumor
- Salt pepper appearance of skull
- SCFE may be seen
- Rarely AVN

Short 4th metacarpal is seen in pseudohypoparahtyroidism

Milkman's/Increment fractures also known as looser's zones or osteoid zones are psudofractures seen in osteomalacia most commonly femur neck. These are also seen in Hereditary Hypophosphatasia, Paget's disease and Fibrous Dysplasia.

Rugger Jersey Spine

- Rugger jersey spine is produced by alternating regions of dense bone and areas of central vertebral radiolucencies.
- Causes of Rugger jersey spine are:
  i. Renal osteodystrophy due to hyperparathyroidism & osteosclerosis
  ii. Osteopetrosis

SCURVY (VIT C: DEFICIENCY)

Scurvy: Deficiency of Vitamin C, causing defect in osteoid formation.

Note: In Rickets—Rosary is Round and non-tender, and in Scurvy it is sharp and tender.

Radiological Feature

- Osteopenia (ground glass appearance) (1st sign) with thinning of cortex (Pencil thin cortex).
- Metaphysis maybe deformed or fractured.
- Frankel's line (zone of provisional calcification increases in width and opacity) due to failure of resorption of calcified cartilage and stands out compared to the severely osteopenic metaphysis.
- Scurvy line or scorbutic zone (Trummerfeld zone) is radiolucent transverse band adjacent to the dense provisional zone.
- Margins of the epiphysis appears relatively sclerotic, termed ringing of epiphyses or Wimberger's Ring sign - Important.
- Lateral metaphyseal spur (Pelkan spur) at ends of metaphysis is produced by outward projection of zone of provisional calcification and periosteal reaction.
- Corner or angle sign is peripheral metaphyseal cleft.
- Subperiosteal hemorrhage. (Lower end of femur and tibia)

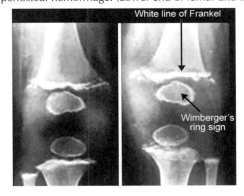

Fig. 21.17.2: Scurvy (Sclerosed margins of epiphysis)

Note: Wimberger Corner Sign: Congenital Syphilis

Note: White line of Frankel is also seen in healing rickets, lead poisoning and methotrexate therapy.

OSTEOPOROSIS-DEXA for Diagnosis

- T score less than -2.5 is osteoporosis
- Osteoporosis with a fracture is severe osteoporosis

Osteoporosis is most common cause for kyphosis

- Z Score = Age + Sex + Race matched

Up to age of 70, Colle's fracture is most common fracture in osteoporotic patient; and after 70 years age Hip fracture is most common fracture. But overall vertebra is the commonest area affected > hip > Colle's.

- Bone mineral density in Hemiplegic patient is reduced maximum in Humerus.

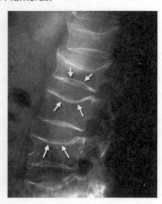

Fig. 21.17.3: X-ray of osteoporotic spine: **Codfish vertebra (Biconcave vertebra)**

Treatment

1. Drug used in osteoporosis.
   Inhibit resorption: **Bisphosphonates, denosumab, calcitonin, estrogen, SERMS, gallium nitrate.**
2. Stimulate formation: Teriparatide (PTH analogue), calcium, calcitriol, fluorides.
3. Both actions: Strontium Ranelate.

   Bisphosphonates use for prolonged periods in osteoporosis increases incidence of hip fractures which are assessed by X-rays.

- The drug of choice for osteoporosis (senile/post-menopausal) – bisphosphonates
- The drug of choice for bisphosphonate resistant osteoporosis-Teriparatide

Fluorosis causes interosseous membrane ossification and increased density in skull vault.
- Dental changes
- Secondary hyperparathyroidism

Infantile Cortical Hyperostosis—Caffey's Disease.

Hypervitaminosis D and A can cause bone abnormalities.

PAGET'S DISEASE/OSTEITIS DEFORMANS

It is characterized by excessive disorganized bone turnover, that encompasses excessive osteoclastic activity initially followed by disorganized excessive new bone formation. It is the osteoclast that appear larger and irregular whereas osteoblast are relatively normal. Bones have mosaic pattern.

- Genetic infection by paramyxovirus (measles and respiratory syncytial virus) has been linked.
- The sites most commonly involved are—**pelvis, tibia, followed by skull, spine, clavicle and femur**
- Paget's disease affects >50 years onwards.
- Affects men more commonly
- Pain is most common presenting symptom
- Limb look bent and feels thick, and skin is unduly warm due to high vascularity hence the name osteitis deform. Skull show frontal bossing and platybasia.

Complications:

1. Cranial nerve ~ 2nd, 5th, 7th, 8th palsy is seen.
2. Nerve compression and spinal stenosis is seen.
3. *Deafness due to nerve compression > otosclerosis*
4. *High output cardiac failure, Hypercalcemia (if immobilized)*
5. *Osteosarcoma (<1%) cases (poorest prognosis)*

Diagnosis

A. Serum calcium and phosphate levels are usually normal.
B. Increased marker of bone formation (e.g. S. alkaline phosphatase and S. Osteocalcin) (**ALP levels are used for monitoring Paget's**)
C. Increased markers of bone resorption
   - Urinary deoxypyridinoline (24 hours assessment) is most valuable.
   - Skull X-ray reveal "cotton wool" or osteoporosis circumscripta, thickening of diploic area. **Increasing Hat Size!**
   - Vertebral cortical thickening at superior and inferior end plates creates a picture frame vertebrae and diffuse sclerosis causing ivory vertebrae
   - Pelvic radiograph show sclerotic iliopectineal line (Brim sign), fusion or disruption of sacroiliac joints, etc.
   - Blade of grass lesion/Flame appearance is seen in Paget's

Treatment

Bisphosphonates are drug of choice and calcitonin is used to relieve pain.

ACHONDROPLASIA MOST COMMON DISPROPORTIONATE DWARFISM

- A primary defect of endochondral bone formation. Autosomal dominant (but 80% are spontaneous mutations). The effect of excessive growth hormone on the mature skeleton.
- They have normal intelligence, trident hand and starfish hand.
- Short interpedicular distance, bullet shaped vertebra, champagne glass pelvis.
- Hooked vertebra are seen in Achondroplasia, Osteogenesis imperfecta, congenital hypothyroidism.

CLEIDOCRANIAL DYSOSTOSIS

- It is an autosomal dominant (AD) disorder caused by CBFA1 gene on chromosome 6 p 21 responsible for osteoblast specific transcription factor and regulation of osteoblastic differentiation. In this disorder bones formed by intramembranous ossification are abnormal (primarily clavicles, cranium and pelvis). — *Absent clavicle.*

Morquios syndrome has most severe skeletal abnormalities amongst Mucopolysaccharidoses.

OSTEOGENESIS IMPERFECTA/LOBSTEIN VROLIK'S/BRITTLE BONE DISEASE

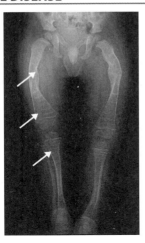

Fig. 21.17.4: Osteogenesis imperfecta

- Osteogenesis Imperfecta/Lobstein Vrolik's/Brittle Bone Disease.
- It is a genetic disorder of connective tissue determined by quantitative and/or qualitative defect in type I collagen formation.
- It is inherited from a parent in autosomal dominant (AD) fashion, may occur as spontaneous mutation, or rarely as autosomal recessive (AR) trait.
- Any fracture pattern maybe seen, and no particular fracture pattern is specifically diagnostic. Fractures heal at a normal rate. Lower limb fractures are more common than upper limb. Femur is commonest bone fractured followed by tibia.
- Hyper laxity of ligaments, with resultant hypermobility of joint is common.
- Rarely recurrent dislocation of patella, radial head and hip joint dislocation and DDH can occur.

Radiological Feature

- Wormian bones, are detached portions of primary ossification centers of adjacent membrane bones. These are seen in skull X-ray. To be significant, it should be more than 10 in number, measure at least 6 mm x 4 mm, and be arranged in general mosaic pattern.
- Ring shaped epiphysis is seen in osteogenesis imperfecta
- Wormian bones are present in osteogenesis imperfecta, other bone dysplasias such as cleidocranial dysplasia, congenital hypothyroidism, and some trisomies.

Ocular Involvement

- "Blue or grey sclerae", is because of **uveal pigment showing through thin collagen layer.**
- Saturn's ring is white sclera immediately surrounding the cornea.

Dentinogenes Imperfecta/Crumbling of Teeth: "Dentine Affected"

- The enamel is essentially normal, as it is of ectodermal origin, not mesenchymal.
- The lower incisors, which erupt first are more severely affected.

- Susceptible to malignant hyperthermia during general anesthesia.
- Sillence classification: Type I to IV.

AD Type I and IV/AR Type II and III

Treatment

- Bisphosphonates (Decreases Osteoclastic bone resorption): One of the few indications of Bisphosphonates is growing age.
- Zebra strip sign is seen on Bisphosphonates therapy.
- Ideal treatment replace *COLIA1* or *COLIA2* gene.

OSTEOPETROSIS

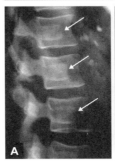 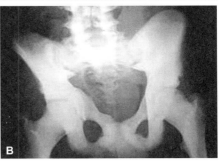

Figs. 21.17.5A and B: (A) X-ray of osteopetrotic bone—bone with in a bone appearance (B) X-ray of osteopetrotic bone—marble bone

Marble bone disease or Albers Schonberg disease.

Etiopathology

- It is a diaphyseal dysplasia characterized by failure of bone resorption due to functional deficiency of osteoclast.
- Inheritance depends on form of disease: Malignant osteopetrosis (congenital form) is autosomal recessive (AR, 11q 13) and late onset Osteopetrosis tarda (adolescence /adult form) is AD (1P 21).

Clinical Presentation

- Severe infections esp. Mandible
- Extramedullary hematopoiesis causing hepatosplenomegaly.
- Cranial nerve palsies (Bony Overgrowth of Cranial Foramen) 2nd, 7th and 8th - blindness and deafness
- Pathological fractures
- Radiological hallmark is increased radiopacity of bones. There is no distinction between cortical and cancellous bone, because intramedullary canal is filled with bone
- Endobones (os in os or bone with in bone appearance) and rugger jersey spine
- Treatment is bone marrow transplant
- **Muscle most commonly affected by congenital absence is Pectoralis major**
- **Dripping candle wax-Melorheostosis.**

Coarse Trabecular Pattern-HOP-G

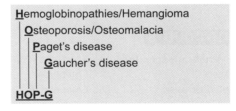

'Bone within a Bone' Appearance NanNha GOPALS

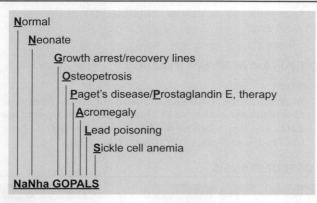

NaNha GOPALS
- **N**ormal
- **N**eonate
- **G**rowth arrest/recovery lines
- **O**steopetrosis
- **P**aget's disease/**P**rostaglandin E, therapy
- **A**cromegaly
- **L**ead poisoning
- **S**ickle cell anemia

Short Metacarpal (s) or Metatarsal (s)-TIP

TIP
- **T**urner's syndrome
- **I**diopathic
- **P**seudohypoparathyroidism/**P**osttraumatic/**P**ostinfarction

Erlenmeyer Flask Deformity GOL POT—It is flask like deformity of lower end of femur

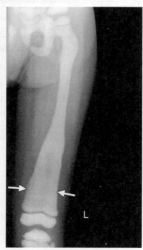

GOL-POT
- **G**aucher's disease
- **O**steopetrosis
- **L**ead poisoning
- **P**yle's disease (metaphyseal dysplasia)
- **O**steodysplasty (Melnick – Needles syndrome)
- **T**halassemia

STUDENTS DOUBTS

1. Ivory Vertebra is seen in? *(PGI Nov 2018)*
   - A. Pagets
   - B. Osteporosis
   - C. Osteopetrosis
   - D. Osteomalaia
   - E. Hyper PTH

Ans. is 'A' Pagets

Ivory vertebra causes are:

LIMPHO
- **L**ymphoma
- **I**nfections (TB)
- **M**edulloblastoma/Metastases
- **P**agets
- **H**emangioma
- **O**steosarcoma/Osteoblastoma

2. Hyperphosphatemia is seen in: *(PGI May 2017)*
   - A. Vitamin D intoxication
   - B. Renal failure
   - C. Fanconi's anemia
   - D. Tumor lysis syndrome
   - E. Hyperparathyroidism

Ans. is 'A' Vitamin D intoxication; 'B' Renal failure; & 'D' Tumor lysis syndrome

Hyperphosphatemia: ↑PO_4^{3-} Levels are associated with:
  a. Increased oral intake
  b. Vitamin D intoxication
  c. Renal failure
  d. Hypoparathyroidism
  e. Pseudohypoparathyroidism
  f. Tumor calcinosis
  g. Tumor Lysis Syndrome
  h. Rhabdomyolysis
  i. Acute hemolysis

3. A patient on bisphosphonate therapy needs to take the following precaution: *(AIIMS Nov 2015)*
   - A. Stay upright after the tablet
   - B. Take the table with milk
   - C. Take the tablet after food
   - D. Take the tablet at bedtime

Ans. is 'A' Stay upright after the tablet

4. What are diastatic fractures? Most common bone associated?

Ans. Diastatic fractures are fractures are separation of cranial bones at sutures.

5. Bony abnormality seen in incontinentia pigmenti.

Ans. Bony abnormalities are Hemivertebra, scoliosis, spina bifida, syndactyly and absent hands.

6. Is shepherd crook deformity characteristic of fibrous dysplasia? Or is seen elsewhere.

Ans. Bone softening disorders like osteogensis imperfecta, Pagets or fibrous dysplasia, all can cause Shepherd Crook deformity but it is most characteristically described for Fibrous Dysplasia.

7. Sir, OSMIC ACID is used for

Ans. Actually not used now but was used earlier for chemical synovectomy often in Hemophilia. Also remember chymopapain is used for chemonucleosis that is chemical degradation of nucleus pulposus in case of disc prolapse, this also is not used now.

8. Sir, Shohl's solution is used in

Ans. Sodium citrate + citric acid used in rickets associated with renal tubular acidosis

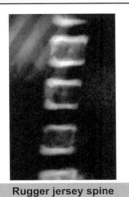
Rugger jersey spine
Chronic renal failure
osteopetrosis

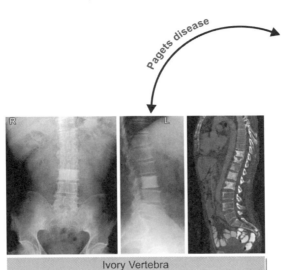
Ivory Vertebra

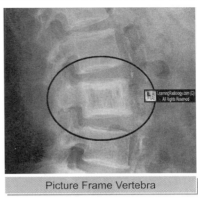
Picture Frame Vertebra

Pagets disease

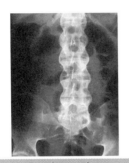
Bamboo spine
Ankylosing spondylitis

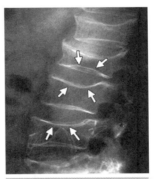
Codfish vertebrae

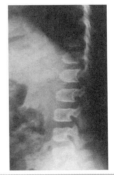
Bullet nose vertebra
Achondroplasia

9. **Sir, Stoss regimen:**

Ans. Treatment schedule for rickets in which Vit D is administered where total of 6 lakh units of vitamin D are given and then on X-rays radiological sign of calcification is noticed.

10. **Sir, Not seen in osteopetrosis:**
    A. Compression of cranial Nerve
    B. Osteomyelitis of mandible
    C. Pancytopenia
    D. Delayed healing of bone

Ans. is 'D' Delayed healing of bone

Cranial nerve compression due to bone encroachment on formina may occur.

Osteomyelitis of the mandible is common due to pancytopenia

Bone encroachment on marrow results in bone marrow failure with resultant pancytopenia.

Fractures usually heal at slower rates in osteopetrosis but few studies have shown fracture healing is normal

Thus all 4 options are correct in case we have to choose one it will be delayed healing of fracture as there is no debate about other features.

11. **A doubt sir, In which condition is Windswept deformity seen? some books say RA, others say Rickets? American authors have published RA, British have published Rickets ... which one to pick sir?**

Ans. Both diseases have wind swept deformity Rickets at knees and at hand in RA but classically it has been named for rickets. It is called as tackle deformity also.

Thus pick up Rickets!

Orthopedics Quick Review

NEET PATTERN

1. Increase bone density with hyperostosis seen in skeletal fluorosis is likely to occur when fluorine concentration in drinking H_2O is above: *(AI 2016)*
   A. 6 ppm	B. 10 ppm
   C. 15 ppm	D. 20 ppm

   Ans. is 'B' 10 ppm

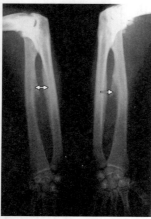

Fig. 21.17.6: Ossification of interosseous membrane seen in fluorosis

2. Neurofibromatosis type 1 most common skeletal abnormality is:
   A. Scoliosis	B. Kyphosis
   C. Anencephaly	D. Celery stalk appearance

   Ans. is 'A' Scoliosis

3. Brown tumor are seen in:
   A. Hyperthyroidism	B. Lead toxicity
   C. Hyperparathyroidism	D. Hypoparathyroidism

   Ans. is 'C' Hyperparathyroidism

4. Mosaic pattern of bone is seen in:
   A. Osteogenesis Imperfecta	B. Osteopetrosis
   C. Paget's Disease	D. Scurvy

   Ans. is 'C' Paget's Disease

18. PEDIATRIC ORTHOPEDICS

Coxa Vara

It is reduced angle between neck and shaft of femur due to some growth anomaly at upper femoral epiphysis (infantile type) or secondary to various other pathologies (acquired).

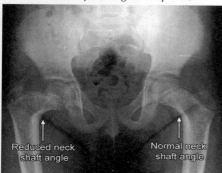

Fig. 21.17.7: Coxa Vara

Congenital Coxa Vara

Clinical

- Painless limp in a child who has just started walking
- Shortening-Limitation of abduction and internal rotation.

Radiological

- Separate triangle of bone in infero-medial part of metaphysis called as Fair Bank's triangle.
- Hilgenreiner's epiphyseal angle; angle between horizontal line joining center (triradiate cartilage) of each hip (Hilgenreiner's line) and line parallel to physis; the normal angle is about 30º.

Treatment (based on HE Angle) – Hilgenreiner's Epiphyseal Angle

- > 40º but < 60º Observation
- > 60º or if shortening is progressive. Subtrochanteric valgus osteotomy

LEGG-CALVE-PERTHES DISEASE/ OSTEOCHONDRITIS DEFORMANS JUVENILIS/ COXA PLANA

It can be defined as osteonecrosis of the proximal femoral epiphysis in a growing child caused by poorly understood (non genetic) factors.

Pathogenesis

Clinical Presentation

- **May be Self-limiting**
- **Bilateral in 10-20% cases**
- 4–8 years of age
- Most frequent symptom is limp that is exacerbated by activity and alleviated with rest.
- 2nd most frequent complaint is pain.
- Abduction (especially in flexion) is nearly always limited and usually internal rotation also. When the hip is flexed it may go into obligatory external rotation (catterall's sign) and knee points towards axilla. (Normally goes towards midclavicular region)
- Head at Risk sign have been described for perthes.

Investigation

- MRI is the investigation of choice.
- On X-rays lateral subluxation of femoral head may be seen, fragmented head with Gage sign, sagging rope sign and Mushroom shaped head.

Management

The main aim of treatment is containment of femoral head in acetabulum. Nonsurgical containment is achieved by orthotic braces All braces abduct the affected hip, most allow for hip flexion, and some control rotation of the limb. Broomstick or petrie cast issued.

Surgical containment is through (1) Femoral varus derotation osteotomy, (2) Chiari osteotomy and cheilectomy (surgically removing protuding fragments of femoral head usually anterolateral).

SLIPPED CAPITAL FEMORAL EPIPHYSIS ADOLESCENT

During a period of rapid growth, **due** to weakening of upper femoral physis and shearing stress from excessive body weight, there is upward and anterior movement of femoral neck on the capital epiphysis. So **the epiphysis is located primarily posteriorly and medially relative to the femoral neck.** So in reality epiphysis does not slip.

Aetiology

- The cause is unknown in vast majority of patients.
- Many of the patients are either **fat and sexually immature or excessively thin and tall.**
- Endocrinopathies such as Hypothyroidism (most common) Growth hormone excess caused by growth hormone deficiency conditions treated by growth hormone administration.
- Chronic renal failure (Hyperparathyroidism)
- Primary hyperparathyroidism
- Pan hypopituitarism associated with intracranial tumors
- Craniopharyngioma
- MEN 2 B
- Turner's syndrome
- Klinefelters syndrome
- Rubinstein Taybi syndrome
- Prior pelvic irradiation
- Many a times it presents in growth spurt.

Pathogenesis and Pathology

Slip occurs through **hypertrophic zone of growth plate** classically in obese hypogonadal male (adiposo genital syndrome)

Clinical Picture

M > F

- An adolescent child (boys 13–15 and girls 11–13) typically overweight or very thin and tall presents with pain some times and Antalgic limp, with the affected side held in a position of increased external rotation, (turning out of leg). Restriction of internal rotation, abduction and flexion.
- A classical sign is tendency of thigh to rotate in to progressively more external rotation, as the affected hip is flexed called as Axis deviation. (Similar to Perthes)
- Chondrolysis (Destruction of Cartilage) and avascular necrosis are possible complications.

Investigation

A line drawn tangential to superior femoral neck **(Klein's line)** on AP view will intersect a portion the lateral capital epiphysis normally. With typical posterior displacement of capital epiphysis this line will intersect a smaller portion of the epiphysis or not at all **Trethowans sign.**

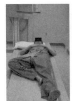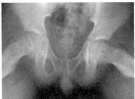

Fig. 21.18.1: Frog leg lateral view

MRI is useful investigation for diagnosis.

Treatment

SCFE is usually a progressive disease that requires prompt surgical treatment. Acute slips, if unstable may be gently reduced before fixation but there are chances of AVN.

Developmental Dysplasia of Hip (DDH)-shallow acetabulum

DDH is failure of maintenance of femoral head due to malformations of acetabulum or femur. **Twin pregnancy does not increase the risk.**

Clinical Diagnosis

BAAHARLO! "DAD", i.e. Barlow's Test—Dislocation by Adduction (DAd).

Thus in Barlows we dislocate hip joint.-Provocative test

IInd part – Now the hip is abducted and pulled. This will cause 'clunk' indicating reduction of hip.

Some consider only 1st part as Barlow's test

Ortolani's Test – the first two alphabets O and R (Ortolani for Reduction) and for Reduction we do abduction of hip. It is similar to 2nd part of Barlow's test.

Short limb as shown by—Higher buttock folds, Galeazzi or Allis sign is lowering of knee on affected side in a lying child with hip and knees flexed.

Trendelenberg's test, telescopy and vascular sign of Narath is positive.

Radiological Features

- Acetabular index increases and CE angle reduces in DDH.
  Alpha angle decreases and Beta angle increases with increasing severity in DDH (Measured on USG)
  Von rosen sign is positive
  Perkins line and Hilgenreiners lines help in diagnosis
  MRI is investigation of choice

Treatment Plan of DDH

Neonate and Young Child (1–6 month) –Closed reduction, Pavlik harness, (Bachelor cast is also used)

6–18 months -open reduction is carried out

18–36 months

Open reduction + femoral rotation osteotomy   pelvic osteotomy

Walking Child (3–6 years)

Open reduction (anterolateral approach) and femoral shortening with **Acetabular reconstruction procedure:** (Salter's,—Most commonly done), (Chiari's pelvic displacement—Salvage procedure and Pemberton osteotomy—Best Corrections).

6–10 years: treatment should be avoided (fear of AVN), in bilateral DDH, in unilateral same as above.

>11 years: in cases of painful hips due to Osteoarthritis, THR may be done (but should be delayed till skeletal maturity).

- Traumatic dislocation of distal femoral epiphysis anterior and lateral

Congenital Dislocation of Knee-hyper extension (genu recurvatum) is the most common presentation

Genu Valgum—the commonest cause of genu valgum (knock knee) is idiopathic > rickets.

Note: Usually OA Causes Genu Varum and RA causes Genu Valgum.

Blount's Disease-The triad of Blount's is Tibia vara, Genu Recurvatum (hyperextension), and internal tibial torsion (internal rotation of tibia).

Metaphysio diaphyseal angle is measured and angle more than 11 degrees require close observation.

Rocker Bottom Foot

Rocker bottom foot, is a foot with a convex plantar surface with a apex of convexity at the talar head is due to wrong correction of CTEV or oblique talus.

Treatment is Grice Procedure.

CLUB FOOT/CONGENITAL TALIPES EQUINO VARUS (CTEV)

Pirani/Dimeglio scoring is for CTEV

Pirani Scoring

Look	Feel	Move
Lateral border (0 to 1)	Talar head (0 to 1)	Equinus (0 to 1)
Medial crease (0 to 1)	Heel (0 to 1)	
Posterior crease (0 to 1)		0 (normal) → 6 (worse)

Cavus increased plantar arch
  Adduction (Adduction of forefoot and mid foot.)
    Varus or Inversion (Inversion of fore, mid and hind foot.)
      Equinus (Equinus (plantar flexion) of ankle)

CAVE (Order of Correction of CTEV)

- Kites angle – AP view talocalcaneal angle.
- Normal value is 20–40 degrees (decreased in CTEV).

Treatment is <1 year cast (starting from birth), Ponsetti method tenotomy of tendoachilles is carried out.

1–3 years Soft tissue release-Posteromedial soft tissue release (Turcos)

But in children older than 3 years of age lateral column shortening procedures are often performed in conjunction with posteromedial soft tissue release.

3–8 years

Soft tissue release together with shortening of lateral side of foot by

Evan - Dillwyn Procedure (i.e. resection and fusion of calcaneocuboid joint)

Dwyer's osteotomy of calcaneum is done to correct calcaneal varus in > 5 years.

8–10 years

Wedge Tarsectomy is done as deformity is more and requires multiple bones to be removed.

> 10 years

Triple arthrodesis is necessary for recurrent or persistent clubfoot deformity in older children (chronic cases). It is best done at > 10 years of age when foot growth is complete and the bones are ossified to achieve good fusion.

It involves fusion of three joints: **TN:** Talo-Navicular; **TC:** Talo-Calcaneal; **CC:** Calcaneo-Cuboid

- **Dennis Brown splint** is used and it encourages abduction and dorsiflexion of foot
- **Thomas designed CTEV Shoes**

Note: CTEV has high chances of recurrence till 7 years of age, hence recurrence is prevented by use of Dennis Brown splint at night and CTEV shoes during day time in a walking child

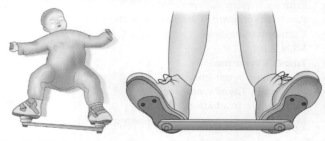

Fig. 21.18.2: Dennis Brown splint

Atypical Clubfoot

Short great toe/Sole Crease
 Hyperextended great toe/Heel crease
  Others (AMC, NF, Spina Bifida)
   Rigid feet
    Tight heel
SHORT CALF

Pollicization is transposition of finger to replace (reconstruct) absent thumb done in Radial Club hand (absent radius)

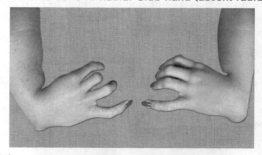

Madelung deformity involves distal radius.

Congenital torticollis Sternocleidomastoid is involved

90% cases resolve by 1 year.

It is not always present at birth (May present up to 3 months).

Fractures in Children

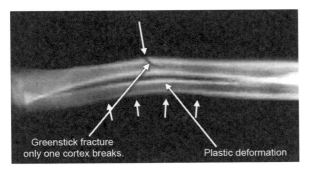

Fig. 21.18.3: Greenstick fracture and plastic deformation

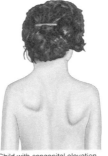

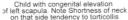
Child with congenital elevation of left scapula. Note Shortness of neck on that side tendency to torticollis

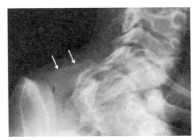
Radiograph shows omovertebral bone (arrows) connection scapula to spinous processes of cervical vertebrae via osteochondral joint (J)

- Salter-Harris type ii is Thurston Holland sign
- Remodeling potential in children

Remodelling of bone is best (maximum) for metaphyseal angulation deformity and least (worst) for diaphyseal rotation deformity.

Toddler's Fracture

It is a fracture in ambulatory child (9 months –3 years).

It is spiral or oblique fracture of lower 2/3 of tibia (Undisplaced). Fibula and periosteum is intact. The mode of trauma is twisting injury.

- **Epiphyseal dysgenesis/Fragmented/Punctate epiphysis hypothyroidism**

Klippel-Feil Syndrome

Kippel-Feil Syndrome is congenital fusion of one or more cervical vertebrae presenting with classical triad of low hair line, short 'web' neck (prominence of trapezius muscle), and limited neck motion seen in 50% cases.

Sprengel shoulder is associated with Spina Bifida, Klippel-Feil Syndrome and Scoliosis.

Note: Usually Skeletal disorders are Autosomal Dominant and Inborn errors of metabolism are Autosomal Recessive.

- Scoliosis least progression is seen in block vertebra
- Scoliosis deformity is assessed by –Cobb's angle
- Turn buckle cast is used for scoliosis
- Rissers cast is used for idiopathic scoliosis
- Scoliosis is Assessed in Forward Flexion (Postural Scoliosis Disappears)
- Peroneus tendons are evertors.

Congenital Pseudoarthrosis

Pseudoarthrosis

It is a false joint that may develop after a fracture that has not united properly due to inadequate immobilization.

If a nonunion allows for too much motion along the fracture gap, the central portion of the callus undergoes cystic degeneration and the luminal surface can actually become lined by synovial like cells, creating a false joint filled with clear fluid-known as pseudoarthrosis.

Most Common Cause of Pseudoarthrosis

Idiopathic> Neurofibromatosis (NF- 1) **(Actually an association, not a cause).**

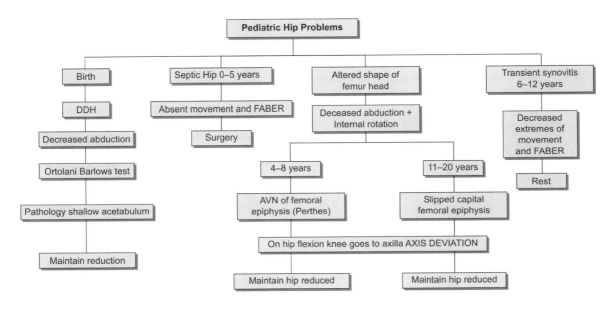

Marfan Syndrome: Fibrillin 1 defect

1. There is increase in the height (Disproportionate)
2. The limbs are long and there is arachnodactyly (fingers and hand are long and have spider like appearance)
3. Scoliosis is seen
4. Pectus excavatum/Pectus carinatum
5. Hyperlaxity
6. High-arched palate
7. Pes planus
8. Hammer toes
9. Early OA is a features
10. Ghent criterion is used for Marfan syndrome

Duchenne Muscular Dystrophy

1. X-linked Recessive (Xp 21)
2. Dystrophin gene mutation is seen
3. Boys (more common)
4. Average age of presentation is 4 years
5. Patient is Unable to walk by 12 years of age
6. Average life span is 26 years
7. Proximal muscle weakness is seen
8. Contractures of Achilles and Hamstring is seen
9. Pseudohypertrophy of calf and tongue is seen
10. Gait—patient is usually a toe walker
11. There is increase in Lumbar Lordosis
12. Scoliosis is seen
13. Gower's sign (patient climbs on himself)
14. Cardiomyopathy and congestive heart failure is seen
15. There is increase in Creatine Kinase and EMG shows Muscle damage. definitive diagnosis is by gene studies

Fascioscapulohumeral Dystrophy

- Face (facial muscle weakness) + Scapula (Winging) + Humerus (Limitation of overhead activity) defects are seen
- AD (Chromosome 4)
- Progressive disease

■ Pyle's disease is Metaphyseal Dysplasia.

STUDENTS DOUBTS

1. The following pelvic X-ray was seen in a patient. All the following signs will be present except: *(AIIMS May 2016)*

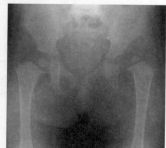

 A. Ortolani
 B. Barlow
 C. Narath
 D. Gaenslen

Ans. is 'D' Gaenslen's Test

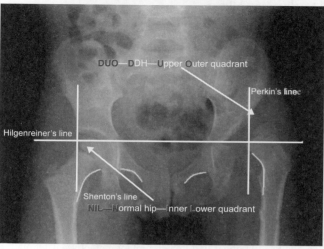

DUO—DDH—Upper Outer quadrant
Perkin's line
Hilgenreiner's line
Shenton's line
NIL—Normal hip—Inner Lower quadrant

2. Radiological Feature of CTEV is
 A. Convergence of talus and calcaneum in AP and Lateral view
 B. Parallelism of talus and calcaneum in AP and lateral view
 C. Excessive divergence of talus and calcaneum in lateral view
 D. Excessive divergence of talus and calcaneum in AP and lateral view

Ans. is 'B' Parallelism of talus and calcaneum in AP and lateral view

3. In Slipped Capital Femoral Epiphysis, slipping occurs at which zone.

Ans. 5 zones of growth plate are:
 – Zone of resting cartilage of growth plate
 – Zone of proliferation –rapid synthesis of collagen requiring vitamin C it is affected in scurvy
 – Zone of hypertrophy-thickest and weakest zone involved in fractures or epiphyseal slip (Slipped Capital Femoral Epiphysis)
 – Zone of maturing cartilage of growth plate (Vitamin D Dependent affected in Rickets)
 – Zone of provisional calcification
 In SCFE the zone of hypertrophy is affected

4. Sir, What is the most common cause of genu recurvatum in children?

Ans. Congenital dislocation of knee called as genu recurvatum is the most common congenital cause and otherwise Blounts disease is the most common cause in less than 3 years of age. Blounts disease is a triad of Tibia vara, genu recurvatum and internal tibial torsion.

5. Blounts if we have to choose between genu varum and tibia vara what should be preferred

Ans. Blounts is infantile tibia vara (<3 years) that's a preferred answer over genu varum.

6. Sir, What is the treatment of congenital talipes equino varus at birth a and why it is called clubfoot?

Ans. CTEV is called as clubfoot as it resembles club, stick used to play golf.

Regarding treatment of CTEV at birth

Now the principles of Ponseti are followed and they recommend manipulation and cast as soon as possible after birth right on day 1.

7. Sir, What is the most preferred treatment for CTEV in adults.

Ans. Triple Arthrodesis that is surgical fusion of 3 joints – Talonavicular, Talocalcaneal and calcaneocuboid.

NEET PATTERN

1. Pirani scoring is used for
   A. CTEV
   B. DDH
   C. Perthes Disease
   D. Slipped capital femoral epiphysis

Ans. is 'A' CTEV

2. Dennis Brown splint encourages:
   A. Dorsiflexion and Abduction
   B. Plantar Flexion and Abduction
   C. Dorsiflexion and adduction
   D. Plantar flexion and adduction

Ans. is 'A' Dorsiflexion and Abduction

3. Tenotomy of which tendon is carried out in Ponseti method:
   A. Tendoachilles
   B. Tibialis Posterior
   C. Tibialis Anterior
   D. Flexor Hallucis Longus

Ans. is 'A' Tendoachilles

4. CTEV which is not a component?
   A. Adduction   B. Varus
   C. Equinus   D. Dorsiflexion

Ans. is 'D' Dorsiflexion

The defect in tibia or fibula

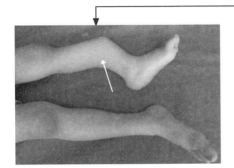
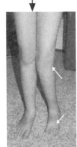
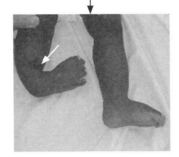
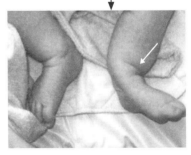

Congenital pseudoarthrosis of tibia
Congenital pseudoarthrosis of tibia there is anterolateral bowing.

Fibular hemimelia
Fibular hemimelia—this is the most common hemimelia the patient presents with limb length discrepancies, valgus at knee, hypoplastic lateral structures, ankle deformity (equinovalgus) and absent or hypoplastic fourth or fifth toe

Tibial hemimelia
Tibial hemimelia—this is a very rare hemimelia the patient presents with limb length discrepancies, varus at knee, hypoplastic medial structures, ankle deformity (equinovarus) and absent or hypoplastic first to third toe

Posteromedial bowing of tibia
Posteromedial bowing of tibia. This condition is the least severe of the four conditions. The deformity is often self-resolving.

19. OSTEOCHONDRITIS DISSECANS AND AVASCULAR NECROSIS

- It is a poorly understood disorder, which leads to softening and separation of a portion of joint surface; resulting in development of small segment of necrotic bone in joint.
- Seen in second decade of life.
- Knee (lower-lateral part of medial femoral condyle) is the most commonly affected joint. Elbow (capitulum) is 2nd common.
- Patient is usually adolescent male, presents with intermittent ache and swelling, localized tenderness and **Wilson's sign** (i.e. pain is felt in extension of flexed knee in medial rotation, but not in lateral rotation).
- The best X-ray view is intercondylar (tunnel view- 30 degrees knee flexion).
  MRI can make early diagnosis of cartilaginous lesions.

O' Driscoll '4R' for Treatment

1. Relief by physiotherapy and pain control modalities few lesions can resolve over time
2. Resect
   Excision if small fragment
3. Replace the joint surface
4. Restore the cartilage lesion

   Fixation with headless screws (Herbert Screw) and protected weight bearing till union.

   If lesion < 2 cm² – Autologous Chondrocyte Transplantation that is cartilage cells are grown in artificial media and then transplanted into cartilage defect.

   Microfracture technique or abrasion arthroplasty – Making drill holes at the base of lesion causing regeneration of fibrocartilage and filling the defect of hyaline cartilage (in normal joint). Thus it is substituting for hyaline cartilage by fibrocartilage.

Types of Osteochondritis

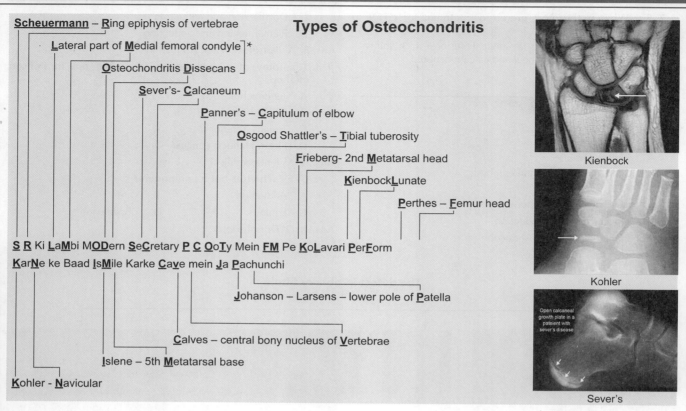

- Scheuermann – Ring epiphysis of vertebrae
- Lateral part of Medial femoral condyle *
- Osteochondritis Dissecans
- Sever's – Calcaneum
- Panner's – Capitulum of elbow
- Osgood Shattler's – Tibial tuberosity
- Frieberg – 2nd Metatarsal head
- Kienbock – Lunate
- Perthes – Femur head
- Johanson – Larsens – lower pole of Patella
- Calves – central bony nucleus of Vertebrae
- Islene – 5th Metatarsal base
- Kohler – Navicular

S R Ki LaMbi MODern SeCretary P C OoTy Mein FM Pe KoLavari PerForm
KarNe ke Baad IsMile Karke Cave mein Ja Pachunchi

Kienböck disease has negative ulnar variance.

AVASCULAR NECROSIS

Head of femur (most common)

Incidence of AVN in fracture neck Femur - Subcapital > transcervical > basicervical.

Most important lateral epiphyseal branch of medial circumflex femoral artery

Scaphoid (proximal pole AVN) - because blood supply distal to proximal

Talus (Body)

Lunate

AVN of Femur head

Idiopathic (Chandler's disease) – most common variety.

Note: Think AVN as an answer if mentioned any disease for which steroids are given, e.g. Nephrotic syndrome or pemphigus vulgaris.

Ficat and arlet staging/university of Pennsylvania staging.

Limitation of abduction and internal rotation (HIV positive on therapy with decreased abduction and internal rotation consider AVN as an answer)

Sectoral sign clinically

Crescent sign on X-rays

MRI (Investigation of Choice) – Double line sign

Bone scan shows Donut/Doughnut sign.

Treatment

1. Early stages protected weight bearing.
2. Pre collapse stage – core decompression to decrease intraosseous pressure in femoral head (**Intraosseous Pressure** Normal 10–20 mm Hg it is 3–4 times in AVN) drill holes are made in femoral head this procedure also opens the channels for vascular ingrowths and it is also supplemented with bone grafting (Vascular or non vascular) or electrical stimulation or Bone Morphogenic Proteins.
3. Muscle Pedicle graft—Quadratus femoris (Meyer's)/ Tensor fascia lata graft can be fixed in femoral head to augment vascularity. They can also be used in non-union.
4. Rotational osteotomy—To get the intact part of femoral head in acetabulum weight bearing area (anterolateral aspect of femur head) this is an extensive procedure requiring vascular repair along with it.
5. Arthritis/Collapse of femoral head – Total hip replacement one of the very commonly done procedure as most patients present at stage of arthritis.

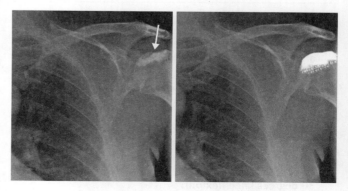

Fig. 21.19.1: Avascular necrosis of humeral head—Snow Cap Sign

1. A 70 yrs male patient has single well defined lytic lesion of skull. The patient had no other complaint and urine examination had no abnormality. What is the most likely diagnosis? *(NEET Pattern 2019)*

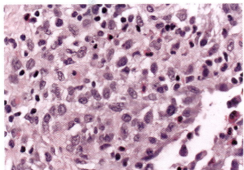

   A. Langerhans cell histiocytosis (LCH)
   B. Localized myeloproliferative disorder
   C. Generalized myeloproliferative disorder
   D. Tumor of Osteoblasts

Ans. is 'A' Langerhans cell histiocytosis (LCH)

Causes of Lytic Lesions in Skull
• Metastasis
• Eosinophilic granuloma and epidermoid
• Lymphoma/Langerhans cell histiocytosis
• Tuberculosis
• Hyperparathyroidism
• Osteomyelitis
• Radiation
• Multiple myeloma

Multiple Myeloma will present with systemic feature and multiple lesions. On skull they show punched out lytic lesions. Localised Myeloproliferative disorder (Plasmacytoma) will have single lesion without systemic features.

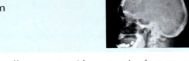

Plasmacytoma: sheets of plasma cells (arrow)

Plasmacytoma
- Solitary bone lesion.
- May occur in spine, pelvis, skull, ribs or femur.
- No plasmacytosis in marrow, no other clinical manifestations of myeloma.
- ABSENCE OF hypercalcemia, renal failure, anemia or additional bone lesions.
- MICROSCOPY:
- The tumor is composed of neoplastic plasma cells.

Langerhans cells histiocytosis (Eosinophilic granuloma)

Langerhans Cell Histiocytosis: Its solitary lesion Eosinophilic Granuloma presents with single lytic lesion with bevelled margins.

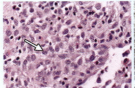 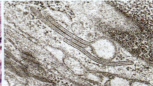

Langerhans cells histiocytosis: Langerhans cells with coffee bean nuclei (arrow)	**Langerhans cells histiocytosis:** Tennis racket shape Birbeck granules.

- May present as solitary lytic lesion or mutisystemic involvement.
- In the skull, presents as lytic lesion of bone.
- Histiocytic cells (Langerhans cells), admixed eosinophils, plasma cells, giant cells.
- Langerhans cells—oval nuclei with longitudinal grooves resembling coffee bean
- IHC: CD1a +, S100 +
- Electron microscopy (EM): Birbeck granules. Tennis racket shaped organelles in cytoplasm.

Osteoblastic proliferation will create bone matrix on biopsy. The osteoblastic tumors are not causes of lytic lesion on skull.

2. A 10 year old present with ankle pain. X-ray has Lytic Lesion with sclerotic rim at calcaneum. Following HPE findings were seen. What is your diagnosis: *(AIIMS Nov 2018)*

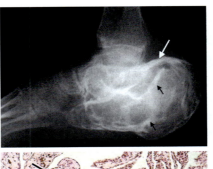

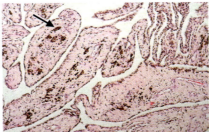

   A. Ochronosis
   B. Hemophilic Pseudotumor
   C. Pigmented Villo Nodular Synovitis (PVNS)
   D. Mycetoma

Ans. is 'B' Hemophilic Pseudotumor

Ochronosis usually presents with lesions in spine. Calcification of Intervertebral discs. The urine turns back on standing. The presentation looks unlikely.

Hemophilia most commonly affects knee joint and ankle joint in children. On xray lytic lesion in bone can be seen and on biopsy hemosiderin laden cells can be seen.

Hemosiderotic Synovitis

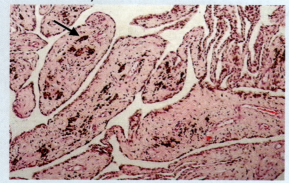

Hemosiderotic synovitis: Villous projections of synovium with hemosiderin pigment (arrow)

- Occurs in chronic intraarticular bleeding. E.g. Hemophilia.

MICROSCOPY:
- Fine villous projections may be present.
- Hemosiderin pigment is present.
- No Proliferation of mononuclear cells
- No multinucleated giant cells

Pigmented Villonodular Synovitis

Pigmented Villo Nodular Synovitis causes swelling of joints most commonly knee. It is a benign lesion of synovium. On biopsy proliferating hyperphotic synovium with popillary projections is seen.

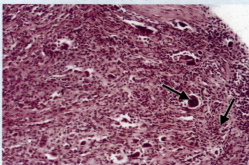

Pigmented villonodular synovitis: Proliferating mononuclear cells with multinucleated giant cells (thin arrow) and hemosiderin (thick arrow)

- Benign lesion of synovium.
- Usually occurs in knee joint.

MICROSCOPY
- Proliferating Hyperplastic synovium with papillary projections.
- Consists of mononuclear cells, multinucleated giant cells, foamy cells and hemosiderin containing macrophages.

Mycetoma will present with draining sinuses. On MRI dot in circle sign is seen. The presentation is unlikely.

Common Mistakes in Few Books

	Incorrect Information	Correct
Investigation for stress fracture	CT Scan	MRI
Earliest change of OM on X-ray	Periosteal Reaction	Loss of soft tissue plane
Earliest change of T.B. spine on X-ray	Reduced Disc space	Loss of curvature of spine
Nerve involved in Supracondylar fracture humerus	Median, Radial Nerve	Anterior Intervenous nerve > Median > Radial > Ulnar nerve
CTEV Cast	Below knee	Above knee
Hangman's fracture	Pedicle/Lamina of C2	Pars inter-articularis of C2
Most common bone to fracture at Birth	Humerus	Clavicle
Rolando fracture	Extra-articular fracture base of 1st metacarpal	Intra-articular fracture of base of 1st metacarpal
Lisfranc's dislocation	Inter-tarsal injury	Tarsometatarsal injury
Fracture Healing last 2 Stages	Remodelling-Modelling	Consolidation → Remodelling
GCT	1/3 malignant	About 5% malignant
Pulsatile bone tumor	GCT	Osteosarcoma > GCT
Tumor with Hyperglycemia	Multiple Myeloma	Chondrosarcoma > Multiple Myeloma
ACL Deficiency difficulty in Walking	Uphill	Downhill
Stress fracture most common site in metatarsal	Shaft	Neck
Scaphoid fracture most common complication	Avascular Necrosis	Nonunion
Fracture Neck Femur most common complication	Nonunion	Avascular Necrosis
Ulnar paradox	Low ulnar Nerve palsy	High ulnar nerve palsy
Most common fracture in elderly	Intertrochanteric	Colle's

MEDMIRACLE
The Learning APP To Help Crack PGMEE With Ease

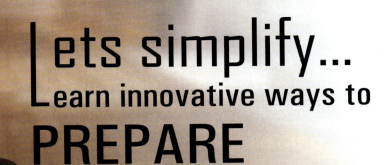

Lets simplify...
Learn innovative ways to
PREPARE

Under The Guidance of Dr. Thameem Saif & Dr. Apurv Mehra

An Initiative by NEET & AIIMS Toppers
Students Who Have Crossed The Stream Know The Secrets

Precise Content @ Lowest Price

Q. Bank
16000+ High Yield Authentic Questions Balanced Proportion of Repeat & New Questions
High Yielding Explanations

Unlimited Tests
Grand Tests, Subject Wise Tests, Exam Mock Tests Image Base Tests with ECG's & Slides
Detailed Performance Analysis To Access & Improve Your Result

Notes
Precise Exam Oriented Updated Content Arranged Topic Wise For
All 19 Subjects

Videos & Audio Lessons
400+ Hours On Conceptual Topics For All 19 Subjects
High Definition With Excellent Sound Quality
By MedMiracle Team of 19 Subject Specialist

Pearl of the day
Important Updates Tables and Images
Not To Be Missed

Talk to MedMiracle Mentors
Get Answers To All Your Academic Queries
by Medmiracle Mentors

Special Offer
MedMiracle Complete Pack - 12 months subscription
With Complimentary Apps **Worth Rs. 7000/-**
1. Dr. Gobind Rai Garg APP (Rs. 4000)
2. Dr. Apurv Mehra ODD APP (Rs. 3000)
★ Complimentary Apps Valid Only On Limited Subscriptions ★

To Avail Rs. 2000 Discount
Apply Code | Type OPQR + Last 5 Digits of Your Phone No
For Example: My Phone No:-(xxxxx64864)
Code: OPQR64864

Special Offer For All OPQR 7th Ed. Buyer & Dr. Apurv's Students
Rs 2000 Discount on MedMiracle Subscriptions
Call/Whatsapp : 8800222009

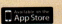

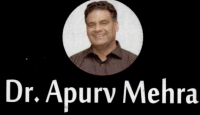

Dr. Apurv Mehra

Dr. Apurv Mehra strives hard to fulfill the dream imbibed into his soul by His Grandparents **Smt. Vidyavati Mehra & Shri Jeevan Ram Mehra** to establish a system where he could spread the torch of knowledge to all & provide high end ethical medical care at the footsteps of all human beings across the divisions of the society. **Vidya Jeevan Orthopedic Centre, Ortho Dhoom Dhadaka & Medmiracle** are the initial steps towards realization of their dreams. Its working principle is on the lines His Grandmother would often read to him...

हो गई है बर्फ पर्बत सी, अब पिघलनी चाहिए हर पर्बत से हिमालय जैसी गंगा जरूर निकली चाहिए
मेरे सीने मे नही, तो तेरे सीने में सही, हो कहीं भी आग लेकिन, इंसानियत की आग जरूर जलनी चाहिए

Vidya (Knowledge)

Dr. Apurv Mehra - Leading Faculty of Orthopedics
Highly Motivational And Inspirational Speaker
Sharing The Torch Of Knowledge

Jeevan (Life)

Dr. Apurv Mehra Youngest Orthopedic Surgeon for Computer Navigation Joint Replacements & Knee Arthroscopy at Max Superspeciality Hospitals, Patparganj & Vaishali, Delhi His Approach To Complex Surgical Issues Makes Him A Standout In Knee Arthoplasty & Ligament Reconstructions.

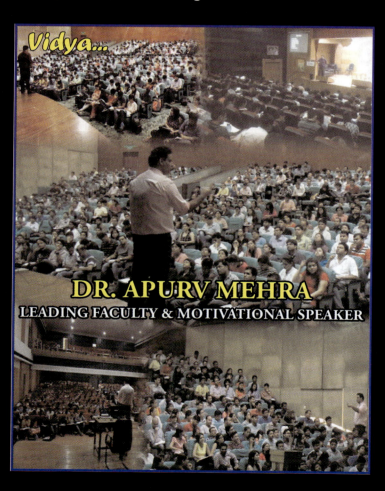

Vidya...
DR. APURV MEHRA
LEADING FACULTY & MOTIVATIONAL SPEAKER

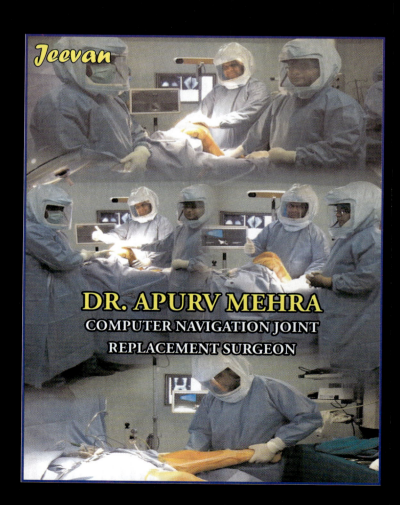

Jeevan
DR. APURV MEHRA
COMPUTER NAVIGATION JOINT REPLACEMENT SURGEON

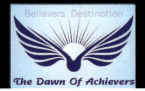

Believers Destination
The Dawn of Achievers

God has been kind to us and our students...
32 ODD sessions in 2018

ORTHO DHOOM DHADAKA
• Ignites Faith   • Helps to Achieve   • Builds Trust

GLIMPSES OF ODD 2018

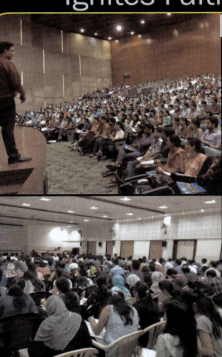
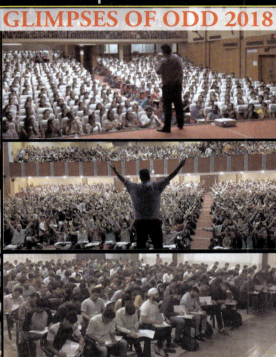
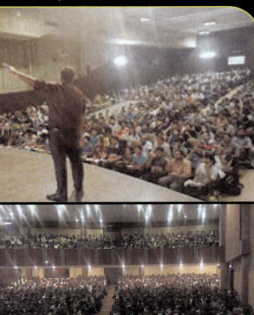

ODD STUDENTS WHO HONORED US

Dr. Umang Arora – Rank 1 AIIMS Nov. 2018
Thank you Sir! Great experience to be guided by You, everything you taught was of immense help in the exam

Dr. Sarthak Wadhera – Rank 1 PGI Nov. 2018
Thank you Sir for the amazing lecture & your unique style of teaching with great mnemonics. The program very well justifies its name-dhoom dhadaka.

Dr. Pavan Gabra – Rank 2 PGI Nov. 2018 & Rank 5 AIIMS Nov. 2018
Excellent informative class, wonderful mnemonics & awesome booklet helped in quick revision in just few hours. Thank you Sir

Dr. Rahul Nema – Rank 3 AIIMS Nov. 2018
Sir your vision on important topics is unmatchable. Could easily answer all the questions you had marked as important for last minute revision. Thank you Sir for the awesome booklet

Dr. Sarvesh Goyal – Rank 4 AIIMS Nov. 2018
Sir you cleared all the concepts in the 2 day session. Just revising what you taught with the ODD Booklet helped me answer all the questions. Thank you Sir

Dr. Shivam Bansal – Rank 3 AIIMS Nov. 2018, Rank 6 PGI Nov. 2018
Thank you Sir. Your interactive way of teaching helped me retain all the concepts for long. You notes are so high yield could easily revise with the help of images in the booklet. Thank you Sir

Dr. Piyush Aggarwal – Rank 9 AIIMS Nov. 2018
Thank you Sir for the great lecture. Revising your notes & the booklet was enough to answer all Ortho questions

Register for ODD Get Dr. Apurv Mehra's Orthopedics App Worth Rs. 3000/- Free
ODD Helpline No: 8800222009

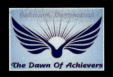

Believers Destination
The Dawn of Achivers

ODD 2.0 SCHEDULE 2019

To Register Log Onto : www.drapurv.com

Register for ODD Get Dr. Apurv Mehra's Orthopedics App Worth Rs. 3000/- Free

FEBRUARY TO APRIL

- ★ BANGALORE : 9th & 10th February
- ★ AHMEDABAD : 16th & 17th February
- ★ RAJKOT : 23rd & 24th February
- ★ DELHI : 2nd & 3rd March
- ★ MUMBAI : 16th & 17th March
- ★ HYDERABAD : 23rd & 24th March
- ★ DELHI-2 : 2nd & 3rd April
- ★ CHENNAI : 6th & 7th April
- ★ NAGPUR : 13th & 14th April
- ★ THRISSUR : 17th & 18th April
- ★ KOLKATA : 27th & 28th April

MAY TO SEPTEMBER

- ★ AURANGABAD : 20th & 21st June
- ★ PATNA : 6th & 7th July
- ★ MUMBAI : 13th & 14th July
- ★ Hyderabad -2 : 20th & 21s July
- ★ Delhi-3 : 27th & 28th July
- ★ PUNE : August
- ★ Thrissur : August
- ★ Chennai : September
- ★ Delhi : September
- ★ Bhopal : September

For Final dates Log on to www.drapurv.com
Join facebook page: Apurv Mehra For Updates

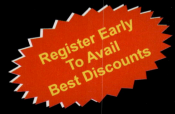
Register Early To Avail Best Discounts

For Discounts • Group • Toppers • Old ODD Student
Call / Whatsapp To 9999664864 / 8800222009
For Updates Join ⓕ Facebook Page: Apurv Mehra
Mail Your Queries To drapurv@medmiracle.in

REGD. OFFICE:- Vidya Jeevan Ortho Pedics Centre, 28, Vigyan Vihar, Near Yamuma Sports Complex (Gate No

Timings: Monday To Saturday: 9 Am To 9 Pm (Sunday Through Appointment Only)
(To Reach us enter Vigyan Vihar on Google Maps)

HISTORY REMEMBERS THOSE WHO CREATE HISTORY

AIIMS / NEET / PGI / JIPMER Toppers
are ODD Students
Who Made Us Proud
(2014 To 2017)

Rank 1- AIIMS November 2017, Dr. Archana Sasi, Delhi February ODD 2.0 Student 2017

Dear Dr. Apruv Mehra Sir, **ODD Concepts, Mnemonics & ODD Booklet Perfect For Last Minute ORTHO Revision**
I'd like to thank you for your help during my preparation for AIIMS PG 2017.I had attended your two day ODD Class in February this year. It was very comprehensive and covered all the topics that were asked this time around. The handbook provided as part of the class is very high yield and is perfect for last minute ortho revision. I've always found ORTHO to be a volatile subject and very memory-based so having attended ODD being so concise yet complete was definitely a boon. Thank you once again !

Rank 2- AIIMS November 2017, Dr.Vishnu Prasad, Delhi February ODD 2.0 Student 2017

Hi Apruv Sir, Vishnu Prasad here. I'm glad to inform you that I secured Rank 2 in AIIMS Nov PG Entrance. I would like to thank your awesome class and motivation. The odd, which I had attended during my internship, made orthopaedics revision very easy for me. **Thanks to ODD and your OPQR book. I could solve all questions on ORTHO with ease**. Please keep inspiring us always.

Rank 3-AIIMS Nov 2017,Dr.Shubham Aggarwal, Delhi ODD Student 2017

Dear Dr.Apurv Mehra Sir, I bagged the third rank in November AIIMS PG and I wish to thank you for your contribution in my success. **I attended your class in 2015 and again in 2016 as it was such an immense help. Your classes ensured that Orthopedics as a subject was not a worry** while I was preparing for entrance and I loved how you inspired me when my confidence was waning. Also, I must say that your **Orthopedics Quick Review Book is amazing. Specially the chapter summarizing entire orthopaedics.**

Rank 6-NEET 2016, Dr.Swasti Pathak, Delhi ODD March Student 2016

ODD was the first lecture I attended before starting for my PG preparation and it was more than enough. **ODD triggered in me a fire to excel in my preparation.** It not only taught me orthopaedics but also oriented me on my approach to other subjects.

Rank 8-JIPMER November 2017, Dr. Ashwati Neena Satheesh, Thrissur ODD 2.0 Student 2017

When I walked out of the 2 day ODD session, I realized the extend of **ODD "Jadoo" (Magic), the student friendly ODD & high yield oriented- ODD Booklet** speaks volume of the time and dedication sir has put into ODD.

Dr. Deeksha Bhalla – Rank 1 PGI May 2016 & Rank 18 AIIMS May 2016, Delhi ODD Student 2016

Coming in contact with Apurv Sir and ODD was a turning point in my preparation. Sir's revolutionary and out-of- the-box approach to the subject, as well as to the process as a whole completely changed my perspective. There is no unnecessary complicating the course material, infact sir broke it up into diagrams, mnemonics and even jingles which one can never forget(one of those was even playing in my head during the exam) and so made sure the ODD booklet was the one I went back to all time, so much so that I was often asked if ortho was the only subject in the entrance. The programme also taught many of us to get out of our mediocrity trained mind sets and aim for the top, reinforcing priorities again and again. I feel indebted to Sir, and I hope he continuesto work miracles for generations of aspirants to come like he did for me. Long live ODD!

Dr. Aashir Kaul – Rank 1 PGI Nov. 2016 & Rank 5 AIIMS Nov. 2016, Delhi ODD Student 2016

Apart from being the best way to revise the entire subject of Orthopedics in a day, ODD motivated me to pursue my dreams. OPQR is undoubtedly the best reference material for orthopaedics as far as any PG Entrance Exam in the country is concerned. Thank You Apruv Sir

Dr. Shivani Kapila – Rank 6 AIIMS Nov. 2016, Delhi ODD Student 2016

I feel very blessed to have attended ODD right at the start of my preparatory year. It gave me the much needed initial acceleration on which I maintained momentum for the rest of the year. The class is very interactive and all the information penetrates the skull and stays in long term memory, especially due to Sir's mnemonics. The ODD notes are excellent for a quick revision of ORTHO in 2-3 hours, especially because of the accompanying pictures. I would highly recommend the class to my juniors. It was one day very well spent. Thank you very much Sir !

Check Out More Reviews @ www.drapurv.com

Dr. Apurv Mehra's Orthopedics App - Food For Your Soul

Most trusted App for Orthopedics preparation

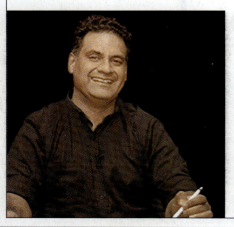
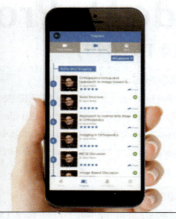

• ✓ PGMEE   • ✓ FMGE

- Chapter Wise Video Lectures according to significan
- Image Based Teaching To Understand Concepts
- Test With Video Discussions
- Includes the famous three hour complete revision vi session

More Than 15000+ Downloads in three months

Dear Students
I Have Prepared This Schedeule to Integrate My Book Orthopedics Quick Review (OPQR) With My ODD App

To understand concepts watch the video lectures while reading OPQR

Days	Videos of App (Units/Topics)	Watch Time of Video in App	Text from Orthopedics Quick Review (OPQR) Dr Apurv Mehra	
Day 1 (8 Hours)	Chapter 1 - Imaging for Orthopedics	165 minutes	Chapter 1 - Imaging for Orthopedics	(Page 1-6)
	Chapter 2 - Infection of Bone and Joints	83 minutes	Chapter 2 - Infection of Bone and Joints	(Page 7-16)
	Chapter 3 - Tuberculosis of Bone and Joints	56 minutes	Chapter 3 - Tuberculosis of Bone and Joints	(Page 17-24)
	Total time for videos on Day 1	5 hours	Total Time for Book on Day 1	3 hours
Day 2 and 3 (16 Hours)	Chapter 4 - Orthopedics Oncology	160 minutes	Chapter 4 - Orthopedics Oncology	(Page 25-50)
	Chapter 5 - Fracture and Fracture Healing		Chapter 5 - Fracture and Fracture Healing	(Page 51-60)
	Chapter 6 - Advanced Trauma Life Support	229 minutes	Chapter 6 - Advanced Trauma Life Support	(Page 61-62)
	Chapter 7 - Upper Limb Traumatology		Chapter 7 - Upper Limb Traumatology	(Page 63-91)
	Total time for videos on Day 2 and 3	7 hours	Total Time for Book on Day 2 and 3	9 hours
Day 4 (9 Hours)	Chapter 8 – Spinal Injury		Chapter 8 – Spinal Injury	
	Chapter 9 – Pelvis and Hip Injury	120 minutes	Chapter 9 – Pelvis and Hip Injury	
	Chapter 9 – Pelvis and Hip Injury		Chapter 9 – Pelvis and Hip Injury	
	Chapter 11 – Fracture Management	60 minutes	Chapter 11 – Fracture Management	
	Chapter 12 – Amputations	60 minutes	Chapter 12 – Amputations	
	Chapter 13 – Sports Injury		Chapter 13 – Sports Injury	(60 pages)
	Total time for videos on Day 4	4 hours	Total Time for Book on Day 4	5 hours
Day 5 and 6 (16 Hours)	Chapter 14 – Neuromuscular Disease	52 minutes	Chapter 14 – Neuromuscular Disease	
	Chapter 15 – Peripheral Nerve Injury	90 minutes	Chapter 15 – Peripheral Nerve Injury	
	Chapter 16 – Joint Disorders	77 minutes	Chapter 16 – Joint Disorders	
	Chapter 17 – Metabolic Disorders of Bone	260 minutes	Chapter 17 – Metabolic Disorders of Bone	(86 pages)
	Total time for videos on Day 5 and 6	8 hours	Total Time for Book on Day 5 and 6	8 hours
Day 7 (8 Hours)	Chapter 18 – Pediatric Orthopedics		Chapter 18 – Pediatric Orthopedics	
	Chapter 19 – Osteochondritis and Avascular Necrosis	3 hours	Chapter 19 – Osteochondritis and Avascular Necrosis	
			Chapter 21 – Summary of Orthopedics	(35 pages)
	Total time for videos on Day 7	3 hours	Total Time for Book on Day 7	5 hours
Revision1 (2 days) Total 16 hours	Day 1 (from the Book 8 hours) OPQR: Summary of Orthopedics + Highlighted MCQ: 1 day		Day 2 (from the App 8 hours) Image Based Revision + MCQ discussion: 6 hours Complete Revision of Orthopedics App: 4 hours	
Revision 2 (1 day) Total 8 Hours	Chapter 21- Summary of Orthopedics – OPQR : 4 hours			
	Complete Revision of Orthopedics App : 4 hours			
Revision 3 Last 7 days before the Exam	Chapter 21- Summary of Orthopedics – OPQR : 4 hours			

To Subscribe log onto : https://apurvmehra.prepladder.com

To know more call on 8800222009